Mathematical Modelling in Animal Nutrition

This book is dedicated to the memory of

Ransom Leland (Lee) Baldwin, V
1935–2007

Honorary Research Fellow in the Centre for Nutrition Modelling

Instructor, mentor and friend to many of us.

Mathematical Modelling in Animal Nutrition

Edited by

James France

Centre for Nutrition Modelling
University of Guelph
Canada

and

Ermias Kebreab

National Centre for Livestock and Environment
University of Manitoba
Canada

Centre for Nutrition Modelling
University of Guelph
Canada

www.cabi.org

CABI is a trading name of CAB International

CABI Head Office
Nosworthy Way
Wallingford
Oxfordshire OX10 8DE
UK

Tel: +44 (0)1491 832111
Fax: +44 (0)1491 833508
E-mail: cabi@cabi.org
Website: www.cabi.org

CABI North American Office
875 Massachusetts Avenue
7th Floor
Cambridge, MA 02139
USA

Tel: +1 617 395 4056
Fax: +1 617 354 6875
E-mail: cabi-nao@cabi.org

A catalogue record for this book is available from the British Library, London, UK.

Library of Congress Cataloging-in-Publication Data

Mathematical modelling in animal nutrition / edited by J. France and E. Kebreab.
p. cm.
Includes bibliographical references and index.
ISBN 978-1-84593-354-8 (alk. paper)
1. Animal nutrition--Mathematical models. I. France, J. II. Kebreab, E. III. Title.

SF95.M337 2008
636.08'52015118--dc22

2007026969

ISBN: 978 1 84593 354 8

Typeset by AMA DataSet Ltd, UK.
Printed and bound in the UK by Biddles Ltd, King's Lynn.

Contents

Contributors

O. AlZahal, *Department of Animal and Poultry Science, University of Guelph, Guelph, Ontario, N1G 2W1, Canada.*

T. Archbold, *Department of Animal and Poultry Science, University of Guelph, Guelph, Ontario, N1G 2W1, Canada.*

A.G. Assis, *Embrapa, National Dairy Cattle Research Centre, Rua Eugenio do Nascimento 610, Dom Bosco, Juiz de Fora, MG, CEP 36038-330, Brazil. Present address: Pole of Excellence in Dairying, Rua Tenete de Freitas 116, Santa Terezinha, Juiz de Fora, MG, CEP 36045-560, Brazil.*

J.L. Atkinson, *Centre for Nutrition Modelling, Department of Animal and Poultry Science, University of Guelph, Guelph, Ontario, N1G 2W1, Canada.*

R.L. Baldwin (deceased), *formerly Department of Animal Science, University of California, Davis, CA, USA.*

A. Bannink, *Division Nutrition and Food, Animal Sciences Group, Wageningen University Research Centre, Lelystad, The Netherlands.*

S.H. Birkett, *Department of Systems Design Engineering, University of Waterloo, Waterloo, Ontario, Canada.*

W. Brindle, *Animal Nutrition and Health Department, Scottish Agricultural College, West Mains Road, Edinburgh, EH9 3JG, UK.*

D.P. Bureau, *Fish Nutrition Research Laboratory and Centre for Nutrition Modelling, Department of Animal and Poultry Science, University of Guelph, Guelph, Ontario, N1G 2W1, Canada.*

O.F. Campos, *Embrapa, National Dairy Cattle Research Centre, Rua Eugenio do Nascimento 610, Dom Bosco, Juiz de Fora, MG, CEP 36038-330, Brazil.*

J.P. Cant, *Centre for Nutrition Modelling, Department of Animal and Poultry Science, University of Guelph, Guelph, Ontario, N1G 2W1, Canada.*

L.A. Crompton, *Animal Science Research Group, School of Agriculture, Policy and Development, University of Reading, Whiteknights, PO Box 237, Reading, RG6 6AR, UK.*

C.F.M. de Lange, *Centre for Nutrition Modelling, Department of Animal and Poultry Science, University of Guelph, Guelph, Ontario, N1G 2W1, Canada.*

M.S. Dhanoa, *Institute of Grassland and Environmental Research, Plas Gogerddan, Aberystwyth, Ceredigion, SY23 3EB, UK.*

R.S. Dias, *Centre for Nutrition Modelling, Department of Animal and Poultry Science, University of Guelph, Guelph, Ontario, N1G 2W1, Canada.*

J. Dijkstra, *Animal Nutrition Group, Wageningen Institute of Animal Sciences, Wageningen University, PO Box 338, 6700 AH Wageningen, The Netherlands.*

M.Z. Fan, *Centre for Nutrition Modelling, Department of Animal and Poultry Science, University of Guelph, Guelph, Ontario, N1G 2W1, Canada.*

J. France, *Centre for Nutrition Modelling, Department of Animal and Poultry Science, University of Guelph, Guelph, Ontario, N1G 2W1, Canada.*

W.J.J. Gerrits, *Animal Nutrition Group, Wageningen Institute of Animal Sciences, Wageningen University, PO Box 338, 6700 AH Wageningen, The Netherlands.*

M.D. Hanigan, *Department of Dairy Science, Virginia Tech, 2080 Litton Reaves, Blacksburg, VA, USA.*

K. Hua, *Fish Nutrition Research Laboratory, Department of Animal and Poultry Science, University of Guelph, Guelph, Ontario, N1G 2W1, Canada.*

R.L. Huang, *Institute of Subtropical Agricultural Research, The Chinese Academy of Sciences, Changsha, Hunan Province, China 410125.*

E. Kebreab, *National Centre for Livestock and Environment, Department of Animal Science, University of Manitoba, Winnipeg, Manitoba, R3T 2N2, Canada.*

B. Kerrigan, *54-2979 River Road, RR3 Chemainus, British Columbia, V0R 1K3, Canada; Centre for Nutrition Modelling, Department of Animal and Poultry Science, University of Guelph, Guelph, Ontario, N1G 2W1, Canada.*

A. Kramer, *Department of Animal Sciences, Wageningen University, 6700 HB Wageningen, The Netherlands.*

M.R. Kramer, *Information Technology Group, Wageningen University, PO Box 17, 6700 AA Wageningen, The Netherlands.*

I. Kyriazakis, *Animal Nutrition and Health Department, Scottish Agricultural College, West Mains Road, Edinburgh, EH9 3JG, UK and Faculty of Veterinary Medicine, University of Thessaly, 43100 Karditsa, Greece.*

J.E. Las, *Department of Animal and Poultry Science, University of Guelph, Guelph, Ontario, N1G 2W1, Canada.*

S. Leeson, *Centre for Nutrition Modelling, Department of Animal and Poultry Science, University of Guelph, Guelph, Ontario, N1G 2W1, Canada.*

T.J. Li, *Institute of Subtropical Agricultural Research, The Chinese Academy of Sciences, Changsha, Hunan Province, China 410125.*

G. Lopez, *Department of Animal and Poultry Science, University of Guelph, Guelph, Ontario, N1G 2W1, Canada.*

S. López, *Departamento de Producción Animal, Universidad de León, 24071 León, Spain.*

B.W. McBride, *Centre for Nutrition Modelling, Department of Animal and Poultry Science, University of Guelph, Guelph, Ontario, N1G 2W1, Canada.*

S. Miller, *Department of Animal and Poultry Science, University of Guelph, Guelph, Ontario, N1G 2W1, Canada.*

J.A.N. Mills, *School of Agriculture, Policy and Development, University of Reading, Earley Gate, PO Box 237, Reading, RG6 6AR, UK.*

P.C.H. Morel, *Institute of Food, Nutrition and Human Health, Massey University, Palmerston North, New Zealand.*

P.J. Moughan, *Riddet Centre, Massey University, New Zealand.*

N.E. Odongo, *Centre for Nutrition Modelling, Department of Animal and Poultry Science, University of Guelph, Guelph, Ontario, N1G 2W1, Canada.*

C.C. Palliser, *Dexcel Ltd, Hamilton, New Zealand.*

D.P. Poppi, *Schools of Animal Studies and Veterinary Science, The University of Queensland 4072, Brisbane, Australia.*

F. Qiao, *Department of Animal and Poultry Science, University of Guelph, Guelph, Ontario, N1G 2W1, Canada.*

J. Rapai, *Department of Land Resource Science, University of Guelph, Guelph, Ontario, N1G 2W1, Canada.*

J.W. Reijs, *Animal Nutrition Group, Wageningen Institute of Animal Sciences, Wageningen University, Wageningen, The Netherlands.*

T.C. Rideout, *Department of Animal and Poultry Science, University of Guelph, Guelph, Ontario, N1G 2W1, Canada.*

A.G. Rius, *Department of Dairy Science, Virginia Polytechnic Institute and State University, Blacksburg, VA 24061, USA.*

F.B. Sandberg, *Animal Nutrition and Health Department, Scottish Agricultural College, West Mains Road, Edinburgh, EH9 3JG, UK.*

Y. Shen, *Department of Animal and Poultry Science, University of Guelph, Guelph, Ontario, N1G 2W1, Canada.*

A.K. Shoveller, *Department of Animal and Poultry Science, University of Guelph, Guelph, Ontario, N1G 2W1, Canada.*

K. Swanson, *Centre for Nutrition Modelling, Department of Animal and Poultry Science, University of Guelph, Guelph, Ontario, N1G 2W1, Canada.*

J.H.M. Thornley, *Centre for Nutrition Modelling, Department of Animal and Poultry Science, University of Guelph, Ontario, N1G 2W1, Canada.*

D.M.S.S. Vitti, *Animal Nutrition Laboratory, Centro de Energia Nuclear na Agricultura, Caixa Postal 96, CEP 13400-970, Piracicaba, SP, Brazil.*

C. Wagner-Riddle, *Department of Land Resource Science, University of Guelph, Guelph, Ontario, N1G 2W1, Canada.*

J. Wang, *National Institute of Animal Sciences, The Chinese Academy of Agricultural Sciences, Beijing, China 100094.*

Z.R. Wang, *College of Animal Science, Xinjiang Agricultural University, Urumqi, Xinjiang Uigur Autonomous Region, China 830052.*

Z.Y. Wang, *College of Wildlife Resources, Northeast Forestry University, Harbin, Heilongjiang Province, China 150040.*

C.B. Yang, *Department of Animal and Poultry Science, University of Guelph, Guelph, Ontario, N1G 2W1, Canada.*

Y.L. Yin, *Institute of Subtropical Agricultural Research, The Chinese Academy of Sciences, Changsha, Hunan Province, China 410125.*

Foreword

If you are walking in the woods and pick up a pine cone, you will observe the precision with which the individual scales spiral about the axis. Imagining the tip of each scale to be a dot, and connecting the dots in various directions, you generate mathematically precise curvatures that botanists refer to as orthostichies and parastichies. Their precision is so reliable that these lines would unerringly indicate where additional scales would be located were the cone longer. This is quantitative biology in its most visible and, in this case, most aesthetic form.

From the time of scientists such as Thomas Huxley and others, biologists have sought mathematical descriptions of how organisms go about their business of nutrition, growth and reproduction. Particularly with respect to nutrition, where precise measurements of inputs, outputs, respiration and growth can be made, concepts of energy balance and health in response to diet have been developed. During the past few decades, mathematicians with little or no biological training have been able to uncover measurable and predictive features of organisms, and biologists with little or no mathematics have been drawn to the application of mathematics to provide validation of the similarities and differences they observe. While it is more difficult to predict a physiological response to a dietary change than it is to predict where the next scale on a pine cone would be, mathematical analyses are beginning to permit with greater certainty the modelling of how nutrition and phenotype are related.

This is a book about animals, primarily the dairy cow and other domestic species, written by a remarkable group of scientists who create a seamless interface between biology and mathematics. The authors of the chapters are all Faculty Members or Honorary Research Fellows of the recently established Centre for Nutrition Modelling at the University of Guelph. This book marks the creation of the Centre. The subjects the authors address are profoundly important for human and animal well-being on our planet. Our dependence upon livestock for milk, eggs, meat and other products has justifiably aligned animal scientists, geneticists and nutritionists around the challenges of having productive, efficient and healthy animal populations. The Holstein dairy cow is the archetype example. It is arguably one of the most specialized domestic species on the planet, and one that I suspect has been subjected to more mathematical analysis than any other creature. It is premature to say that the dairy cow is the pine cone of animal agriculture, but the work described here moves us significantly in that direction.

Lastly, many of the contributions in this book were developed with students. I dedicate this brief foreword to a botany professor who was my mentor many years ago and who taught me about the wonders of plant development. The authors of this volume similarly need to be commended for the efforts they are making to ensure that there will be a next generation of people who will be able to understand animal nutrition in what will undoubtedly be a changing and more complex world.

Alan Wildeman
Vice-President Research
University of Guelph

Acknowledgement

J. France and E. Kebreab are Canada Research Chairs in Biomathematics in Animal Nutrition and in Modelling Sustainable Agricultural Systems, respectively. The authors wish to thank the Canada Research Chairs Programme for its support.

1 Introduction

J. FRANCE[1] AND E. KEBREAB[1,2]

[1]Centre for Nutrition Modelling, Department of Animal and Poultry Science, University of Guelph, Canada; [2]National Centre for Livestock and Environment, Department of Animal Science, University of Manitoba, Canada

The subject of nutrition concerns the nature of feeds and feed nutrients and the needs of animals for these substances. According to Webster's Dictionary, nutrition is 'the series of processes by which an organism takes in and assimilates food for promoting growth and replacing worn or injured tissues'. It is an applied science and, therefore, a multidisciplinary one. According to the popular textbook by Lloyd *et al.* (1978), the subject of nutrition is 'a montage of several scientific disciplines grouped around the age-old arts of homemaking and husbandry'. This 'montage of scientific disciplines' includes physiology, biochemistry, microbiology and, among others, mathematics. Mathematical modelling is concerned with applications of mathematics to real-world problems and processes, such as those encountered in subjects like animal nutrition.

Traditionally, quantitative research into animal nutrition, as in many other areas of biology, has been empirically based and has centred on statistical analysis of experimental data. While this has provided much of the essential groundwork, more attention has been given in recent years to improving our understanding of the underlying mechanisms that govern the processes of digestion and metabolism, and this requires an increased emphasis on theory and mathematical modelling. The primary purpose of each of the subsequent chapters of this book, therefore, is to promulgate quantitative approaches concerned with elucidating mechanisms in a particular area of the nutrition of ruminants, pigs, poultry, fish or pets. Given the diverse scientific backgrounds of the contributors of each chapter (the chapters in the book are arranged according to subject area), the imposition of a rigid format for presenting mathematical material has been eschewed, though basic mathematical conventions are adhered to. Before considering each area, however, it is necessary to review the role and practice of mathematical modelling and to overview the different mathematical approaches that may be adopted.

Role and Practice of Mathematical Modelling

Modelling is a central and integral part of the scientific method. As phrased eloquently by Arturo Rosenbluth and Norbert Weiner, 'the intention and result of a scientific inquiry is to obtain an understanding and control of some part of the universe. No substantial part of the universe is so simple that it can be grasped and controlled without abstraction. Abstraction consists in replacing the part of the universe under consideration by a model of similar but simpler structure. Models, formal or intellectual on the one hand, or material on the other, are thus a central necessity of scientific procedure' (Rosenbluth and Weiner, 1945). Models therefore provide us with representations that we can use. They provide a means of applying knowledge and a means of expressing theory and advancing understanding (i.e. operational models and research models). They are simplifications, not duplications of reality. To quote from an editorial that appeared in the *Journal of the American Medical Association*, 'a model, like a map, cannot show everything. If it did, it would not be a model but a duplicate. Thus, the classic definition of art as *the purgation of superfluities* also applies to models and the model-maker's problem is to distinguish between the superfluous and the essential' (Anon., 1960). This is, of course, an affirmation of Occam's Razor, that entities are not to be multiplied beyond necessity.

To appreciate fully the role of mathematical modelling in the biological sciences, it is necessary to consider the nature and implications of organizational hierarchy (levels of organization) and to review the types of models that may be constructed.

Organizational hierarchy

Biology, including animal nutrition, is notable for its many organizational levels. It is the existence of the different levels of organization that give rise to the rich diversity of the biological world. For the animal sciences, a typical scheme for the hierarchy of organizational levels is shown in Table 1.1. This scheme can be continued in both directions and, for ease of exposition, the different levels are labelled ..., $i + 1$, i, $i - 1$, ... Any level of the scheme can be viewed as a system, composed of subsystems lying at a lower level, or as a subsystem of higher-level systems. Such a hierarchical scheme has some important properties:

1. Each level has its own concepts and language. For example, the terms of animal production such as *plane of nutrition* and *live weight gain* have little meaning at the cell or organelle level.

2. Each level is an integration of items from lower levels. The response of the system at level i can be related to the response at lower levels by a reductionist scheme. Thus, a description at level $i - 1$ can provide a mechanism for behaviour at level i.

3. Successful operation of a given level requires lower levels to function properly, but not necessarily vice versa. For example, a microorganism can be extracted from the rumen and can be grown in culture in a laboratory so that it is

Table 1.1. Levels of organization.

Level	Description of level
$i + 3$	Collection of organisms (herd, flock)
$i + 2$	Organism (animal)
$i + 1$	Organ
i	Tissue
$i - 1$	Cell
$i - 2$	Organelle
$i - 3$	Macromolecule

independent of the integrity of the rumen and the animal, but the rumen (and, hence, the animal) relies on the proper functioning of its microbes to operate normally itself.

Three categories of model are briefly considered in the remainder of this chapter: teleonomic, empirical and mechanistic. In terms of this organizational hierarchy, teleonomic models usually look upwards to higher levels, empirical models examine a single level and mechanistic models look downwards, considering processes at a level in relation to those at lower levels.

Teleonomic modelling

Teleonomic models (see Monod, 1975, for a discussion of teleonomy) are applicable to apparently goal-directed behaviour and are formulated explicitly in terms of goals. They usually refer responses at level i to the constraints provided by level $i + 1$. It is the higher-level constraints that, via evolutionary pressures, can select combinations of the lower-level mechanisms, which may lead to apparently goal-directed behaviour at level i. Currently, teleonomic modelling plays only a minor role in biological modelling, though this role might expand. It has not, as yet, been applied to problems in animal nutrition and physiology, though it has found some application in plant and crop modelling (Thornley and France, 2007).

Empirical modelling

Empirical models are models in which experimental data are used directly to quantify relationships and are based at a single level (e.g. the whole animal) in the organizational hierarchy discussed above. Empirical modelling is concerned with using models to describe data by accounting for inherent variation in the data. Thus, an empirical model principally sets out to describe and is based on observation and experiment, and not necessarily on any preconceived biological theory. The approach derives from the philosophy of empiricism and generally adheres to the methodology of statistics.

Empirical models are often curve-fitting exercises. As an example, consider modelling voluntary feed intake in a growing, non-lactating ruminant. An empirical approach to this problem would be to take a data set and fit a linear regression equation, possibly:

$$I = a_0 + a_1 W + a_2 \frac{dW}{dt} + a_3 D \qquad (1.1)$$

where I denotes intake, W is live weight, D is a measure of diet quality and a_0, a_1, a_2 and a_3 are parameters.

We note that in Eqn 1.1, level i behaviour (intake) is described in terms of level i attributes (live weight, live weight gain and diet quality). As this type of model is principally concerned with prediction, direct biological meaning cannot be ascribed to the equation parameters and the model suggests little about the mechanisms of voluntary feed intake. If the model fits the data well, the equation might be extremely useful, though it is specific to the particular conditions under which the data were obtained and so the range of its predictive ability will be limited.

Mechanistic modelling

Mechanistic models are process based and seek to understand causation. A mechanistic model is constructed by looking at the structure of the system under investigation, dividing it into its key components and analysing the behaviour of the whole system in terms of its individual components and their interactions with one another. For example, a simplified mechanistic description of intake and nutrient utilization for a growing pig might contain five components, namely two body pools (protein and fat), two blood plasma pools (amino acids and other carbon metabolites) and a digestive pool (gut fill), and include interactions such as protein and fat turnover, gluconeogenesis from amino acids and nutrient absorption. Thus, the mechanistic modeller attempts to construct a description of the system at level i in terms of the components and their associated processes at level $i - 1$ (and possibly lower) in order to gain an understanding at level i in terms of these component processes. Indeed, it is the connections that interrelate the components that make a model mechanistic. Mechanistic modelling follows the traditional philosophy and reductionist method of the physical and chemical sciences.

Model evaluation

Model evaluation is not a wholly objective process. Models can be perceived as hypotheses expressed in mathematics and should therefore be subject to the usual process of hypothesis evaluation. To quote Popper, 'these *conjectures* are controlled by criticism; by attempted *refutations*, which include several critical tests. They may survive these tests, but they can never be positively justified . . . by bringing out our mistakes it makes us understand the difficulties of the problem we are trying to solve' (Popper, 1969). A working scientific hypothesis must therefore be subjected to criticism and evaluation in an attempt to refute it. In the Popperian sense, the term *validation* must be assumed to mean a failed attempt at falsification, since models cannot be proved valid, but only invalid. Validation is thus best avoided.

Following Popper's analysis, the predictions of a model should be compared with as many observations as possible. However, there is often a lack of suitable data to compare predictions with observations, because the available data are used to estimate model parameters and hence cannot be used to evaluate the model independently, or because the entities simply have not or cannot be measured experimentally. We refute the opinion of some referees and editors that a model is valuable if, and only if, its predictions are fully accurate. The evaluation of research models depends on an appraisal of the total effort, within which mathematical modelling serves to provide a framework for integrating knowledge and formulating hypotheses. For applied models, evaluation involves comparison of the results of the new model and of existing models in a defined environment (the champion–challenger approach). In all cases, the objectives of a modelling exercise should be examined to assess their legitimacy and to what extent they have been fulfilled.

Mathematical Approaches

At this point in our discussion, it is important to give a correct picture of the nature of mathematics. Mathematics is often seen as a kind of tool, as the handmaiden of science and technology. This view fails to acknowledge or reflect the potential role of mathematics in science and technology as an integral part of the basic logic underlying the previewing and developmental imagination which drives these vital disciplines. The use of the word *tool* to describe mathematics is, we submit, pejorative. Tools operate on materials in a coercive way by cutting, piercing, smashing, etc. Mathematics is used in a completely non-coercive way, by appealing to reason, by enabling us to see the world more clearly, by enabling us to understand things we previously failed to understand.

Mathematics itself is an umbrella term covering a rich and diverse discipline. It has several distinct branches, e.g. statistics (methods of obtaining and analysing quantitative data based on probability theory), operational research (methods for the study of complex decision-making problems concerned with the best utilization of limited resources) and applied mathematics (concerned with the study of the physical world and includes, for example, mechanics, thermodynamics, theory of electricity and magnetism). The mathematical spectrum is illustrated in Fig. 1.1.

Statistics has had a major influence on research in animal nutrition, and in applied biology generally, and is well understood by biologists. This is hardly surprising given that many of the techniques for the design and analysis of experiments were pioneered in the 1920s to deal with variability in agricultural field experiments and surveys caused by factors beyond the control of investigators,

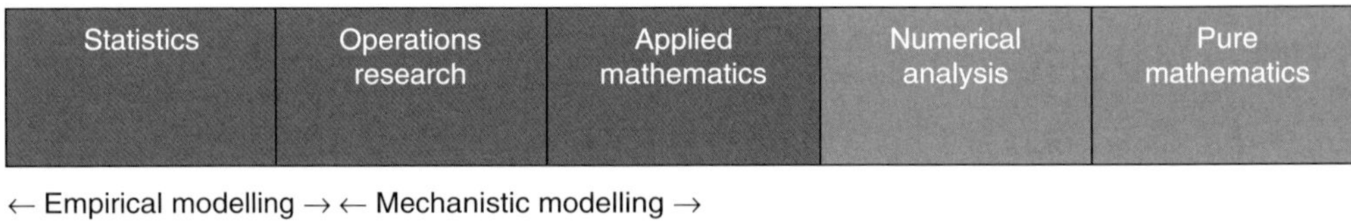

Fig. 1.1. A mathematical spectrum.

such as the weather and site differences. Other pertinent branches of mathematics, such as applied mathematics and operational research, are less well understood. In the rest of this chapter, we explore a key paradigm from each of these three branches, viz. the regression and the linear programming (LP) paradigms from statistics and operational research, respectively, and the rate:state formalism of applied mathematics (biomathematics).

Regression paradigm

Linear multiple regression models pervade applied biology. The mathematical paradigm assumes there is one stochastic variable Y and q deterministic variables $X_1, X_2, ..., X_q$, and that $E(Y \mid X_1, X_2, ..., X_q)$, the expected value of Y given $X_1, X_2, ..., X_q$, is linearly dependent on $X_1, X_2, ..., X_q$:

$$E(Y| X_1, X_2, ..., X_q) = \beta_0 + \beta_1 X_1 + \beta_2 X_2 + ... + \beta_q X_q, \tag{1.2}$$

and the variance $V(Y \mid X_1, X_2, . . ., X_q)$ is constant:

$$V(Y| X_1, X_2, ..., X_q) = \sigma^2.$$

Y is known as the dependent variable, $X_1, X_2, ..., X_q$ as the independent variables, and the equation:

$$Y = \beta_0 + \beta_1 X_1 + \beta_2 X_2 + ... + \beta_q X_q,$$

as the regression equation. The parameters $\beta_1, \beta_2, ..., \beta_q$ are the partial regression coefficients.

It is convenient to write Eqn 1.2 in the form:

$$E(Y| X_1, X_2, ..., X_q) = \widetilde{\beta}_0 + \beta_1 (X_1 - \bar{x}_1) + \beta_2 (X_2 - \bar{x}_2) + ... + \beta_q (X_q - \bar{x}_q),$$

where the $\bar{x}_i$s are computed from the n observations $(y_1, x_{11}, x_{21}, ..., x_{q1})$, $(y_2, x_{12}, x_{22}, ..., x_{q2})$, ..., $(y_n, x_{1n}, x_{2n}, ..., x_{qn})$ as, e.g. $\bar{x}_1 = \sum_{j=1}^{n} x_{1j} / n$. The sum of squares of the y_js from their expectations is, therefore:

$$S(\widetilde{\beta}_0, \beta_1, ..., \beta_q) = \sum_{j=1}^{n} [y_j - \widetilde{\beta}_0 - \beta_1 (x_{1j} - \bar{x}_1) - \beta_2 (x_{2j} - \bar{x}_2) - ... - \beta_q (x_{qj} - \bar{x}_q)]^2,$$

and the least squares estimates of the parameters $\widetilde{\beta}_0, \beta_1, \beta_2, \ldots, \beta_q$ are the solutions of the normal equations:

$$\frac{\partial S}{\partial \widetilde{\beta}_0} = \frac{\partial S}{\partial \beta_1} = \frac{\partial S}{\partial \beta_2} = \ldots = \frac{\partial S}{\partial \beta_1} = 0.$$

Parameter β_0 can be determined knowing $\widetilde{\beta}_0$. A linear multiple regression model (reference Chapter 2 on digestibility) is linear in the parameters β_1, $\beta_2, \ldots, \beta_q$. A non-linear model that can be transformed into a form which is linear in the parameters (e.g. by taking natural logarithms) is said to be intrinsically linear. Draper and Smith (1998) is recommended reading on regression methods.

Many of the models regularly applied in animal nutrition are large systems of linked regression equations, e.g. current feed evaluation systems, typically divested of their standard errors and correlation coefficients and often embedded in spreadsheet software such as Microsoft Excel© (Microsoft Office 2007, Seattle, Washington). Despite mathematical shortcomings and biological limitations (e.g. in the case of feed evaluation systems, their factorial nature, and hence limited representation of energy–protein interactions, their failure to predict product composition accurately, etc.), such models have proved, and will continue to prove, highly successful in the practice of animal nutrition (Theodorou and France, 2000).

LP paradigm

An LP problem has three quantitative aspects: an objective; alternative courses of action for achieving the objective; and resource or other restrictions. These must be expressed in mathematical terms so that the solution can be calculated. The mathematical paradigm is:

$$\min Z = \sum_{j=1}^{q} c_j X_j, \text{[objective]}$$
$$\sum_{j=1}^{q} a_{ij} X_j \geq \text{ or } \leq b_i; i = 1,2,\ldots,m, \text{ [constraints]}$$
$$X_j \geq 0; j = 1,2,\ldots,q, \text{ [non-negativity conditions]}$$

where Z is the objective function and the X_js are decision variables. The c_js, a_{ij}s and b_is ($b_i \geq 0$) are generally referred to as costs, technological coefficients and right-hand-side values, respectively. The paradigm is generally solved using a simplex algorithm (see Thornley and France, 2007).

This formalism is much less restrictive than it first appears. For example, maximization of an objective function is equivalent to minimizing the negative of that function; an equality constraint can be replaced by entering it as both a $\geq$ and a $\leq$ constraint; and any real variable can be expressed as the difference between two positive variables. Also, there are various extensions of this paradigm that allow, for example: examination of the way the optimal solution changes as one or more of the coefficients varies (parametric programming); non-linear functions of single variables to be accommodated (separable programming); decision variables to take integer values (integer programming); the objective of an activity or enterprise to be expressed in terms of targets or goals, rather than in terms of optimizing a single criterion (goal programming); and multiple objective functions to be considered (compromise programming). Further description of these techniques can be found in Thornley and France (2007).

Typical applications in animal nutrition include: formulating feed compounds and least-cost rations; allocating stock to feeding pens; etc. – see Thornley and France (2007) for details.

Rate:state formalism

Differential equations are central to the sciences and act as the cornerstone of applied mathematics. It is often claimed that Sir Isaac Newton's great discovery was that they provide the key to the 'system of the world'. They arise within biology in the construction of dynamic, deterministic, mechanistic models. There is a mathematically standard way of representing such models called the rate:state formalism. The system under investigation is defined at time t by q state variables: X_1, X_2, ..., X_q. These variables represent properties or attributes of the system, such as visceral protein mass, quantity of substrate, etc. The model then comprises q first-order differential equations, which describe how the state variables change with time:

$$\frac{dX_i}{dt} = f_i(X_1, X_2, ..., X_q; \mathbf{S});\ i = 1,2,...,q, \tag{1.3}$$

where $\mathbf{S}$ denotes a set of parameters and the function f_i gives the rate of change of the state variable X_i.

The function f_i comprises terms which represent the rates of processes (with dimensions of state variable per unit time), and these rates can be calculated from the values of the state variables alone with, of course, the values of any parameters and constants. In this type of mathematical modelling, the differential equations are constructed by direct application of scientific law based on the Cartesian doctrine of causal determinism (e.g. the law of mass conservation, the first law of thermodynamics), or by application of a continuity equation derived from more fundamental scientific laws. The rate:state formalism is not as restrictive as first appears because any higher-order differential equation can be replaced by, and a partial differential equation approximated by, a series of first-order differential equations.

If the system under investigation is in steady state, solution to Eqn 1.3 is obtained by setting the differential terms to zero and manipulating algebraically to give an expression for each of the components and processes of interest. Radioisotope data, for example, are usually resolved in this way and, indeed, many of the time-independent formulae presented in the animal nutrition literature are likewise derived (reference Chapter 12 on protein turnover; Chapter 16 on phosphorus metabolism). However, in order to generate the dynamic behaviour of any model, the rate:state equations must be integrated.

For the simple cases, analytical solutions are usually obtained. Such models are widely applied in digestion studies to interpret time-course data from marker and *in vitro* experiments where the functional form of the solution is fitted to the data using a curve-fitting procedure (reference Chapter 3 on non-linear functions). This enables biological measures such as mean retention time and extent of digestion in the gastrointestinal tract to be calculated from the estimated parameters.

For the more complex cases, only numerical solutions to the rate:state equations can be obtained (reference Chapter 4 on dynamic growth models). This can be conveniently achieved by using one of the many computer software packages available for tackling such problems. Such models are used to simulate complex digestive and metabolic systems (reference Chapter 6 on interpreting metabolite exchange; Chapter 7 on protozoal metabolism). They are normally used as tactical research tools to evaluate current understanding for adequacy and, when current understanding is inadequate, help identify critical experiments. Thus, they play a useful role in hypothesis evaluation and in the identification of areas where knowledge is lacking, leading to less ad hoc experimentation. Also, a mechanistic simulation model is likely to be more suitable for extrapolation than an empirical model, as its biological content is generally far richer (reference Chapter 5 on intake regulation; Chapter 8 on methane emissions; Chapter 22 on lactation potential; Chapter 23 on Molly).

Sometimes, it is convenient to express a differential equation as an integral equation; for example Eqn 1.3 may be written:

$$X_i = X_i(0) + \int_0^t f_i(X_1, X_2, \ldots, X_q; \mathbf{S})\mathrm{d}t; i = 1,2,\ldots,q,$$

where $X_i(0)$ denotes the initial (zero time) value of X_i. Integral equations arise not only as the converse of differential equations, but also in their own right. For example, the response of a system sometimes depends not just on the state of the system per se, but also on the form of the input. Input P and output U might then be related by the convolution (or Faltung) integral:

$$U(t) = \int_0^t P(x)W(t-x)\mathrm{d}x = P(t) * W(t),$$

where x is a dummy variable ranging over the time interval zero to the present time t during which the input has occurred and W is a weighting function which weights past values of the input to the present value of the output. The symbol * denotes the convolution operator. Integral equations are much less common in biology than differential equations, though they occur as convolution integrals in areas such as tracer kinetics. Further discussion of these issues can be found in Thornley and France (2007).

Conclusions

The first step in the application of scientific precepts to a problem is to identify objectives. Next, appropriate information is collated to generate theories and hypotheses, which are subsequently tested against observations. Mathematical models, particularly process-based ones, provide a useful means of integrating knowledge and formulating hypotheses (reference Chapter 18 on pathogen challenges; Chapter 21 on nutritional strategies). Thus, mathematical modelling is an integral part of a research programme, with the experimental and modelling objectives highly interrelated.

The mathematical expression of hypotheses in models forms a central role in a research programme. Kuhn (1963) stresses the importance of research performed by scientists within a scientific discipline which slowly but steadily increases knowledge, and the more rapid progress which from time to time is achieved by efforts of scientists in a true interdisciplinary manner. Progress in modelling depends on a variety of approaches and ideas. Thus, while further refinements of models may provide knowledge that is of value in its own right, that value is greatly enhanced if these refinements can be related to the interaction between observations resulting from experiments and from simulations. Modelling increases the efficiency and effectiveness of experiments with animals and enhances progress in understanding and controlling the nutrition of animals (reference Chapter 24 on sugarcane fed to dairy cattle).

Data are being generated at a rapidly increasing rate as a consequence of advances in technology, computing and engineering (reference Chapter 9 on supporting measurements; Chapter 10 on data capture; Chapter 17 on methodological considerations). Also, the climate within which animal nutrition (and animal science generally) operates has become increasingly turbulent. Consequently, each unit of data generated receives less attention from the experimentalist now than would have been the case in past years. Thus, data mining and manipulation provide increasing opportunity for mathematical modelling through, for example, meta-analysis (St-Pierre, 2001). It is perhaps an obligation that such opportunity be grasped in order to make more effective use of scarce research funds.

Biological research, if it is to remain truly relevant, must be undertaken at several levels of generality, e.g. cell, tissue or organ, whole organism, population. There is much more to biology than just molecular science. This chapter has identified different modelling approaches, i.e. teleonomic, empirical and mechanistic modelling, and different mathematical paradigms drawn from various branches of mathematics. No approach or paradigm is advocated as being universally superior; no one has a monopoly on wisdom. It is noteworthy that the chapters in this book cover ruminant, swine, poultry, fish and pet nutrition (reference Chapter 11 on simple-stomached animals; Chapter 13 on pets; Chapter 14 on swine; Chapter 15 on broilers; Chapter 19 on beef cattle; Chapter 20 on fish). It is, after all, a truism that those modelling ruminant nutrition have things to learn from their counterparts working, for example, in swine nutrition and vice versa (reference Chapter 25 on ruminal digestion and pig growth). Thus, scientific pluralism, not just across animal species but also across levels of generality and types of modelling, should be a pillar for future development of the activity of animal nutrition modelling. This book, hopefully, represents a step in that direction.

Acknowledgement

We thank Dr John Thornley for many useful discussions over a number of years.

References

Anon. (1960) Working models in medicine. *Journal of the American Medical Association* 174, 407–408.

Draper, N.R. and Smith, H. (1998) *Applied Regression Analysis*, 3rd edn. Wiley, New York.

Kuhn, T.S. (1963) *The Structure of Scientific Revolutions*. University Press, Chicago, Illinois.

Lloyd, L.E., McDonald, B.E. and Crampton, E.W. (1978) *Fundamentals of Nutrition*, 2nd edn. W.H. Freeman and Company, San Francisco, California.

Monod, J. (1975) *Chance and Necessity*. Collins/Fount, London.

Popper, K.R. (1969) *Conjecture and Refutations. The Growth of Scientific Knowledge*, 3rd edn. Routledge and Kegan Paul, London.

Rosenbluth, A. and Weiner, N. (1945) The role of models in science. *Philosophical Science* 12, 316–321.

St-Pierre, N.R. (2001) Integrating quantitative findings from multiple studies using mixed model methodology. *Journal of Dairy Science* 84, 741–755.

Theodorou, M.K. and France, J. (2000) *Feeding Systems and Feed Evaluation Models.* CAB International, Wallingford, UK.

Thornley, J.H.M. and France, J. (2007) *Mathematical Models in Agriculture, Quantitative Methods for the Plant, Animal and Ecological Sciences*, 2nd edn. CAB International, Wallingford, UK, xvii + 906pp.

2 Linear Models for Determining Digestibility

M.S. Dhanoa,[1] S. López[2] and J. France[3]

[1]Institute of Grassland and Environmental Research, Aberystwyth, UK;
[2]Departamento de Producción Animal, Universidad de León, Spain;
[3]Centre for Nutrition Modelling, Department of Animal and Poultry Science, University of Guelph, Canada

Introduction

One of the main challenges for animal nutritionists is to find the statistical relationship between variables, attempting to define the possible causal relation between them (i.e. to which extent one variable affects or even causes the other) and to predict the value of one variable from a different variable that can be measured more easily. One of the variables is always random and of particular interest, is often called the response or dependent variable and is denoted by y. The other variable can be random or fixed and is primarily used to predict or explain the behaviour of y, is called the argument, explanatory or independent variable and is usually denoted by x. When both variables show some association (i.e. values of both variables seem to vary together), it can be assumed that there is some mathematical relationship between them that can be represented as $y = f(x)$, where f is some mathematical formula representing the functional relation between the two variables. The mathematical form for the relationship can be a linear function, and many processes in biology can be well described by linear models, either because the process is inherently linear or more likely because, over a short range, any process can be well approximated by a linear model. Non-linear modelling is reviewed in Chapter 3 of this book.

A brief overview of linear regression will be presented in this chapter, followed by an appraisal examining the use of linear models to estimate digestibility, one of the main components of the nutritive value of feedstuffs, and hence one of the most studied variables in quantitative animal nutrition.

Linear Regression

It is not the aim of this section to deal with an in-depth description of linear regression, just to provide a concise introduction to place the topic in context.

A more detailed description can be found in any classical statistics textbook (Steel and Torrie, 1980; Fox, 1997; Draper and Smith, 1998; Kleinbaum *et al*., 1998; Seber and Lee, 2003; Kaps and Lamberson, 2004; Motulsky and Christopoulos, 2004; Harrell, 2006).

Linear regression attempts to model the relationship between two variables by fitting a linear equation to observed data. Before a linear equation is fitted to experimental data, it is important to determine whether or not there is a relationship between the variables of interest. A scatterplot of the response (y-axis) against the explanatory (x-axis) variable may already indicate a specific trend (increasing or decreasing) of covariation between both variables. A valuable measure of the statistical association between two variables is the Pearson correlation coefficient. If the association between the proposed explanatory and dependent variables is not significant, then fitting a linear regression equation to the data probably will not provide a useful model.

The equation of any straight line may be written in the form:

$$y = a + bx,$$

where x is the independent ('input') variable and y is the dependent ('output') variable. The term independent variable suggests that its value can be chosen at will, whereas the dependent variable is an effect of x, i.e. causally dependent on the independent variable, as in a stimulus–response or input–output model. For a value of x, this functional linear relation assigns a value to y. Parameter b is called the regression coefficient and represents the slope or steepness of the line quantifying the change in y for each unit change in x (Fig. 2.1).

Thus, it is expressed in the units of the y-variable divided by the units of the x-variable. If the slope is positive, y increases as x increases. If the slope is negative, y decreases as x increases. Parameter a is the intercept (the value of y when $x = 0$) or the point where the line crosses the y-axis (Fig. 2.1). In some situations, especially when the model is formulated to represent a relationship of cause and

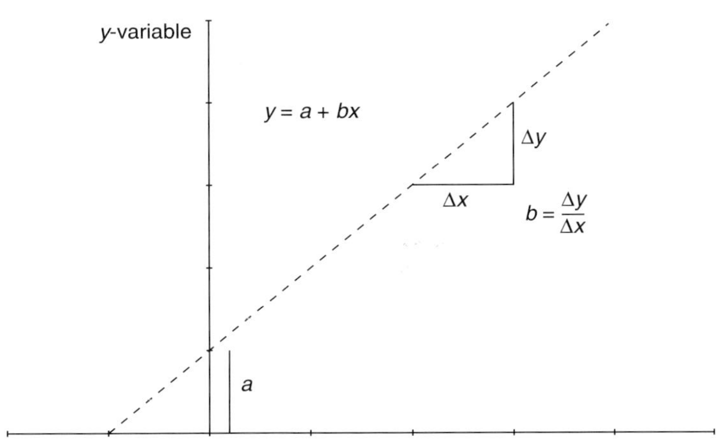

Fig. 2.1. Graphical representation of a straight line of slope b and y-intercept a.

effect, the slope and/or intercept has some biological meaning. However, in many cases there is not any causal relation at all and the linear regression line is used as a standard equation to find new values of y from x, or x from y. In this latter case, the linear model is highly empirical.

There are other linear models apart from the equation for a straight line. Polynomial and multiple regression equations are linear models, even though the resulting function may not be a straight line. A polynomial equation has the general form:

$$y = a + b_1x + b_2x^2 + b_3x^3 + \ldots + b_nx^n,$$

where n is the degree of the polynomial and b_1, b_2, b_3, ..., b_n are the partial regression coefficients. If $n = 1$, the model is a first-order polynomial equation, which is identical to the equation for a straight line. If $n = 2$, it is a second-order or quadratic equation; if $n = 3$ it is a third-order or cubic equation, and so on. A second- or higher-order equation will result in a curved graph of y versus x (different depending on values of b_1, b_2, b_3 ...), but polynomial equations cannot be considered strictly non-linear models as, when x and the other parameters are held constant, a plot of any parameter (b_1, b_2, b_3 ...) versus y will be linear. Therefore, from a mathematical point of view, the polynomial equation is considered a linear model. Polynomial regression can be useful to create a standard curve for interpolation, or to create a smooth curve for graphical analysis (spline lines), but these equations are rarely useful for describing biological and chemical processes.

Multiple regression fits a model that defines y as a function of two or more independent (x_1, x_2, x_3, ..., x_n) variables to data, in the general form:

$$y = a + b_1x_1 + b_2x_2 + b_3x_3 + \ldots + b_nx_n,$$

where b_1, b_2, b_3, ..., b_n are the partial regression coefficients. For example, a model might define a biological response as a function of both time and nutrient concentration. The graphical representation of this model would be (n + 1)-dimensional (a straight line if $n = 1$, or a surface if $n = 2$). Even though the function may not be a straight line, these models are considered 'linear' because, if the unknown parameters are considered to be variables and the explanatory variables are considered known coefficients corresponding to those 'variables', then the problem becomes a system of linear equations that can be solved for the values of the unknown parameters. In these functions, each explanatory variable is multiplied by an unknown parameter, there is at most one unknown parameter with no corresponding explanatory variable, and all of the individual terms are summed in the final function form, resulting in a linear combination of the parameters. In statistical terms, any function that meets these criteria is a 'linear function'. According to this definition, other functions such as:

$$y = a + b\,z(x),$$

where $z(x)$ may represent any mathematical function of x (as, for example, $z(x) = \ln(x)$) will also be linear in the statistical sense, for they are linear in the parameters, though not with respect to the observed explanatory variable, x. In this case, it is useful to think of $z(x)$ as a new independent variable, formed by modifying the original variable x. Indeed, any linear combination of functions

$z(x)$, $g(x)$, $h(x)$ ... is a linear regression model. In contrast, a segmented model with two or more straight lines meeting at certain breakpoints, although linear in appearance, has to be solved by non-linear regression.

In general, the goal of linear regression is to find the line that best predicts y from x. The most common method for fitting a regression line is the method of least squares. This method calculates the best-fitting line for the observed data by minimizing the sum of the squares of the vertical deviations from each data point to the line (if a point lies on the fitted line exactly, then its vertical deviation is 0). Goodness-of-fit of the linear regression analysis can be assessed using the square of the correlation (r^2) between the predictor and response variables, usually referred to as the coefficient of determination; that is the proportion of a sample variance of a response variable that is 'explained' by the predictor variable (x) or the fraction of the variation that is shared between x and y. Examination of residuals (deviations from the fitted line to the observed values) allows investigation of the validity of the assumption that a linear relationship exists between two variables. If the assumptions of linear regression have been met and the model is satisfactory for the experimental data, there should be no discernible trend or pattern in the distribution of the residuals, so that the scatterplot should not vary with x and the residuals should be randomly scattered above and below the line at $y = 0$ without large clusters of adjacent points that are all above or all below that line.

Estimates of the unknown parameters obtained from linear least squares regression are the optimal estimates from a broad class of possible parameter estimates, and good results can be obtained with relatively small data sets. The theory associated with linear regression is well understood and allows for construction of different types of easily interpretable statistical intervals for predictions, calibrations and optimizations. On the other hand, the main disadvantages of linear least squares are limitations in the shapes that linear models can assume over long ranges, possibly poor extrapolation properties and sensitivity to outliers. Whenever a linear regression model is fitted to a group of data, the range of the data should be carefully observed. Attempting to use a regression equation to predict values outside this range (extrapolation) is often inappropriate, and may yield unreliable results.

Linear modelling has been used extensively in animal nutrition; therefore, it would prove exceptionally challenging to summarize its applications in a single chapter. Thus, a detailed review of the multiple features of animal nutrition in which linear models have been applied is beyond the scope of this chapter. The next sections will focus on the application of linear models in determining and predicting feed digestibility. This is a key concept in feed evaluation and can be used as an excellent example to illustrate the derivation and application of linear models, given the different approaches used to characterize nutrient balance in the digestive tract and to predict digestibility based on the implementation of mathematically linear equations.

Feed Digestibility

Digestibility is a quantitative concept to define the efficiency of digestion of a feed in the gastrointestinal (GI) tract assessing the quantities in which nutrients are absorbed from a given feedstuff after being digested. In theory, digestibility is the proportion of an ingested nutrient that is digested and absorbed (McDonald *et al.*, 2002). However, as it is impossible to collect and measure what is digested and absorbed from the feed, any fraction of the feed that does not appear in the faeces (i.e. disappears during its passage through the digestive tract) can be considered digested and absorbed. Thus, digestibility is most accurately defined as that portion which is not excreted in the faeces and which is assumed as having been absorbed by the animal.

Along with other feed attributes (chemical composition) and the efficiency of metabolic utilization of nutrients by the animal, digestibility is one of the components defining the nutritive value of feeds for the animal (Raymond, 1969). For most feedstuffs, the incomplete digestion of feeds in the GI tract represents the main loss of nutrients during feed utilization by the animal, and it is also the main source of variation in the nutritive value, being responsible for the major differences among feedstuffs (Raymond, 1969). Therefore, feed digestibility is one of the essential concepts in animal nutrition, and its determination and estimation is of remarkable importance in the field of feed evaluation.

The reference method to measure digestibility is based on total faecal collection when the animal receives the test feed (*in vivo* digestibility, *DMD*). However, this method is expensive, laborious and time-consuming, so a number of alternatives have been investigated to predict feed digestibility from feed composition or laboratory measurements. In most cases, these approaches are based on empirical linear models of the form:

$$DMD = \alpha + \beta_1 x_1 + \beta_2 x_2 + \beta_3 x_3 + \ldots + \beta_n x_n,$$

where α is the intercept, $\beta_1, \beta_2, \beta_3, \ldots, \beta_n$ are parameters and $x_1, x_2, x_3, \ldots, x_n$ are the predictors. The estimates of α and $\beta_1, \beta_2, \beta_3, \ldots, \beta_n$ may depend on the method used, animal species, forage type and other conditioning treatments.

In vivo digestibility

Feed evaluation has become much more detailed since the middle of the 20th century and dry matter digestibility is one of the oldest measures of forage feeding quality. The earliest digestibility feeding trials were conducted at Weende Experimental Station at the University of Göttingen, Germany around 1860 (Schneider and Flatt, 1975). Detailed description of principles and procedures specific to forages may be found in some literature reviews (Schneider and Flatt, 1975; Wainman, 1977; Minson, 1990; McDonald *et al.*, 2002). Processing any feed to extract energy and nutrients by the animal's ingestive and whole-tract digestive systems can produce a range of values of digestibility. Some of the factors that influence digestibility include species, breed, sex, age and maturity of the host animal and harvesting, season, maturity, drying, freeze-drying, freezing and conservation of the forage. Uncontrollable biological and meteorological factors can also affect the digestibility measurements (Givens and Moss, 1994; Rymer, 2000).

Determination of digestibility – direct approach

A digestion trial involves a record of the nutrients consumed and total collection of the faeces which correspond to that particular intake. Procedures for measuring feed intake and methods of collecting faeces are described in detail by different authors (Schneider and Flatt, 1975; Cammell, 1977; Minson, 1981, 1990; Cochran and Galyean, 1994; Rymer, 2000; McDonald *et al*., 2002).

Let the total daily intake of food by an animal be I (g dry matter (DM) day^{-1}) equal to:

$$I = f_{off} - f_{ref},$$

where f_{off} and f_{ref} are the amounts of feed offered to and refused (orts) by the animal, respectively, both in g DM day^{-1}. If faecal output corresponding to that particular intake is F (g DM day^{-1}), then the amount of DM digested and absorbed (A, g DM day^{-1}) can be calculated by difference as:

$$A = I - F,$$

and the apparent whole-tract digestibility of DM (DMD, g digested g^{-1} ingested) is given by the simple equation:

$$DMD = \frac{I - F}{I} = 1 - \frac{F}{I}. \qquad (2.1)$$

I and F are functionally related by the identity:

$$F = g(I) = (1 - DMD)I,$$

where g denotes an arbitrary, monotonically increasing function of I. The coefficient (1 – DMD) represents the apparent indigestibility (i.e. the proportion of feed that is collected and measured in faeces) of DM, which is denoted by R and equals:

$$R = \frac{F}{I}.$$

Similarly, digestibility of any feed component (also called partial digestion coefficient) can be calculated if the composition of feed ingested and faeces voided is known. Let the dietary intake of a component x be I_x (g of x day^{-1}) and its output in the faeces be F_x (g of x day^{-1}). I_x and F_x can be calculated as:

$$I_x = I \times C_{xi}, \quad \text{and}$$
$$F_x = F \times C_{xf}, \quad \text{respectively,}$$

where C_{xi} and C_{xf} are the concentrations of component x in the feed consumed and in faeces, respectively, both in g of x g^{-1} DM. Apparent digestibility of component x, D_x (g digested g^{-1} ingested), is given by the equation:

$$D_x = \frac{I_x - F_x}{I_x} = 1 - \frac{F_x}{I_x}.$$

Apparent indigestibility of x (R_x) will be:

$$R_x = \frac{F_x}{I_x} = \frac{FC_{xf}}{IC_{xi}} = R\frac{C_{xf}}{C_{xi}} \quad (\text{i.e. } R_x C_{xi} = RC_{xf}),$$

and therefore D_x can be calculated from DMD as:

$$1 - D_x = (1 - DMD)\frac{C_{xf}}{C_{xi}}, \quad \text{giving}$$

$$D_x = \frac{C_{xi} - (1 - DMD)C_{xf}}{C_{xi}}. \tag{2.2}$$

For any component x, the digestible nutrient content of the DM in the feed (d_x, in g of digestible x kg^{-1} DM) is calculated from the equation:

$$d_x = C_{xi} \times D_x = \frac{I_x}{I} \times \frac{I_x - F_x}{I_x} = \frac{I_x - F_x}{I}, \quad \text{or}$$

$$d_x = C_{xi} - (1 - DMD)C_{xf}.$$

The digestible organic matter (OM) content of forages has been used widely (the so-called D value) as an indicator of their energy value (Minson, 1990), because of the close relationship between OM digestibility and digestible energy concentration of forages:

$$D\,\text{value} = d_{OM} = C_{OM} \times D_{OM} = \frac{I_{OM} - F_{OM}}{I}.$$

Determination of digestibility – indirect approaches

The direct approach for determining feed digestibility is only suitable for feeds or mixtures which constitute the entire diet of the animal and can be fed alone, providing feed intake can be controlled and total faecal output can be collected and recorded. In a practical situation, this is not always possible and some alternatives to the direct method have been developed to measure digestibility under those specific conditions.

DIGESTIBILITY BY DIFFERENCE OR REGRESSION. Some feedstuffs cannot be fed alone as they may cause digestive disorders in the animal. For instance, starchy concentrates, if fed alone, may cause a drastic drop in rumen pH outside the optimum range for microbial fermentation and can cause ruminal acidosis (Van Soest, 1994). A feedstuff with a high fat content may also affect microbial activity in the rumen. Thus, these feedstuffs can only be fed in combination with other ingredients (such as forages) to prevent potential detrimental effects. The digestibility of these feedstuffs that cannot be fed alone can be estimated by difference or by regression (Schneider and Flatt, 1975; Rymer, 2000; McDonald *et al.*, 2002).

A feedstuff which cannot be fed alone will be called the supplementary feed, whereas the other ingredient of the mixture will be called the basal feed, and this should be a feedstuff that can be fed alone and of known digestibility (D_b) measured in a previous or subsequent digestion trial. In estimating the supplementary feed digestibility (D_s) by difference, a digestion trial is conducted in which the animals are fed a diet with known proportions (s and b, both in g DM feed g^{-1} DM diet) of supplementary and basal feeds, respectively. Let the daily DM intake of diet be I,

$$I = sI + bI.$$

The corresponding faecal output for that intake is F, but faeces from each feed cannot be distinguished. However, as the basal feed digestibility (D_b) is known, the faecal output from this feed (F_b) can be estimated as:

$$F_b = bI(1 - D_b).$$

Then faecal output from the supplement can be estimated by difference as:

$$F_s = F - F_b = F - bI(1 - D_b),$$

and the supplementary feed digestibility (D_s) can be calculated as:

$$D_s = \frac{sI - [F - bI(1 - D_b)]}{sI}.$$

This equation may be used to estimate the digestibility of the DM, or of any nutritional component of the supplementary feed. This indirect approach is based on the assumption that there are no interactions or associative effects between both feedstuffs (basal and supplementary) when each is fed in a mixed ration, and thus the digestibility of the basal feed is the same if fed alone or if included in the total mixed ration.

Digestibility of the supplement can also be estimated by linear regression. In this case, a number of mixed rations are formulated, varying the proportions of supplementary and basal feeds, and the digestibility of each mixed ration is determined by the direct approach. Then, digestibility values recorded are regressed against the proportion of supplementary feed in each diet and, assuming there are no associative effects between the two feeds, a straight line can be reasonably fitted to the data (Fig. 2.2). The intercept of the equation (parameter a) represents the digestibility of the basal feed (digestibility when the proportion of supplementary feed is zero) and the extrapolated value for the proportion of supplementary feed in the diet equal to unity (i.e. supplement is the only ingredient of the ration) corresponds to the digestibility coefficient for the supplementary feed (Fig. 2.2).

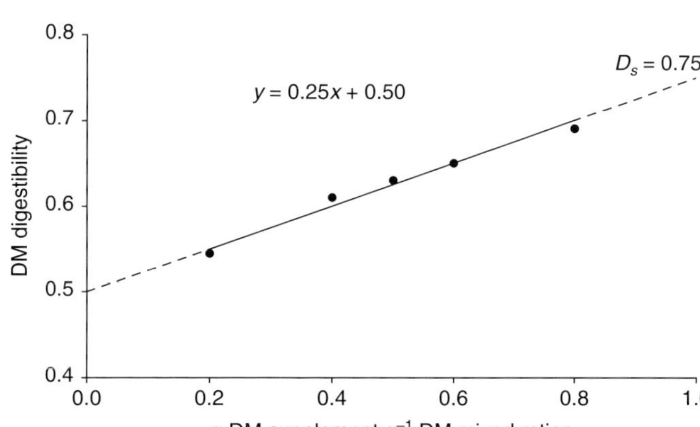

Fig. 2.2. Determination of digestibility of a supplementary feed (D_s) by regression.

INDICATOR METHOD. There are other situations, such as when animals are grazing or fed as a group, when none of the above methods can be used, mainly because it is impossible to measure the intake of each individual. In these situations, digestibility can still be measured if the feed consumed by the animal contains some substance which is known to be completely indigestible (Van Soest, 1994; McDonald *et al.*, 2002). This substance is termed an *indicator* and the method is based on the assumption that, as the indicator is completely indigestible, there should be complete faecal recovery of this substance (i.e. the quantities of indicator ingested with the feed (I_m) and collected in faeces (F_m) are equal),

$$I_m = F_m, \quad \text{or} \quad IC_{mi} = FC_{mf},$$

where C_{mi} and C_{mf} (both in g indicator g^{-1} DM) are the concentrations of indicator in the feed consumed by and in the faeces of each animal, respectively.

From this assumption, the ratio between both concentrations gives an estimate of digestibility (Penning and Johnson, 1983; Bartiaux-Thill and Oger, 1986; Krysl *et al.*, 1988; Van Soest *et al.*, 1992). Let digestibility of the indicator be D_m and, according to the definition of indicator, $D_m = 0$ (it is a completely indigestible substance). Then, applying Eqn 2.2 for the partial digestion coefficient of any component:

$$D_m = \frac{C_{mi} - (1 - DMD)C_{mf}}{C_{mi}} = 0$$

Solving this equation,

$$DMD = 1 - \frac{C_{mi}}{C_{mf}} = \frac{C_{mf} - C_{mi}}{C_{mf}}. \qquad (2.3)$$

From Eqn 2.2, and using Eqn 2.3 for *DMD*, the digestibility of any feed component x can be calculated as:

$$D_x = \frac{C_{xi} - [1 - (1 - C_{mi} / C_{mf})]C_{xf}}{C_{xi}} = 1 - \frac{C_{mi}C_{xf}}{C_{mf}C_{xi}}.$$

The accuracy of this method relies on complete faecal recovery of the indicator. If this condition is not met, but the faecal recovery of an indicator (denoted as F_m / I_m and in units of g indicator in faeces g^{-1} indicator ingested) is constant and can be quantified, then a correction can be applied to Eqn 2.3 for the estimation of *DMD* from the concentrations of indicator in feed and faeces (Schneider and Flatt, 1975):

$$DMD = 1 - \frac{F_m}{I_m}\frac{C_{mi}}{C_{mf}}.$$

Apart from being completely indigestible (showing complete faecal recovery), an ideal indicator substance (also called marker) should be inert, innocuous, with a similar passage rate through the GI as the digesta and easily and accurately measurable in feed and faeces (Warner, 1981; Van Soest, 1994). An internal indicator is a substance possessing these properties that is a natural constituent of the feed. Some naturally occurring substances that have been used as indicators to estimate apparent digestibility in pasture animals are lignin, indigestible neutral detergent fibre (NDF) or acid detergent fibre (ADF), silica, acid-insoluble ash or chromogens (Van Soest, 1994; Rymer, 2000). External markers or indicators are substances that are added to the diet, such as stains, dyes, plastic and rubber, metal oxides (the most commonly used material is chromic oxide, Cr_2O_3), rare earths and other mordants, some isotopes, etc. (Van Soest, 1994; Rymer, 2000), and have been used mainly to estimate faecal output and in experiments to obtain information about rumen volume, rates of passage or digesta flow. More recently, waxes consisting of long-chain n-alkanes have been used, with the advantage that they include a wide range of substances with different chain lengths. Some of these waxes are already contained in herbaceous plants (internal) and some are not usually present in feedstuffs but can be added as external markers (Dove and Mayes, 1991; Mayes and Dove, 2000).

The indicator method (also called the ratio technique) may also be used to estimate feed intake in grazing animals (Greenhalgh, 1982; Penning and Johnson, 1983; Van Soest, 1994; Peyraud, 1998; Mayes and Dove, 2000). From Eqn 2.1, intake (g DM day^{-1}) equals:

$$I = \frac{F}{1 - DMD}.$$

Faecal output can be measured under grazing conditions by total collection of faeces using a bag attached to the animal by a harness (Cordova *et al.*, 1978). *DMD* can be measured in a previous experiment by harvesting herbage from the sward and conducting a digestion trial controlling feed intake and faeces production. If this digestion trial is conducted indoors, intake and faecal output in the trial are denoted as $I^{(i)}$ and $F^{(i)}$, respectively. Similarly, faecal output collected in the grazing trial (outdoors) is denoted as $F^{(o)}$, and feed intake $I^{(o)}$ can be estimated as:

$$I^{(o)} = F^{(o)} \frac{I^{(i)}}{F^{(i)}}.$$

This procedure, however, has major drawbacks and alternative approaches have been proposed. A small sample of pasture can be collected and *in vitro* or *in situ* techniques (see below) used to estimate *DMD*. The main difficulty is to obtain a representative sample of the herbage grazed, and animals with oesophageal fistulae have been used. Another option is to use an internal indicator for estimating *DMD* from the ratio of the concentrations of the substance in herbage and in faeces (Penning and Johnson, 1983; Bartiaux-Thill and Oger, 1986). If all faecal output (*F*) is collected in bags and recorded, then intake (*I*) can be estimated from these concentrations according to Eqn 2.3 as:

$$I = \frac{FC_{mf}}{C_{mi}}.$$

Furthermore, an external indicator can be used to estimate faecal output to avoid the inconvenience of total collection using harnesses (Peyraud, 1998). When an external marker (such as Cr_2O_3) is administered continuously or frequently to reach a steady concentration of marker in faeces, then faecal output can be calculated as follows:

$$F = \frac{D_{mi}}{C_{mf}},$$

where D_{mi} is the quantity of marker dosed daily (g day^{-1}) (Krysl *et al.*, 1988; Peyraud, 1998). A dual marker approach using an internal indicator (*i* superscript) to estimate digestibility and an external indicator (*e* superscript) to estimate faecal output will allow feed intake in grazing animals to be estimated:

$$I = \frac{D_{mi}^{(e)}}{C_{mf}^{(e)}} \frac{C_{mf}^{(i)}}{C_{mi}^{(i)}}.$$

Apparent and true digestibility

It is assumed in calculating digestibility that the amount of nutrient digested and absorbed in the alimentary tract is equal to the difference between the amount of nutrient ingested by the animal and the amount voided in faeces. Thus, it is assumed that any substrate ingested in the feed and not appearing in faeces has been digested and absorbed. In ruminants, however, gases such as methane produced from fermentation of carbohydrates represent material from the ingested feed that is not absorbed, as the gases are lost by eructation (McDonald *et al.*, 2002). This loss may cause slight overestimation of digestible OM content of ruminant feedstuffs.

In the calculation of digestibility, it is also assumed that faeces are composed entirely of undigested feed components. Faeces, however, contain in addition other substances of endogenous (digestive enzymes, waste substances secreted into the gut, sloughed cells) or microbial (contained in microorganisms flowing with the digesta from either the forestomachs or the hindgut) origin (Van Soest *et al.*, 1992; Van Soest, 1994). Therefore:

$$F = Ind + M_f,$$

where *Ind* (g day^{-1}) is the indigested feed residue contained in faeces and M_f (g day^{-1}) the metabolic microbial and endogenous matter in the faeces. When digestibility is calculated assuming the amount of substrate absorbed is the balance between feed intake (*I*) and total faecal output (*F*), the value estimated (Eqn 2.1) is termed the apparent digestibility coefficient (Colburn *et al.*, 1968; Van Soest, 1994). To calculate the true digestibility coefficient, the amount of nutrient absorbed is the difference between feed intake and the respective indigested residues from the diet escaping digestion and excreted in faeces exclusive of metabolic and endogenous products (Colburn *et al.*, 1968; Van Soest, 1994). The indigested feed residue contained in faeces cannot be distinguished in the faecal output, but can be estimated by difference as:

$$Ind = F - M_f.$$

Then, true digestibility ($D^{(t)}$, g digested g^{-1} ingested) is:

$$D^{(t)} = \frac{I - Ind}{I} = \frac{I - (F - M_f)}{I}.$$

If apparent digestibility is denoted as $D^{(a)}$, then:

$$D^{(t)} = D^{(a)} + \frac{M_f}{I},$$

so the coefficient of true digestibility is always higher than that of apparent digestibility if there is a metabolic loss in faeces (Van Soest, 1994). Similarly, for any feed component x, true digestibility is:

$$D_x^{(t)} = D_x^{(a)} + \frac{M_{xf}}{I_x},$$

where M_{xf} is the amount of metabolic nutrient x excreted in faeces (g day^{-1}). Whereas the metabolic faecal matter contains significant concentrations of protein and lipids, there should not be metabolic faecal loss of fibre or structural carbohydrates (cellulose). These latter compounds are only of plant origin and, for them, apparent and true digestibility coefficients are equal (Van Soest, 1994).

The difference between apparent and true digestibility is of especial significance for crude protein (CP) (Souffrant, 1991; Darragh and Hodgkinson, 2000). The nitrogen of non-dietary origin excreted in faeces is termed the *metabolic faecal nitrogen* (*MFN*) and is considered to be related directly to the DM intake (Van Soest, 1994; McDonald *et al.*, 2002). For the same DM intake, *MFN* is related to the amount of indigestible matter contained in the diet (Schneider and Flatt, 1975). Different procedures have been used to estimate *MFN*, among others the determination of faecal nitrogen from animals on a nitrogen-free diet or using rations with a completely digestible protein (true digestibility of protein is assumed or known to be 100%), measuring the increment in faecal nitrogen obtained when dietary nitrogen is increased or using stable isotope tracer techniques to differentiate metabolic and indigestible feed nitrogen in faeces (Souffrant, 1991; Zebrowska and Buraczewski, 1998; Danfaer and Fernandez, 1999). One of the procedures is based on the close relationship between apparent digestibility of protein and the CP content of feedstuffs (Mitchell, 1942; Van Soest, 1994). Both variables are positively correlated and the relationship follows a curved trend because the decline observed in digestibility as CP content decreases is more drastic with low-nitrogen feedstuffs (Fig. 2.3). With these feedstuffs, *MFN* is the main nitrogenous fraction of the faecal matter and may even account for a greater quantity than the N intake, leading to a negative apparent digestibility coefficient (Schneider and Flatt, 1975). As the CP content of forages approaches zero, apparent digestibility tends to minus infinity, resulting in a typical hyperbolic curve that can be represented by the equation:

$$D_{CP}^{(a)} = \alpha - \frac{\beta}{C_{CPi}},$$

where $D_{CP}^{(a)}$ is apparent digestibility of CP, C_{CPi} is CP content of feed ingested and α (upper asymptote) and β are parameters. If all terms in the equation are multiplied by C_{CPi}, then a linear model is derived:

$$D_{CP}^{(a)} C_{CPi} = d_{CP} = \alpha C_{CPi} - \beta,$$

where d_{CP} is the digestible CP content of feedstuff (g kg^{-1} DM). In this equation, both parameters (α and β) have biological meaning. The slope α represents the true digestibility coefficient of the protein ($D_{CP}^{(t)}$, g CP truly digested g^{-1} CP ingested), whereas the intercept β represents faecal excretion of protein (g CP kg^{-1} DM)

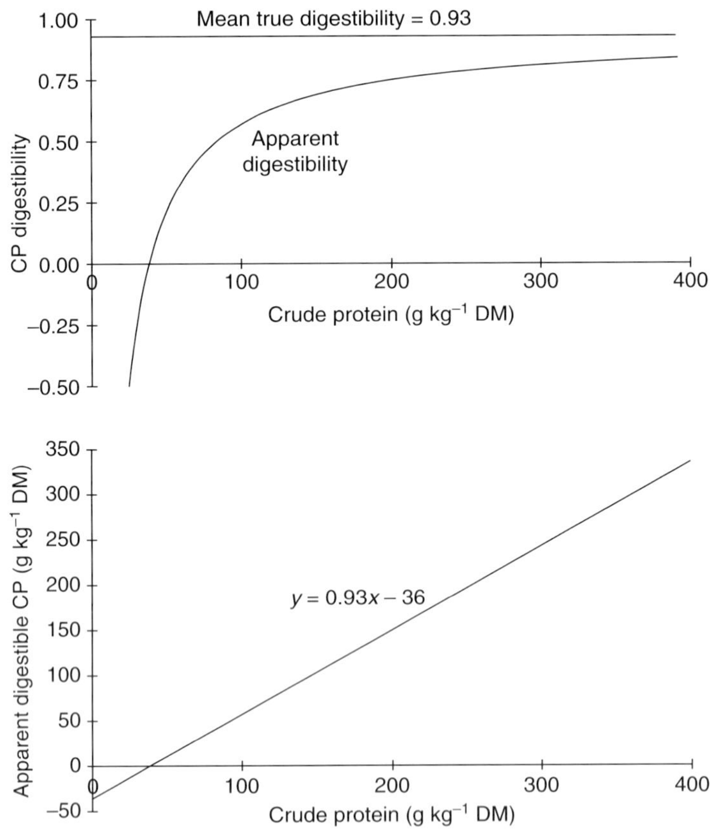

Fig. 2.3. Relation between apparent or true digestibility of crude protein (CP) and CP concentration in the diet (upper figure) and between apparent digestible protein and CP contents of the diet (lower figure), showing the regression analysis technique to estimate true digestibility and endogenous faecal output (adapted from Van Soest, 1994).

when protein intake is zero. This parameter is an estimate of the excretion of metabolic protein in faeces (i.e. $6.25 \times NMF$). Thus:

$$d_{CP} = D_{CP}^{(t)} C_{CPi} - 6.25 \times NMF.$$

This procedure has been called the regression analysis technique to estimate true digestibility and endogenous faecal output (Van Soest, 1994) and has been used not only for protein, but also to study digestive availability of minerals (such as calcium or phosphorus) for which there is an important contribution of the metabolic component to total faecal output, and thus apparent digestibility is of little meaning (McDonald *et al.*, 2002).

This regression approach has also been used to discern feed fractions or entities that show uniform true digestibility over a wide range of feedstuffs (Lucas, 1964). For these fractions, it is enough to know their contents in a given feed to predict also the digestible and indigestible portions of that specific nutrient (Van Soest, 1994).

Feed fractions showing variable true digestibilities across different types of feeds are regarded as 'non-ideal'. To implement this approach, the regression analysis technique is applied to a given feed component or entity (CP, cell contents, NDF, cellulose, lignin, etc.) and for different types of feedstuffs (forage legumes or grasses, concentrates), testing independent regressions for homogeneity of slopes, that is, to determine whether or not the slopes of individual regressions can be considered to be estimates of a common regression coefficient (that represents true digestibility). Van Soest (1994) described in detail this method and its applications and called it the Lucas uniformity test. This author also summarized the results obtained when the linear model was used to study the behaviour of different feed fractions. Lignin (Fig. 2.4) may be considered as an ideal fraction, giving an equation that confirms it can be considered an indigestible fraction (slope = –0.02) in all feedstuffs. Protein and cell contents (neutral detergent solubles) show important metabolic faecal fractions and high true digestibilities. As for cell contents, true digestibility is not significantly less than complete (slope = 0.98 ± 0.02) and the intercept must estimate the net metabolic loss of total feed DM, as there cannot be cell wall of endogenous origin in faeces. In ruminants, true digestibility of CP would be in the range 0.92–0.95 and the endogenous fraction would be between 36 and 39 g protein kg^{-1} DM intake. Finally, structural carbohydrates are the principal non-ideal components of feeds, showing different true digestibilities for different classes of feedstuffs. The cellulose test shows different regressions for grasses and legumes, with a significant difference for the pooled regression which showed a large standard error, demonstrating the lack of uniformity.

Prediction of digestibility

In vivo digestibility trials are dependent on the use of animals and are hence expensive, laborious and time-consuming, requiring considerable amounts of the test feed. Therefore, the capacity of these trials is rather limited and large-scale evaluation or ranking of feeds is not practical. This is why some laboratory alternatives have been adopted and the results obtained from easier and less expensive routine tests can be related back to the *in vivo* situation using linear regression models. Prediction of feed digestibility from compositional or *in vitro* information has become a necessity in all feeding systems. A predictor of forage nutritive value is a quality-related characteristic of the forage that can be measured in the laboratory by simple methods. Using analytical results and digestibility values determined by feeding trials for a number of standard representative feeds, multiple regression equations can be derived statistically and used to predict the digestibility of other samples. A large number of different equations for predicting OM digestibility of forages from a variety of explanatory variables are provided in the literature. In these equations, forage digestibility (Table 2.1) is predicted from: (i) botanical features (including leafiness, botanical composition, growth or maturity stage), also considering the harvesting and preservation conditions; (ii) chemical composition; (iii) physical properties (density, spectrum for near-infrared reflectance); (iv) *in vitro* measurements of

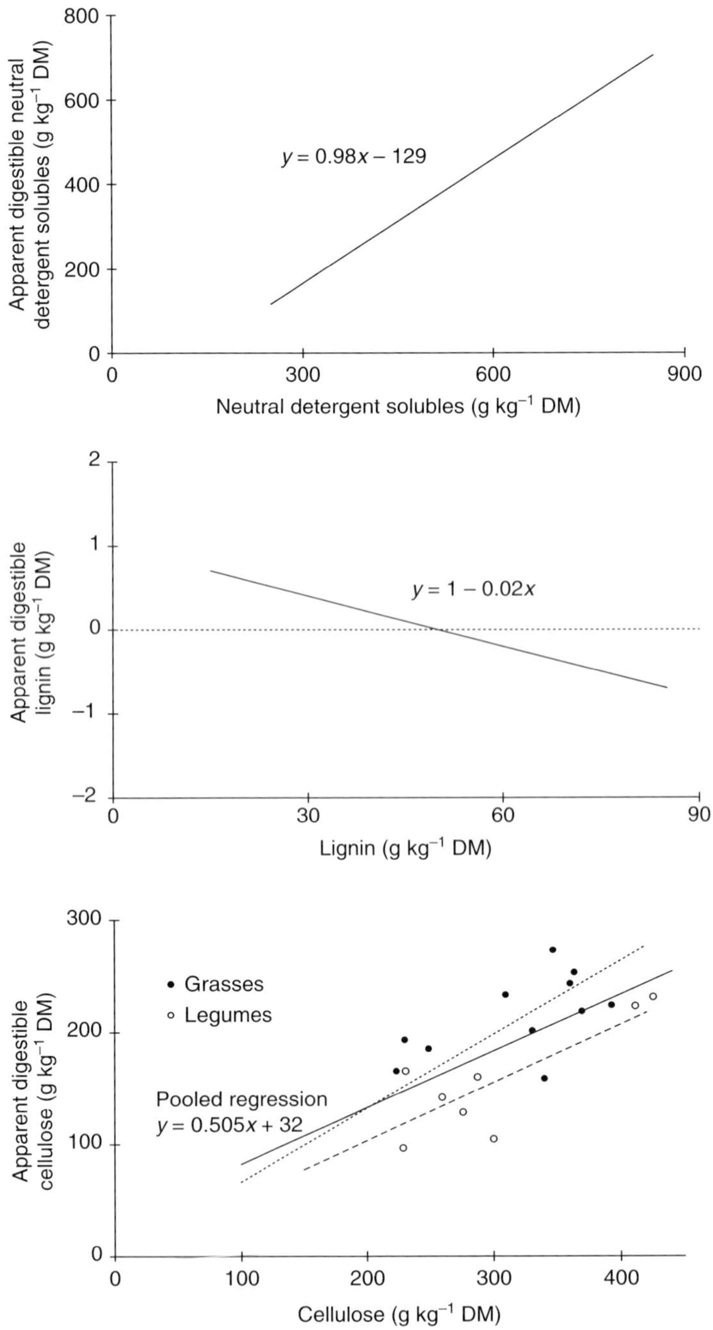

Fig. 2.4. Application of the regression analysis technique in the test for uniform feed fractions (Lucas method), showing how neutral detergent solubles and lignin can be considered ideal uniform fractions, whereas cellulose is a representative example of a non-ideal fraction (adapted from Van Soest, 1994).

Table 2.1. Ranges in correlation coefficients and in residual standard deviations (RSD)† associated with the prediction of *in vivo* digestibility from various predictors.

	Range in correlation coefficient	Range in RSD (g digested g^{-1} ingested)
Chemical composition		
Crude protein	+0.44 to +0.79	0.020 to 0.065
NDF	–0.45 to –0.80	0.024 to 0.051
ADF	–0.75 to –0.88	0.036 to 0.090
Lignin	–0.61 to –0.83	0.043
Alternative methods of estimating digestibility		
In vitro digestibility[a]	+0.94	0.016
Enzymatic	+0.94 to +0.99	0.018 to 0.032
In situ	+0.98	0.010 to 0.030
NIR	+0.95	0.006 to 0.027

† Data combined from Minson (1990), Carro *et al.* (1994) and Van Soest (1994).
[a]Tilley and Terry (1963).

digestibility (using either buffered rumen fluid or enzymatic solutions); or (v) *in situ* disappearance coefficients (Reed and Goe, 1989; ILCA, 1990; Minson, 1990; Hvelplund *et al.*, 1995; Kitessa *et al.*, 1999; Adesogan, 2002).

Most of these equations are based purely on the statistical relationship between variables and the performance of regression methods facilitated by improved computing facilities, resulting sometimes in equations without biological meaning. One of the consequences of this empirical approach is that the large numbers of equations available in the literature differ significantly in the predicting variables, in the regression coefficients for the same predictors and in the estimated prediction error. Diverse equations have been obtained for separate classes of feeds and forages, and different laboratories may use different equations for the same combination of predicted and explanatory variables. These empirical prediction equations are a consequence of the specific data set used in their construction, so that they are only useful when the situation to be predicted is mirrored by the original data set. Thus, these equations have a variable degree of unreliability, due to environmental and species variation, interactions among plant species in mixed forages and difficulty in accounting for basic cause–effect relationships between ruminal digestion and plant composition (Chesson, 1993; Van Soest, 1994). Any error in estimating digestibility is passed along to, and constitutes the largest error in, the final estimate of nutritive value of the forage. Despite these criticisms, empirical equations are widely used in feed evaluation systems.

Prediction from chemical composition of feeds

Forage components ultimately control digestibility and availability of nutrients, giving rise to a close relationship between chemical composition and digestibility.

With feeds that vary little in composition, little variation in digestibility is expected, whereas feeds showing large differences in composition (some forages) show significant variability in digestibility. In this latter case, digestibility can be predicted with an acceptable degree of accuracy from some of the chemical components (Schneider and Flatt, 1975; Andrieu *et al.*, 1981; Minson, 1982; Barber *et al.*, 1984; Fonnesbeck *et al.*, 1984; Andrieu and Demarquilly, 1987; CSIRO, 1990; AFRC, 1993; NRC, 1996).

In general, feed digestibility is positively correlated with CP content, mainly because more digestible feeds have higher CP content. There is also a significant and positive relationship between CP digestibility and CP content of feedstuffs (Fig. 2.3). The fractions crude fibre (CF) and nitrogen-free extract (NFE) determined in the Weende analysis system show less consistent and more variable (across different types of feedstuffs) correlations with digestibility (Schneider and Flatt, 1975), mainly because the analysis system fails to separate structural and non-structural carbohydrates into CF and NFE, respectively. This loose, unrealistic (with some feedstuffs, correlations with digestibility are negative for NFE and positive for CF) and variable relationship with digestibility indicates that these fractions may be of little nutritional significance, and it is one of the reasons why the system has been abandoned and replaced progressively by the detergent system proposed by Van Soest (1967). In these chemically based methods, feed DM is partitioned into cell contents (simple sugars, protein, non-protein nitrogenous compounds, lipids, organic acids, pectins and soluble minerals), which are completely digestible, and cell wall (cellulose, hemicellulose and lignin), being more or less digestible depending on the degree of lignification (Van Soest, 1967). Determination of NDF and ADF fractions of a feed has become routine laboratory analysis. Digestibility shows negative correlations with NDF and, especially, with ADF and lignin and, with some feeds, these correlations reach a high level of statistical significance (Morrison, 1976; Minson, 1990; Van Soest, 1994). A negative association between acid-detergent insoluble nitrogen (ADIN) and CP digestibility has been substantiated, mainly because ADIN in most feeds appears to be essentially indigestible (Van Soest and Mason, 1991; Van Soest, 1994).

On the basis of these statistical correlations, a number of empirical equations have been derived to predict digestibility from chemical composition. Usually, the equations are different for each class of feedstuff and the variables are selected stepwise using multiple regression procedures to determine the statistical improvement attained when an additional variable is included in the model.

Some equations have been proposed to adjust the digestibility of individual samples of a feed, using the proximate composition values as the independent variables. These equations are applicable to feeds for which there have been a sufficient number of digestion trials to establish fairly accurate mean values. These equations are of the form:

$$D = \overline{D} + b_1(x_1 - \overline{x_1}) + b_2(x_2 - \overline{x_2}) + b_3(x_3 - \overline{x_3}) + \ldots + b_n(x_n - \overline{x_n}),$$

where D is the digestibility coefficient of an individual sample of the feed to be predicted, x_1, x_2, x_3, ..., and x_n are the contents (g kg^{-1} DM) of nutritive fractions

1, 2, 3, ... and n in that specific sample, $\overline{D}, \overline{x_1}, \overline{x_2}, \overline{x_3}$, and $\overline{x_n}$ are the average digestibility and nutrient contents of the feed (for instance, tabulated values) and b_1, b_2, b_3, ... and b_n are the regression coefficients. Schneider and Flatt (1975) provided values of these partial regression coefficients for adjusting digestibility values to proximate composition of feeds for cattle and sheep.

However, in most cases only the proximate composition is known and few or no digestibility data of that specific feedstuff are available. Equations have been developed for estimating digestibility from the chemical composition of the given feed, which are generally in the form:

$$D = a + b_1x_1 + b_2x_2 + b_3x_3 + \ldots + b_nx_n,$$

where D is the digestibility coefficient to be predicted, x_1, x_2, x_3, ... and x_n are the contents (g kg^{-1} DM) of nutritive fractions 1, 2 , 3, ... and n in that feed, a is a constant and b_1, b_2, b_3, ... and b_n are the partial regression coefficients (Schneider and Flatt, 1975; Weiss, 1994). The values of these parameters are specific for the class of feed under consideration and for each animal species. Thus, different equations need to be used for each type of feed and each animal species.

In these two latter approaches, purely empirical equations are used and the nutritionist should be aware of the limitations of such approaches, mainly because predictive equations are only accurate if used under conditions similar to those from which calibration data were obtained. Alternatively, theoretically based equations or summative models have been proposed (Goering and Van Soest, 1970; Van Soest *et al.*, 1992; Weiss *et al.*, 1992) based on the partitioning of feed DM into two basic fractions, one which is completely available (cell contents or neutral detergent solubles, NDS) and one which is not (cell wall or NDF) (Van Soest, 1994):

$$DM = NDS + NDF,$$

and thus, in terms of concentrations in the DM (g kg^{-1} DM), $C_{NDS} + C_{NDF} = 1$. In the summative equation, it is assumed that DMD can be calculated from the digestibility of its fractions as:

$$DMD = D_{NDS}C_{NDS} + D_{NDF}C_{NDF} - M_f = D_{NDS}(1 - C_{NDF}) + D_{NDF}C_{NDF} - M_f.$$

From the regression analysis (Lucas test), constant values for M_f of 0.129 g g^{-1} DM and for NDS true digestibility (D_{NDS}) of 0.98 (not significantly different from unity) can be assumed, leaving D_{NDF} as the only unknown variable if chemical composition of the feed (NDF content) has been determined. Cell wall digestibility (D_{NDF}) is related to lignification and can be estimated from an empirical equation based on the lignin to ADF ratio (L, g lignin g^{-1} ADF) as:

$$D_{NDF} = -0.105 - 0.789\log(L).$$

Therefore,

$$DMD = 0.98(1 - C_{NDF}) - [0.105 + 0.789\log(L)]C_{NDF} - 0.129.$$

In this simple model, DMD is predicted from the content (C_{NDF}) and composition (L) of cell wall, as the two main factors determining forage digestibility. Summative models are superior to empirical equations when applied to a mixture of forages (legumes and grasses), but are less accurate when applied to a single plant species. These theoretically based models can be expanded to include additional sources of variation, but also require more compositional data than empirical equations.

Near-infrared spectroscopy

Digestibility can be predicted from spectra information obtained from near-infrared (NIR) spectroscopy; a rapid, low-cost and non-destructive analysis that is increasingly used as a routine technique in feed evaluation (Shenk and Westerhaus, 1994; Givens and Deaville, 1999; Deaville and Flinn, 2000; Reeves, 2000). First, a calibration is conducted to establish an equation to predict reference method information (in this case, digestibility) from NIR spectral information:

$$D = a + b_1x_1 + b_2x_2 + b_3x_3 + \ldots + b_nx_n,$$

where D is the digestibility coefficient (reference value), x_1, x_2, x_3, ... and x_n are NIR absorbance values (n is the number of explanatory variables in the model), a is a constant and b_1, b_2, b_3, ... and b_n are scaling factors that relate changes in the x variables to D. The extensive spectral information (absorbance at each wavelength over a given range) can be reduced into a smaller number of independent factors by principal components analysis or by partial least squares. On the other hand, calibrations can be performed directly on the absorbance data, or using data obtained by derivatizing the spectrum (Shenk and Westerhaus, 1994). The accuracy of NIR spectroscopy analysis equations is directly related to the structure and distribution of the selected samples in the calibration set that must be representative of the entire population to be analysed. NIR calibrations for forage have been limited to a single botanical group (a single species, legumes, grasses) or type of forage (silage, hay, fresh herbage), because the calibration error is increased as the set is expanded to include different types of samples.

Calibration statistics using NIR for prediction of chemical composition in forages are superior compared to those achieved for prediction of nutritional attributes such as digestibility. NIR spectroscopy is based on the relationship between spectral characteristics (absorbance at certain wavelengths) and chemical and physical attributes of the sample scanned. Consequently, high accuracy of prediction is expected for single chemical entities that can be determined with high precision (such as protein), and lower accuracy can be anticipated for analytical fractions that are not well-defined compounds (such as lignin), or for indicators of nutritive value that are measured using biological methods (such as digestibility or degradability). In this latter case, the relationship between reference and spectral data is complex and has to be attributed to the association between the NIR spectra and several different chemical entities and physical properties that determine digestibility (Norris *et al.*, 1976; Redshaw *et al.*, 1986; Clark and Lamb, 1991). In addition, animal response as measured by biological methods is subject to increased variability from different sources of experimental and sampling errors (differences between animals, days, etc.), which will affect the performance of the NIR predictions. NIR spectroscopy is a predictive method and, as such, is highly dependent upon the error associated with the reference method and will therefore inherit these errors, in addition to those arising from the photometric technique (Shenk and Westerhaus, 1994; Deaville and Flinn, 2000). Thus, the most accurate predictions can only be achieved with the most accurate reference values, and a higher level of tolerance might be applied when evaluating the prediction statistics of digestibility using NIR spectral data. NIR spectra contain information associated with all chemical entities of a sample and, as digestibility is related to all chemical components, an improved prediction would be expected with NIR spectra compared with individual chemical data (Deaville and Flinn, 2000).

In vitro *alternatives*

A further approach is to reproduce in the laboratory the reactions which take place in the alimentary tract of the animal, recording measurements that may be used as indicators of *in vivo* digestibility. These are called *in vitro* methods and prediction of digestibility has been mainly from end point measurements either of substrate disappearance (gravimetric procedures) or of fermentation end product (gases, volatile fatty acids (VFAs)) formation. These procedures have been reviewed by López (2005).

In vitro procedures to measure digestibility of ruminant feeds are based on the anaerobic fermentation of a sample substrate with medium (buffer solution of composition similar to saliva) and filtered rumen fluid as a source of microbes. The most commonly used method, the two-stage technique for the *in vitro* digestion of forage crops, was proposed by Tilley and Terry (1963). The first stage of this method comprises incubation in buffered rumen fluid for 48 h and, in the second stage, the residue is digested for another 48 h with acid-pepsin. Since the original procedure was published, modifications have been introduced to increase laboratory throughput, precision and accuracy. Of note is the procedure proposed by Goering and Van Soest (1970) in which the second stage is replaced by an extraction in neutral detergent at 100°C for 1 h, so the analysis is substantially shortened. In this latter procedure, it is assumed that, after the first incubation in rumen fluid, all cell contents should be completely digested and, if remaining in the residue for any reason, this 'digested' fraction of the residue is removed by extraction with neutral detergent. The extraction also washes out any microbial debris in the residue, leaving only the wholly indigestible fraction of the feed sample incubated. Thus, Van Soest (1994) suggests that the latter procedure gives true *in vitro* digestibility, in contrast to the Tilley and Terry procedure, which gives a value more related to apparent *in vivo* digestibility (Fig. 2.5). Both procedures have been standardized to reduce the influence of several sources of error and allow large-scale evaluation of forage feeds, while taking into account some of the factors that influence digestibility, predicting *in vivo* digestibility with a high degree of accuracy. Obviously, these techniques yield a single digestibility for each feedstuff, though *in vivo* the value may be affected by level of feed intake and diet composition. Many studies have shown strong statistical correlations ($r > 0.9$) between *in vivo* and *in vitro* digestibility data (Osbourn and Terry, 1977; Marten and Barnes, 1980; Weiss, 1994; Minson, 1998). A strong correlation does not necessarily mean that *in vitro* digestibility

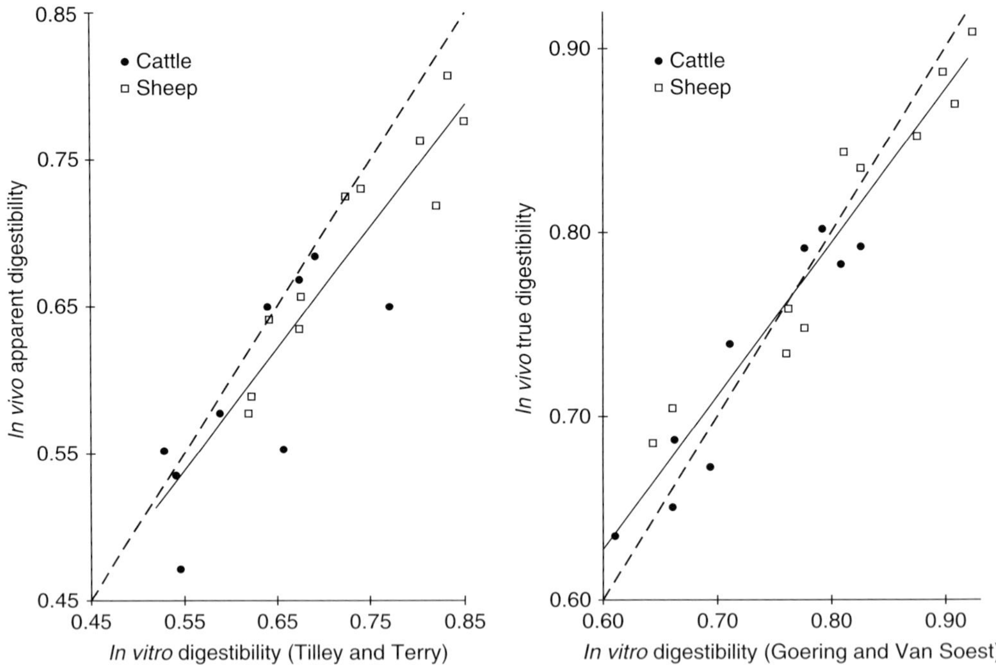

Fig. 2.5. Prediction of apparent and true *in vivo* digestibility from different *in vitro* digestibility methods (Tilley and Terry, 1963, and Goering and Van Soest, 1970, respectively). The dashed line is the mean diagonal ($y = x$) or line of equality (adapted from Van Soest, 1994).

equals *in vivo* values (Fig. 2.5); usually, an equation must be derived to convert *in vitro* data to *in vivo* digestibility (Fig. 2.6). For some forages, however, a high degree of reproducibility can be attained and both values are very similar, so that, when a linear model is fitted regressing *in vivo* against *in vitro* digestibilities, a slope parameter not significantly different from unity has been observed (Terry *et al.*, 1978; Van Soest, 1994). Prediction error can be reduced considerably by using different regression equations for different forage species (Minson and McLeod, 1972; Weiss, 1994; Minson, 1998).

The need for developing methods that do not use rumen fluid as the inoculum led to the proposal of procedures using enzyme (cellulase, hemicellulase) preparations instead. For a detailed review of the sourcing and use of enzymes, see Jones and Theodorou (2000). Earlier versions of these preparations were not sufficiently effective in degrading more mature herbage samples. Search for better cellulases continued and Jones and Hayward (1975) found solubility of dried grasses in *Trichoderma* cellulase to be highly correlated with *in vivo* digestibility. These authors modified their procedure by including pepsin pretreatment of samples (Jones and Hayward, 1975). A high correlation with *in vivo* digestibility has also been observed if a neutral detergent extraction, under reflux at 100°C, is used as a pretreatment prior to incubation with a fungal cellulase (Roughan and Holland, 1977; Dowman and Collins, 1982). Enzyme solubility (*ES*, g digested

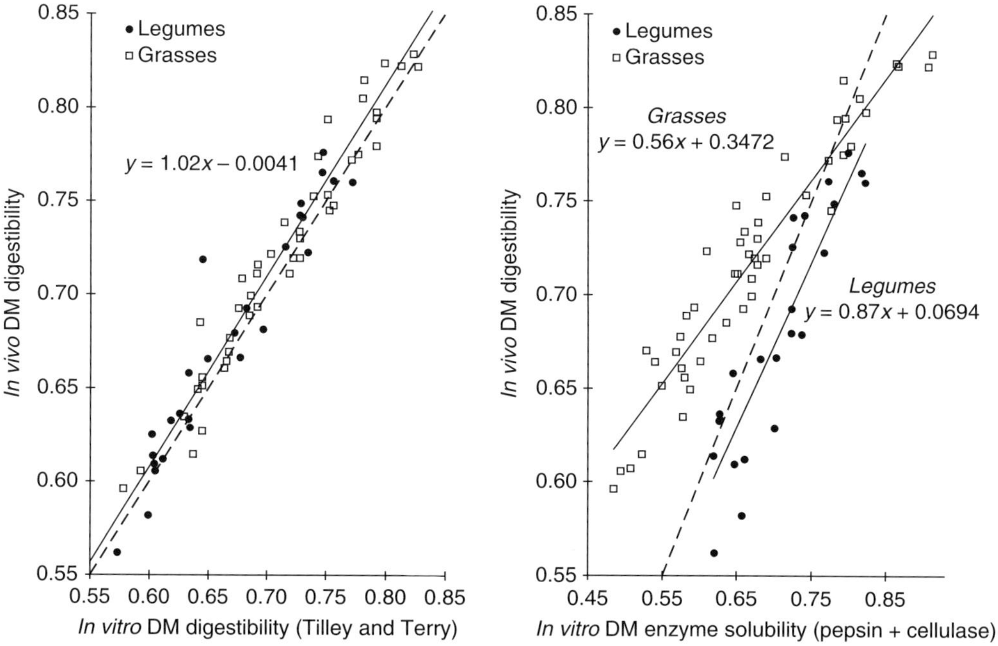

Fig. 2.6. Prediction of *in vivo* digestibility from *in vitro* digestibility using rumen fluid (Tilley and Terry, 1963) or an enzymatic procedure (pepsin + cellulase). The dashed line is the mean diagonal ($y = x$) or line of equality (adapted from Terry *et al.*, 1978).

g^{-1} incubated) recorded by these procedures is always lower than *in vivo* digestibility (*DMD*), requiring calibration using a linear equation (Fig. 2.6) of the form:

$$DMD = \alpha' + \beta' ES,$$

with different values for α' and β', depending on the type of forage (β' ranging from 0.56 for grasses to 1.05 for lucerne) (Terry *et al.*, 1978; Jones and Theodorou, 2000). Slope values significantly lower than unity suggest some lack of reproducibility, so that enzyme solubility values are useful as relative values for comparisons between forages, but a prediction equation is required to obtain estimates of *in vivo* digestibility (Marten and Barnes, 1980; Jones and Theodorou, 2000).

In recent decades, a method based on the incubation of the sample in buffered rumen fluid recording the volume of fermentation gas at different times after inoculation of the *in vitro* culture has been used extensively for feed evaluation and rumen fermentation studies (Theodorou *et al.*, 1994; Williams, 2000; López, 2005; Makkar, 2005). Menke *et al.* (1979) reported a high correlation between digestible OM content of forages and gas production *in vitro* ($r = 0.96$). It is important to understand that the technique assumes that the gas produced in batch cultures is just the consequence of fermentation of a given amount of substrate, and the major assumption in gas production equations is that the rate at which gas is produced is directly proportional to the rate at which substrate is degraded (France *et al.*, 2000). The degraded substrate can be used not only for production of fermentation gas, but also for synthesis of microbial matter or of VFAs. Therefore, two feedstuffs showing the same substrate degradability after incubation *in vitro* may give rise to a different production of fermentation gas, if the degraded substrate is used more efficiently (fermentation gas is a loss) to form VFA or microbial matter. The concept of fermentation efficiency (mg of degraded substrate ml^{-1} of fermentation gas production) has been introduced (Blümmel *et al.*, 1997) to represent this partitioning of the substrate degraded and to compare feedstuffs. A number of empirical equations have been proposed to predict *in vivo* digestibility and energy value of ruminant feedstuffs from chemical components and gas production after 24 h of incubation as the independent variables (Menke and Steingass, 1988; Chenost *et al.*, 2001). For example, OM digestibility (OMD) of forages can be predicted with an acceptable degree of accuracy ($R^2 > 0.9$) from gas production (GP) at 24 h and the crude protein (C_{CP}) and ash (C_{ash}) contents:

$$OMD = 14.9 + 0.889\,GP + 0.045\,C_{CP} + 0.065\,C_{ash}.$$

In gas production studies, there is potential to reduce dependence on rumen liquor as the inoculum source by using faeces and many studies have shown encouraging results (El Shaer *et al.*, 1987; Omed *et al.*, 2000; Dhanoa *et al.*, 2004). The main problem with the *in vitro* gas production technique is lack of standardization (in comparison with gravimetric *in vitro* digestibility methods), despite the large number of possible sources of variation, so that different procedures are used in different laboratories (Williams, 2000; López, 2005), making comparison of results obtained at various sites infeasible and rendering it impossible to establish a general calibration equation valid for any situation.

The in situ *method*

In this case, digestion studies are conducted in the rumen of a living animal, instead of simulating rumen conditions in the laboratory, hence the term *in situ*. The disappearance of substrate is measured when an undegradable porous bag containing a small amount of the feedstuff is suspended in the rumen of a cannulated animal and incubated for a particular time interval (Ørskov *et al.*, 1980). The feed is thus exposed directly to the ruminal environment.

The technique is based on the assumption that disappearance of substrate from the bags represents actual substrate degradation by the rumen microbes and their enzymes. However, not all the matter leaving the bag has been previously degraded and some of the residue remaining in the bag is not really undegradable matter of feed origin. Furthermore, the bag can be considered an independent compartment in the rumen, with the cloth representing a 'barrier' that on one side allows for the degradation of the feed to be assessed without mixing with the rumen contents, but on the other side implies an obstacle for simulating actual rumen conditions inside the bag. Finally, some methodological aspects require standardization for the technique to be considered precise and reproducible. The influence of the different sources of variation (bag and sample characteristics, dietary effects, microbial contamination of the residue, etc.) on disappearance measurements have been investigated extensively and reviewed since the early 1980s and a number of technical and methodological recommendations have been made (Ørskov *et al.*, 1980; Huntington and Givens, 1995;

Vanzant *et al.*, 1998; Broderick and Cochran, 2000; Nozière and Michalet-Doreau, 2000; Ørskov, 2000; López, 2005).

The history of *in situ* studies can be traced back to Quin *et al.* (1938) when silk bags were used, although the method gained widespread application when Ørskov and McDonald (1979) suggested its use to determine protein degradability in the rumen. However, the technique has been used as a means to predict feed digestibility in ruminants (Van Keuren and Heinemann, 1962; Demarquilly and Chenost, 1969; Nocek, 1988; Judkins *et al.*, 1990; Flachowsky and Schneider, 1992; Carro *et al.*, 1994; Nozière and Michalet-Doreau, 2000), although there are not many comparisons between *in situ* data and corresponding *in vivo* values. DM or OM disappearance at a given incubation time in the rumen is used as an end point measurement (gravimetric) that can be used as predictor of digestibility. In this case, the main issue is the need to select an appropriate period of incubation, as no single end point will be correct for all circumstances. *In situ* DM disappearance after 12–24 h of incubation shows a significant correlation with DM intake, whereas disappearances at longer incubation times (36–72 h) are better correlated with DM and OM digestibility (Judkins *et al.*, 1990; Flachowsky and Schneider, 1992; Carro *et al.*, 1994), and Demarquilly and Chenost (1969) reported several linear equations to estimate OM *in vivo* digestibility (y) from *in situ* DM disappearance after 48 h of incubation (x), of the form (Fig. 2.7):

$$y = \alpha + \beta x.$$

Equations are different for each botanical group (legumes or grasses) and for each type of forage (fresh herbage, hay or silage). Depending on the type of feedstuffs studied, *in situ* disappearance values after 48 h may be fairly similar to (Flachowsky and Schneider, 1992) or substantially higher than (Judkins *et al.*, 1990) *in vivo* DM digestibility values. Nevertheless, both are strongly correlated

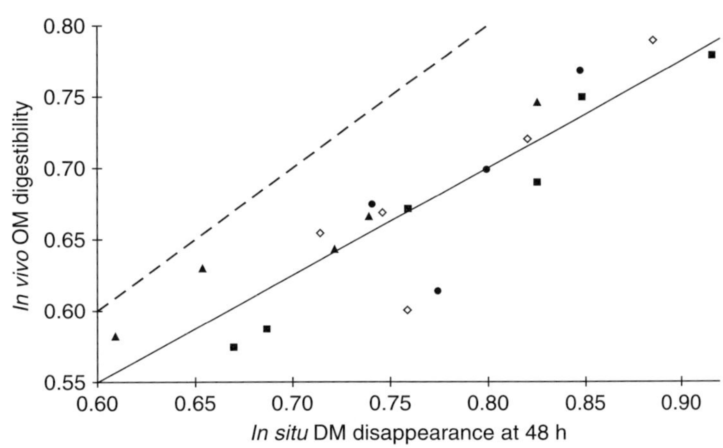

Fig. 2.7. Prediction of *in vivo* digestibility from *in situ* disappearance values after 48 h of incubation in the rumen. The dashed line is the mean diagonal ($y = x$) or line of equality (adapted from Demarquilly and Chenost, 1969).

and rank forages rather consistently. Regardless of all its limitations, the *in situ* technique is one of the best ways to access the rumen environment; it is fairly rapid and reproducible and requires minimal equipment. Therefore, it is one of the techniques used most extensively in feed evaluation for ruminants.

Also, an *in situ* mobile bag technique has been proposed to determine intestinal digestion in ruminants (Hvelplund, 1985; de Boer *et al.*, 1987). Samples of feed or residues after incubation in the rumen are weighed into small polyester bags, which are introduced directly into the abomasum or proximal duodenum and subsequently collected from either the ileum or faeces. Substrate disappearance from the bag is assumed to be due to digestion in the lower tract and an indicator of intestinal digestibility.

Prediction from rumen degradation kinetics

End point feed evaluation procedures discussed above do not provide information on the dynamics of degradation in the rumen and have a main limitation as values are for a unique incubation time. *In vitro* or *in situ* substrate disappearance or *in vitro* gas production can be measured at different incubation times, resulting in characteristic curved profiles showing the time course of fermentation and/or degradation of feedstuffs. Non-linear models can be fitted to these data to estimate kinetic parameters that summarize the information from the curves and are indicators of the rate and extent of degradation of feeds in the rumen (López, Chapter 3, this volume). The most popular model is the exponential equation proposed by Ørskov and McDonald (1979):

$$p = a + b(1 - e^{-ct}),$$

where p is the substrate disappearance at incubation time t and a, b and c are parameters. Other models have been derived using a more mechanistic and compartmental approach, dividing the substrate into three fractions with different kinetic behaviour; namely, a fraction that disappears immediately from the bag and can be assumed to be soluble in the rumen (fraction W or parameter a); a fraction that is insoluble but potentially degradable at a given rate and disappears from the rumen by the processes of both digestion and passage (fraction S or parameter b); and an undegradable fraction that remains in the bag indefinitely and in the rumen disappears only by passage to the lower tract (fraction U) (Fig. 2.8). Fraction S starts to be degraded after a lag time (L) and, thereafter, its degradation kinetics can be represented by a differential equation:

$$\frac{dS}{dt} = -\mu S \qquad t > L,$$

where μ (or parameter c, h^{-1}) is the fractional degradation rate that can be assumed constant (first-order kinetics or exponential model) or vary with time (i.e. $\mu = f(t)$), leading to different non-linear models that can be fitted to degradation profiles varying in shape from diminishing returns to sigmoidal (S-type) (France *et al.*, 1990; Dhanoa *et al.*, 1995; López *et al.*, 1999; López, 2005, Chapter 3, this volume). The degree of sigmoidicity may be an indication of poor feed quality or a poor rumen environment, or a combination of both. A similar approach can be

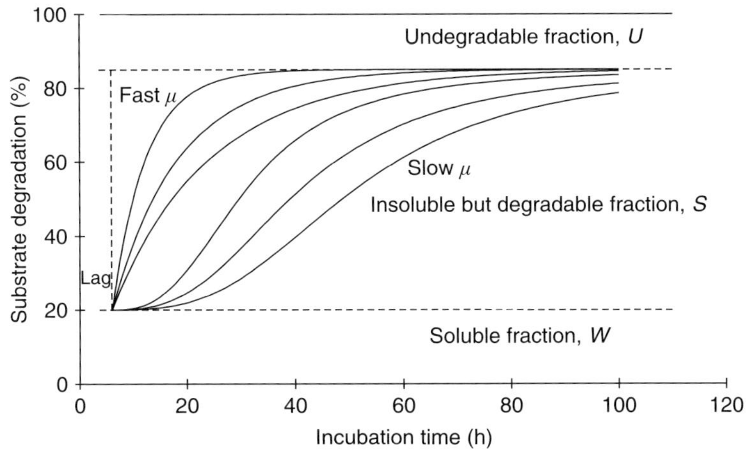

Fig. 2.8. Substrate degradation curves from *in situ* disappearance data, showing the partitioning of the substrate into different fractions (soluble, insoluble but potentially degradable and completely undegradable) and differences in the curve shape as fractional degradation rate (μ) is increased.

used for gas production profiles (France *et al.*, 1993, 2000, 2005; Dhanoa *et al.*, 2000) but, in this case, fractions W and S have to be considered as a single entity.

Some interesting attributes characteristic of each degradation profile can be calculated from the model parameters that indicate the rate of degradation of each feedstuff, such as half-life (time taken for half the S fraction to degrade) or average degradation rate. Although degradation rate can be affected by ruminal factors, under some specific conditions it can also be assumed to be an intrinsic characteristic of each feed (Mertens, 2005).

Assuming degradation kinetics are the same in the bag or in *in vitro* culture as in the rumen proper, the extent of degradation of feeds in the rumen can be calculated taking into account that, in this case, fraction S will disappear by both digestion and passage. Models have been proposed to represent the competition between these two processes in which kinetic parameters for degradation and passage are integrated to estimate whole tract digestibility or actual extent of degradation of feed in the rumen (Blaxter *et al.*, 1956; Waldo *et al.*, 1972). This simple original approach has been extended to the models developed subsequently (López *et al.*, 1999; France *et al.*, 2000, 2005). Extent of degradation in the rumen can be calculated for a given passage rate, which in turn is affected mainly by the type of feed, animal species and the level of feed intake. Fractional passage rate (k, h^{-1}) is estimated using marker kinetics modelling (Chapter 3 of this book). For the simple exponential model, the expression to calculate extent of degradation in the rumen (E, g degraded g^{-1} ingested) from *in situ* or *in vitro* parameters is:

$$E = W + \frac{\mu S e^{-kL}}{\mu + k} = a + \frac{c b e^{-kL}}{c + k}.$$

For other models, such a simple expression cannot be derived, but E can still be determined by numerical integration. This derivation reveals the important role of mathematical modelling in linking data obtained by *in situ* or *in vitro* methods to *in vivo* degradability.

Once the modelling (mostly non-linear) has been completed, meaningful quantities (parameters or functions thereof) can be related back to *in vivo* measurements of digestibility and a working calibration developed (Ørskov, 2000). Most reported studies just correlate model parameters with the *in vivo* quantities, but the use of derived parameters (such as average degradation rate or extent of degradation) may improve the prediction of *in vivo* digestibility. In this sense, the most common conclusion is that rate parameters show a significant correlation with feed intake, whereas extent parameters (potential or effective degradability) are better correlated with digestibility (Ørskov, 2000; Carro *et al.*, 2002). Nevertheless, extent of degradation values is generally lower than whole tract digestibility, mainly because degradability takes into account ruminal processes only, whereas some substrates are further digested in the lower tract.

Prediction from faecal measurements

Under grazing conditions, prediction of digestibility from feed characteristics is highly dependent on collecting a representative sample of herbage. Whereas it is relatively simple to collect a sample of the pasture on offer, it may be far more difficult to take a representative sample of what is actually grazed by the animal. This can happen in any situation where the animal is able to exhibit significant diet selection, with a strong preference for some fractions of the feed on offer. In this case, prediction of digestibility from attributes of the forage fed to the animal may be subject to serious error.

An alternative method is to establish a relationship between forage digestibility and concentration of an indicator substance in the faeces (Peyraud, 1998). Data obtained from conventional *in vivo* digestibility trials with animals in stalls or metabolic cages are used to determine the statistical relationship between digestibility and the chemical composition of faeces. This relationship is represented mathematically by equations (usually linear models) that are then applied to a grazing situation.

This approach was developed in the late 1940s after observing a close relationship between the herbage OM digestibility and the nitrogen content of faeces. Since then, faecal nitrogen has been used as a faecal indicator to predict feed digestibility with highly satisfactory predictive accuracy, being considered a special type of marker 'generated mathematically' (Van Soest, 1994).

Faecal nitrogen is highly correlated with DM intake, due in part to the fact that a significant proportion of total faecal nitrogen is of endogenous and microbial origin (metabolic faecal nitrogen), which is excreted in amounts that are approximately proportional to the amount of DM ingested. Thus, faecal nitrogen could be used as a predictor for estimating herbage intake by grazing ruminants, and Lancaster (1949) indicated that faecal nitrogen would also be related to forage digestibility. Although, initially, it was suggested that the relationship between faecal nitrogen and dietary intake was relatively constant, regardless of the N content of the forages, some early studies showed that forage protein level might have some effect on the amount of faecal nitrogen relative to DM intake. Regression equations developed for forage cut at various times of the year were different, depending on the N content of the forage (Minson, 1990). The method would be expected to be more accurate with low-protein roughages, as the correlation is less significant with forages of higher N content because, with these forages, the proportion of metabolic nitrogen in total faecal nitrogen is decreased.

The relationship between digestibility and faecal nitrogen content (N_f, g N kg^{-1} faecal organic matter) may be fitted by a hyperbolic equation, such as:

$$D_{OM} = \alpha - \frac{\beta}{N_f},$$

where α and β are positive parameters, estimated from regression analysis (Lancaster, 1949; Minson, 1990; Peyraud, 1998). Lancaster (1954) reported a similar formula for predicting OM digestibility of the form:

$$\frac{I_{OM}}{F_{OM}} = \frac{1}{1 - D_{OM}} = \alpha + \beta N_f.$$

As reviewed by Minson (1990), a number of authors have observed a relationship between OM digestibility and faecal nitrogen concentration for temperate forages which approaches a straight line and can be fitted approximately by a linear model ($D_{OM} = \alpha + \beta N_f$); and Chenost (1985) proposed fitting a quadratic polynomial:

$$D_{OM} = \alpha + \beta N_f - \gamma N_f^2.$$

However, there is not a single general equation suitable for all forages and conditions, and many of the equations derived (especially in terms of the value of the slope parameter) are valid only in circumstances similar to those under which calibration data were recorded (Rymer, 2000). Therefore, it has been recommended that different equations be used for a particular plant species, pasture type, geographical location, or even for each cut or harvest season (Greenhalgh and Corbett, 1960; Peyraud, 1998). Anyhow, the technique can result in reasonably accurate prediction of digestibility, as up to 93% of the variation in *in vivo* digestibility can be explained by concentration of faecal nitrogen (Rymer, 2000). Faecal nitrogen gives an estimate of digestibility and intake with an error of about 10–15%, which can be diminished somewhat by calibration with animals stall-fed forage as similar as possible to that grazed (Van Soest, 1994).

Other faecal indicators have been used to predict digestibility, such as chromogen, fibre (ADF), soluble matter or methoxyl concentration in faeces (Wofford *et al.*, 1985; Rymer, 2000), with different degrees of accuracy in estimating herbage DM or OM digestibility. The combined use of several faecal indicators can improve accuracy of prediction and extend applicability of the models.

These methods based on faecal indicators seem to take into account individual variability in digestibility and effects of changes in feed intake on herbage digestibility, but are well suited only for use with forages and not with concentrate feeds.

Concluding Remarks

Given the importance of feed digestibility as an index of nutritional value, a number of alternative procedures have been developed aiming to predict *in vivo* digestibility. Most of these alternatives are effective for screening purposes, providing useful data when the research objective is ranking of feedstuffs or comparing experimental treatments. However, their validity as a means to predict *in vivo* digestibility coefficients accurately is less certain due to a multiplicity of sources of variation, the most influential being methodological. In some of the *in vitro* and other laboratory procedures, there is a lack of standardization between different laboratories, jeopardizing their precision and reproducibility, and thus the possibility of comparing and interpreting data from different origins and of achieving a 'universal' predictive equation valid under any circumstances. The other main handicap is the need for calibration and validation of results against *in vivo* data. Although there is sufficient evidence that all the laboratory and *in situ* data are highly correlated with *in vivo* digestibility, not many suitable prediction equations are available because of lack of *in vivo* data on the same feedstuffs. Ruminant nutritionists must thus be aware of the limitations of each of the predictive approaches.

References

Adesogan, A.T. (2002) What are feeds worth? A critical evaluation of selected nutritive value methods. In: *Proceedings 13th Annual Florida Ruminant Nutrition Symposium*. University of Florida, Gainesville, Florida, pp. 33–47.

AFRC (1993) *Energy and Protein Requirements of Ruminants*. CAB International, Wallingford, UK.

Andrieu, J. and Demarquilly, C. (1987) Valeur nutritive des fourrages: tables et prévision. *Bulletin Technique CRZV Theix, INRA* 70, 61–73.

Andrieu, J., Demarquilly, C. and Wegat-Litre, E. (1981) Tables de prévision de la valeur alimentaire des fourrages. In: *Prévision de la Valeur Nutritive des Aliments des Ruminants*. INRA Publications, Versailles, France, pp. 345–580.

Barber, W.P.B., Adamson, A.H. and Altman, J.F.B. (1984) New methods of feed evaluation. In: Haresign, W. and Cole, D.J.A. (eds) *Recent Advances in Animal Nutrition*. Butterworths, London, pp. 161–176.

Bartiaux-Thill, N. and Oger, R. (1986) The indirect estimation of the digestibility in cattle of herbage from Belgian permanent pasture. *Grass and Forage Science* 41, 269–272.

Blaxter, K.L., Graham, N.McC. and Wainman, F.W. (1956) Some observations on the digestibility of food by sheep, and on related problems. *British Journal of Nutrition* 10, 69–91.

Blümmel, M., Makkar, H.P.S. and Becker, K. (1997) *In vitro* gas production: a technique revisited. *Journal of Animal Physiology and Animal Nutrition* 77, 24–34.

Boer, G. De, Murphy, J.J. and Kennelly, J.J. (1987) Mobile nylon bag for estimating intestinal availability of rumen undegradable protein. *Journal of Dairy Science* 70, 977–982.

Broderick, G.A. and Cochran, R.C. (2000) *In vitro* and *in situ* methods for estimating digestibility with reference to protein degradability. In: Theodorou, M.K. and France,

J. (eds) *Feeding Systems and Feed Evaluation Models*. CAB International, Wallingford, UK, pp. 53–85.

Cammell, S.B. (1977) *Equipment and Techniques used for Research into the Intake and Digestion of Forages by Sheep and Calves*. Grassland Research Institute Technical Report No. 24, Hurley, UK.

Carro, M.D., López, S., Gonzalez, J.S. and Ovejero, F.J. (1994) Comparison of laboratory methods for predicting digestibility of hay in sheep. *Small Ruminant Research* 14, 9–17.

Carro, M.D., López, S., González, J.S., Ovejero, F.J. and Ranilla, M.J. (2002) *In vitro* methods as predictors of voluntary intake and digestibility of hays fed to sheep. *Australian Journal of Agricultural Research* 53, 471–479.

Chenost, M. (1985) Estimation de la digestibilité de l'herbe ingérée au pâturage à partir de l'azote fécal et de quelques autres paramètres fécaux. *Annales de Zootechnie* 34, 205–228.

Chenost, M., Aufrère, J. and Macheboeuf, D. (2001) The gas-test technique as a tool for predicting the energetic value of forage plants. *Animal Research* 50, 349–364.

Chesson, A. (1993) Mechanistic models of forage cell wall degradation. In: Jung, H.G., Buxton, D.R., Hatfield, R.D. and Ralph, J. (eds) *Forage Cell Wall Structure and Digestibility*. ASA-CSSA-SSSA, Madison, Wisconsin, pp. 347–376.

Clark, D.H. and Lamb, R.C. (1991) Near infrared reflectance spectroscopy: a survey of wavelength selection to determine dry matter digestibility. *Journal of Dairy Science* 74, 2200–2205.

Cochran, R.C. and Galyean, M.L. (1994) Measurement of *in vivo* forage digestion by ruminants. In: Fahey, G.C. Jr (ed.) *Forage Quality, Evaluation, and Utilization*. ASA-CSSA-SSSA, Madison, Wisconsin, pp. 613–643.

Colburn, M.W., Evans, J.L. and Ramage, C.H. (1968) Apparent and true digestibility of forage nutrients by ruminant animals. *Journal of Dairy Science* 51, 1450–1457.

Cordova, F.J., Wallace, J.D. and Pieper, R.D. (1978) Forage intake by grazing livestock: a review. *Journal of Range Management* 31, 430–438.

CSIRO (1990) *Feeding Standards for Australian Livestock. Ruminants*. CSIRO Publications, Melbourne, Australia.

Danfaer, A. and Fernandez, J.A. (1999) Developments in the prediction of nutrient availability in pigs: a review. *Acta Agriculturae Scandinavica Section A – Animal Science* 49, 73–82.

Darragh, A.J. and Hodgkinson, S.M. (2000) Quantifying the digestibility of dietary protein. *Journal of Nutrition* 130, 1850S–1856S.

Deaville, E.R. and Flinn, P.C. (2000) Near infrared (NIR) spectroscopy: an alternative approach for the estimation of forage quality and voluntary intake. In: Givens, D.I., Owen, E., Axford, R.F.E. and Omed, H.M. (eds) *Forage Evaluation in Ruminant Nutrition*. CAB International, Wallingford, UK, pp. 301–320.

Demarquilly, C. and Chenost, M. (1969) Étude de la digestion des fourrages dans le rumen par la méthode des sachets de nylon. Liaison avec la valeur alimentaire. *Annales de Zootechnie* 18, 419–436.

Dhanoa, M.S., France, J., Siddons, R.C., López, S. and Buchanan-Smith, J.G. (1995) A non-linear compartmental model to describe forage degradation kinetics during incubation in polyester bags in the rumen. *British Journal of Nutrition* 73, 3–15.

Dhanoa, M.S., López, S., Dijkstra, J., Davies, D.R., Sanderson, R.S., Williams, B.A., Sileshi, Z. and France, J. (2000) Estimating the extent of degradation of ruminant feeds from a description of their gas production profiles observed *in vitro*: comparison of models. *British Journal of Nutrition* 83, 131–142.

Dhanoa, M.S., France, J., Crompton, L.A., Mauricio, R.M., Kebreab, E., Mills, J.A.N., Sanderson, R., Dijkstra, J. and López, S. (2004) A proposed method to determine the extent of degradation of a feed in the rumen from the degradation profile obtained with the *in vitro* gas production technique using feces as the inoculum. *Journal of Animal Science* 82, 733–746.

Dove, H. and Mayes, R.W. (1991) The use of plant wax alkanes as marker substances in studies of the nutrition of herbivores: a review. *Australian Journal of Agricultural Research* 42, 913–952.

Dowman, M.G. and Collins, F.C. (1982) The use of enzymes to predict the digestibility of animal feeds. *Journal of the Science of Food and Agriculture* 33, 689–696.

Draper, N.R. and Smith, H. (1998) *Applied Regression Analysis*, 3rd edn. Wiley, New York.

Flachowsky, G. and Schneider, M. (1992) Influence of various straw-to-concentrate ratios on *in sacco* dry matter degradability, feed intake and apparent digestibility in ruminants. *Animal Feed Science and Technology* 38, 199–217.

Fonnesbeck, P.V., Wardeh, M.F. and Harris, L.E. (1984) *Mathematical Models for Estimating Energy and Protein Utilization of Feedstuffs*, Bulletin 508. Utah State University, Logan, Utah.

Fox, J. (1997) *Applied Regression Analysis, Linear Models and Related Methods*. Sage Publications, Thousand Oaks, California.

France, J., Thornley, J.H.M., López, S., Siddons, R.C., Dhanoa, M.S., Van Soest, P.J. and Gill, M. (1990) On the two-compartment model for estimating the rate and extent of feed degradation in the rumen. *Journal of Theoretical Biology* 146, 269–287.

France, J., Dhanoa, M.S., Theodorou, M.K., Lister, S.J., Davies, D.R. and Isac, D. (1993) A model to interpret gas accumulation profiles associated with *in vitro* degradation of ruminant feeds. *Journal of Theoretical Biology* 163, 99–111.

France, J., Dijkstra, J., Dhanoa, M.S., López, S. and Bannink, A. (2000) Estimating the extent of degradation of ruminant feeds from a description of their gas production profiles observed *in vitro*: derivation of models and other mathematical considerations. *British Journal of Nutrition* 83, 131–142.

France, J., López, S., Kebreab, E., Bannink, A., Dhanoa, M.S. and Dijkstra, J. (2005) A general compartmental model for interpreting gas production profiles. *Animal Feed Science and Technology* 123–124, 473–485.

Givens, D.I. and Deaville, E.R. (1999) The current and future role of near infrared reflectance spectroscopy in animal nutrition: a review. *Australian Journal of Agricultural Research* 50, 1131–1145.

Givens, D.I. and Moss, A.R. (1994) Effect of breed, age and bodyweight of sheep on the measurement of apparent digestibility of dried grass. *Animal Feed Science and Technology* 46, 155–162.

Goering, M.K. and Van Soest, P.J. (1970) *Forage Fiber Analysis (Apparatus, Reagents, Procedures and Some Applications)*. Agricultural Handbook No. 379, Agricultural Research Service, USDA, Washington, DC.

Greenhalgh, J.F.D. (1982) An introduction to herbage intake measurements. In: Leaver, J.D. (ed.) *Herbage Intake Handbook*. The British Grassland Society, Reading, UK, pp. 1–10.

Greenhalgh, J.F.D. and Corbett, J.L. (1960) The indirect estimation of digestibility of pasture herbage. 1. Nitrogen and chromogen as faecal index substance. *Journal of Agricultural Science, Cambridge* 55, 371–376.

Harrell, F.E. Jr (2006) *Regression Modelling Strategies with Applications to Linear Models, Logistic Regression, and Survival Analysis Series*, 2nd edn. Springer, Berlin.

Huntington, J.A. and Givens, D.I. (1995) The *in situ* technique for studying the rumen degradation of feeds: a review of the procedure. *Nutrition Abstracts and Reviews Series B (Livestock Feeds and Feeding)* 65, 63–93.

Hvelplund, T. (1985) Digestibility of rumen microbial protein and undegraded protein estimated in the small intestine of sheep and by *in sacco* procedure. *Acta Agriculturae Scandinavica Supplement* 25, 132–144.

Hvelplund, T., Andrieu, J., Weisbjerg, M.R. and Vermorel, M. (1995) Prediction of the energy and protein value of forages for ruminants. In: Journet, M., Grenet, E., Farce, M.H., Theriez, M. and Demarquilly, C. (eds) *Recent Developments in the Nutrition of Herbivores*. INRA Editions, Paris, pp. 205–227.

ILCA (International Livestock Centre for Africa) (1990) *Livestock Systems Research Manual.* Working Paper 1, Vol. 1. ILCA, Addis Ababa.

Jones, D.I.H. and Hayward, M.V. (1975) The effect of pepsin pretreatment of herbage on the prediction of dry matter digestibility from solubility in fungal cell cellulase solutions. *Journal of the Science of Food and Agriculture* 26, 711–718.

Jones, D.I.H. and Theodorou, M.K. (2000) Enzyme techniques for estimating digestibility. In: Givens, D.I., Owen, E., Axford, R.F.E. and Omed, H.M. (eds) *Forage Evaluation in Ruminant Nutrition*. CAB International, Wallingford, UK, pp. 155–173.

Judkins, M.B., Krysl, L.J. and Barton, R.K. (1990) Estimation of diet digestibility: a comparison of 11 techniques across six different diets fed to rams. *Journal of Animal Science* 68, 1405–1415.

Kaps, M. and Lamberson, W. (2004) *Biostatistics for Animal Science*. CAB International, Wallingford, UK.

Kitessa, S., Flinn, P.C. and Irish, G.G. (1999) Comparison of methods used to predict the *in vivo* digestibility of feeds in ruminants. *Australian Journal of Agricultural Research* 50, 825–841.

Kleinbaum, D.G., Kupper, L.L., Muller, K.E. and Nizam, A. (1998) *Applied Regression Analysis and other Multivariable Methods*, 3rd edn. Duxbury Press (Brooks/Cole Publishing Company), Pacific Grove, California.

Krysl, L.J., Galyean, M.L., Estell, R.E. and Sowell, B.F. (1988) Estimating digestibility and faecal output in lambs using internal and external markers. *Journal of Agricultural Science, Cambridge* 111, 19–25.

Lancaster, R.J. (1949) Estimation of digestibility of grazed pasture from faeces nitrogen. *Nature, London* 163, 330–331.

Lancaster, R.J. (1954) Measurement of feed intake of grazing cattle and sheep. V Estimation of the feed-to-faeces ratio from the nitrogen content of the faeces of pasture fed cattle. *New Zealand Journal of Science and Technology* 36, 15–20.

López, S. (2005) *In vitro* and *in situ* techniques for estimating digestibility. In: Dijkstra, J., Forbes, J.M. and France, J. (eds) *Quantitative Aspects of Ruminant Digestion and Metabolism*, 2nd edn. CAB International, Wallingford, UK, pp. 87–121.

López, S., France, J., Dhanoa, M.S., Mould, F. and Dijkstra, J. (1999) Comparison of mathematical models to describe disappearance curves obtained using the polyester bag technique for incubating feeds in the rumen. *Journal of Animal Science* 77, 1875–1888.

Lucas, H.L. (1964) Stochastic elements in biological models; their sources and significance. In: Gurland, J. (ed.) *Stochastic Models in Medicine and Biology*. University of Wisconsin Press, Madison, Wisconsin, pp. 355–383.

McDonald, P., Edwards, R.A., Greenhalgh, J.F.D. and Morgan, C.A. (2002) *Animal Nutrition*, 6th edn. Pearson Education Ltd, Harlow, UK.

Makkar, H.P.S. (2005) *In vitro* gas methods for evaluation of feeds containing phytochemicals. *Animal Feed Science and Technology* 123–124, 291–302.

Marten, G.C. and Barnes, R.F. (1980) Prediction of energy digestibility of forages with *in vitro* rumen fermentation and fungal enzyme systems. In: Pigden, W.J., Balch, C.C. and Graham, M. (eds) *Standardization of Analytical Methodology for Feeds*. IDCR/IUNS, Ottawa, pp. 61–71.

Mayes, R.W. and Dove, H. (2000) Measurement of dietary intake in free-ranging mammalian herbivores. *Nutrition Research Reviews* 13, 107–138.

Menke, K.H. and Steingass, H. (1988) Estimation of the energetic feed value obtained from chemical analysis and *in vitro* gas production using rumen fluid. *Animal Research and Development* 28, 7–55.

Menke, K.H., Raab, L., Salewski, A., Steingass, H., Fritz, D. and Schneider, W. (1979) The estimation of the digestibility and metabolizable energy content of ruminant feedingstuffs from the gas production when they are incubated with rumen liquor. *Journal of Agricultural Science, Cambridge* 93, 217–222.

Mertens, D.R. (2005) Rate and extent of digestion. In: Dijkstra, J., Forbes, J.M. and France, J. (eds) *Quantitative Aspects of Ruminant Digestion and Metabolism*, 2nd edn. CAB International, Wallingford, UK, pp. 13–47.

Minson, D.J. (1981) The measurement of digestibility and voluntary intake of forages with confined animals. In: Wheeler, J.L. and Mochrie, R.D. (eds) *Forage Evaluation: Concepts and Techniques*. CSIRO, Melbourne, Australia, pp. 159–174.

Minson, D.J. (1982) Effect of chemical composition on feed digestibility and metabolizable energy. *Nutrition Abstracts and Reviews, Series B* 52, 591–615.

Minson, D.J. (1990) *Forage in Ruminant Nutrition*. Academic Press, San Diego, California.

Minson, D.J. (1998) A history of *in vitro* techniques. In: Deaville, E.R., Owen. E., Adesogan, A.T., Rymer, C., Huntington, J.A. and Lawrence, T.L.J. (eds) In vitro *Techniques for Measuring Nutrient Supply to Ruminants*, Occasional Publication No. 22. British Society of Animal Science, Edinburgh, UK, pp. 13–19.

Minson, D.J. and McLeod, M.N. (1972) The *in vitro* technique: its modification for estimating digestibility of large numbers of pasture samples. Division of Tropical Crops and Pastures, Technical Paper No. 8. CSIRO, Melbourne, Australia, pp. 1–15.

Mitchell, H.H. (1942) The evaluation of feeds on the basis of digestible and metabolizable nutrients. *Journal of Animal Science* 1, 159–173.

Morrison, I.M. (1976) New laboratory methods for predicting the nutritive value of forage crops. *World Review of Animal Production* 12, 75–82.

Motulsky, H. and Christopoulos, A. (2004) *Fitting Models to Biological Data Using Linear and Nonlinear Regression. A Practical Guide to Curve Fitting*. Oxford University Press, Oxford, UK.

Nocek, J.E. (1988) *In situ* and other methods to estimate ruminal protein and energy digestibility: a review. *Journal of Dairy Science* 71, 2051–2069.

Norris, H.K., Barnes, R.F., Moore, J.E. and Shenk, J.S. (1976) Predicting forage quality by near infrared reflectance spectroscopy. *Journal of Animal Science* 43, 889–897.

Nozière, P. and Michalet-Doreau, B. (2000) *In sacco* methods. In: D'Mello, J.P.F. (ed.) *Farm Animal Metabolism and Nutrition*. CAB International, Wallingford, UK, pp. 233–253.

NRC (1996) *Nutrient Requirements of Beef Cattle*, 7th edn. National Academic Press, Washington, DC.

Omed, H.M., Lovett, D.K. and Axford, R.F.E. (2000) Faeces as a source of microbial enzymes for estimating digestibility. In: Givens, D.I., Owen, E., Axford, R.F.E. and Omed, H.M. (eds) *Forage Evaluation in Ruminant Nutrition*. CAB International, Wallingford, UK, pp. 135–154.

Ørskov, E.R. (2000) The *in situ* technique for the estimation of forage degradability in ruminants. In: Givens, D.I., Owen, E., Axford, R.F.E. and Omed, H.M. (eds) *Forage Evaluation in Ruminant Nutrition*. CAB International, Wallingford, UK, pp. 175–188.

Ørskov, E.R. and McDonald, I. (1979) The estimation of protein degradability in the rumen from incubation measurements weighted according to rate of passage. *Journal of Agricultural Science, Cambridge* 92, 499–503.

Ørskov, E.R., Hovell, F.D. deB. and Mould, F. (1980) The use of the nylon bag technique for the evaluation of feedstuffs. *Tropical Animal Production* 5, 195–213.

Osbourn, D.F. and Terry, R. (1977) *In vitro* techniques for the evaluation of ruminant feeds. *Proceedings of the Nutrition Society* 36, 219–225.

Penning, P.D. and Johnson, R.H. (1983) The use of internal markers to estimate herbage digestibility and intake. *Journal of Agricultural Science, Cambridge* 100, 127–138.

Peyraud, J.L. (1998) Techniques for measuring faecal flow, digestibility and intake of herbage in grazing ruminants. In: *Techniques for Investigating Intake and Ingestive Behaviour by Farm Animals* (IXth European Intake Workshop). IGER, North Wyke, UK, pp. 39–43.

Quin, J.I., Van der Wath, J.G. and Myburgh, S. (1938) Studies on the alimentary tract of Merino sheep in South Africa. IV. Description of experimental technique. *Onderstepoort Journal of Veterinary Science and Animal Industry* 11, 341–360.

Raymond, W.F. (1969) The nutritive value of forage crops. *Advances in Agronomy* 21, 1–108.

Redshaw, E.S., Mathison, G.W., Milligan, L.P. and Weisenburger, R.D. (1986) Near infrared reflectance spectroscopy for predicting forage composition and voluntary consumption and digestibility in cattle and sheep. *Canadian Journal of Animal Science* 66, 103–115.

Reed, J.D. and Goe, M.R. (1989) Estimating the nutritive value of cereal crop residues: implications for developing feeding standards for draught animals. *ILCA Bulletin* 34, 2–9.

Reeves III, J.B. (2000) Use of near infrared reflectance spectroscopy. In: D'Mello, J.P.F. (ed.) *Farm Animal Metabolism and Nutrition*. CAB International, Wallingford, UK, pp. 185–207.

Roughan, P.G. and Holland, R. (1977) Predicting *in vivo* digestibilities of herbages by exhaustive enzymic hydrolysis of cell walls. *Journal of the Science of Food and Agriculture* 28, 1057–1064.

Rymer, C. (2000) The measurement of forage digestibility *in vivo*. In: Givens, D.I., Owen, E., Axford, R.F.E. and Omed, H.M. (eds) *Forage Evaluation in Ruminant Nutrition*. CAB International, Wallingford, UK, pp. 113–134.

Schneider, B.H. and Flatt, W.P. (1975) *The Evaluation of Feeds through Digestibility Experiments*. The University of Georgia Press, Athens, Georgia.

Seber, G.A.F. and Lee, A.J. (2003) *Linear Regression Analysis*, 2nd edn. Wiley, New York.

El Shaer, H.M., Omed, H.M., Chamberlain, A.G. and Axford, R.F.E. (1987) Use of faecal organisms from sheep for the *in vitro* determination of digestibility. *Journal of Agricultural Science, Cambridge* 109, 257–259.

Shenk, J.S. and Westerhaus, M.O. (1994) The application of near infrared reflectance spectroscopy (NIRS) to forage analysis. In: Fahey, G.C. Jr (ed.) *Forage Quality, Evaluation, and Utilization*. ASA-CSSA-SSSA, Madison, Wisconsin, pp. 406–449.

Souffrant, W.B. (1991) Endogenous nitrogen losses during digestion in pigs. In: Verstegen, M.W.A., Huisman, J. and den Hartog, L.A. (eds) *Digestive Physiology in Pigs* (EAAP Publ. 54). Pudoc, Wageningen, The Netherlands, pp. 147–166.

Steel, R.G.D. and Torrie, J.H. (1980) *Principles and Procedures of Statistics*, 2nd edn. McGraw-Hill, New York.

Terry, R.A., Mondell, D.C. and Osbourn, D.F. (1978) Comparison of two *in vitro* procedures using rumen liquor-pepsin or pepsin-cellulase for prediction of forage digestibility. *Journal of the British Grassland Society* 33, 13–18.

Theodorou, M.K., Williams, B.A., Dhanoa, M.S., McAllan, A.B. and France, J. (1994) A simple gas production method using a pressure transducer to determine the fermentation kinetics of ruminant feeds. *Animal Feed Science and Technology* 48, 185–197.

Tilley, J.M.A. and Terry, R.A. (1963) A two-stage technique for the *in vitro* digestion of forage crops. *Journal of the British Grassland Society* 18, 104–111.
Van Keuren, R.W. and Heinemann, W.W. (1962) Study of a nylon bag technique for *in vivo* estimation of forage digestibility. *Journal of Animal Science* 21, 340–345.
Van Soest, P.J. (1967) Development of a comprehensive system of feed analysis and its application to forages. *Journal of Animal Science* 26, 119–128.
Van Soest, P.J. (1994) *Nutritional Ecology of the Ruminant*, 2nd edn. Cornell University Press, Ithaca, New York.
Van Soest, P.J. and Mason, V.C. (1991) The influence of the Maillard reaction upon the nutritive value of fibrous feeds. *Animal Feed Science and Technology* 32, 45–53.
Van Soest, P.J., France, J. and Siddons, R.C. (1992) On the steady-state turnover of compartments in the ruminant gastrointestinal tract. *Journal of Theoretical Biology* 159, 135–145.
Vanzant, E.S., Cochran, R.C. and Titgemeyer, E.C. (1998) Standardization of *in situ* techniques for ruminant feedstuff evaluation. *Journal of Animal Science* 76, 2717–2729.
Wainman, F.W. (1977) Digestibility and balance in ruminants. *Proceedings of the Nutrition Society* 36, 195–202.
Waldo, D.R., Smith, L.W. and Cox, E.L. (1972) Model of cellulose disappearance from the rumen. *Journal of Dairy Science* 55, 125–129.
Warner, A.C.I. (1981) Rate of passage of digesta through the guts of mammals and birds. *Nutrition Abstracts and Reviews Series B (Livestock Feeds and Feeding)* 51, 789–820.
Weiss, P.E. (1994) Estimation of digestibility of forages by laboratory methods. In: Fahey, G.C. Jr (ed.) *Forage Quality, Evaluation, and Utilization*. ASA-CSSA-SSSA, Madison, Wisconsin, pp. 644–681.
Weiss, W.P., Conrad, H.R. and St. Pierre, N.R. (1992) A theoretically-based model for predicting total digestible nutrient values of forages and concentrates. *Animal Feed Science and Technology* 39, 95–110.
Williams, B.A. (2000) Cumulative gas production technique for forage evaluation. In: Givens, D.I., Owen, E., Axford, R.F.E. and Omed, H.M. (eds) *Forage Evaluation in Ruminant Nutrition*. CAB International, Wallingford, UK, pp. 135–154.
Wofford, H., Holechek, J.L., Galyean, M.L., Wallace, J.D. and Cardenas, M. (1985) Evaluation of fecal indices to predict cattle diet quality. *Journal of Range Management* 38, 450–454.
Zebrowska, T. and Buraczewski, S. (1998) Methods for determination of amino acids bioavailability in pigs – review. *Asian–Australasian Journal of Animal Sciences* 11, 620–633.

3 Non-linear Functions in Animal Nutrition

S. López

Departamento de Producción Animal, Universidad de León, Spain

Introduction

Animal nutritionists are primarily involved in the study of the digestive and metabolic processes regarding the utilization of nutrients. With this aim, the analysis and interpretation of some response functions and time-dependent data are of interest to establish the effects of specific nutrients on processes such as digestion, growth or lactation, or to examine the time course of events. Usually, this sort of data follows a curvilinear pattern that may be represented by a non-linear function. Until only a few decades ago, these functions were solved using approximations entailing linear transformations or graphical procedures, owing to limitations in the computational facilities for non-linear regression. However, more recently, a number of statistical packages have been designed to address this issue, leading to an important advance in all the statistical procedures concerning non-linear regression, and hence a more extended use of non-linear functions to represent physical, chemical or biological processes.

The aims in this chapter are to introduce briefly some of the basic principles of non-linear regression, to present some of the non-linear functions used in animal nutrition to represent time-dependent processes and events and to examine the current and potential use of these functions to describe responses to nutrients.

Non-linear Regression

Regression allows for examining data with a specific model (equation), finding the parameters of a model to best fit a set of data values and separating the systematic pattern or main trend (set of identifiable components or variability explained by the model) from what is left over (random or residual error). Thus, regression is used to describe complex relationships between variables that are somewhat concealed by a large variability originating from a number of potential sources (Draper and Smith, 1998; Thornley and France, 2007).

Non-linear models represent curved relationships and have at least one parameter appearing non-linearly, i.e. the functional form of the equation is not linear with respect to the unknown parameters (Ratkowski, 1983). Non-linear regression is a procedure for fitting any selected equation to data, endeavouring to smooth data, interpolate for unknown values and make observations continuous over the range of values of the explanatory variable (Bates and Watts, 1988; Seber and Wild, 2003). The main advantage of non-linear regression over many other curve-fitting procedures is the broad range of functions that can be fitted. As with other procedures of curve fitting, the goal in non-linear regression is to obtain estimates of parameters that minimize the residual error, measured as the sum of the squares of the distances of the data points to the curve. This is the criterion used by the least squares method (Bates and Watts, 1988; Seber and Wild, 2003), and can be very efficient in using the available information for curve fitting, producing good estimates of the unknown parameters in the model with relatively small data sets and using experimental data (Motulsky and Ransnas, 1987; Draper and Smith, 1998). An alternative to the least squares function is maximum likelihood estimation, which, in successive approximations, results in those values of the parameters which maximize the probability of obtaining that particular set of data (Seber and Wild, 2003).

Unlike linear and multiple regression procedures in which the least squares estimates of the parameters can always be obtained analytically, non-linear regression can be solved only by numerical methods following iterative optimization procedures (Ratkowski, 1983; Bates and Watts, 1988; Seber and Wild, 2003) to compute the parameter estimates that require initial values of the parameters. In successive iterations, these initial values are adjusted so that the residual sum of squares is reduced significantly in each step. Adjustments of the parameter estimates continue until a convergence criterion is met, accepting that from this point only a negligible, if any, improvement in fit to the data is possible. If the residual sum of squares is assumed to be a function of the parameter values, a solution is achieved for that combination of parameter estimates, resulting in a minimum residual sum of squares or in a maximum of the likelihood function. The starting values must be reasonably close to the, as yet, unknown parameter estimates, or the optimization procedure may not converge. Bad starting values can also cause the software to converge to a local minimum, rather than the global minimum that defines the least squares estimates. Several methods or algorithms (steepest descent, Gauss–Newton, Marquardt, simplex algorithm) can be used to find, in each iteration, the adjusted parameter values with which residual variance is significantly decreased (Bates and Watts, 1988; Pykh and Malkina-Pykh, 2001; Seber and Wild, 2003). Some decisions have to be taken before performing curve fitting by non-linear regression, such as the choice of the equation to be fitted, the initial values of the parameters to start the iterative procedure and the constraints on values of these parameters, if differential weighting of data points is required, and the algorithm and convergence criterion to be used (Motulsky and Ransnas, 1987; Bates and Watts, 1988; Seber and Wild, 2003). All these options can be specified in the different computer programs available for non-linear regression.

Once a model has been fitted, it may be important to assess the performance and to compare the fit attained with different non-linear equations, selecting the 'best' regression equation (Motulsky and Ransnas, 1987; Draper and Smith, 1998; Burnham and Anderson, 2002; Motulsky and Christopoulos, 2003). Goodness-of-fit is usually assessed from the residual variance (unexplained by the model), taking into account the number of parameters of the model. The proportion of variance accounted for by the model, residual sum of squares and residual mean squares, and Akaike's and Bayesian information criteria are statistics commonly used to assess goodness-of-fit. The analysis of residual distribution (plots of residuals against the independent variable) is also useful to determine the fitting behaviour of a given equation. Finally, analysis of sensitivity and uncertainty in the value of the parameters (standard error of the parameters, changes observed when parameter values are altered by a specific amount, changes in parameter estimates when a data point is changed or omitted) may be of use in interpreting the results.

Sometimes, data require the use of a non-linear function within a statistical model including both fixed (treatment) and random (experimental unit) effects (Davidian and Giltinan, 1995). These are called non-linear mixed models (both fixed and random effects may have a non-linear relationship to the response variable) and have to be fitted by maximizing an approximation to the likelihood integrated over the random effects (Peek *et al.*, 2002). These models have a wide variety of applications, such as non-linear growth curves or the analysis of longitudinal data (Davidian and Giltinan, 1995; Schinckel and Craig, 2001). Non-linear mixed effects modelling fits the best model to the population as a whole and, at the same time, uses random variation in the parameters to get the best fit for each individual.

Non-linear Functions for Dynamic Processes

Non-linear functions used to represent some time-course events that are an object of study in animal nutrition are presented. The purpose is not an in-depth analysis of each equation or model (for this see Thornley and France, 2007), but to provide just an overview of the large number of diverse functions that have been used to represent dynamic processes such as microbial growth, substrate degradation in the rumen, digesta passage kinetics, somatic growth and milk or egg production. Some reference texts provide a long list of possible mathematical functions (Abramowitz and Stegun, 1964; Ratkowski, 1983; Bates and Watts, 1988; Draper and Smith, 1998; Seber and Wild, 2003; National Institute of Standards and Technology, 2007; Thornley and France, 2007).

Microbial growth

There is a mutual and reciprocal relationship between fermentation and microbial growth kinetics in the digestive tract of herbivores, as microbes obtain their nutrients from the fermentation of feeds, which, in turn, takes place by the action of microbial enzymes (López *et al.*, 2006). In ruminants, the growth of the microbial population also determines the amount of microbial protein reaching the abomasum and duodenum, which is one of the main sources of amino acids to the animal (Van Soest, 1994). Therefore, microbial growth is an important process to be considered in models of microbial fermentation of feeds and of microbial synthesis in the rumen. Different approaches to predict microbial synthesis in the rumen have been reviewed by Dijkstra *et al.* (1998). To understand aspects of the rumen microbial ecosystem, mixed ruminal microorganisms have been grown *in vitro* in batch and continuous cultures (López, 2005). The mathematical equations describing these cultures are helpful in discerning the essential parameters of microbial metabolism and in predicting the partitioning of substrate into microbial biomass and fermentation end products (Dijkstra *et al.*, 1998).

Most of the physical models to study ruminal microbial metabolism have been based on the chemostat, as the rumen is a system of continuous culture of microorganisms. The differential equations describing the dynamics of the chemostat are presented in López *et al.* (2000a). Batch cultures can also be useful to estimate parameters (specific growth rate and lag time) required to study growth under different physical and chemical conditions, to enable the effects of antimicrobials to be investigated, to formulate appropriate microbiological media, or to build prediction models for use in food and fermentation microbiology (McMeekin *et al.*, 1993; Whiting and Buchanan, 1997). Modelling of microbial growth in batch cultures can be applied at various levels. A primary-level model is an equation or function that is used to describe the microbial response (in terms of microbial numbers, concentration of colony-forming units or optical density as an indirect measurement) over time with a characteristic set of parameter values (McMeekin *et al.*, 1993; Whiting, 1995; McMeekin and Ross, 2002). Secondary models predict changes in primary model parameters based on single or multiple environmental conditions and can be useful to establish the conditions (pH, temperature, nutrient type and concentrations) at which microbial growth in the rumen is optimum (maximum growth rate or shortest lag time).

Microbial growth in batch cultures exhibits four different phases: lag phase, growth phase, stationary phase and death phase (Fig. 3.1), and can be represented by the general equation: $dN/dt = \mu N$, where N denotes microbial biomass (in units of mass, optical density, numbers, etc.), t is time (h) and μ is the specific growth rate (h^{-1}), which can be a function of time (López *et al.*, 2004). The rate of change in the log microbial biomass [$\ln(N)$] is then:

$$\frac{d(\ln N)}{dt} = N^{-1}\frac{dN}{dt} = \mu(t). \tag{3.1}$$

If L_0 denotes the value of $\ln(N)$ at time zero, then integrating Eqn 3.1 yields:

$$\ln(N) = L_0 + \int_0^t \mu(t)dt = f(t),$$

giving $\ln(N)$ as a function of time. The relationship between $\ln(N)$ and time follows a characteristic sigmoidal pattern that can be described empirically using

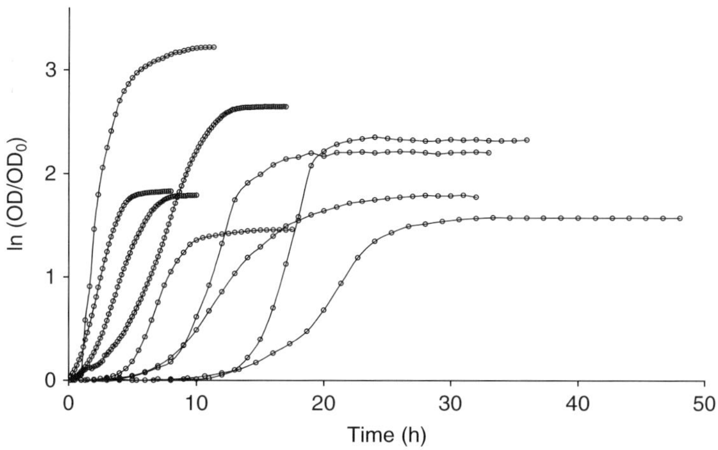

Fig. 3.1. Growth curves of different microbial (bacteria and fungi) species [natural log of optical density versus time].

non-linear functions. The maximum value of μ, μ_{max}, occurs at time t^* (h), which is found by solving $d\mu/dt = 0$. The lag time, T (h), is the intercept of the tangent to the steepest part of the $f(t)$ versus time curve with the curve's lower bound.

Some candidates for $f(t)$ as microbial growth functions are presented in Table 3.1 (López *et al.*, 2004). In this table, λ (h^{-1}) is a rate parameter, υ (dimensionless) is a shape or curvature parameter and L_∞ is the maximum log microbial population size.

Sigmoidal functions that have been used for modelling somatic growth and population dynamics (Thornley and France, 2007) have been also applied to microbial growth (Zwietering *et al.*, 1990; McMeekin *et al.*, 1993; Peleg, 1997; López *et al.*, 2004), allowing for the estimation of descriptive growth parameters (maximum specific growth rate and lag time). However, numbers (colony-forming units) or absorbance units require a logarithmic transformation because of their statistical non-normality and their heteroskedasticity (variance is not uniform over all measurement conditions), so that, if data are not transformed, the regression analysis will be flawed. The use of ln(N) instead of N as the response variable means that the models are not simply expressions of the original growth functions (Zwietering *et al.*, 1990; McMeekin *et al.*, 1993) and thus should be considered modified forms of the original functions (modified Gompertz or logistic). Other sigmoidal functions have been used specifically to describe microbial growth in batch cultures (Baranyi and Roberts, 1995; Buchanan *et al.*, 1997; Swinnen *et al.*, 2004).

Many of these mathematical functions have been used empirically, as the mechanisms governing the process are unknown and difficult to represent by a mechanistic model. Moreover, the μ derived for most of the different candidate equations are explicit functions of time and therefore have to be considered semi- or non-autonomous differential equations when modelling growth (Baranyi *et al.*, 1993). Nevertheless, as the equations seem to mimic reality, it is anticipated that

Table 3.1. Candidate functions for microbial growth in batch cultures.

Linear	$L_0, \quad t \le \tau$ $L_0 + \mu(t-\tau), \quad \tau < t < t_f$ $L_\infty, \quad t \ge t_f$
Logistic	$\dfrac{L_\infty}{1+e^{-\lambda(t-t^*)}}$
Gompertz	$L_\infty \exp[-e^{-\lambda(t-t^*)}]$
von Bertalanffy	$L_0 + (L_\infty - L_0)\left(1-e^{-\lambda t}\right)^{1/\upsilon}$
Richards	$\dfrac{L_\infty}{[1+\upsilon e^{-\lambda(t-t^*)}]^{1/\upsilon}}$
Morgan	$\dfrac{L_0 K^\upsilon + L_\infty t^\upsilon}{K^\upsilon + t^\upsilon}$
Weibull	$L_\infty - (L_\infty - L_0)\exp[-(\lambda t)^\upsilon]$
France	$L_0, t < \tau$ $L_\infty - (L_\infty - L_0)e^{\left[-\lambda(t-\tau)+d\left(\sqrt{t}-\sqrt{\tau}\right)\right]}, t \ge \tau$
Baranyi & Roberts	$L_0 + \mu_{max} t + L_1 - L_2$, where $L_1 = \ln[e^{-\mu_{max} t} - e^{-\mu_{max}(t+T)} + e^{-\mu_{max} T}]$, $L_2 = \ln\left[1 + \dfrac{e^{\mu_{max}(t-T)} + e^{-\mu_{max} T}}{e^{(L_\infty - L_0)}}\right]$

the quantitative concepts and mechanisms underlying some of these expressions will be identified in the future as more understanding is gained.

Microbial growth is highly dependent on the availability of substrate (S). At low substrate concentrations, μ increases linearly with S (i.e. in a first-order manner), whereas, at high S values, μ is independent of S (i.e. μ is a zero-order function of S). The relationship between substrate concentration (S) and specific growth rate (μ) often assumes the form of saturation kinetics, described by the Monod equation (Monod, 1949):

$$\mu = \mu_{max}\left(\frac{S}{K_S + S}\right),$$

where K_S is the saturation coefficient (i.e. the concentration of substrate equal to half that causing saturation). There are other equations to represent this relationship (Blackman, Tessier, Moser, Contois); all of them can be described by a single differential equation (Kargi and Shuler, 1979):

$$\frac{d\upsilon}{dS} = K\upsilon^a(1-\upsilon)^b,$$

where $\upsilon = \mu/\mu_{max}$, S is the rate-limiting substrate concentration and K, a and b are constants with different values for each equation.

Rate and extent of degradation

Kinetic degradation parameters are necessary to predict feed digestibility and protein degradability (López *et al.*, 2000a; López, 2005). The amount of substrate degraded in the rumen is the result of competition between digestion and passage. Several models have been proposed since that of Blaxter *et al.* (1956), in which kinetic parameters for degradation and passage are integrated to estimate the actual extent of degradation of feed in the rumen.

Degradation parameters are usually estimated from degradation profiles (Fig. 3.2) obtained using either the polyester bag technique or the gas production technique (López *et al.*, 2000b; López, 2005). In the first case, a time-course disappearance curve for each feed component is obtained *in situ* by measuring the amount of residue remaining in the bag at several time points. Similar gravimetric methods have been employed in which the feed is incubated *in vitro*, either with buffered rumen fluid or with enzymes (López, 2005). Disappearance curves are used to evaluate the kinetics of degradation of feeds in the rumen, by assuming that disappearance from the bag equals degradation of feed in the rumen. The gas production technique aims to measure the rate of production of fermentation gases, which can be used to predict the rate of feed degradation, assuming that the amount of gas produced reflects the amount of substrate degraded (Dijkstra *et al.*, 2005).

To associate disappearance or gas production curves with digestion in the rumen, models have been developed based on compartmental schemes (France *et al.*, 1990, 2000, 2005), which assume that the feed component comprises at least two fractions: a potentially degradable fraction S and an undegradable fraction U. Fraction S will be degraded at a fractional rate μ (h^{-1}), after a discrete lag time L (h). The dynamic behaviour of the fractions is described by the differential equations:

$$dS/dt = 0, \quad 0 \le t < L, \tag{3.2a}$$

$$= -\mu S, \quad t \ge L, \tag{3.2b}$$

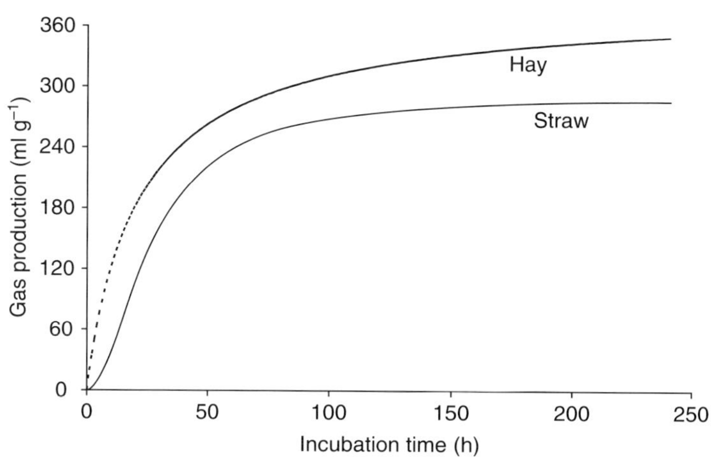

Fig. 3.2. Gas production curves of forages.

$$dU/dt = 0, \quad t \geq 0. \tag{3.2c}$$

Therefore, the parameters to be estimated are the initial size of fraction S, the size of U, the lag time (L) and the fractional degradation rate (μ).

An essential aspect of modelling ruminal degradation concerns the kinetics assumed for the process itself. The models may represent a variety of possible kinetic processes: zero-, first-, or second-order degradation kinetics (Robinson *et al.*, 1986; France *et al.*, 1990), first-order degradation kinetics combined with a first-order lag process (Van Milgen *et al.*, 1991) and fractional degradation rates varying with time (France *et al.*, 1993a, 2000, 2005) or related to microbial activity (France *et al.*, 1990). Some of the models are classical growth functions and can be used, by similarity in the curves' shape, to describe disappearance profiles.

The most commonly used model (Ørskov and McDonald, 1979) assumes first-order kinetics, implying that substrate degraded at any time is proportional to the amount of potentially degradable matter remaining at that time, with constant fractional rate μ. This model has been extensively used owing to its simplicity, but it is not capable of describing the large diversity of degradation profiles (Fig. 3.2). Degradation models which incorporate microbial growth kinetics are in nature sigmoidal (France *et al.*, 1990, 1993a; Van Milgen and Baumont, 1995), indicating the potential inadequacy of simple diminishing returns models to estimate the rate and extent of degradation (Mertens, 2005).

France *et al.* (2000) postulated that μ may vary with time according to different mathematical functions, so that different models (Table 3.2) can be derived to describe either *in situ* disappearance (López *et al.*, 1999) or *in vitro* gas production profiles (France *et al.*, 2000, 2005). Some of these functions are capable of describing both a range of shapes with no inflexion point (diminishing returns behaviour) and a range of sigmoidal shapes in which the inflexion point is variable. It must be pointed out that some models can describe both types of behaviour, depending on the values of certain parameters. On substituting for the function proposed for μ and integrating, Eqn 3.2b yields an equation for the S fraction remaining during the incubation *in situ* or *in vitro* at any time t that can be expressed in the general form:

$$S = S_0 \times [1 - \Phi(t)], \tag{3.3}$$

where S_0 is the zero-time quantity of the S fraction, $\Phi(t)$ is a positive monotonically increasing function with an asymptote at $\Phi(t) = 1$ (Table 3.2) and t is incubation time (h). A discrete lag parameter (L) may be included in models, mainly in those with diminishing returns behaviour, to represent the time interval before degradation commences ($\Phi = 0$ for $t \leq L$). For each function, μ can be obtained from Eqns 3.2b and 3.3 as:

$$\mu = -\frac{1}{S}\frac{dS}{dt} = \frac{1}{(1-\Phi)}\frac{d\Phi}{dt}.$$

This function constitutes the mechanistic interpretation of the degradation processes.

In situ disappearance (D, g g^{-1} incubated) is given by (López *et al.*, 1999):

$$D = W + S_0 - S = W + S_0 \times \Phi(t). \tag{3.4}$$

Table 3.2. Alternative functions for Φ in the general equation of the *in situ* disappearance curve $D = W + S_0 \times \Phi(t)$ (except for parameters W, S_0 and L, the meanings of all the other constants are specific to each model).

Model description	$\Phi(t) =$	Nodes in segmented models
Diminishing returns models		
Segmented model with three spline lines delimited by two nodes or break points, constraining splines 1 and 3 to be horizontal asymptotes	$\frac{c}{S_0}(t-L)$	$L < t \le L + \frac{S_0}{c}$
Simple negative exponential equation (monomolecular, Mitscherlich or first-order kinetics model) with lag phase	$1-e^{-c(t-L)}$	$t > L$
Rational function or inverse polynomial with lag phase, which is a rectangular hyperbola. Also known as the Michaelis–Menten equation in enzyme kinetics	$\frac{t-L}{t-L+K}$	$t > L$
Sigmoidal models		
Lag compartment model, in which lag and degradation are considered compartments both represented by first-order kinetics	$1-\frac{ce^{-\lambda t}-\lambda e^{-ct}}{c-\lambda}$	
Generalized Mitscherlich, which contains a square root time-dependence component (results in monomolecur for $d = 0$)	$1-e^{-c(t-L)-d(\sqrt{t}-\sqrt{L})}$	$t > L$
Generalized Michaelis–Menten (results in Michaelis–Menten if $c = 1$)	$\frac{t^c}{t^c+K^c}$	
Ordinary logistic, autocatalytic or inverse exponential, symmetrical about an inflection point M, which can be calculated from $K = \exp(cM)$	$\frac{1-e^{-ct}}{1+Ke^{-ct}}$	
Gompertz, non-symmetrical about an inflection point M, which can be calculated from $K = \exp[-\exp(cM)]$	$\frac{K-K^{\exp(-ct)}}{K-1}$	
Gompertz, non-symmetrical about an inflection point $M = \frac{1}{c}\ln\left(\frac{c}{b}\right)$	$1-\exp\left[-\frac{b}{c}(e^{ct}-1)\right]$	
Modified Von Bertalanffy	$(1-e^{-ct})^{1/\nu}$	

Similarly, gas production profiles observed *in vitro* can be represented by (France *et al.*, 2000):

$$G = YS_0 \times \Phi(t), \tag{3.5}$$

where G (ml) denotes total gas accumulation to time t and Y (ml gas g^{-1} degradable DM) is a constant yield factor (Dijkstra *et al.*, 2005). These functions assume a single degradable pool S. Some models reported in the literature are termed dual- or multiple-pool models and include a number n of degradable pools, each with a different size and a different fractional degradation rate. Substrate disappearance or gas production profiles can be described by additive functions, each representing one of the degradable pools:

$$D = W + \sum_{i=1}^{n} S_{0_i} \Phi_i(t), \text{and} \, G = \sum_{i=1}^{n} Y_i S_{0_i} \Phi_i(t),$$

where n is the number of pools, S_{0_i} is the initial size of each pool i and $\Phi_i(t)$ is the mathematical function representing the degradation of pool i (Groot *et al.*, 1996). Sometimes, these models are over-parameterized and can be fitted only if a large number of data points are available.

Rates of degradation and passage can be combined to calculate the extent of degradation of the substrate in the rumen (France *et al.*, 1990, 1993a). In the rumen, if S is the amount of potentially degradable substrate remaining which is subjected to both passage and degradation, the rate of disappearance of S is given by:

$$\begin{aligned} \frac{dS}{dt} &= -kS, \quad t < L, \\ &= -(k + \mu)S, \quad t \geq L, \end{aligned}$$

where k (h^{-1}) is the fractional rate of passage from the rumen and is assumed constant. To obtain S, the solutions of these differential equations are:

$$\begin{aligned} S &= S_0 e^{-kt}, \quad t < L, \\ S &= S_0 e^{-kt} \times (1 - \Phi), \quad t \geq L. \end{aligned}$$

Using these equations, the extent of degradation in the rumen (E, g degraded g^{-1} ingested) is given by the equations:

$$E = \frac{W + \int_L^{\infty} \mu S dt}{W + S_0 + U} = \frac{W + kS_0 \int_L^{\infty} \Phi e^{-kt} dt}{W + S_0 + U},$$

for *in situ* disappearance profiles (López *et al.*, 1999), and:

$$E = \frac{\int_L^{\infty} \mu S dt}{S_0 + U} = \frac{kS_0 \int_L^{\infty} \Phi e^{-kt} dt}{S_0 + U},$$

for *in vitro* gas production profiles (France *et al.*, 2000, 2005).

These equations provide a general expression for calculating the extent of degradation, which is applicable to any model expressed in the form of Eqns 3.4 and 3.5. As expressions for ruminal extent of degradation for various models have been worked out (López *et al.*, 1999; France *et al.*, 2000), testing more flexible models will contribute to enhancing our understanding of degradation and fermentation kinetics, leading to better diet formulation and animal nutrition.

Passage of digesta through the gastrointestinal tract

Residence time in the gastrointestinal (GI) tract or in one of its compartments, usually expressed as the mean retention time (MRT) and calculated as the reciprocal of fractional rate of passage (Warner, 1981; Faichney, 2005), is an important parameter affecting feed intake, extent of substrate degradation (thus, feed digestibility and fermentation end products) and microbial growth and efficiency in the rumen.

Passage kinetics are usually studied using digesta markers, substances contained in the feed itself (internal markers) or added to the feed (external markers), which are indigestible (not absorbed) and physically similar and intimately associated with the digesta, should not affect or be affected by the GI tract or the microbial population and should be determined by a specific and sensitive analytical method (Warner, 1981).

Markers are administered orally or intraruminally as a pulse dose, as regular and frequent multiple doses or as a continuous infusion. Then, samples of digesta are collected in the rumen, abomasum, small intestine or in faeces at different times after marker administration and digesta kinetics are estimated from the plots of marker concentration in digesta or faeces (μg of marker g^{-1} DM) against time (h). Most usually, marker concentration curves are non-linear.

One of the earliest approaches to estimating MRT in the rumen was applied to the liquid phase and based on a simple single-compartment scheme, assuming instantaneous, continuous and complete mixing in the compartment, steady-state conditions (constant inflow, outflow and compartment size) and mass action dilution turnover (first-order kinetics). Thus, following cessation of a continuous infusion or a single dose of a marker into the rumen (i.e. the compartment), the disappearance of the marker from the compartment (Fig. 3.3) can be described by the simple exponential model:

$$C_t = C_0 e^{-kt},$$

where C_t is the concentration of marker (mg l^{-1}) in the compartment at time t (h), C_0 is the initial concentration of marker (mg) and k is the fractional dilution rate (h^{-1}), equivalent to the fractional outflow rate of the liquid digesta. This equation can be transformed yielding a linear equation on a logarithmic scale (log[C_t] versus time) and thus k can be estimated by simple linear regression. However, more accurate estimates of C_0 and k can be obtained by fitting the exponential model to multiple values recorded over a series of times after dosing.

Rumen volume (V, l) can be calculated from C_0 and k as $V = D/C_0$, where D (mg) is the amount of marker administered as a pulse dose, or as $V = I/(kC_i)$

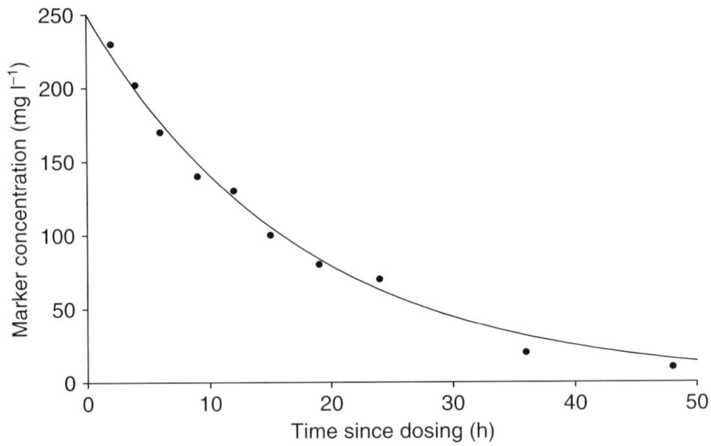

Fig. 3.3. Concentration decay of marker in rumen liquid digesta.

when marker is infused continuously in the rumen, and digesta are sampled after stopping that infusion, where I (mg h^{-1}) is the infusion rate of marker and C_i is the steady concentration of marker reached just before cessation of the infusion.

Fluid flow from the reticulo-rumen (F, h^{-1}) can be estimated as $F = kV$. However, steady-state conditions are not usually observed in the rumen and the model is not always applicable. Limitations of this simple approach to studying digesta outflow from the rumen have been widely recognized (Warner, 1981; Ellis *et al.*, 1994; Faichney, 2005). Nevertheless, the model has been used extensively in marker studies (such as digesta markers or isotopes) to estimate pool size and flows into and from a compartment, providing steady-state conditions are prevalent.

Rate of passage of particulate matter has usually been studied using the faecal marker excretion technique, based on the assumption that, after a single oral or intraruminal dose of marker, the cumulative effects of marker retention in the various sections of the GI tract will result in a characteristic pattern of marker excretion in faeces (Fig. 3.4), with an initial lag phase followed by an ascending part that can show diminishing returns or sigmoidal behaviour and a final descending part after a maximum peak that shows a characteristic exponential decay. A satisfactory mathematical description of the faecal excretion curve can be achieved by fitting different non-linear equations. From the parameters of these functions, mean retention time and rate of passage of the digesta in the different sections of the GI tract (in particular in the rumen) can be calculated.

Equations used to describe such a family of curves have been derived from multi-compartmental models of digesta flow. These models assume the existence of mixing compartments and flow segments between the sites of dosing and sampling. In the mixing compartments, digesta are retained for some time, whereas, in the flow segments, transit of digesta may occur by non-mixing displacement, leading to some delay in the flow of marker between two compartments. Flow segments can be incorporated into the model as discrete time lags.

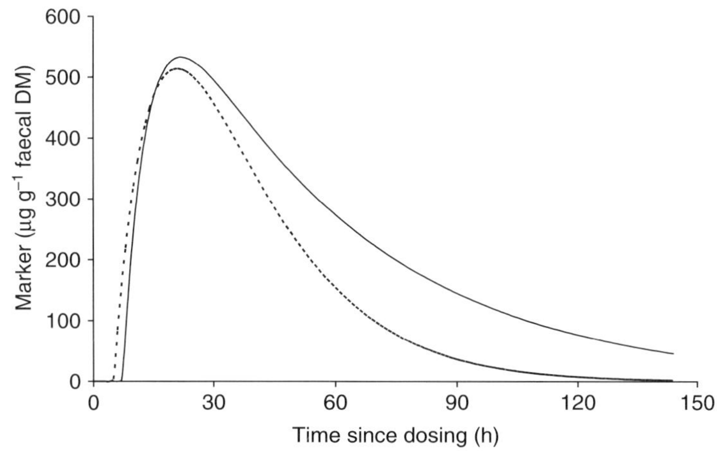

Fig. 3.4. Faecal marker excretion curves for sheep.

Using this approach, Blaxter *et al.* (1956) developed a three-pool (rumen, abomasum and faeces) model, with a constant lag time (τ, h) representing the flow of digesta through the lower tract (between abomasum and faeces). The solution of the model to describe the rate of appearance of marker in faeces (y, μg marker g^{-1} faecal DM) resulted in the non-linear function:

$$y = 0, \quad 0 \le t < \tau,$$
$$= \frac{k_1 k_2}{(k_2 - k_1)}[e^{-k_1(t-\tau)} - e^{-k_2(t-\tau)}], \quad t \ge \tau,$$

where k_1 and k_2 (h^{-1}) are rate constants representing the fractional rates of passage through the rumen (slow pool) and the abomasum (fast pool), respectively. This equation cannot be used when $k_1 = k_2$ and, in this case, curves can be described with the alternative equation provided by Grovum and Williams (1973). Fitting the model by non-linear regression has the difficulty that in many cases k_1 tends to equal k_2, and thus the iterative process fails to converge. Grovum and Williams (1973) proposed a graphical procedure to fit the model by regressing natural log-transformed faecal marker concentrations against time and estimating k_1 as the slope of the straight line resulting from the descending part of the original curve. They also identified the compartments as the reticulo-rumen and caecum/proximal colon and suggested calculating mean retention time in the rumen as $1/k_1$ and total mean retention time in the GI tract as $1/k_1+1/k_2+\tau$.

France *et al.* (1985) performed a unifying mathematical analysis of the use of compartmental models with and without time lags, deriving equations for models with a different number of compartments (3 or 4 mixing compartments) and for the generalized *n*-compartmental model. Discrete or distributed time lags were incorporated into the model. From the generalized multi-compartmental model, and assuming first-order kinetics in the flows between consecutive compartments, Dhanoa *et al.* (1985) proposed a multiplicative equation containing a single exponential term and a double exponential term for describing faecal outflow rate:

$$y = Ae^{-k_1 t} \exp[-(n-2)e^{-(k_2-k_1)t}],$$

where n is the number of compartments in the model, k_1 and k_2 are rate constants for the two compartments of the GI tract having the longest retention times (most probably rumen and caecum) and A is a scale parameter dependent on k_1, k_2 and n. This non-linear equation has been used extensively in digesta flow studies in ruminants, being able to fit a wide range of data successfully. Estimation of parameters enables several useful biological measures to be evaluated, including rumen MRT.

The general n-pool model derived by France *et al.* (1985) is closely related to the gamma function and its derivation. In the models described so far, it is assumed that fractional flow rates (the ks) are constant, assuming first-order kinetics. Matis (1972) suggested that, in some compartments, fractional rates could be variable with time, so that the probability for escape of a particle increases with its residence time in the compartment. Matis (1972) proposed the use of a gamma distribution of residence times to derive a stochastic model incorporating the time dependency of particle passage through the rumen. France *et al.* (1985) suggested a compartmental derivation of this model (dividing the rumen into two compartments) or using an alternative scheme including a time lag exponentially distributed. Pond *et al.* (1988) extended the stochastic approach of Matis (1972), deriving one- and two-compartmental models, assuming digesta kinetics in one of the compartments would be time-dependent following a gamma distribution. As a result, various non-linear equations were derived assuming different gamma residence time distributions, according to the family of integer gamma functions denoted by Gn, with n corresponding to the order of the gamma function. For a single-compartment model, the generalized equations derived were:

$$D_t = D_0 e^{-\lambda(t-\tau)} \sum_{i=0}^{n-1} \left[\frac{\lambda^i (t-\tau)^i}{i!} \right], \tag{3.6}$$

where D_t is the dose of marker remaining in the compartment at time t after dosing, D_0 is the initial dose of marker, λ is the rate parameter for gamma-distributed residence times, τ is a discrete time delay and n is order of time dependency, and

$$C_t = \frac{C_0}{\bar{k}} \frac{\lambda^n (t-\tau)^{n-1} e^{-\lambda(t-\tau)}}{(n-1)!},$$

where C_t is the concentration of marker in the material leaving the compartment at time t after dosing, C_0 is the initial concentration of marker in the compartment, λ is the rate parameter for gamma-distributed residence times, τ is a discrete time delay, n is order of time dependency and $\bar{k}$ is mean flow rate (average fractional outflow rate), equal to $c \times \lambda$, where c is a constant having a different value for each order of time dependency (Pond *et al.*, 1988). For $n = 1$ (G1), the fractional rate of passage is constant over time, resulting in the model assuming linear kinetics.

The two-compartment model included a gamma time dependency (G*n*) into one of the compartments, whereas digesta kinetics in the other compartment was assumed to follow first-order kinetics (G1), resulting in the following generalized equations:

$$D_t = D_0 \left\{ \delta^n e^{-k(t-\tau)} + e^{-\lambda(t-\tau)} \sum_{i=0}^{n-1} \left[\frac{(1-\delta^{n-i})\lambda^i (t-\tau)^i}{i!} \right] \right\},$$

where D_t, D_0, τ and n are as in Eqn 3.6, k is the fractional rate of passage for the time-independent compartment, λ is the rate parameter for gamma-distributed residence times and $\delta = \lambda/(\lambda - k)$, and:

$$C_t = C_0 \left\{ \delta^n e^{-k(t-\tau)} - e^{-\lambda(t-\tau)} \sum_{i=1}^{n} \left[\frac{\delta^i \lambda^{n-i} (t-\tau)^{n-i}}{(n-i)!} \right] \right\},$$

where k, λ, δ, τ and n are as above, C_t is the concentration of marker in the material leaving the last compartment at time t after dosing and C_0 is the initial concentration of marker in the compartment where the marker is dosed. Although these two-compartment models do not specify the order or relative size of the two sequential compartments, Pond *et al.* (1988), based on the estimates of the parameters, pointed out that the time-dependent process would be consistently associated with the faster turnover compartment, so that k would be the slow rate of passage. Thus, ruminal retention time is calculated as $1/k$ and total tract mean retention time as $1/k + n/\lambda + \tau$.

More advanced aspects of digesta flow were considered by France *et al.* (1993b) and Thornley *et al.* (1995), who investigated the effects of diffusion and viscosity on faecal excretion patterns of markers in ruminants by considering a two-compartment model of the GI tract comprising a pure mixing pool and a second compartment exhibiting streamline flow.

Growth

In animals not subjected to major feeding restrictions, the plot of live weight against age or time results in a characteristic sigmoidal growth curve, consisting of three differentiated parts: an initial self-accelerating phase, an intermediate linear phase and a final self-decelerating phase which fades out as the animal reaches maturity (Fig. 3.5). Inflection of the growth pattern seems to occur in many farm species soon after puberty. Growth rate (weight gain per unit of time, usually in g or kg day^{-1}) varies with age, increasing during the self-accelerating phase until reaching a maximum in the intermediate phase, when it is relatively constant. In the last phase, the growth rate decreases progressively to zero, reaching a final plateau when the animal achieves mature or asymptotic body weight, maintaining a relatively stable weight with changes attributed to the availability of feed, the demands of the reproductive cycle and the season of the year. This is the general pattern for somatic growth, although there may be some inevitable (at birth, weaning or puberty) or occasional (owing to seasonal or

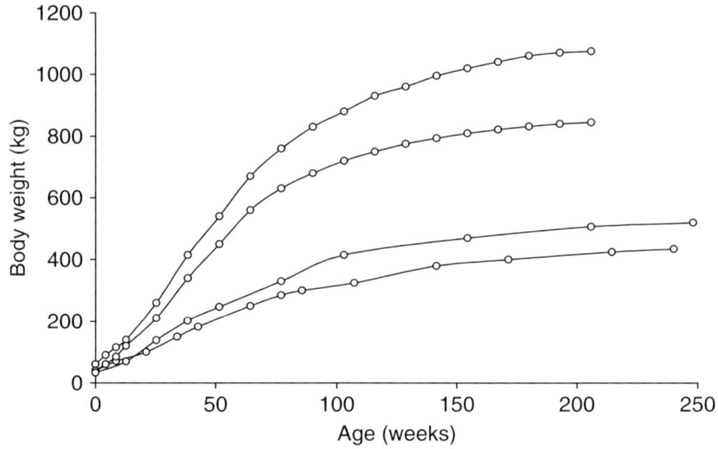

Fig. 3.5. Growth curves of four breeds of cattle.

environmental factors, feed shortage, compensatory growth, productive or reproductive cycles, etc.) deviations from the prevalent sigmoidal trend (Swatland, 1994; Lawrence and Fowler, 2002). There may also be some circadian (daily) periodicity in growth rate, or even erratic spurts of growth. One difficulty in describing growth is separating the long-term sigmoid pattern from short-term deviations. The growth curves of meat animals raised under commercial conditions may appear as a relatively linear slope, because the maximum growth rate occurs within the commercial growing period, and the sigmoid shape becomes apparent only if animals are kept beyond a typical market weight. This biologically distinct period of linear growth may be isolated from its sigmoidal context to improve the fit of predicted curves to actual data.

Growth functions have been widely used to provide a mathematical description of time-course data on the growth of an organism, an organ, a tissue or a population of organisms. Growth curves of a wide variety of species were similar when scaled appropriately for mature size (Taylor, 1980). A large number of growth equations or functions have been reported (Turner *et al.*, 1976; Ricker, 1979; Parks, 1982; Ratkowski, 1983; Simondon *et al.*, 1992; Gill and Oldham, 1993; Zeide, 1993; France *et al.*, 1996; López *et al.*, 2000c; Sainz and Baldwin, 2003; Seber and Wild, 2003; Wellock *et al.*, 2004) trying to describe the somatic growth curve of animals (Table 3.3) best in terms of a few parameters that can be interpreted biologically and used to derive other relevant growth traits. This approach avoids the hazards of independently interpreting a large number of weight–age points that are subject to temporary environmental effects, errors of measurement and random environmental influences (Fitzhugh, 1976). Fitting a curve with sufficient data for each individual would be expected to smooth out the random deviations. Parameters estimated after fitting growth functions can be useful to understand how genetic and environmental factors affect growth attributes, to identify alternative strategies to improve the efficiency of meat production, to assess the genetic merit and

Table 3.3. Growth equations, where W is body weight (kg), t is age (time since birth) and W_0 and W_f are initial and asymptotic weights, respectively (except for the parameters W_0 and W_f, the meaning of all the other constants is specific to each model).

Equation	Functional form
Linear growth	$W = W_0 + bt$
Polynomials	$W = W_0 + b_1t + b_2t^2 + \ldots + b_nt^n$
Ratio of polynomials	$W = \dfrac{W_0 + b_1t + b_2t^2 + \ldots + b_it^i}{W_0 + b_1t + b_2t^2 + \ldots + b_nt^n}$
Count	$W = W_0 + bt + c\ln(t+1)$
Reed	$W = a + bt + c\ln(t+1) + \dfrac{d}{t+1}$
	$W = a + bt + c\ln(t+1) + \dfrac{d}{t+1} + \dfrac{e}{(t+1)^2}$
Wingerd	$W = W_0 + bt + c\sqrt{t}$
Exponential	$W = W_0e^{kt}, \quad 0 \le t \le t_f,$
	$= W_f, \quad t > t_f$
Kouchi	$W = W_0 + bt^c$
Monomolecular/ Mitscherlich	$W = W_f - (W_f - W_0)e^{-kt}$
	$W = W_f(1 - e^{-kt}), if\ W_0 = 0$
Brody	$W = W_0e^{k_1t}, \quad 0 \le t \le t^*,$
	$= W_f - (W_f - W^*)e^{-k_2(t-t^*)} \quad t \ge t^*$
Wan's generalized monomolecular	$W = W_f - \dfrac{1}{\dfrac{b}{W_f} + \left(\dfrac{1}{W_f - W_0} - \dfrac{b}{W_f}\right)\exp(kt)}$
Exponential quadratic	$W = W_0\exp\left[k\left(t - \dfrac{at^2}{2}\right)\right]$
Gaussian	$W = W_0 + (W_f - W_0)(1 - e^{-kt^2})$
Exponential polynomials	$W = W_0\exp(a_1t + a_2t^2 + a_3t^3 + \ldots)$
France	$W = 0, \quad t < T$
	$= W_f - (W_f - W_0)\exp[-k(t-T) + 2c(\sqrt{t} - \sqrt{T})], \quad t \ge T$
Peal–Reed	$W = \dfrac{W_f}{1 + be^{-(k_1t + k_2t^2 + k_3t^3)}}$
Logistic/Verhulst/ Robertson	$W = \dfrac{W_0W_fe^{kt}}{W_f - W_0 + W_0e^{kt}} \qquad W = \dfrac{W_f}{1 + e^{-k(t-t^*)}}$
	$W = \dfrac{W_0W_f}{W_0 + (W_f - W_0)e^{-kt}}$

(Continued)

Table 3.3 *Continued.*

Equation	Functional form
Gompertz	$W = W_0 \exp\left[\frac{a}{k}(1-e^{-kt})\right]$ $W = W_f \exp\left[-e^{-k(t-t^*)}\right]$
	$W = W_f \exp\left[-\frac{a}{k}e^{-kt}\right]$
Jolicoeur's generalized Gompertz	$W = W_0 + (W_f - W_0)\exp\left[-b\exp\left(\frac{1}{k_1 t} - k_2 t\right)\right]$
Sloboda	$W = W_f \exp[-b\exp(-kt^c)]$
Chanter	$W = \frac{W_0 B}{W_0 + (B - W_0)\exp\left[-\frac{\alpha}{k}(1-e^{-kt})\right]}$, where $B = \frac{W_f W_0(e^{a/k} - 1)}{W_0 e^{a/k} - W_f}$
Von Bertalanffy	$W = [W_f^{\,n} - (W_f^{\,n} - W_0^{\,n})e^{-kt}]^{1/n}$ $W = W_f[1 - ne^{-k(t-t^*)}]^{1/n}$
Special case of Von Bertalanffy	$W = [W_f^{1/3} - (W_f^{1/3} - W_0^{1/3})e^{-kt}]^3$
Modified Von Bertalanffy	$W = W_0 + (W_f - W_0)(1-e^{-kt})^{1/n}$
Richards/ Chapman	$W = \frac{W_0 W_f}{[W_0^{\,n} + (W_f^{\,n} - W_0^{\,n})e^{-kt}]^{1/n}}$ $W = \frac{W_f}{[1 + ne^{-k(t-t^*)}]^{1/n}}$
Schnute and Richards	$W = \frac{W_f}{\left[1 + be^{-kt^p}\right]^{1/n}}$
Turner's generic growth function	$W = \frac{W_f}{\{1 + [1 + bnp(t - t^*)]^{-1/p}\}^{1/n}}$
Turner's hyperlogistic	$W = \frac{W_f}{1 + [1 + bp(t - t^*)]^{-1/p}}$
Turner's hyperGompertz	$W = W_f \exp\{-[bp(t - t^*)]^{-1/p}\}$
Schumacher	$W = W_0 \exp\left[\frac{kt_0 t}{t + t_0}\right]$ $W = W_0 \exp\left[\frac{t}{t + t_0}\ln\left(\frac{W_f}{W_0}\right)\right]$
Schumacher/ Johnson	$W = W_f \exp\left[-\frac{kt_0^{\,2}}{t + t_0}\right]$ $W = W_f \exp\left[-\frac{2t^*}{t}\right]$
Schumacher	$W = W_0 + (W_f - W_0)\exp\left[\frac{1}{kt}\right]$
Korf/Lundqvist-Matern	$W = W_f \exp(-kt^{-c})$
Michaelis–Menten (rectangular hyperbola)	$W = \frac{W_0 K + W_f t}{K + t}$
Hill/Morgan–Mercer–Flodin/ López	$W = \frac{W_0 K^n + W_f t^n}{K^n + t^n}$

(*Continued*)

Table 3.3 *Continued.*

Equation	Functional form
Levakovic	$W = W_f\left[\frac{t^n}{K' + t^n}\right]^c$
Log-logistic	$W = W_f - \frac{W_f - W_0}{1 + \exp[n\ln(kt)]} = W_f - \frac{W_f - W_0}{1 + (kt)^n}$
Weibull/Janoscheck	$W = W_f - (W_f - W_0)\exp[-(kt)^n]$
Bridges	$W = W_0 + W_f\{1 - \exp[-(kt^n)]\}$
Power function	$W = W_f(W_0 / W_f)^{\left[\frac{1}{1+(kt)^n}\right]}$
Stannard	$W = \frac{W_f}{\left[1 + \left(\sqrt[n]{\frac{W_f}{W_0}} - 1\right)e^{-kt}\right]^n}$ $\quad W = \frac{W_f}{[1 + \theta e^{-ct/n}]^n}$
Overman and Scholtz	$W = W_f + W_0\left[1 - \frac{\mathrm{erf}\frac{t - t^*}{n} + \mathrm{erf}\frac{t^*}{n}}{1 + \mathrm{erf}\frac{t^*}{n}}\right]$
Hyperbolastic 1	$W = \frac{W_f}{1 + b\exp[-cW_f t - d\,\mathrm{arcsin\,h}(t)]}$
Hyperbolastic 2	$W = \frac{W_f}{1 + b\,\mathrm{arcsin\,h}[\exp(-cW_f t^n)]}$
Hyperbolastic 3	$W = W_f - b\exp[-ct^n - \mathrm{arcsin\,h}(dt)]$
Segmented model	$W = a\exp\left[\frac{k_1}{2}(t - t_0)^2 + k_0(t - t_0)\right], \quad t \le t_0,$ $= a\exp\left[\frac{k_2}{2}(t - t_0)^2 + k_0(t - t_0)\right], \quad t > t_0$

growth potential of meat animals, to estimate nutrient requirements of animals based on their expected daily weight gain or to make management, husbandry and marketing decisions.

The term 'growth function' is generally used to denote an analytical function which can be written as a single equation connecting body weight (W) to time (t), as in the general form $W = f(t)$, where f denotes some functional relationship. Some of these equations have been derived from the integration of mathematical functions representing the changes in the growth rate over time (i.e. $\mathrm{d}W/\mathrm{d}t = f'(t)$). The use of growth functions is quite empirical, as the form of the function f is usually chosen by simply selecting the equation providing a closer fit to the observed data (Brown *et al.*, 1976; Simondon *et al.*, 1992; Fekedulegn *et al.*,

1999; López *et al.*, 2000c; Behr *et al.*, 2001). However, derivatives of the commonly used functions do not always describe the corresponding mean growth-rate curve and complex curvilinear functions do not help to explain the nature of growth unless some biological meaning may be attached to their terms. Some functions that have been used to predict growth are based on deterministic differential equations that seek a biological interpretation. Ideally, a growth function should represent some underlying physiological or biochemical mechanisms or constraints ruling the growth process. For example, autocatalysis results in exponential growth, limited nutrient gives rise to an asymptote and senescence or differentiation may cause diminishing growth rates and asymptotic behaviour (Thornley and France, 2007). Such growth functions can be expressed in the 'rate is a function of state' form:

$$\frac{\mathrm{d}W}{\mathrm{d}t} = g(W),$$

where g denotes a function of W as a state variable. An equation in this latter form is preferred as it can usually have some biological plausibility and interpretation (in metabolic terms) and its parameters may be meaningful, providing some mechanistic description of growth, unlike equations in which growth rate is a purely empirical function of time. However, growth is the result of the integration of several different biological processes, so it seems naïve to represent such a complex phenomenon by a single differential equation or analytical function standing for a given mechanism. In fact, many growth functions are derived from differential equations in which growth rate is a function φ of both W and t:

$$\frac{\mathrm{d}W}{\mathrm{d}t} = \varphi(W,t).$$

Explicitly time-dependent (also called non-autonomous) differential equations make the model more empirical and decrease its scientific interpretability. Therefore, if possible, the defining differential equation should be in the form $\mathrm{d}W/\mathrm{d}t = g(W)$. Thornley and France (2007) developed a two-compartment model considering growth as a process in which material from a substrate compartment (S) is transferred to a second compartment (body mass, W) without loss. The model results in the general 'rate is a function of state' differential equation, and assumptions concerning how growth rate ($\mathrm{d}W/\mathrm{d}t$) depends on W and S enable different growth functions to be derived.

Different polynomial functions have been suggested to fit growth data, but the growth functions most extensively used are non-linear and belong to two main groups: exponential polynomials and asymptotic functions. In turn, asymptotic growth may be represented by diminishing returns functions (negative exponential, hyperbolic equations), by sigmoidal functions or by segmented or piecewise models with an abrupt cut-off at the upper asymptote (Turner *et al.*, 1976; Ricker, 1979; Ratkowski, 1983; Koops, 1986; France *et al.*, 1996; Whittemore and Green, 2001; Seber and Wild, 2003). The simplest sigmoidal functions are characterized by a fixed inflection point (occurring at a fixed proportion of asymptotic weight, W_f), such as the logistic function (symmetric around an inflexion point at 0.5 W_f) or the Gompertz model (asymmetric around an inflection point at W_f/e). More complex and flexible sigmoidal functions are capable of describing either diminishing returns or sigmoidal patterns and, in this latter case, the inflexion point may be variable, occurring at any weight or time. These are considered nested or generalized models, as they encompass other simpler functions as specific parameters adopt certain values (Turner *et al.*, 1976; Tsoularis and Wallace, 2002). A classical example is the Richards function, which, for some given values of its parameters, may result in the monomolecular, logistic, Gompertz or Von Bertalanffy equations (Table 3.3; Thornley and France, 2007).

Along with the traditional growth functions, other approaches have been proposed to study longitudinal data and growth, such as repeatability models, neural network models, infinite-dimensional models, covariance functions and random regression models (including orthogonal Legendre polynomials, segmented polynomials (spline functions) or sine and cosine functions as approximations to Fourier series) (Arango and Van Vleck, 2002).

As body weight increases, the weights of all organs, tissues and chemical components also increase, but at different rates. The relationship of the weight of each component to body weight appears to be curvilinear and has been represented by allometric equations, such as the exponential equation of Huxley (Huxley, 1924; Huxley and Teissier, 1936) or the quadratic polynomial of Butterfield (Butterfield, 1988). Differentiation of the allometric equations allows the composition of gains in empty body weight to be determined for any particular live weight (Gill and Oldham, 1993; Thornley and France, 2007).

Milk production

A classical non-linear curve is the representation of the time course of lactation. The lactation curve of the dairy cow (daily milk yield in kg against time in days) shows a rapid increase in yield after parturition to a peak a few weeks later, followed by a gradual decline until the cow is dried off about 10 months after calving, giving a dry period of about 8 weeks (Fig. 3.6). A similar trend has been observed in other ruminant species (sheep and goats), although the shape of the curve may be slightly different, with a less sharp profile (a lower peak) and a faster or slower decline in the descending part of the curve.

A number of mathematical equations have been proposed to describe the lactation curve, with the aim to fit them to milk yield data and to obtain estimates of some important performance features, such as initial yield after parturition, time to peak and production at that peak (maximum yield), duration of the lactation, total yield per lactation and persistency, defined either as extent to which peak yield is maintained or rate of decline in milk production after peak (Masselin *et al.*, 1987; Thornley and France, 2007). Thus, accurate description of lactation curves has an important relevance to the dairy livestock industry for

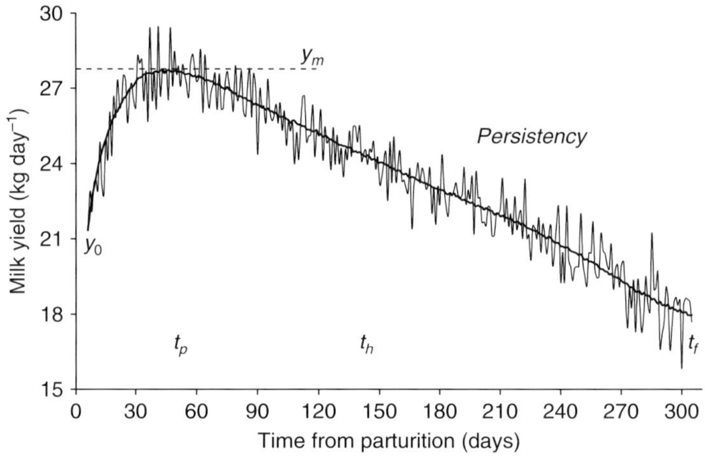

Fig. 3.6. Lactation curve in a dairy cow (fitted and recorded yields).

research, breeding and management, providing interesting information for determining nutrient allowances for lactating animals, estimating total yield per lactation from incomplete records and forecasting herd performance. Lactation equations represent a useful tool for developing and evaluating mechanistic models, aimed at explaining the main features of the milk production pattern in terms of known biology of the mammary gland during pregnancy and lactation.

Milk secretion seems to be influenced by two interdependent processes, representing the activities of secretory cell growth and death in the udder (Dijkstra *et al.*, 1997; Thornley and France, 2007). Both processes seem to be responsible for the changes in milk yield over the lactation cycle, leading to the characteristic shape of the lactation curve. Hence, a multiplicative form of two functions is usually adopted in many of the equations proposed to describe the lactation curve. Rook *et al.* (1993) presented a general form of the equation for the lactation curve, in which daily milk yield (y, kg) was represented by:

$$y = a\phi_1(t)\phi_2(t),$$

where a is a positive scalar, $\phi_1(t)$ is a positive monotonically increasing function, $\phi_2(t)$ is a monotonically decreasing function, with unit initial value and an asymptote at $\phi_2(t) = 0$, and t is time since the start of lactation. $\phi_1(t)$ may thus be envisaged as a growth curve and $\phi_2(t)$ as a regression curve. Papajcsik and Bodero (1988) and Rook *et al.* (1993) suggested several alternative functions as candidates for $\phi_1(t)$ and $\phi_2(t)$ (Table 3.4). Some of the functions considered candidates for $\phi_1(t)$ have been used to model asymptotic growth. Combinations of different alternative candidates for $\phi_1(t)$ with those for $\phi_2(t)$ will result in some of the various equations found in the literature to describe lactation curves.

An account of some time-dependent functions proposed to describe the lactation curve in dairy cows, sheep and goats is given in Table 3.5. A large number of equations have been reported (Masselin *et al.*, 1987; Papajcsik and Bodero, 1988; Morant and Gnanasakthy, 1989; Beever *et al.*, 1991; Sherchand *et al.*,

Table 3.4. Alternative functions for $\phi_1(t)$ and $\phi_2(t)$ in the general equation for the lactation curve $y = a\phi_1(t)\phi_2(t)$.

$\phi_1(t) =$	Power	t^b
	Mitscherlich	$1-be^{-kt}$
	Michaelis–Menten	$\dfrac{1}{1+\dfrac{b}{k+t}}$
	Generalized saturation kinetics	$\dfrac{1}{1+\dfrac{b}{k+t^n}}$
	Logistic	$\dfrac{1}{1+be^{-kt}}$
	Gompertz	$b\exp[(-\ln b)(1-e^{-kt})]$
	Hyperbolic tangent	$\dfrac{1+\tanh(b+kt)}{2}$
	Natural logarithm	$\ln(bt)$
	Arctangent	$\arctan(bt)$
$\phi_2(t) =$	Exponential	e^{-ct}
	Inverse straight line	$\dfrac{1}{1+ct}$
	Inverse hyperbolic cosine	$\dfrac{1}{\cosh(ct)}$

1995; Olori *et al.*, 1999; Landete-Castillejos and Gallego, 2000; Silvestre *et al.*, 2006; Thornley and France, 2007), ranging from simple linear functions (to fit only the declining phase of the lactation) to complex multiphasic models with a large number of parameters. Equations are presented attempting to group them according to their functional form. Most of the equations are empirical models, based on the similarity between observed lactation profiles and the fitted curves achieved with each equation. For instance, growth functions, such as logistic and Gompertz, written in their differential form and expressed as a function of time, have potential application as lactation equations, because the lactation curve is similar to the plot of growth rate (daily weight gain) against time (Thornley and France, 2007).

The function most widely applied to describe lactation curve has been the incomplete gamma equation proposed by Wood (1967): $y_t = at^be^{-ct}$, where y_t is rate of milk production (kg day^{-1}) at time t (day) since parturition and a, b and c are positive parameters. The model is not given to a realistic mechanistic representation, although it can be developed from a rather speculative interpretation as summarized by Thornley and France (2007). Parameters a, b and c of the equation cannot easily be interpreted, but can be used to derive useful approximations of some interesting features of the lactation, namely length of lactation, total milk yield, time to maximum yield and the average relative rate of decline after peak yield (an indicator of persistency). These calculations are explained in detail by Thornley and France (2007).

Table 3.5. Equations used to describe the lactation curve, where Y_t is milk yield (kg day^{-1}), t is time of lactation (day) and the other symbols are for parameters that define the scale and shape of the curve.

Equation	Functional form
(a) Polynomial functions	
Simple linear	$Y_t = a - bt$
Quadratic	$Y_t = a + bt - ct^2$
(b) Polynomials combined with other functions	
Hyperbolic	$Y_t = a + b/t$
Nelder (inverse polynomial)	$Y_t = \dfrac{t}{a + bt + ct^2}$
Ratio of polynomials	$Y_t = \dfrac{a(t+b)}{(t+b)^2 + c^2}$
Singh and Gopal	$Y_t = a - bt + d\ln(t)$
	$Y_t = a + bt + ct^2 + d\ln(t)$
Guo and Swalve	$Y_t = a + b\sqrt{t} + c\log(t)$
Ali and Schaeffer	$Y_t = a + bt + ct^2 - d\log(t) - k[\log(t)]^2$
(c) Exponential functions	
Gaines or Brody (declining exponential)	$Y_t = ae^{-ct}$
Cobby and Le Du – double exponential	$Y_t = a(1 - e^{-dt})e^{-bt} = a(e^{-bt} - e^{-ct})$; $c = b + d$
Sikka (parabolic exponential)	$Y_t = ae^{(bt - ct^2)}$
Cobby and Le Du	$Y_t = a(1 - e^{-ct}) - bt$
Wilmink	$Y_t = a + be^{-kt} + ct$
Morant and Gnanasakthy	$Y_t = a\exp\left(-bt + ct^2 + \dfrac{d}{t}\right)$
Emmans and Fisher	$Y_t = a\exp[-e^{d-bt}]e^{-ct}$
Dijkstra	$Y_t = a\exp\left[\dfrac{b}{c}(1 - e^{-ct}) - dt\right]$
Pollott	$Y_t = \left[a_1\Big/\left(1 + \dfrac{1-b}{b}e^{-ct}\right) - a_2\Big/\left(1 + \dfrac{1-d}{d}e^{-gt}\right)\right](1 - e^{-ht})$
(d) Gamma function and modified equations	
Wood	$Y_t = at^be^{-ct}$
Jenkins and Ferrell	$Y_t = at\,e^{-ct}$
Dhanoa	$Y_t = at^{kc}e^{-ct}$
Sauvant and Fehr	$Y_t = d + at^be^{-ct}$
Schneeberger	$Y_t = a(t - t_0)^be^{-c(t-t_0)}$
(e) Multiphasic models	
Molina and Boschini (linear modal)	$Y_t = a - b\lvert t - t_p\rvert$
Piecewise or segmented model	$Y_t = a, \quad 0 \le t < t_p,$
	$= a - k(t - t_p), \quad t > t_p.$

(*Continued*)

Table 3.5. *Continued.*

Equation	Functional form
Piecewise or segmented model	$Y_t = a, \quad 0 \le t < t_p,$ $= a\exp[-k(t - t_p)], \quad t > t_p.$
Piecewise or segmented model	$Y_t = a + ct, \quad 0 \le t < t_p,$ $= a + ct_p, \quad t_p \le t \le t_d,$ $= a + ct_p - k(t - t_d), \quad t > t_d.$
Grossman and Koops, 1988 (multiphasic and biphasic models)	$Y_t = \sum_{i=1}^{p} [a_i b_i \{1 - \tanh^2[b_i(t - c_i)]\}]$ $Y_t = a_1 b_1 \{1 - \tanh^2[b_1(t - c_1)]\} + a_2 b_2 \left\{1 - \tanh^2\left[b_2(t - c_2)\right]\right\}$
Weigel (modified Grossman and Koops, 1988)	$Y_t = d\{1 - \tanh^2[b(t^k - c)]\}$ $Y_t = d_1\{1 - \tanh^2[b_1(t^k - c_1)]\} + d_2\{1 - \tanh^2[b_2(t - c_2)]\}$
Grossman *et al.*, 1999 (two intersecting straight lines with a smooth transition)	$Y_t = a + bt + k\ln(d + e^{ct})$
Grossman *et al.*, 1999 (three intersecting straight lines with a smooth transition – generalized lactation persistency model)	$Y_t = a + bt - \frac{b}{k_1}\ln(d + e^{k_1 t}) + \frac{g}{k_2}\ln(h + e^{k_2 t})$
Grossman *et al.*, 1999 (three intersecting straight lines with a smooth transition – simplified lactation persistency model)	$Y_t = at - a\ln(b + e^t) + c\ln(d + e^t)$
Grossman and Koops, 2003	$Y_t = \frac{a}{1 + e^{-(t - c_1)/b_1}} - \frac{p_2 a}{1 + (0.5e^{-(t - c_2)/b_2})^2} - \frac{p_3 a}{1 + e^{-(t - c_3)/b_3}}$ $- \frac{p_4 a}{(1 + 0.5e^{-(t - c_4)/b_4})^2}$

Mechanistic models derive a mathematical function for the lactation curve from differential equations representing some of the biological processes of lactation (e.g. mammary gland growth and regression, hormone levels or nutrient flow). The equations derived by Dijkstra *et al.* (1997) and by Pollott (2000) fall into this category.

Recently, there has been considerable interest in modelling individual test-day records for genetic evaluation of dairy cattle as a replacement for the traditional use of estimated accumulated 305-day yields (Jensen, 2001; Powell and Norman, 2006). Test-day models are designed to estimate genetic parameters from the relationship between milk yield and different sources of variation (fixed and random effects), using random regression models and covariance functions (Swalve, 1995, 2000; Van Bebber *et al.*, 1997; Meyer, 1998; Jensen, 2001; Schaeffer, 2004). With the development of these statistical models used in genetic evaluation, interest has been renewed in the analysis of lactation curves, because one of the main factors is days in milk (stage of lactation) and thus test-day models need to incorporate effects such as the general shape of the lactation curve or the different variation of test-day yields depending on time from parturition (Swalve, 2000; Jensen, 2001). A number of approaches have been proposed for the effect of the lactation curve to be accounted for in these models, such as using the parametric equations shown in Table 3.5, Legendre orthogonal polynomials (Brotherstone *et al.*, 2000; Schaeffer, 2004), autoregressive models (Carvalheira *et al.*, 2002), stochastic and Bayesian models (Rekaya *et al.*, 2000) or cubic splines (White *et al.*, 1999).

Egg production

Another classical non-linear curve is the time course of egg production in laying poultry, particularly in commercial laying hens. Typically, the curve is a representation of the average production rate of a flock of birds (Fig. 3.7), plotting the average percentage of birds in the flock laying an egg on a daily basis (i.e. *eggs* × 100/(7 × *birds*); where *eggs* is the total number of eggs laid in the flock each week and *birds* is the total number of hens in the flock) against time (either in weeks of age or in weeks after onset of laying). This plot results in a smooth curve, with an initial increase to a peak and a subsequent steady decrease to the end of the production period (Leeson and Summers, 1997). The curve is very similar to the lactation curve and several equations have been used to describe it,

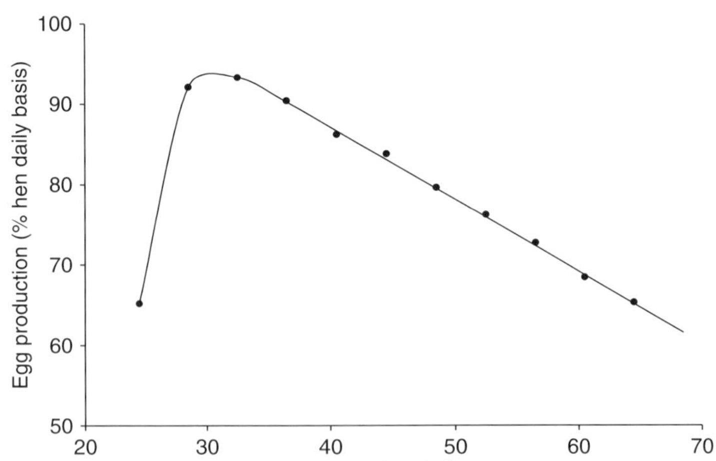

Fig. 3.7. Egg production curve for a commercial laying hen (fitted and recorded values).

some of them similar to those used to fit lactation data (Thornley and France, 2007). Some of the models have been derived to represent the production cycle of each individual hen. Although the general pattern of this curve is similar, the discrete nature of the variable (number of eggs laid by a given hen weekly) results in a decreasing part of the curve with several successive descending steps or phases (Grossman and Koops, 2001).

Similarly to the lactation curve, the whole egg production curve with the increasing and decreasing egg output periods may be represented mathematically by equations including two functions in a multiplicative form (Narushin and Takma, 2003). Logistic, Mitscherlich and other somatic growth functions have been the preferred functions to represent the increasing section of the curve, whereas the second declining section has been reported to be represented by linear or curvilinear (exponential or polynomial) functions. Other approaches to modelling the egg production curve include cyclic functions, segmented polynomials and smoothed intersecting straight lines (Grossman and Koops, 2001). An account of different equations found in the literature (Gavora *et al.*, 1982; Fialho and Ledur, 1997; Narushin and Takma, 2003) is provided in Table 3.6.

Different comparative studies have concluded that performance of most of these equations fitting egg production data is satisfactory, attaining a similar goodness-of-fit with all functions. However, only the McMillan equation offers a compartmental interpretation of the biological process, considering egg production as a two-stage, sequential process, consisting of a primordial stage and a developing stage, and assuming all flows between pools and out of the system obey mass action kinetics (McMillan, 1981).

Nutrient Response Functions

Response functions

One of the goals of modelling is to describe cause–effect relationships with an operator of transition or 'input–output' function. Every system has a response to each possible combination of environmental conditions or factors that directly affect processes or characteristics of the system. Given the system, the magnitude (and kind) of its response depends on the levels of factors at a particular time. The resultant relationship between environmental factors and system response is described with the response functions (Pykh and Malkina-Pykh, 2001; Motulsky and Christopoulos, 2003).

Assuming there are n influencing factors with a significant impact on the process under study, these factors may be designated as vector $x = (x_1, x_2, ..., x_n)$, where each factor x_i has a real value within the interval $x_i = (x_i^{min}, x_i^{max})$, called the tolerance interval and delimited by the minimal and maximal values of the given factor. The point (on the interval) x_i^{opt} at which the characteristic under study reaches the maximal value is called the optimal point for the given factor x_i. The function F representing the changes observed in the system's process or

Table 3.6. Equations used to describe the egg production curve, where Y_t is a measure of laying performance for a flock (egg production rate) or for an individual bird (eggs per week, per clutch or per month), t is time (bird's age or time from onset of laying) and the other symbols are for parameters that define the scale and shape of the curve.

Equation	Functional form
Simple linear (only for the declining phase)	$Y_t = a - bt$
Polynomials (3rd or 4th order)	$Y_t = a + bt + ct^2 + dt^3 + gt^4$
Narushin and Takma (ratio of polynomials)	$Y_t = \dfrac{at^3 + bt^2 + ct + d}{t^2 + ft + g}$
Adams and Bell	$Y_t = \dfrac{a}{1 + bc^t} - d(t - g)$
Lokhorst	$Y_t = \dfrac{100}{1 + ab^t} - (ct^2 + dt + f)$
McMillan, 1981 (double exponential)	$Y_t = a(e^{-bt} - e^{-ct})$
McMillan *et al.*, 1970 (compartmental model)	$Y_t = a(1 - be^{-ct}))e^{-kt}$
Minder and McMillan	$Y_t = a\dfrac{(1 - e^{-ct})}{c}e^{-kt}$
Gavora (Wood or gamma function)	$Y_t = at^b e^{-ct}$
Modified gamma function	$Y_t = a(t - t_0)^b e^{-c(t - t_0)}$
McNally	$Y_t = at^b e^{-ct + d\sqrt{t}}$
Yang (logistic-curvilinear)	$Y_t = \dfrac{ae^{-ct}}{1 + e^{-k(t-b)}}$
Kovalenko and Tribat (exponential of a 2nd- or 3rd-order polynomial)	$Y_t = \exp(a + bt + ct^2 + dt^3)$
Multiphasic models	
Fialho and Ledur (piecewise or segmented model)	$Y_t = a - 3a\left(\dfrac{t_p - t}{t_p}\right)^2 + 2a\left(\dfrac{t_p - t}{t_p}\right)^3, \quad 0 \le t < t_p,$ $= a - c(t - t_p), \quad t \ge t_p$
Grossman *et al.*, 2000 (three intersecting straight lines with a smooth transition – simplified egg production persistency model for the flock)	$Y_t = a\left(\dfrac{b}{t_2 - t_1}\right)\left[\ln\left(\dfrac{e^{t/a} + e^{t_1/a}}{1 + e^{t_1/a}}\right) - \ln\left(\dfrac{e^{t/a} + e^{t_2/a}}{1 + e^{t_2/a}}\right)\right]$ $+ ac\ln\left(\dfrac{e^{t/a} + e^{(t_2+p)/a}}{1 + e^{(t_2+p)/a}}\right)$
Grossman *et al.*, 2000 (simplified egg production persistency model for an individual bird)	$Y_t = \dfrac{b}{t_2}t - a\dfrac{b}{t_2}\ln\left(\dfrac{e^{t/a} + e^{t_2/a}}{1 + e^{t_2/a}}\right)$ $+ ac\ln\left(\dfrac{e^{t/a} + e^{(t_2+p)/a}}{1 + e^{(t_2+p)/a}}\right)$
Grossman and Koops, 2001	$Y_t = a\left(\dfrac{1 - e^{-t}}{1 + e^{-t}}\right) - b\left(\dfrac{1 - e^{-t}}{1 + e^{-(t-c)}}\right)$

characteristic y as a result of varying the levels of the active factors $x_1, x_2, \ldots, x_n$ is called the response function (Pykh and Malkina-Pykh, 2001) of the system:

$$y = F(x_1, x_2, \ldots, x_n).$$

This is a generalized response function in which all the influencing factors are accounted for. A partial response function represents a single active factor (i.e. with a single explanatory variable $y = f_i(x_i)$). In many cases, the plot of the partial response function $f_i(x_i)$ to the varying levels of factor x_i is non-linear with an upper asymptote. The parametric form of the function has to be selected, if possible, from prior knowledge of the system or from measurements of input–output data (paired values of y and $x_1, x_2, \ldots, x_n$) obtained in experimental trials. In this latter case, the function may well be capable of interpolating within the range of observations, but cannot be considered fully predictive. The mathematical form of the response function may be variable. Some responses are linear, but others show clear non-linear trends that can only be represented by non-linear equations. Most of these equations are basically the same functions cited above for time-course data, the explanatory variable being the level of the factor studied instead of time (Motulsky and Christopoulos, 2003).

Response functions in animal nutrition

The response function method is a basic approach for investigating dose–effect relationships (Motulsky and Christopoulos, 2003) and, within the field of nutrition, to establish the response to the supply of energy, protein or other nutrients (AFRC, 1991). The classical approach in feeding trials has been to investigate the effects of varying intake levels of specific nutrients on animal performance. In these trials, one factor (a specific nutrient) is changed, while others are held as constant as possible (ILCA, 1990). In general, animal response obeys the Liebig principle of limiting factors (law of minimum), so that performance is completely determined by the level of a particular nutrient which is at the lowest concentration relative to its optimum amount (Thornley and France, 2007). In most cases, the expected response is characterized by a minimum threshold of the nutrient, below which the process concerned cannot proceed (e.g. minimum dose of vitamin or mineral sufficient to prevent clinical signs of deficiency), an optimum at which the rate of response is greatest (e.g. level associated with the maximum performance response) and a maximum level above which the process may be inhibited (e.g. dose from which a vitamin or mineral becomes toxic to the animal) (Pykh and Malkina-Pykh, 2001). Thus, before reaching the level of toxicity, the production response of most animals to most nutrients is subject to the law of diminishing returns, so that, after an initial increase in marginal returns, there is a diminishing rate of return so that the additional output yielded by each additional unit of an input (marginal physical product) will fall as the total amount of the input rises (holding all other inputs constant). This results in a typical curvilinear and asymptotic profile described by some non-linear or segmented functions (Thornley and France, 2007). Some representative examples of response functions used in animal nutrition will be briefly described.

In a typical feeding trial, different groups of animals are fed at different levels of energy or protein intake to ascertain the level that promotes an intended level of performance (Thornley and France, 2007). In growing animals, the response function is daily weight gain (Fig. 3.8), whereas, in dairy animals, the target function is milk yield or composition. This approach has been used to predict animal performance at a given feeding level and to assess nutrient requirements of the animal (AFRC, 1991; Whittemore *et al.*, 2001a,b). Dietary energy or protein requirement may be considered as that amount which will provide a high enough level of energy or protein to permit maximal economic return for the production unit (maximum growth rate or milk yield and feed efficiency). In the case of dairy cows, there are also a number of studies which report the effect of concentrate level in the ration on feed intake, milk yield and weight changes over extended periods of time (Walker *et al.*, 2004). The common trend in these relationships is an increase in performance with increasing dietary or energy intake up to a certain level; thereafter increases in intake produce no further increase in yield. However, this general pattern is not always that consistent, because nutritional reserves of the animal may be sufficient in the short term to allow normal health and yield even if the diet is inadequate, thus concealing the actual response to dietary nutrients. Energy and protein supplied with feed can also be used for different purposes, and thus, in dairy cows, response to supplements of energy added to the diet is negatively curvilinear in the case of milk yield and positively curvilinear in the case of live weight gain. Finally, animal performance (weight gain or milk yield) may not reflect the actual energy or protein retained in products (milk, eggs) or body tissues (Oldham, 1995; Reynolds and Beever, 1995; Satter and Dhiman, 1995).

Therefore, response functions have been used to represent the relationship between energy or nutrient retention in body tissues or in milk and energy or nutrient intake (Fig. 3.9). A classical relationship is that between energy balance (or retention) and metabolizable energy (ME) intake (Fig. 3.10), one of the bases of energy–feeding systems. The rate of energy retention by the growing animal is

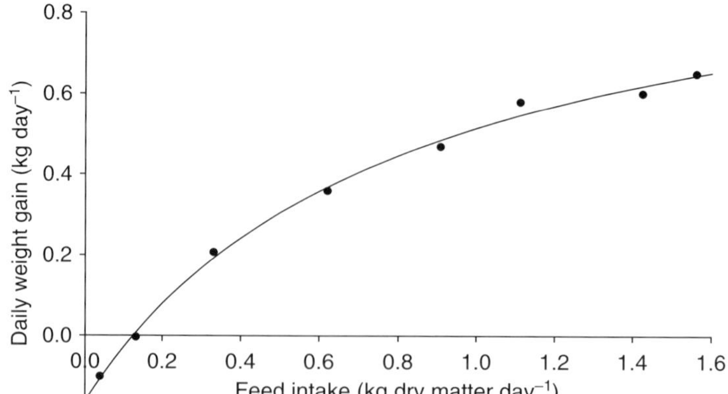

Fig. 3.8. Effects of varying feed intake on growth rate of an animal.

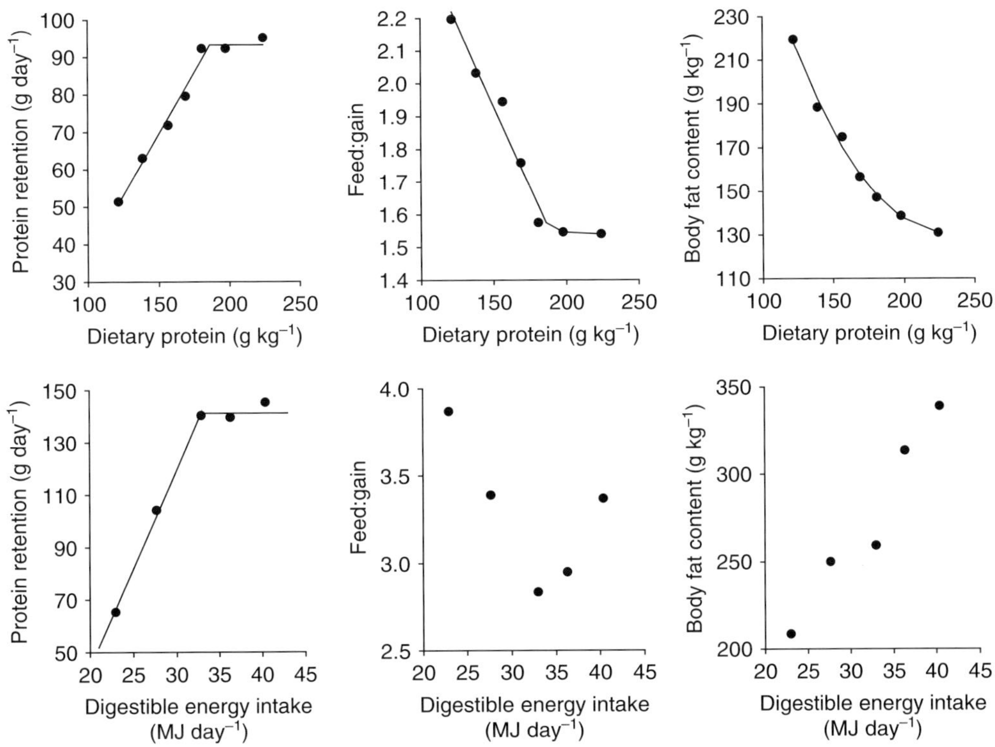

Fig. 3.9. Response curves in growing pigs: effects of dietary protein content and digestible energy intake on pig performance (Campbell, 1988).

non-linearly related to the level of ME intake, as successive increments in daily intake result in progressively smaller increments in daily energy retention in body weight gain (Blaxter, 1989; Van Milgen *et al.*, 2000). Blaxter and Wainman (1961) approximated this non-linear relationship with a segmented model involving two straight lines intersecting at zero energy retention. The intercept at zero ME intake represents the net energy requirements for maintenance (i.e. fasting metabolism), the intersection at zero energy balance represents the ME required for maintenance, the slope of the line below maintenance represents the efficiency of utilization of ME for maintenance and the slope above maintenance represents the efficiency of utilization of ME for growth and fattening. In the case of lactating animals, the relationship between milk energy output and ME intake has traditionally been assumed to be linear, assuming similar efficiencies of utilization of ME for maintenance and lactation. The intercept of this plot is fasting metabolism. Although conceptually it is convenient to envisage a difference in the efficiency of utilization of ME below and above maintenance, it has been argued whether there should be an abrupt bend or whether the relationship should be represented by a smooth curve. This relationship (net energy versus ME intake) can be described in both cases using the Mitscherlich equation, assuming the response obeys the law of diminishing returns (slope of the curve

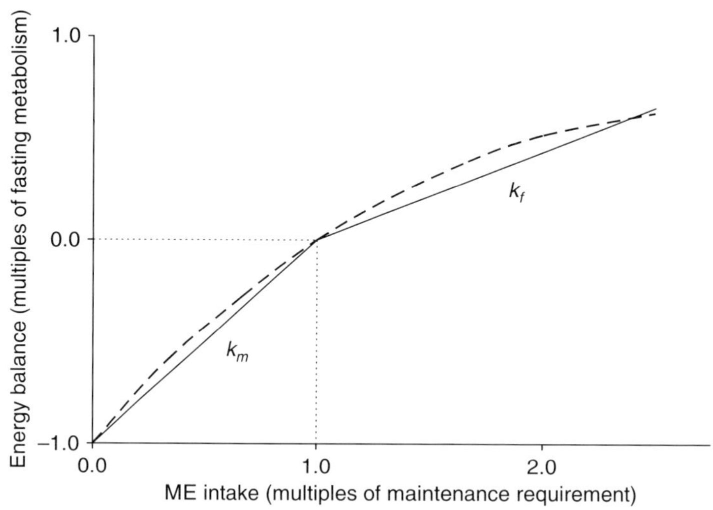

Fig. 3.10. Change in energy balance of the animal in relation to its metabolizable energy (ME) intake.

is continuously decreasing). Finally, assuming that over any segment of the response curve there may be an increasing slope, France *et al.* (1989), for growing animals, and Kebreab *et al.* (2003), for lactating dairy cows, have proposed some sigmoidal functions (logistic, Gompertz) for situations in which the law of diminishing returns does not apply to the rate of energy retention across the whole range of intakes.

A similar approach has been used for protein evaluation of feeds and assessment of protein and amino acid requirements of animals. Diets are used which are accepted as satisfactory in all respects other than protein, and then nitrogen balance is determined at different levels of protein intake (Black *et al.*, 1986; Campbell, 1988; Satter and Dhiman, 1995). Initially, the response is linear and increasing up to reaching a plateau (abrupt threshold), representing the greatest nitrogen retention that can be achieved under those experimental conditions (Fig. 3.11). The intercept at zero protein intake represents the net amount of nitrogen required for maintenance (i.e. endogenous losses), protein intake at zero nitrogen balance represents the amount of dietary protein required for maintenance and the slope is the efficiency of utilization of dietary protein, a combined assessment of protein digestibility (fraction which is absorbed) and biological value (fraction of absorbed protein which is retained) (Fuller, 1988). It is important to point out that this response is observed for a given level of energy intake and that, as energy supply is increased, the animal is able to respond to further increments of protein, reaching higher asymptotic values up to achieving the animal's potential for protein retention (Black *et al.*, 1986; Campbell, 1988; Whittemore *et al.*, 2001b). Response to a given essential amino acid follows a similar pattern (Black *et al.*, 1986; Boorman and Ellis, 1996; Waterlow, 1996). The utilization of an essential amino acid is assessed by giving diets containing different levels of the amino acid in question, but equal levels of the remaining

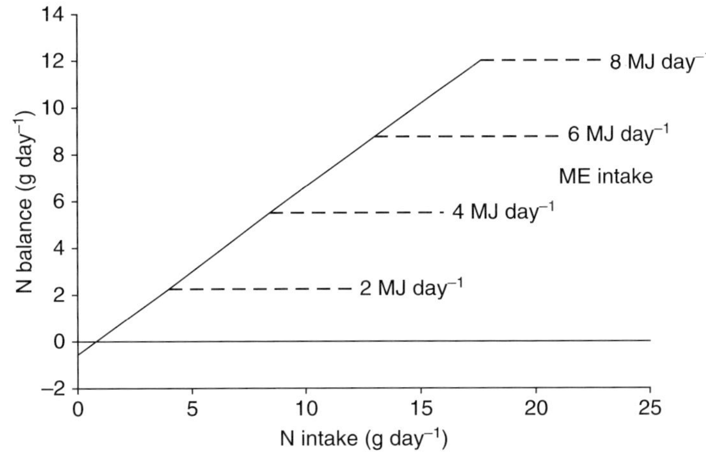

Fig. 3.11. Relationship between N balance and N intake at different metabolizable energy intakes in growing pigs.

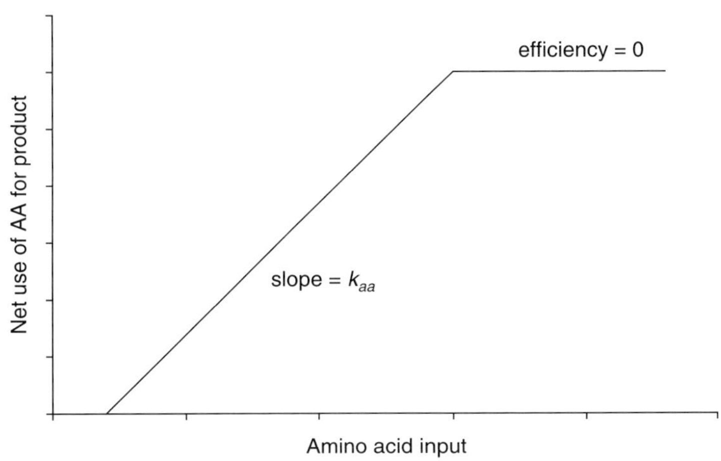

Fig. 3.12. Net use of amino acid for product (milk, tissue) in response to change in input of one amino acid.

amino acids, and measuring N retention or amino acid recovery in body tissues or products (milk). The simplest model for such a response is that of the broken stick (Oldham, 1987), in which an increment of the amino acid is converted to product at the limiting efficiency and, beyond a certain point, there is no further response (conversion efficiency = 0) as amino acid supply exceeds the capacity of the animal to use it (Fig. 3.12). The efficiency of use of a dietary amino acid for protein accretion is a combined estimate of its digestibility and availability (the fraction of the amino acid which is in a utilizable form), so that amino acid availability can be calculated providing its true digestibility is known (Fuller, 1988). Before reaching the maximum response, it is assumed that utilization of the amino acid is not constrained by other features of the diet or animal, whereas, upon reaching the upper asymptote, use of the amino acid is constrained because the animal's potential for protein retention is achieved, or protein synthesis is limited by the supply of energy or another amino acid (Fuller, 1988). Apart from the segmented model using straight lines, polynomial (quadratic), exponential and Mitscherlich functions have been suggested as more realistic to describe the diminishing returns pattern. Using these response functions, protein and amino acid requirements are established as the minimum intakes, which would certainly prove adequate for maximum N retention and thus maximum growth rate or milk yield. Similar response functions can be applied to determine dietary requirements of most minerals and vitamins (McDonald *et al.*, 2002).

Towards animal response models

Two different means of system representation are of interest, namely the input–output relation method and the state–variable method (Rand, 2004; Thornley and France, 2007). The approach described in the previous section is based on phenomenological whole-animal response (input–output method), and has been used extensively in animal nutrition to assess nutrient requirements and efficiency of utilization of feed energy and nutrients (protein, amino acids, micronutrients) for a particular type of animal in terms of stated economic goals and measurable animal characteristics. Then, once a performance target is established, energy and nutrient requirements to meet that target are drawn up and a ration is devised to match supply and demand for energy and then balanced for protein, minerals and vitamins (Beever *et al.*, 2000; McDonald *et al.*, 2002). Although most current feeding systems follow this strategy, it is increasingly recognized that the approach is prone to a number of weaknesses (AFRC, 1991; Beever *et al.*, 2000; López *et al.*, 2000a).

First, nutrient utilization from feed intake (input) for retention in animal tissue or in any product such as milk or eggs (output) is a complex phenomenon involving a number of processes at different levels (organic, cellular, molecular). Despite its simplicity, it seems likely that this approach is too empirical and aggregated, trying to describe such complexity with just a single equation to represent nutrient utilization at a single level (whole-animal) and ignoring all the nutrient fluxes at lower hierarchical levels of biological organization. With this approach, an observed response may apply only to a specific set of environmental, physiological, genetic and dietary conditions (Thornley and France, 2007). At this level, responses to nutrient supply provide information about animal requirements and effects on the amount of product expected at a given intake, but little is known about the effects on product composition (López *et al.*, 2000a).

The approach also focuses on response to a specific nutrient, whereas response may be affected significantly by the multiple interactions among different nutrients. Interactions of factors result in modifications of the response to changes in levels of one factor as a result of varying levels of another factor or factors (Boorman and Ellis, 1996; St-Pierre and Thraen, 1999). The combined response to two factors has to be represented by a three-dimensional response surface. Furthermore, energy is considered as a single entity, but energy is contained in specific nutrients and its utilization depends on the nature of the chemical compounds in which it is contained and their metabolic use (López *et al.*, 2000a).

The response to a given nutrient may not be wholly expressed when the animal uses its body reserves to make up for any dietary deficiency (Oldham, 1995; Reynolds and Beever, 1995). On the other hand, this simple model assumes that dietary nutrients ingested above maintenance are used almost exclusively for weight gain (growing animals) or milk production (lactating animals). However, nutrients may follow different alternative pathways. For example, amino acids are not used for protein synthesis only; they can be used as glucogenic substrates or degraded to obtain energy. The nature of the end products of digestion, as well as their influence on hormonal activity, is important to reconcile the partition of energy or protein utilization between milk and body tissue (Oldham, 1995).

Although, initially, this approach seeks to maximize the efficiency of conversion of feed to animal product, in practice, levels recommended to support maximum rates of production can be exceeded without toxicity, until incremental benefits are just offset by incremental costs. Regardless of the diminishing rate of return at high levels of intake, it may be justified in practice to feed more than the recommended standards, depending upon the financial benefit accruing from the increased yield relative to the cost of increasing nutrient supply, so the level of nutrient considered optimal may depend greatly upon price ratios. This strategy does not take into account the higher excretion of wasteful products such as N or P that may be detrimental to the environment, or the incidence of digestive or metabolic disorders in the animal concomitant with such high levels of intake (AFRC, 1991; St-Pierre and Thraen, 1999).

The principal tool of the input–output method is the transfer function, but this does not include any information concerning the internal structure of the system and its behaviour. However, response functions are only as good as our conceptual understanding of the system and the data used in the development of the model. The current challenge for modellers within the field of animal nutrition seems to move from a requirement (input–output) to a response (state–variable) system (AFRC, 1991; Thornley and France, 2007), developing models in which specific nutrients, metabolic pools and compartments are identified and a flow structure is defined to represent fluxes of nutrients between different pools and processes, along with exchange with the environment (feed intake, products, excretion of waste compounds), with the final target of predicting the response to dietary changes at the whole-animal level (AFRC, 1991; Beever *et al.*, 2000). Analysis of the response for each of the nutritional processes at cellular and molecular levels should increase our understanding of the underlying biochemical and physiological processes and allow identification of the primary factors affecting animal production. The response to nutrients depends on many factors concerned with the animal, the feed and the environment, and some of these must be included as explicit variables in the model, but, if all possible interactions are considered, the system will probably become too complex. With these models, it will be possible to address important issues other than just level of production, such as nutritional constraints to product composition or quality, excretion of waste products and nutrition-related disorders affecting animal health and welfare.

References

Abramowitz, M. and Stegun I. (1964) *Handbook of Mathematical Functions with Formulas, Graphs and Mathematical Tables*. National Bureau of Standards and US Government Printing Office, Washington, DC (reprinted with corrections in 1972).

AFRC (1991) Technical committee on responses to nutrients, Report No. 7, Theory of response to nutrients by farm animals. *Nutrition Abstracts and Reviews, Series B: Livestock Feeds and Feeding* 61, 683–722.

Arango, J.A. and Van Vleck, L.D. (2002) Size of beef cows: early ideas, new developments. *Genetics and Molecular Research* 1, 51–63.

Baranyi, J. and Roberts, T.A. (1995) Mathematics of predictive food microbiology. *International Journal of Food Microbiology* 26, 199–218.

Baranyi, J., Roberts, T.A. and McClure, P. (1993) A non-autonomous differential equation to model bacterial growth. *Food Microbiology* 10, 43–59.

Bates, D.M. and Watts D.G. (1988) *Nonlinear Regression Analysis and Its Applications*. Wiley, New York.

Beever, D.E., Rook, A.J., France, J., Dhanoa, M.S. and Gill, M. (1991) A review of empirical and mechanistic models of lactational performance by the dairy-cow. *Livestock Production Science* 29, 115–130.

Beever, D.E., France, J. and Alderman, G. (2000) Prediction of response to nutrients by ruminants through mathematical modelling and improved feed characterization. In: Theodorou, M.K. and France, J. (eds) *Feeding Systems and Feed Evaluation Models*. CAB International, Wallingford, UK, pp. 275–297.

Behr, V. de, Hornick, J.L., Cabaraux, J.F., Alvarez, A. and Istasse, L. (2001) Growth patterns of Belgian Blue replacement heifers and growing males in commercial farms. *Livestock Production Science* 71, 121–130.

Black, J.L., Campbell, R.G., Williams, I.H., James, K.J. and Davies, G.T. (1986) Simulation of energy and amino acid utilisation in the pig. *Research and Development in Agriculture* 3, 121–145.

Blaxter, K.L. (1989) *Energy Metabolism in Animals and Man*. Cambridge University Press, Cambridge, UK.

Blaxter, K.L. and Wainman, F.W. (1961) The utilisation of food by sheep and cattle. *Journal of Agricultural Science, Cambridge* 57, 419–425.

Blaxter, K.L., Graham, N.McC. and Wainman, F.W. (1956) Some observations on the digestibility of food by sheep, and on related problems. *British Journal of Nutrition* 10, 69–91.

Boorman, K.N. and Ellis, G.M. (1996) Maximum nutritional response to poor-quality protein and amino acid utilisation. *British Poultry Science* 37, 145–156.

Brotherstone, S., White, I.M.S. and Meyer, K. (2000) Genetic modelling of daily milk yield using orthogonal polynomials and parametric curves. *Animal Science* 70, 407–415.

Brown, J.E., Fitzhugh, H.A. Jr and Cartwright, T.C. (1976) A comparison of nonlinear models for describing weight–age relationships in cattle. *Journal of Animal Science* 42, 810–818.

Buchanan, R.L., Whiting, R.C. and Damert, W.C. (1997) When is simple good enough? A comparison of the Gompertz, Baranyi, and three-phase linear models for fitting bacterial growth curves. *Food Microbiology* 14, 313–326.

Burnham, K.P. and Anderson, D.R. (2002) *Model Selection and Multimodel Inference: A Practical Information–Theoretic Approach*, 2nd edn. Springer-Verlag, New York.

Butterfield, R.M. (1988) *New Concepts of Sheep Growth*. The Department of Veterinary Anatomy, University of Sydney, Sydney, Australia.

Campbell, R.G. (1988) Nutritional constraints to lean tissue accretion in farm animals. *Nutrition Research Reviews* 1, 233–253.

Carvalheira, J., Pollak, E.J., Quaas, R.L. and Blake, R.W. (2002) An autoregressive repeatability animal model for test-day records in multiple lactations. *Journal of Dairy Science* 85, 2040–2045.

Davidian, M. and Giltinan, D.M. (1995) *Nonlinear Models for Repeated Measurement Data*. Chapman and Hall, New York.

Dhanoa, M.S., Siddons, R.C., France, J. and Gale, D.L. (1985) A multicompartmental model to describe marker excretion patterns in ruminant faeces. *British Journal of Nutrition* 53, 663–671.

Dijkstra, J., France, J., Dhanoa, M.S., Maas, J.A., Hanigan, M.D., Rook, A.J. and Beever, D.E. (1997) A model to describe growth patterns of the mammary gland during pregnancy and lactation. *Journal of Dairy Science* 80, 2340–2354.

Dijkstra, J., France, J. and Davies, D.R. (1998) Different mathematical approaches to estimating microbial protein supply in ruminants. *Journal of Dairy Science* 81, 3370–3384.

Dijkstra, J., Kebreab, E., Bannink, A., France, J. and López, S. (2005) Application of the gas production technique in feed evaluation systems for ruminants. *Animal Feed Science and Technology* 123–124, 561–578.

Draper, N.R. and Smith, H. (1998) *Applied Regression Analysis*, 3rd edn. Wiley, New York.

Ellis, W.C., Matis, J.H., Hill, T.M. and Murphy, M.R. (1994) Methodology for estimating digestion and passage kinetics of forages. In: Fahey, G.C. Jr (ed.) *Forage Quality, Evaluation, and Utilization*. American Society of Agronomy, Crop Science Society of America and Soil Science Society of America, Madison, Wisconsin, pp. 682–756.

Faichney, G.J. (2005) Digesta flow. In: Dijkstra, J., Forbes, J.M. and France, J. (eds) *Quantitative Aspects of Ruminant Digestion and Metabolism*, 2nd edn. CAB International, Wallingford, UK, pp. 49–86.

Fekedulegn, D., Mac Siurtain, M.P. and Colbert, J.J. (1999) Parameter estimation of nonlinear growth models in forestry. *Silva Fennica* 33, 327–336.

Fialho, F.B. and Ledur, M.C. (1997) Segmented polynomial model for estimation of egg production curves in laying hens. *British Poultry Science* 38, 66–73.

Fitzhugh, H.A. Jr (1976) Analysis of growth curves and strategies for altering their shape. *Journal of Animal Science* 42, 1036–1051.

France, J., Thornley, J.H.M., Dhanoa, M.S. and Siddons, R.C. (1985) On the mathematics of digesta flow kinetics. *Journal of Theoretical Biology* 113, 743–758.

France, J., Dhanoa, M.S., Cammell, S.B., Gill, M., Beever, D.E. and Thornley, J.H.M. (1989) On the use of response functions in energy-balance analysis. *Journal of Theoretical Biology* 140, 83–99.

France, J., Thornley, J.H.M., López, S., Siddons, R.C., Dhanoa, M.S., Van Soest, P.J. and Gill, M. (1990) On the two-compartment model for estimating the rate and extent of feed degradation in the rumen. *Journal of Theoretical Biology* 146, 269–287.

France, J., Dhanoa, M.S., Theodorou, M.K., Lister, S.J., Davies, D.R. and Isac, D. (1993a) A model to interpret gas accumulation profiles associated with *in vitro* degradation of ruminant feeds. *Journal of Theoretical Biology* 163, 99–111.

France, J., Thornley, J.H.M., Siddons, R.C. and Dhanoa, M.S. (1993b) On incorporating diffusion and viscosity concepts into compartmental-models for analysing faecal marker excretion patterns in ruminants. *British Journal of Nutrition* 70, 369–378.

France, J., Dijkstra, J. and Dhanoa, M.S. (1996). Growth functions and their application in animal sciences. *Annales de Zootechnie* 45, 165–174.

France, J., Dijkstra, J., Dhanoa, M.S., López, S. and Bannink, A. (2000) Estimating the extent of degradation of ruminant feeds from a description of their gas production profiles observed *in vitro*: derivation of models and other mathematical considerations. *British Journal of Nutrition* 83, 131–142.

France, J., López, S., Kebreab, E., Bannink, A., Dhanoa, M.S. and Dijkstra, J. (2005) A general compartmental model for interpreting gas production profiles. *Animal Feed Science and Technology* 123–124, 473–485.

Fuller, M.F. (1988) Methods of protein evaluation for non-ruminants. In: Ørskov, E.R. (ed.) *Feed Science, World Animal Science, B4*. Elsevier, Amsterdam, pp. 81–101.

Gavora, J.S., Liljedahl, L.E., McMillan, I. and Ahlen, K. (1982) Comparison of three mathematical-models of egg-production. *British Poultry Science* 23, 339–348.

Gill, M. and Oldham, J.D. (1993) Growth. In: Forbes, J.M. and France, J. (eds) *Quantitative Aspects of Ruminants' Digestion and Metabolism*. CAB International, Wallingford, UK, pp. 383–403.

Groot, J.C.J., Cone, J.W., Williams, B.A., Debersaques, F.M.A. and Lantinga, E.A. (1996) Multiphasic analysis of gas production kinetics for *in vitro* fermentation of ruminant feeds. *Animal Feed Science and Technology* 64, 77–89.

Grossman, M. and Koops, W.J. (1988) Multiphasic analysis of lactation curves in dairy-cattle. *Journal of Dairy Science* 71, 1598–1608

Grossman, M. and Koops, W.J. (2001) A model for individual egg production in chickens. *Poultry Science* 80, 859–867.

Grossman, M. and Koops, W.J. (2003) Modeling extended lactation curves of dairy cattle: a biological basis for the multiphasic approach. *Journal of Dairy Science* 86, 988–998.

Grossman, M., Hartz, S.M. and Koops, W.J. (1999) Persistency of lactation yield: a novel approach. *Journal of Dairy Science* 82, 2192–2197.

Grossman, M., Gossman, T.N. and Koops, W.J. (2000) A model for persistency of egg production. *Poultry Science* 79, 1715–1724.

Grovum, W.L. and Williams, V.J. (1973) Rate of passage of digesta in sheep. 4. Passage of marker through the alimentary tract and the biological relevance of rate-constants derived from the changes in concentration of marker in faeces. *British Journal of Nutrition* 30, 313–329.

Huxley, J.S. (1924) Constant differential growth-ratios and their significance. *Nature* 114, 895–896.

Huxley, J.S. and Teissier, G. (1936) Terminology of relative growth. *Nature* 137, 780–781.

ILCA (International Livestock Centre for Africa) (1990) *Livestock Systems Research Manual*, Vol. 2. ILCA, Addis Ababa.

Jensen, J. (2001) Genetic evaluation of dairy cattle using test-day models. *Journal of Dairy Science* 84, 2803–2812.

Kargi, F. and Shuler, M.L. (1979) Generalized differential specific rate equation for microbial-growth. *Biotechnology and Bioengineering* 21, 1871–1875.

Kebreab, E., France, J., Agnew, R.E., Yan, T., Dhanoa, M.S., Dijkstra, J., Beever, D.E. and Reynolds, C.K. (2003) Alternatives to linear analysis of energy balance data from lactating dairy cows. *Journal of Dairy Science* 86, 2904–2913.

Koops, W.J. (1986) Multiphasic growth curve analysis. *Growth* 50, 169–177.

Landete-Castillejos, T. and Gallego, L. (2000) The ability of mathematical models to describe the shape of lactation curves. *Journal of Animal Science* 78, 3010–3013.

Lawrence, T.L.J. and Fowler, V.R. (2002) *Growth of Farm Animals*, 2nd edn. CAB International, Wallingford, UK.

Leeson, S. and Summers, J.D. (1997) *Commercial Poultry Production*, 2nd edn. University Books, Guelph, Ontario, Canada.

López, S. (2005) *In vitro* and *in situ* techniques for estimating digestibility. In: Dijkstra, J., Forbes, J.M. and France, J. (eds) *Quantitative Aspects of Ruminant Digestion and Metabolism*, 2nd edn. CAB International, Wallingford, UK, pp. 87–121.

López, S., France, J., Dhanoa, M.S., Mould, F. and Dijkstra, J. (1999) Comparison of mathematical models to describe disappearance curves obtained using the polyester bag technique for incubating feeds in the rumen. *Journal of Animal Science* 77, 1875–1888.

López, S., Dijkstra, J. and France, J. (2000a) Prediction of energy supply in ruminants, with emphasis on forages. In: Givens, D.I., Owen, E., Omed, H.M. and Axford, R.F.E. (eds) *Forage Evaluation in Ruminant Nutrition*. CAB International, Wallingford, UK, pp. 63–94.

López, S., France, J., Dijkstra, J. and Dhanoa, M.S. (2000b) Models to interpret degradation profiles obtained from *in vitro* and *in situ* incubation of ruminant feeds. In: McNamara, J.P., France, J. and Beever, D.E. (eds) *Modelling Nutrient Utilization in Farm Animals*. CAB International, Wallingford, UK, pp. 73–86.

López, S., France. J., Gerrits, W.J.J., Dhanoa, M.S., Humphries, D.J. and Dijkstra, J. (2000c) A generalized Michaelis–Menten equation for the analysis of growth. *Journal of Animal Science* 78, 1816–1828.

López, S., Prieto, M., Dijkstra, J., Dhanoa, M.S. and France, J. (2004) Statistical evaluation of mathematical models for microbial growth. *International Journal of Food Microbiology* 96, 289–300.

López, S., Prieto, M., Dijkstra, J., Kebreab, E., Dhanoa, M.S. and France, J. (2006) Functions for microbial growth. In: Kebreab, E., Dijkstra, J., Bannink, A., Gerrits, W.J.J. and France, J. (eds) *Nutrient Digestion and Utilization in Farm Animals: Modelling Approaches*. CAB International, Wallingford, UK, pp. 54–68.

McDonald, P., Edwards, R.A., Greenhalgh, J.F.D. and Morgan, C.A. (2002) *Animal Nutrition*, 6th edn. Pearson Education Ltd, Harlow, UK.

McMeekin, T.A. and Ross, T. (2002) Predictive microbiology: providing a knowledge-based framework for change management. *International Journal of Food Microbiology* 78, 133–153.

McMeekin, T.A., Olley, J.N., Ross, T. and Ratkowsky, D.A. (1993) *Predictive Microbiology: Theory and Application*. Wiley, New York.

McMillan, I. (1981) Compartmental model analysis of poultry egg-production curves. *Poultry Science* 60, 1549–1551.

McMillan, I., Fitz-Earle, M. and Robson, D.S. (1970) Quantitative genetics of fertility I. Lifetime egg production of *Drosophila melanogaster* – Theoretical. *Genetics* 65, 349–353.

Masselin, S., Sauvant, D., Chapoutot, P. and Milan, D. (1987) Les modèles d'ajustement des courbes de lactation. *Annales de Zootechnie* 36, 171–206.

Matis, J.H. (1972) Gamma-time dependency in Blaxter's compartment model. *Biometrics* 28, 597–602.

Mertens, D.R. (2005) Rate and extent of digestion. In: Dijkstra, J., Forbes, J.M. and France, J. (eds) *Quantitative Aspects of Ruminant Digestion and Metabolism*, 2nd edn. CAB International, Wallingford, UK, pp. 13–47.

Meyer, K. (1998) Estimating covariance functions for longitudinal data using random regression models. *Genetics Selection Evolution* 30, 221–240.

Monod, J. (1949) The growth of bacterial cultures. *Annual Review of Microbiology* 3, 371–394.

Morant, S.V. and Gnanasakthy, A. (1989) A new approach to the mathematical formulation of lactation curves. *Animal Production* 49, 151–162.

Motulsky, H.J. and Christopoulos, A. (2003) *Fitting Models to Biological Data Using Linear and Nonlinear Regression. A Practical Guide to Curve Fitting.* GraphPad Software Inc., San Diego, California.

Motulsky, H.J. and Ransnas, L.A. (1987) Fitting curves to data using nonlinear regression: a practical and nonmathematical review. *FASEB Journal* 1, 365–374.

Narushin, V.G. and Takma, C. (2003) Sigmoid model for the evaluation of growth and production curves in laying hens. *Biosystems Engineering* 84, 343–348.

National Institute of Standards and Technology (2007) Digital Library of Mathematical Functions, http://dlmf.nist.gov/ (accessed 9 December 2007).

Oldham, J.D. (1987) Efficiencies of amino acid utilisation. In: Jarrige, R. and Alderman, G. (eds) *Feed Evaluation and Protein Requirement Systems for Ruminants.* Commission of the European Communities, Luxembourg, pp. 171–186.

Oldham, J.D. (1995) Protein requirements and responses: a United Kingdom perspective. In: Lawrence, T.L.J., Gordon, F.J. and Carson, A. (eds) *Breeding and Feeding the High Genetic Merit Dairy Cow.* BSAS, Edinburgh, UK, pp. 21–29.

Olori, V.E., Brotherstone, S., Hill, W.G. and McGuirk, B.J. (1999) Fit of standard models of the lactation curve to weekly records of milk production of cows in a single herd. *Livestock Production Science* 58, 55–63.

Ørskov, E.R. and McDonald, I. (1979) The estimation of protein degradability in the rumen from incubation measurements weighted according to rate of passage. *Journal of Agricultural Science, Cambridge* 92, 499–503.

Papajcsik, I.A. and Bodero, J. (1988) Modelling lactation curves of Friesian cows in a sub-tropical climate. *Animal Production* 47, 201–207.

Parks, J.R. (1982) *A Theory of Feeding and Growth of Animals.* Springer-Verlag, Berlin.

Peek, M.S., Russek-Cohen, E., Wait, D.A. and Forseth, I.N. (2002) Physiological response curve analysis using nonlinear mixed models. *Oecologia* 132, 175–180.

Peleg, M. (1997) Modeling microbial populations with the original and modified versions of the continuous and discrete logistic equations. *Critical Reviews in Food Science and Nutrition* 37, 471–490.

Pollott, G.E. (2000) A biological approach to lactation curve analysis for milk yield. *Journal of Dairy Science* 83, 2448–2458.

Pond, K.R., Ellis, W.C., Matis, J.H., Ferreiro, H.M. and Sutton, J.D. (1988) Compartment models for estimating attributes of digesta flow in cattle. *British Journal of Nutrition* 60, 571–595.

Powell, R.L. and Norman, H.D. (2006) Major advances in genetic evaluation techniques. *Journal of Dairy Science* 89, 1337–1348.

Pykh, Y.A. and Malkina-Pykh, I.G. (2001) *The Method of Response Function in Ecology.* WIT Press, Southampton, UK.

Rand, W.M. (2004) Variability in planning and assessment: statistical considerations and models. *Journal of Nutrition* 134, 1610S–1616S.

Ratkowski, D.A. (1983) *Nonlinear Regression Modeling.* Marcel Dekker, New York.

Rekaya, R., Carabano, M.J. and Toro, M.A. (2000) Bayesian analysis of lactation curves of Holstein-Friesian cattle using a non-linear model. *Journal of Dairy Science* 86, 2691–2701.

Reynolds, C.K. and Beever, D.E. (1995) Energy requirements and responses: a United Kingdom perspective. In: Lawrence, T.L.J., Gordon, F.J. and Carson, A. (eds) *Breeding and Feeding the High Genetic Merit Dairy Cow*. BSAS, Edinburgh, UK, pp. 31–41.

Ricker, W.E. (1979) Growth rates and models. In: Hoar, W.S., Randall, D.J. and Brett, J.R. (eds) *Fish Physiology*, Vol. VIII. Academic Press, New York, pp. 677–743.

Robinson, P.H., Fadel, J.G. and Tamminga, S. (1986) Evaluation of mathematical models to describe neutral detergent residue in terms of its susceptibility to degradation in the rumen. *Animal Feed Science and Technology* 15, 249–271.

Rook, A.J., France, J. and Dhanoa, M.S. (1993) On the mathematical-description of lactation curves. *Journal of Agricultural Science, Cambridge* 121, 97–102.

St-Pierre, N.R. and Thraen, C.S. (1999) Animal grouping strategies, sources of variation, and economic factors affecting nutrient balance on dairy farms. *Journal of Animal Science* 77 (Suppl. 2), 72–83.

Sainz, R.D. and Baldwin, R.L. (2003) Modeling and growth. In: Scanes, C.G. (ed.) *Biology of Growth of Domestic Animals*. Iowa State Press/Blackwell, Ames, Iowa, pp. 214–219.

Satter, L.D. and Dhiman, T.R. (1995) Protein and energy requirements and responses: a United States perspective. In: Lawrence, T.L.J., Gordon, F.J. and Carson, A. (eds) *Breeding and Feeding the High Genetic Merit Dairy Cow*. BSAS, Edinburgh, UK, pp. 43–50.

Schaeffer, L.R. (2004) Application of random regression models in animal breeding. *Livestock Production Science* 86, 35–45.

Schinckel, A.P. and Craig, B.A. (2001) Nonlinear mixed effects model for swine growth. 2001 Purdue Swine Research Reports, pp. 20–25.

Seber, G.A.F. and Wild, C.J. (2003) *Nonlinear Regression*. Wiley, New York.

Sherchand, L., McNew, R.W., Kellogg, D.W. and Johnson, Z.B. (1995) Selection of a mathematical model to generate lactation curves using daily milk yields of Holstein cows. *Journal of Dairy Science* 78, 2507–2513.

Silvestre, A.M., Petim-Batista, F. and Colaco, J. (2006) The accuracy of seven mathematical functions in modeling dairy cattle lactation curves based on test-day records from varying sample schemes. *Journal of Dairy Science* 89, 1813–1821.

Simondon, K.B., Simondon, F., Delpeuch, F. and Cornu, A. (1992) Comparative study of five growth models applied to weight data from Congolese infants between birth and 13 months of age. *American Journal of Human Biology* 4, 327–335.

Swalve, H.H. (1995) Test-day models in the analysis of dairy production data – a review. *Archiv für Tierzucht – Archives of Animal Breeding* 38, 591–612.

Swalve, H.H. (2000) Theoretical basis and computational methods for different test-day genetic evaluation methods. *Journal of Dairy Science* 83, 1115–1124.

Swatland, H.J. (1994) *Structure and Development of Meat Animals and Poultry*. Technomic Publishing Co. Inc., Lancaster, Pennsylvania.

Swinnen, I.A.M., Bernaerts, K., Dens, E.J.J., Geeraerd, A.H. and Van Impe, J.F. (2004) Predictive modelling of the microbial lag phase: a review. *International Journal of Food Microbiology* 94, 137–159.

Taylor, St C.S. (1980) Live-weight growth from embryo to adult in domesticated mammals. *Animal Production* 31, 223–235.

Thornley, J.H.M. and France, J. (2007) *Mathematical Models in Agriculture: Quantitative Methods for the Plant, Animal and Ecological Sciences*, 2nd edn. CAB International, Wallingford, UK.

Thornley, J.H.M., France, J., Dhanoa, M.S. and Siddons, R.C. (1995) The effects of diffusion and viscosity on ruminant faecal excretion of markers in a simple compartmental model. *British Journal of Nutrition* 74, 747–763.

Tsoularis, A. and Wallace, J. (2002) Analysis of logistic growth models. *Mathematical Biosciences* 179, 21–55.

Turner, M.E., Bradley, E., Kirk, K. and Pruitt, K. (1976) A theory of growth. *Mathematical Biosciences* 29, 367–373.

Van Bebber, J., Reinsch, N., Junge, W. and Kalm, E. (1997) Accounting for herd, year and season effects in genetic evaluations of dairy cattle: a review. *Livestock Production Science* 51, 191–203.

Van Milgen, J. and Baumont, R. (1995) Models based on variable fractional digestion rates to describe ruminal *in situ* digestion. *British Journal of Nutrition* 73, 793–807.

Van Milgen, J., Murphy, M.R. and Berger, L.L. (1991) A compartmental model to analyze ruminal digestion. *Journal of Dairy Science* 74, 2515–2529.

Van Milgen, J., Quiniou, N. and Noblet, J. (2000) Modelling the relation between energy intake and protein and lipid deposition in growing pigs. *Animal Science* 71, 119–130.

Van Soest, P.J. (1994) *Nutritional Ecology of the Ruminant*, 2nd edn. Cornell University Press, Ithaca, New York.

Walker, G.P., Dunshea, F.R. and Doyle, P.T. (2004) Effects of nutrition and management on the production and composition of milk fat and protein: a review. *Australian Journal of Agricultural Research* 55, 1009–1028.

Warner, A.C.I. (1981) Rate of passage of digesta through the guts of mammals and birds. *Nutrition Abstracts and Reviews Series B (Livestock Feeds and Feeding)* 51, 789–820.

Waterlow, J.C. (1996) The requirements of adult man for indispensable amino acids. *European Journal of Clinical Nutrition* 50 (Suppl. 1), S151–S179.

Wellock, I.J., Emmans, G.C. and Kyriazakis, I. (2004) Describing and predicting potential growth in the pig. *Animal Science* 78, 379–388.

White, I.M.S., Thompson, R. and Brotherstone, S. (1999) Genetic and environmental smoothing of lactation curves with cubic splines. *Journal of Dairy Science* 82, 632–638.

Whiting, R.C. (1995) Microbial modeling in foods. *Critical Reviews in Food Science and Nutrition* 35, 464–494.

Whiting, R.C. and Buchanan, R.L.B. (1997) Predictive modelling. In: Doyle, M.P., Beuchat, L.R. and Montville, T.J. (eds) *Food Microbiology Fundamentals and Frontiers*. American Society for Microbiology Press, Washington, DC, pp. 728–739.

Whittemore, C.T. and Green, D.M. (2001) Growth of the young weaned pig. In: Varley, M.A. and Wiseman J. (eds) *The Weaner Pig – Nutrition and Management*. CAB International, Wallingford, UK, pp. 1–15.

Whittemore, C.T., Green, D.M. and Knap, P.W. (2001a) Technical review of the energy and protein requirements of growing pigs: energy. *Animal Science* 73, 199–215.

Whittemore, C.T., Green, D.M. and Knap, P.W. (2001b) Technical review of the energy and protein requirements of growing pigs: protein. *Animal Science* 73, 363–373.

Wood, P.D.P. (1967) Algebraic model of the lactation curve in cattle. *Nature, London* 216, 164–165.

Zeide, B. (1993) Analysis of growth equations. *Forest Science* 39, 594–616.

Zwietering, M.H., Jongenburger, I., Rombouts, F.M. and van't Riet, K. (1990) Modeling of the bacterial growth curve. *Applied and Environmental Microbiology* 56, 1875–1881.

4 Interesting Simple Dynamic Growth Models

J.H.M. THORNLEY

Centre for Nutrition Modelling, Department of Animal and Poultry Science, University of Guelph, Canada

Introduction

Growth functions have had an important role in animal nutrition partly, if not largely, because the growth equations are analytically soluble (Thornley and France, 2007). Analytical models can be of great heuristic value. However, there are some quite simple models without analytical solutions which are, nevertheless, rather instructive. Using a computer and suitable software, numerical solutions are now usually easy to obtain, readily permitting exploration and understanding of the model's equations. Some of these simple models are extensions of growth models, and some explore new ground. The intention is to illustrate the consequences of various biological assumptions in leading to models which may be valuable in phenomenological or semi-empirical nutritional studies.

Autocatalytic Growth with Substrate Limitation

Autocatalytic growth is the key starting point for many nutritional studies of animals and their parts. The basic growth equation is:

$$\frac{dW}{dt} = \mu W. \tag{4.1}$$

W (kg) denotes weight and μ (day^{-1}) specific growth rate. μ may reflect (a spatial) average or local substrate concentration, S (M) (M denotes concentration with units of 10^3 mol m^{-3} = mol dm^{-3} – use of the name 'molar' is not recommended due to possible confusion with 'molar' referring to quantities of substance; Royal Society, 1975), which may be quite dynamic, determined by supply–demand considerations. Define dependence of μ in Eqn 4.1 on S by:

$$\mu = \mu_{max} \frac{S^q}{K^q + S^q}. \tag{4.2}$$

μ_{max} (day^{-1}) is the maximum value of μ ($S \to \infty$); K (M) is the value of substrate S for half-maximal rate. Parameter q permits sigmoidal ($q > 1$), as well as non-sigmoidal ($q \le 1$), including the Michaelis–Menten ($q = 1$), substrate responses to be explored.

Assume that substrate (S) is converted into product (W) without loss. Conservation gives:

$$W + S = W_0 + S_0 = W_f. \tag{4.3}$$

W_0 and S_0 are the time $t = 0$ values of W and S. With Eqns 4.2 and 4.3, Eqn 4.1 becomes (substituting $S = W_f - W$):

$$\frac{dW}{dt} = \mu_{max} W \frac{(W_f - W)^q}{K^q + (W_f - W)^q}. \tag{4.4}$$

Eqn 4.4 cannot, in general, be integrated, except for particular q values [$q = 0$ (unlimited growth), 1 (Michaelis–Menten growth), 2]. Also, for $W_f \to \infty$, exponential growth with specific growth rate μ_{max} is recovered. With $K \to \infty$, $\mu_{max} \to \infty$, μ_{max}/K^q = constant c (mass^{-q}/time), then a modified logistic growth equation is recovered:

$$\frac{dW}{dt} = cW(W_f - W)^q. \tag{4.5}$$

Eqn 4.5 is identical to the logistic if $q = 1$.

Figure 4.1a illustrates responses of Eqn 4.4 when $q = 1$, with K varying. In each case, μ_{max} is adjusted so that the initial slope is the same. For the logistic ($K \to \infty$), the inflexion point is at half the asymptote. For other K-values, weight at inflexion can have higher values and approaches the asymptote as $K \to \infty$. However, time of inflexion varies little.

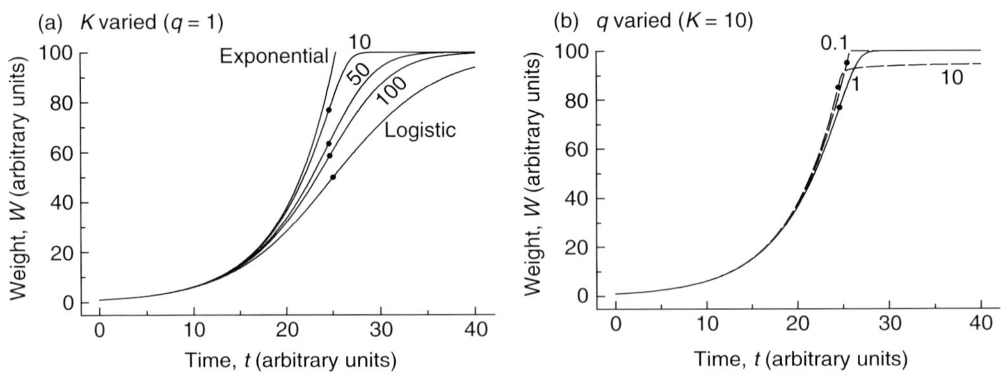

Fig. 4.1. Autocatalytic growth with sigmoidal Michaelis–Menten-like substrate limitation (Eqn 4.4). Curves have the same initial dry weight ($W_0 = 1$), asymptote $W_f = 100$ and initial slope (μ_{max} is adjusted to achieve this). (a) K is varied with $q = 1$. Unlimited exponential growth is obtained with $W_f = 1 \times 10^{10}$; $\mu_{max} = 0.18165$. The logistic limit has $K = 1 \times 10^9$ and $\mu_{max} = 0.18349 \times 10^7 = 0.18165K/99$. (b) q is varied with $K = 10$. Filled circles show inflexion points.

Figure 4.1b shows the effect of varying sigmoidicity parameter q. Again, all initial slopes are the same. For small q, exponential growth proceeds almost until the asymptote is attained. For high q, exponential growth is followed by slow approach to the asymptote. Weights at inflexion are at a high fraction of the final asymptote. The solid curve in Fig. 4.1b is the same as the $K = 10$ curve in Fig. 4.1a.

Delaying Growth

Growth requires substrate and machinery to convert substrate into dry weight. Growth rate can be influenced either through substrate provision or by modulating constants representing machinery (e.g. μ_{max} of Eqn 4.2). This section illustrates how delays can be represented in the logistic and Gompertz growth equations.

Delayed logistic

A simple empirical approach to delayed action on growth rate function, g, is to assume a discrete delay:

$$\text{if } t \le \tau, \text{then } g(W,t) = \frac{dW}{dt} = 0 \tag{4.6}$$

else $g(W,t) =$ function of W and t.

t is the time variable, τ a delay time. The logistic equation is:

$$\frac{dW}{dt} = \mu_0 W\left(1 - \frac{W}{W_f}\right), \tag{4.7}$$

where W (kg) is dry weight, μ_0 (day^{-1}) is a growth rate parameter and W_f (kg) is final dry weight. Eqns 4.6 and 4.7 lead to:

$$t < \tau, W = W_0; t \ge \tau, W = \frac{W_0 W_f}{W_0 + (W_f - W_0)e^{\mu(t-\tau)}}. \tag{4.8}$$

In Eqn 4.8, the usual logistic growth curve is shifted right by τ along the time axis, but with unchanged shape.

However, a discrete time delay is abrupt, which may be biologically unrealistic for some applications. A gamma function can provide a flexible delay function which, in the limit, approaches a step function. Figure 4.2a illustrates the compartmental scheme which gives rise to the gamma function. There are n compartments with state variables $y_1, \ldots, y_n$. An irreversible reaction with the same rate constant k applies to all n variables. If, at time $t = 0$, $y_1 = 1$ and $y_2, \ldots, y_n = 0$, then, at time t, y_n is given by:

$$y_n(t) = \frac{(kt)^{n-1} e^{-kt}}{(n-1)!}. \tag{4.9}$$

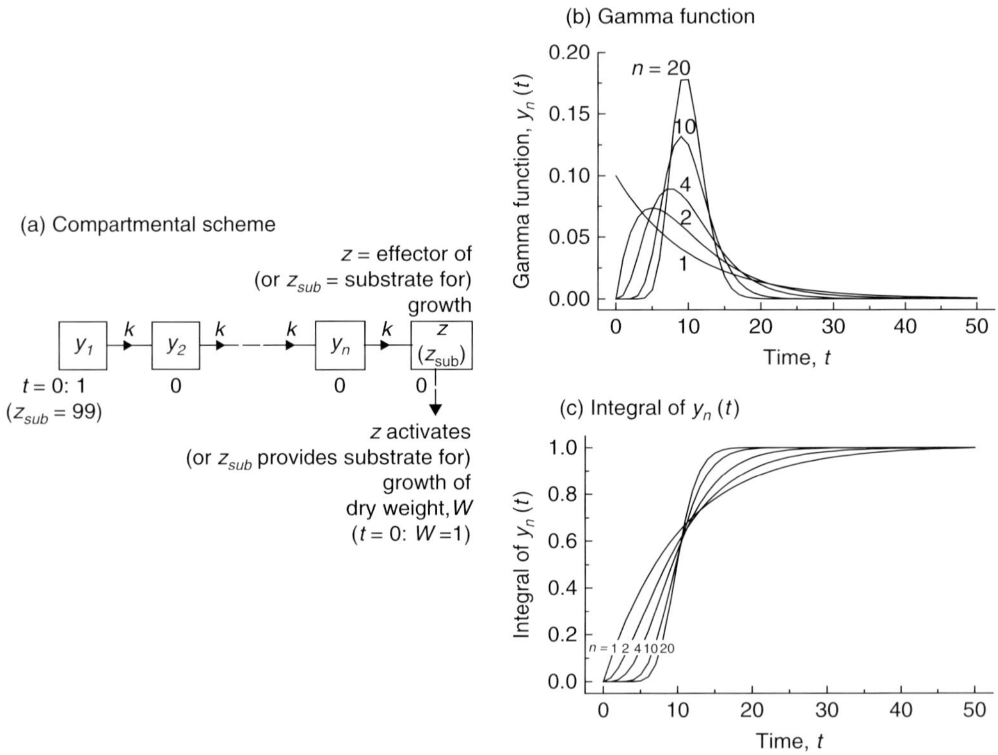

Fig. 4.2. Delayed growth using a compartmental scheme to give a gamma delay. Pools y_1 to y_n all have the same exit rate constant, k. Pool z is where accumulation of a biochemical effector might occur (Figs 4.2a and 4.3a). Alternatively, this pool can be regarded as containing substrate, which is consumed in growth (z_{sub}). Pool initial values are given on the $t = 0$ line. (99) refers to the initial value of y_1 when growth substrate is supplied to pool y_1; a value of 99 causes the final weight W_f to be $99 + W_0 = 100$ (Eqn 4.12, Fig. 4.3d) when substrate is converted to dry weight without loss. W_0 is initial ($t = 0$) value of weight W.

The rate at which material accumulates in compartment z (Fig. 4.2a) is ky_n and, with Eqn 4.9, this gives:

$$z_n(t) = k\int_0^t y_n \, \mathrm{d}t = \int_0^t \frac{k^n t^{n-1} e^{-kt}}{(n-1)!} \, \mathrm{d}t. \qquad z_n(\infty) = 1 \tag{4.10}$$

Equations 4.9 and 4.10 are drawn in Fig. 4.2b and c. z_n is closely related to the incomplete gamma function (Thornley and France, 2007, glossary, Eqn G80; to transform $z_n(t)$ into $\gamma_3(\nu, n)$, substitute $kt = \nu$ in Eqn 4.10).

Mean time of arrival in the nth compartment, τ, is:

$$\tau = \langle t \rangle = \frac{\int_{t=0}^{\infty} t y_n \, \mathrm{d}t}{\int_{t=0}^{\infty} y_n \, \mathrm{d}t} = \frac{n}{k}. \tag{4.11}$$

Equation 4.11 is valuable for relating n and k to known delays. Assuming that the last compartment, z (Fig. 4.2), is a non-metabolized effector of logistic growth, then the two-state variable problem for logistic growth plus a delay becomes:

$$\frac{dz}{dt} = ky_n(t) = \frac{k^n t^{n-1} e^{-kt}}{(n-1)!}. \quad t = 0,\ z = 0.$$
$$\frac{dW}{dt} = z(t)\mu W\left(1 - \frac{W}{W_f}\right). \quad t = 0,\ W = W_0 = 1. \tag{4.12}$$

μ (day^{-1}) is a specific growth rate constant. W_f is the final dry weight. Initial dry weight is W_0.

Equations 4.12 were integrated numerically to give solutions for z (the growth toggle) and dry weight W. This was carried out for various values of delay parameters n and k with n/k = constant = τ = 20 to give a constant average delay of 20 time units (Eqn 4.11). A discrete delay (Eqn 4.6) is approximated by taking a high value of n (100). Results are shown in Fig. 4.3a and c. Figure 4.3a illustrates effector pool z, which toggles logistic growth. The consequential effect on dry weight W (Fig. 4.3c) shows that early growth is increased as the delay becomes less abrupt (decrease n, the number of compartments). However, dry weight is small in this region and, in practical terms, there may be little gain from using a more complicated gamma-delay formulation rather than the simpler discrete delay (Eqn 4.6).

If pool z is treated as a substrate consumed by growth rather than as a non-metabolized effector of growth, then z no longer has the simple time course given by Eqns 4.12 (Fig. 4.3a). Equations 4.12 become (writing z_{sub} for the substrate pool):

$$\frac{dz_{sub}}{dt} = (W_f - W_0)k\, y_n(t) - \frac{dW}{dt};$$
$$\frac{dW}{dt} = \mu W \frac{z_{sub}}{W_f}. \tag{4.13}$$
$$t = 0,\ z_{sub} = 0,\ W = W_0 = 1.$$

z_{sub} replaces z. The ($W_f - W_0$) term supplies the correct amount of substrate to the z_{sub} pool (Fig. 4.2) so that, when all substrate is converted to dry weight, final dry weight is W_f (z varies between 0 and 1). The second equation is based on the logistic equation, replacing S by z_{sub} (Thornley and France, 2007, equation 5.16a). Results are shown in Fig. 4.3b and d. Substrate z_{sub} now decreases to zero, rather than approaching an asymptote of 99, which would be the case if substrate were not consumed. The early behaviour of dry weight is little different (cf. Fig. 4.3c and d), but the approach to the asymptote is far slower in Fig. 4.3d because substrate is running out.

This approach to delaying growth can be applied to many growth functions in animal nutrition.

Delayed Gompertz

The Gompertz equation is truly remarkable because it has three 'morphs'. First, it can be written in 'open' form:

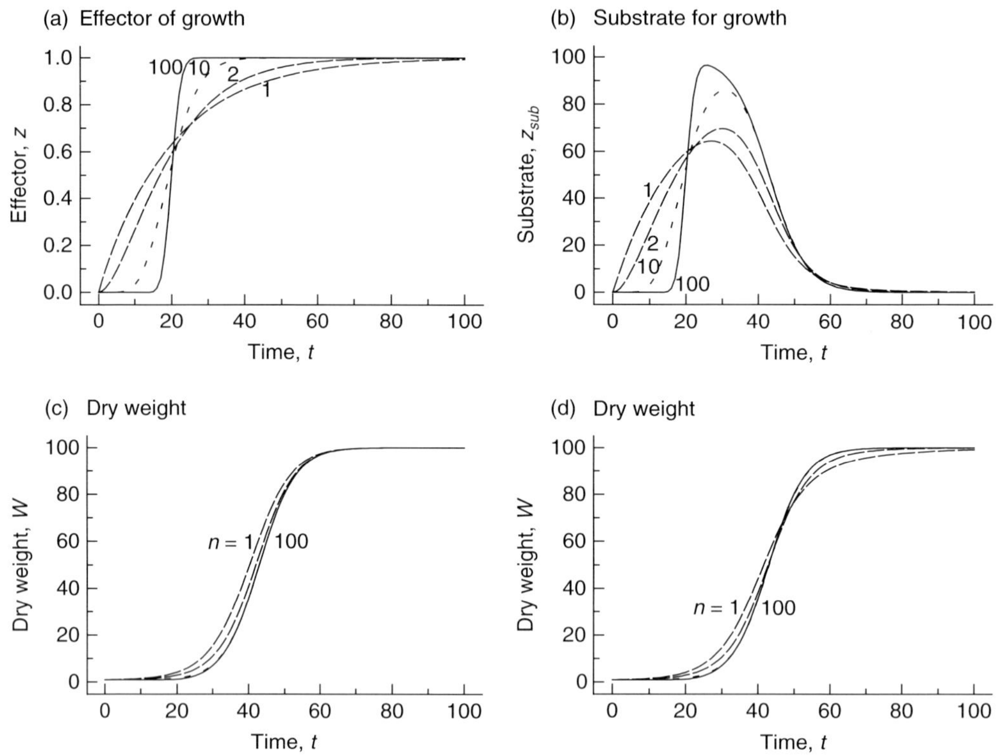

Fig. 4.3. Effects of a gamma delay are illustrated with reference to logistic growth and the two schemes in Fig. 4.2. In all cases, the delay time $\tau = 20$. Logistic Eqn 4.8 parameters are $W_0 = 1$, $\mu = 0.2$, $W_f = 100$. Gamma delay parameters are $n = 100, 10, 2, 1$ as indicated with $k = 5, 0.5, 0.1, 0.05$, respectively, so that $n/k = \tau = 20$ is constant (Eqn 4.11). (a) Non-metabolized growth effector z. (b) Substrate for growth z_{sub}. (c) Dry weight W given by Eqn 4.12 with z effecting growth. (d) Dry weight W given by Eqn 4.13, with z_{sub} as the metabolized substrate for growth.

$$\frac{\mathrm{d}W}{\mathrm{d}t} = \mu_0\left[1 - \frac{D}{\mu_0}\ln\left(\frac{W}{W_0}\right)\right]. \tag{4.14}$$

W_0 (kg) is initial weight, μ_0 (day^{-1}) initial specific growth rate, and D (day^{-1}) a parameter reflecting rate of development or differentiation. 'Open' because final weight depends on values of parameters μ_0 and D during the simulation, and these may depend on growth conditions.

Second, it can be written in targeted form:

$$\frac{\mathrm{d}W}{\mathrm{d}t} = DW\ln\left(\frac{W_f}{W}\right). \tag{4.15}$$

Final dry weight W_f (kg) is preordained.

Last, and possibly giving the most insight, the open form of Eqn 4.14 can be written as a two-state variable problem:

$$\frac{dW}{dt} = \mu W,$$
$$\frac{d\mu}{dt} = -D\mu.$$
$$D = 0.05\ \text{day}^{-1},\ t = 0 : W = W_0 = 1\ \text{kg}, \mu = \mu_0 = 0.230259\ \text{day}^{-1}. \tag{4.16}$$

With these parameter values, final weight $W_f = W_0 \exp(\mu_0/D) = 100$ kg. Weight at inflexion $W^* = W_f/e$ (e = 2.718).

A problem with the Gompertz is that specific growth rate begins declining immediately at $t = 0$ and the inflexion point is a low fraction of final weight. It may be useful to delay the onset of development, which causes the specific growth rate to decline. Arguably, this is biologically what happens in many organisms. A recipe for this is suggested.

An extra state variable is added to the usual two-state variable formulation of the Gompertz, so that Eqn 4.16 becomes:

$$\frac{dW}{dt} = \mu W,$$
$$\frac{d\mu}{dt} = -D\mu,$$
$$\frac{dD}{dt} = k(D_{max} - D). \tag{4.17}$$
$$k = 0.02, D_{max} = 0.05\ \text{day}^{-1}$$
$$t = 0 : W = W_0 = 1\ \text{kg}, \mu = \mu_0 = 0.096217\ \text{day}^{-1},$$
$$D = D_0 = 0\ \text{day}^{-1}.$$

The extra rate constant, k, determines how quickly D (development) moves towards the value D_{max}, which causes specific growth rate μ to decrease. The value of μ_0, with the given values of k and D_{max}, gives rise to an asymptotic dry weight of 100 kg. For the same asymptote, this value of μ_0 is less than that of Eqn 4.16 because delaying the developmental decrease in specific growth rate causes overall growth to be increased.

Some analysis of Eqn 4.17 is possible, giving:

$$D = D_{max}(1 - e^{-kt}).$$
$$\mu = \mu_0 \exp\left[-D_{max}\left(t - \frac{1 - e^{-kt}}{k}\right)\right]. \tag{4.18}$$
$$\frac{dW}{dt} = \mu_0 W \exp\left[D_{max}\left(t - \frac{1 - e^{-kt}}{k}\right)\right].$$

The third of these equations cannot be integrated analytically. The first equation is related to the gamma function (Eqns 4.9 and 4.10) and, indeed, the approach is similar in that section.

Figure 4.4 illustrates the consequence of delaying development. In Fig. 4.4a, the Gompertz is drawn with the parameters in Eqn 4.16; the Gompertz with

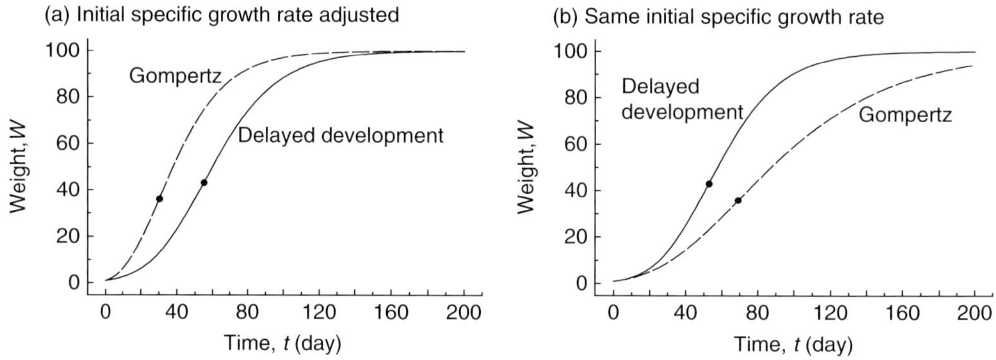

Fig. 4.4. Gompertz with delayed development. Initial weight and final asymptote are 1 and 100 kg in all cases. (a) Gompertz Eqn 4.16 parameters: $\mu_0 = 0.2303$, $D = 0.05$ day^{-1}; Gompertz with delayed development Eqn 4.17 parameters: $\mu_0 = 0.09622$, $k = 0.02$, $D_{max} = 0.05$ day^{-1}. Final development rates (D and D_{max}) are the same, but initial growth rates (μ_0) differ. (b) Gompertz Eqn 4.16 parameters: $\mu_0 = 0.1$, $D = 0.02171$ day^{-1}; Gompertz with delayed development Eqn 4.17 parameters: $\mu_0 = 0.1$, $k = 0.02$, $D_{max} = 0.05329$ day^{-1}. Initial growth rates are the same, but final development rates differ. Inflexion points are indicated by •.

delayed development is drawn with the parameters in Eqn 4.17; these parameter sets give the same asymptote, but the initial specific growth rate is less for delayed development (given by μ_0 in each case). In Fig. 4.4b, initial specific growth rate $\mu_0 = 0.1$ day^{-1} is the same for both curves (Eqns 4.16 and 4.17); for the Gompertz Eqn 4.16, $D = 0.0217147$ day^{-1} to give asymptote $W_f = 100$ kg; for delayed development as in Eqn 4.17, $k = 0.02$ day^{-1}, but D_{max} is increased to 0.053294 so that development occurs at a higher rate after being delayed; this also gives $W_f = 100$ kg. In both cases, with delayed development the inflexion point occurs at a higher fraction of asymptotic dry mass.

The delay method used in Eqn 4.17 can be extended using more compartments (differential equations).

Square Root-Time Growth Equation

Here a rate:state equation is described in which growth is, optionally, diminishing returns throughout, or initially autocatalytic with an inflexion point, but where dry weight, W, is *asymptotically* always proportional to the square root of time, t. Dry weight growth rate is:

$$\frac{dW}{dt} = \frac{c^2}{2(W + K_1)} \frac{W}{(W + K_2)}; t = 0, W = W_0 = 1 \text{ kg}. \qquad (4.19)$$
$$c^2 = 100 \text{ kg}^2 \text{ day}^{-1}, K_1 = 20, K_2 = 20 \text{ kg}.$$

c^2, K_1 and K_2 are parameters. W_0 is the initial value of W. A tentative interpretation of this equation is suggested below at the end of this section.

Note first that, assuming $K_1 = K_2 = 0$:

$$\frac{\mathrm{d}W}{\mathrm{d}t} = \frac{c^2}{2W}, \qquad (4.20)$$
$$\therefore W = \sqrt{W_0^2 + c^2 t}.$$

For $c^2 t \gg W_0$, Eqn 4.20 becomes:

$$W = c\sqrt{t}. \qquad (4.21)$$

This is the simplest of the possibilities offered by Eqn 4.19.

A second possibility is obtained if it is assumed that K_1 (or K_2) = 0 and writing K_2 (or K_1) = K, then:

$$\frac{\mathrm{d}W}{\mathrm{d}t} = \frac{c^2}{2W}\frac{W}{K+W}; \; t = 0, W = W_0. \qquad (4.22)$$
$$W = -K + \sqrt{(K + W_0)^2 + c^2 t}.$$

$\mathrm{d}W/\mathrm{d}t$ decreases monotonically as W increases and there is no inflexion point. At large t, $W \rightarrow c\sqrt{t} - K$.

Returning to Eqn 4.19, integration yields:

$$c^2 t = W^2 - W_0^2 + 2(K_1 + K_2)(W - W_0) + 2K_1 K_2 \ln\left(\frac{W}{W_0}\right)$$
$$= (W + K_1 + K_2)^2 - (W_0 + K_1 + K_2)^2 + 2K_1 K_2 \ln\left(\frac{W}{W_0}\right). \qquad (4.23)$$

Equation 4.23, essentially for $t(W)$, is not soluble analytically for $W(t)$. For large t, $W \rightarrow c\sqrt{t} - K_1 - K_2$.

Differentiating Eqn 4.19 and equating to zero gives the point of inflexion at (t^*, W^*) with:

$$W^* = \sqrt{K_1 K_2}. \qquad (4.24)$$

t^* is obtained by substituting $W = W^*$ into Eqn 4.23.

Figure 4.5 illustrates Eqn 4.19 for various values of K_1 and K_2. With, say, $K_2 = 0$, then increasing K_1 decreases the asymptote ($c\sqrt{t}$) by K_1. There is no non-zero inflexion point if either K_1 or $K_2 = 0$ (Eqn 4.24) (top two curves). In the next three curves, both weight and time at inflexion increase (Eqns 4.24 and 4.23). In the bottom three curves, weight at inflexion is the same, but time of inflexion increases.

Last, consider a tentative biological interpretation of Eqn 4.19. Growth is regarded as resulting from the product of substrate provision and growth machinery activity. An organism growing linearly in one dimension could have a substrate transport path of length proportional to weight, supplying substrate at a rate proportional to inverse weight; this could correspond to the $1/(W + K_1)$ term. The second term, $W/(W + K_2)$, might represent a growth machinery activity which saturates with organism size.

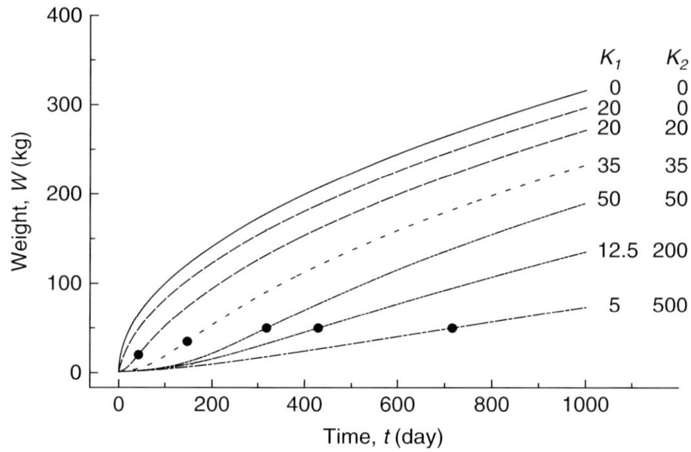

Fig. 4.5. Square root-time growth function (Eqn 4.19). $c^2 = 100$ kg^2 day^{-1}. Values of K_1 and K_2 are as shown. Inflection points are indicated by •.

'Open' Logistic Growth

The three-parameter logistic growth equation may be written:

$$\frac{dW}{dt} = \mu W \left(1 - \frac{W}{W_f}\right). \qquad (4.25)$$

$$\mu = 0.2\,\text{day}^{-1},\ W_f = 100\,\text{kg}, W(t=0) = 1\,\text{kg}.$$

W is weight (state variable), μ a specific growth rate parameter and W_f is final weight. Growth is targeted on a prescribed final weight. For many organisms, final weight depends on conditions during growth. It is easy to modify parameter μ according to nutrition (e.g. with the Michaelis-Menten equation) or temperature (with a temperature function, e.g. Thornley, 1998, Fig. 3.6). However, this merely causes the organism to approach the same final weight faster or slower. It is less obvious how to modify W_f during growth according to actual growth conditions. Early limiting conditions produce a greater effect than late limitation. Degree of limitation is also important. Here, a recipe for such a modification is proposed (Thornley and France, 2005; Thornley *et al.*, 2007).

Equation 4.25 is replaced by two differential equations, now with five parameters:

$$\frac{dW}{dt} = f_{\text{lim}}\mu W \left(1 - \frac{W}{W_f}\right),$$

$$\frac{dW_f}{dt} = -D(1 - f_{\text{lim}})(W_f - W). \qquad (4.26)$$

$$\mu = 0.2\,\text{day}^{-1},\ D = 0.1\,\text{day}^{-1}, f_{\text{lim}} = 1,$$

$$W(t=0) = W_0 = 1\,\text{kg},\ W_f(t=0) = W_{f0} = 100\,\text{kg}.$$

W_f is now a state variable whose initial value (100 kg) assumes no growth limitation. D is a development or differentation rate. f_{lim} is a fraction ($0 \le f_{\text{lim}} \le 1$), which reflects a possible growth limitation. The dW_f/dt equation causes final weight W_f to move towards actual weight W at a rate depending on D times the degree to which growth is limited $(1 - f_{\text{lim}})$. If $f_{\text{lim}} = 1$, there is no growth limitation and W_f does not change from its initial value. If $f_{\text{lim}} = 0$, there is no growth at all. Here, it is assumed, for simplicity, that the same growth-limiting factor f_{lim} occurs in the first and second of Eqn 4.26, affecting specific growth rate and change of asymptote.

While it is possible to eliminate W_f between these two differential equations and obtain a higher-order equation, this is not very helpful. Instead, divide the two differential equations to eliminate dt and integrate (given constant parameters) to give:

$$\frac{W}{W_0} = \left(\frac{W_{f0}}{W_f}\right)^{\mu f_{\text{lim}}/[D(1-f_{\text{lim}})]}. \qquad (4.27)$$

At $t \to \infty$, $W = W_f = W_{max}$ (say), with:

$$W_{max} = \sqrt[\left[1+\frac{\mu f_{\text{lim}}}{D(1-f_{\text{lim}})}\right]]{W_0 W_{f0}{}^{\mu f_{\text{lim}}/[D(1-f_{\text{lim}})]}}. \qquad (4.28)$$

Note that, with constant parameters, the asymptote of organism weight depends on μ/D, as it does in the Gompertz (Thornley and France, 2007, Section 5.5, Eqn 5.27).

Figure 4.6 illustrates the behaviour of the open logistic equation. In Fig. 4.6a, D alone is varied, $f_{\text{lim}} = 0.5$ and other parameters are as in Eqn 4.26. Slow rates of development (D) give little change in final weight due to limitation, whereas if development (D) is more comparable with growth (μ), then final weight can be much depressed. Figure 4.6b simply depicts a changing timescale, as μ and D are varied but maintaining the same ratio and, therefore, asymptote (Eqn 4.28). Figure 4.6c shows the effect of imposing a limitation of $f_{\text{lim}} = 0.5$ at different times with a moderate value of $D = 0.05$ day^{-1}, half the size of $\mu = 0.1$ day^{-1} (Fig. 4.6a). Imposing limitation at 70 days produces a negligible effect, at 50 days, it is noticeable, at 20 and 0 days, final weight is much depressed.

Logistic Equation Modified for Substrate Supply and Product Inhibition

The modifications described in this section lead to an equation with exponential, linear and asymptotic terms. Assume basic logistic growth:

$$\frac{dW}{dt} = \mu_0 \frac{W}{W_f} S. \qquad (4.29)$$

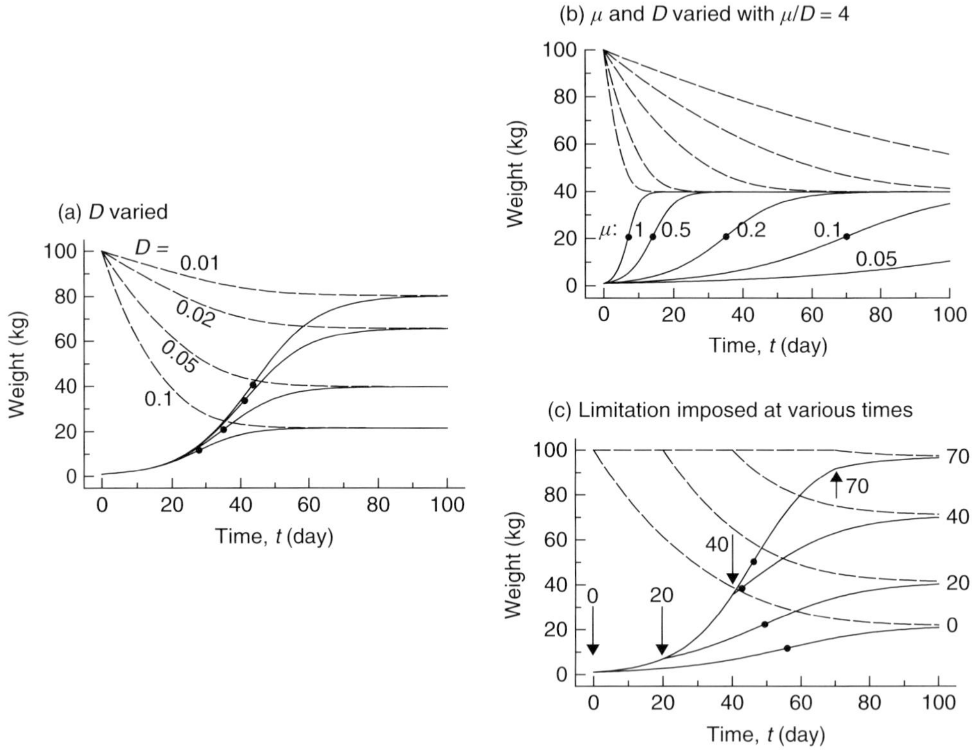

Fig. 4.6. 'Open' logistic growth. The logistic equation is modified to give Eqn 4.26, which give a variable final weight depending on conditions. Solid lines indicate weight W, dashed lines the dynamically varying asymptote, W_f. Inflection points are shown by •. $W_0 = 1$ and $W_{f0} = 100$ kg throughout. (a) $\mu = 0.2$ day^{-1}, $f_{lim} = 0.5$ and D(day^{-1}) as indicated. (b) $f_{lim} = 0.5$, μ (day^{-1}) as indicated, $D = \mu/4$. (c) $\mu = 0.1$, $D = 0.05$ day^{-1}, with $f_{lim} = 0.5$ imposed at the times indicated (day).

Here, W (kg) is weight, t (day) is time, S is substrate (kg) (a variable), μ_0 (day^{-1}) is a specific growth rate parameter and W_f (kg) is final weight. The usual assumption that substrate is converted into dry weight W without loss is made:

$$S + W = W_f. \qquad (4.30)$$

Substituting Eqn 4.30 in Eqn 4.29 gives the standard logistic form:

$$\frac{dW}{dt} = \mu_0 W \frac{W_f - W}{W_f}. \qquad (4.31)$$

$$W(t = 0) = W_0.$$

These equations are modified for Michaelis–Menten substrate dependence and for product inhibition:

$$\frac{dW}{dt} = \mu_0 \frac{W}{W_f} \frac{SK_S}{K_S + S} \frac{J_I}{J_I + I}. \qquad (4.32)$$

K_S is a Michaelis–Menten parameter (kg) and J_I is an inhibition parameter with the same units as inhibitor, I. Note that if $K_S \gg S$ and $J_I \gg I$, then the equation reverts to the logistic. Assume that inhibitor I is generated proportional to dry weight produced, that I is not metabolized and its initial value is zero, so that:

$$I = W - W_0. \tag{4.33}$$

Define a maximum specific growth rate parameter (when $S \to \infty$ and $I \to 0$ in Eqn 4.32) as:

$$\mu_{max} = \frac{1}{W}\frac{\mathrm{d}W}{\mathrm{d}t}(S \to \infty, I \to 0) = \frac{\mu_0 K_S}{W_f}. \tag{4.34}$$

Eliminate S, I and μ_0 from Eqn 4.32 with Eqns 4.30, 4.33 and 4.34 to give:

$$\frac{\mathrm{d}W}{\mathrm{d}t} = \mu_{max} W \frac{W_f - W}{K_S + W_f - W} \frac{J_I}{J_I + W - W_0}. \tag{4.35}$$

Apart from the last factor on the right side, this equation is essentially identical to an equation proposed by Birch (1999, Eqn 11).

Actual specific growth rate μ at time $t = 0$ is (Eqn 4.35):

$$\mu(t = 0) = \frac{1}{W}\frac{\mathrm{d}W}{\mathrm{d}t}(t = 0) = \mu_{max} \frac{W_f - W_0}{K_S + W_f - W_0}. \tag{4.36}$$

This equation enables us to choose a constant initial specific growth rate, $\mu(t = 0)$ and, as parameter K_S is varied, calculate the parameter μ_{max} for use in Eqn 4.35.

Equation 4.35 can be integrated:

$$\begin{aligned}\mu_{\max} t = {} & \left(1 + \frac{K_S}{W_f}\right)\left(1 - \frac{W_0}{J_I}\right)\ln\left(\frac{W}{W_0}\right) + \frac{W - W_0}{J_I} \\ & + \frac{K_S}{W_f}\left(1 + \frac{W_f - W_0}{J_I}\right)\ln\left(\frac{W_f - W_0}{W_f - W}\right).\end{aligned} \tag{4.37}$$

On the right side of the equation, the first term gives exponential growth, the second term linear growth and the last term generates the asymptote, as $W \to W_f$. Although there is no algebraic solution for $W(t)$, when Eqn 4.35 is integrated numerically, then t from Eqn 4.37 gives a useful check on algebraic and numerical accuracy.

By differentiating Eqn 4.35 and equating $\mathrm{d}^2W/\mathrm{d}t^2$ to zero, it can be shown that weight W^* at the inflexion point is given by a root of the quadratic:

$$\begin{aligned}0 &= (J_I - W_0 - K_S)W^2 - 2(J_I - W_0)(K_S + W_f)W + W_f(J_I - W_0)(K_S + W_f). \\ &= aW^2 + bW + c. \\ W^* &= \frac{1}{2a}[-b - \sqrt{(b^2 - 4ac)}].\end{aligned} \tag{4.38}$$

Time of inflexion is obtained by applying Eqn 4.37.

The modified logistic growth curve is drawn in Fig. 4.7 for different values of parameters K_S and J_I (Eqn 4.32). Initial weight (W_0), initial specific growth rate (Eqn 4.36) and asymptote W_f are the same for all curves. In Fig. 4.7a, it can be seen that the weight at the inflexion point (Eqn 4.38) can vary over a considerable (and possibly useful) range. The growth rate (Fig. 4.7b) can be peaked

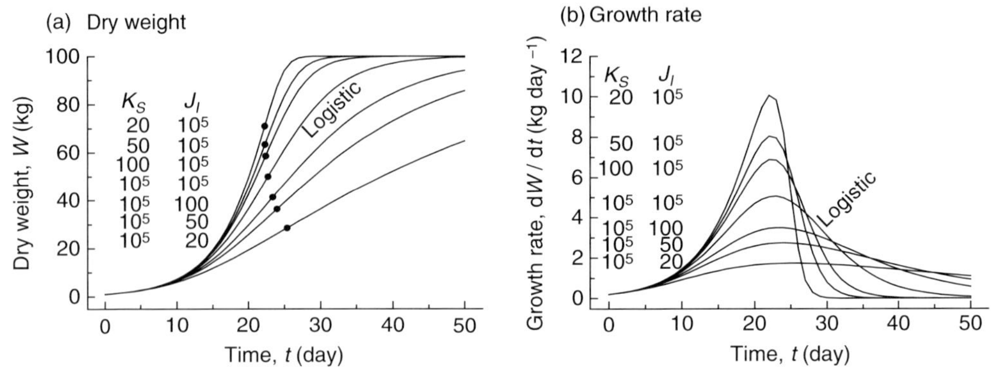

Fig. 4.7. Logistic growth modified for Michaelis–Menten-type substrate response and product inhibition. Constant parameters are: $W_f = 100$, $W_0 = 1$ kg, initial specific growth rate $\mu(t = 0)$ (Eqn 4.36) = 0.2 day^{-1}. J_I and K_S are varied as indicated. For each value of K_S, a value of μ_{max} is obtained with Eqn 4.36 for use in Eqn 4.35. (a) Dry weight, W: Eqn 4.35 is integrated numerically using the fourth-order Runge–Kutta method with $\Delta t = 0.01$ day. Inflection points are indicated by •. (b) Growth rate is calculated with Eqn 4.35.

(high affinity for substrate, low K_S; no inhibition, high J_I) or relatively flat (no response to substrate, high K_S; much product inhibition, low J_I). The latter approximates expo-linear growth.

Compensatory Growth

Many species experience considerable changes in food availability during their lives, varying from near starvation to glut. Perhaps as an adaptation to such conditions, some organisms grow faster when recovering from starvation than during a continuous period of high food availability. This phenomenon is known as 'compensatory' growth. It occurs widely, in vertebrates (Wilson and Osbourn, 1960) and invertebrates (Bradley *et al.*, 1991). It has been reported that, in some species (notably fish), animals provided with variable food supplies can outgrow those to whom food is continuously available (Broekhuizen *et al.*, 1994). Compensatory growth is therefore important when considering both natural and managed populations.

There have been few theoretical studies of the topic. Broekhuizen *et al.* (1994) have made a valuable contribution and our model is based, in part, on their work. Compensatory responses can be variable, depending on species and age, the severity, duration and nature of the nutritional limitation and then the post-limitation conditions. Sometimes, growth appears simply to be delayed, whereas in other cases there is a genuine 'catching up' or even 'overtaking', with intermediate responses also being observed. However, experimentation is often difficult and results rarely speak unambiguously. Key concepts in any theoretical analysis concern intake and maintenance. Some authors have mentioned a variable growth efficiency, although this might be interpreted as a variable maintenance requirement. Our analysis aims to provide a flexible generic framework applicable to a range of such problems.

Model scheme

This is illustrated in Fig. 4.8. There are four state variables, of which three denote weights: of substrate (W_S, kg C), reserves (W_R, kg C) and structure (W_X, kg C). For simplicity, it is assumed that carbon (C) is the significant nutrient. The fourth dimensionless state variable, y, is associated with structure W_X and denotes degree of development or nearness to maturity. Intake ($I_{i\rightarrow S}$, kg C day^{-1}) is into the substrate pool. Substrate can be used for maintenance ($O_{S\rightarrow mai}$, kg C day^{-1}), structural growth (G_X, kg C day^{-1}) or converted into reserves ($O_{S\rightarrow R}$, kg C day^{-1}). Reserves can be converted back into substrate ($O_{R\rightarrow S}$, kg C day^{-1}).

Variables are defined for total weight (W, kg C) and the 'concentrations' of substrate and reserves [S, R, kg substrate C, reserve C (kg structural C)$^{-1}$]:

$$W = W_S + W_R + W_X.$$
$$S = \frac{W_S}{W_X}, R = \frac{W_R}{W_X}. \tag{4.39}$$

Intake

Intake $I_{i\rightarrow S}$ (kg C day^{-1}) is the primary driver of growth. Our model assumes *ad libitum* intake, with:

$$I_{i\rightarrow S} = hc_i W_x^{\,q_i}.$$
$$h = \left(\frac{R_{opt}^{\,q_R} + K_{Rh}^{\,q_R}}{R^{q_R} + K_{Rh}^{\,q_R}} \right)^{q_h}.$$
$$R_{opt} = 1, K_{Rh} = 1\,\text{kg reserve C kg structural C}^{-1}, q_R = 2, q_h = 2. \tag{4.40}$$
$$c_i = 0.1\,(\text{kg C})^{q_i - 1}\,\text{day}^{-1}, q_i = \frac{2}{3}.$$

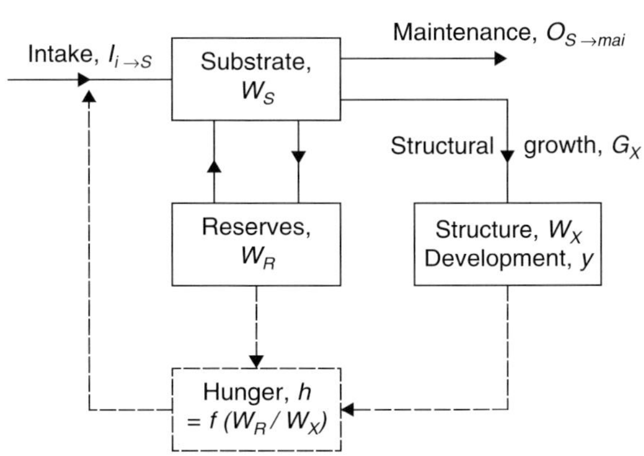

Fig. 4.8. Compensatory growth scheme. The three weight state variables are immediately available substrate (W_S), structural weight (W_X) and reserves (W_R). A developmental state variable y is associated with the structural pool, W_X, and denotes degree of maturity. Solid arrows denote fluxes of matter, dashed arrows, information.

The hunger factor, h, is an empirical dimensionless multiplier, depending on parameters R_{opt} and K_{Rh}, as well as reserve concentration R. When reserve concentration R equals an optimum value R_{opt}, h is unity with no effect on intake, $I_{i\to S}$. If $R = 0$, h takes its maximum value of 4, increasing intake; if $R > R_{opt}$, then $h < 1$, decreasing intake. A q_R of 2 makes the response to R of the quantity in brackets sigmoid about unity; a q_h of 2 amplifies the effect on h. Otherwise, the intake equation is standard. c_i is a constant: an organism of structural weight $W_X = 1$ kg C has an intake of 0.1 kg C day^{-1}. q_i is a dimensionless scaling factor.

Maintenance

How maintenance is represented in a model depends on the level of detail of the model. A biochemical-level model where processes of breakdown, (re-)synthesis, leakage, ion-pumping, etc., are explicit has no need to talk about maintenance. However, at the aggregated level of Fig. 4.8, it is convenient to include a maintenance requirement, recognizing that this is an approximation. We assume that both reserves and structure require maintaining. There is also a choice between representing maintenance as a drain on C substrate (S), as done here, or alternatively, as a degradation (loss) of the components to be maintained (reserves, structure). Representing maintenance as a drain on C substrate requires that maintenance be decreased as the availability of C substrate decreases, otherwise S may be driven negative and the model will fail. Outputs of C substrate for maintenance of reserves and structure ($O_{S\to Rmai}$, $O_{S\to Xmai}$, kg C day^{-1}) are modelled similarly:

$$\begin{aligned}
O_{S\to Rmai} &= c_{Rmai} W_R^{q_{Rmai}} \frac{1}{1 + K_{SRmai}/S}.\\
c_{Rmai} &= 0.02(\text{kg C})^{1-q_{mai}}\,\text{day}^{-1}, q_{Rmai} = 0.75,\\
K_{SRmai} &= 0.005\,\text{kg substance C (kg structural C)}^{-1}.\\
O_{S\to Xmai} &= c_{Xmai} W_X^{q_{Xmai}} \frac{1}{1 + K_{SXmai}/S}.\\
c_{Xmai} &= 0.02(\text{kg C})^{1-q_{mai}}\,\text{day}^{-1}, q_{Xmai} = 0.75,\\
K_{SXmai} &= 0.002\,\text{kg substance C (kg structural C)}^{-1}.
\end{aligned} \tag{4.41}$$

The cs are constants. The qs are dimensionless scaling factors. Maintenance of structure is given a higher priority for C substrate with $K_{SXmai} = 0.002$ than that of reserves ($K_{SRmai} = 0.005$) (the lower the K value, the lower the substrate concentration S at which the process is switched off). Total maintenance requirement is (kg substrate C day^{-1}):

$$O_{S\to mai} = O_{S\to Rmai} + O_{S\to Xmai}. \tag{4.42}$$

Structural growth

This is modelled by means of a modified Gompertz (Thornley and France, 2007, Section 5.5), enabling growth of W_X to be partially decoupled from development (y). Rate of increase of structural weight W_X is:

$$\begin{aligned}
\frac{dW_X}{dt} &= \mu_X W_X \frac{S}{K_{SX} + S} e^{-y}, W_X(t=0) = 1\,\text{kg structural C}.\\
\mu_X &= 0.1\,\text{day}^{-1}, K_{SX} = 0.001\,\text{kg substrate C (kg structural C)}^{-1}.
\end{aligned} \tag{4.43}$$

The low value of K_{SX} gives structural growth a high priority.

Rate of increase of the dimensionless 'developmental' variable y is:

$$\frac{dy}{dt} = k_y \frac{S}{K_{Sy} + S}, \; y(t = 0) = 0.$$
$$k_y = 0.02171\,\text{day}^{-1}, K_{Sy} = 0.001\,\text{kg substrate C (kg structural C)}^{-1}. \quad (4.44)$$

If S = constant, then y increases linearly with time, t, with $y = k_y t$. Note that final weight/initial weight = $\exp(\mu_X/k_y)$ = 100 for the unmodified Gompertz, providing for a 100-fold increase in structural weight. Note also that, with the default values given for parameters K_{SX} and K_{Sy}, the substrate (S) dependence on growth and development are the same, so that changing substrate provision does not alter the asymptote of structural growth.

Structural growth takes substrate from pool W_S. If the carbon efficiency of structural growth is Y_X, then the flux of substrate C required is:

$$O_{S \to X} = \frac{1}{Y_X} \frac{dW_X}{dt}, \; Y_X = 1. \quad (4.45)$$

This causes a C flux to respiration of:

$$\frac{1 - Y_X}{Y_X} \frac{dW_X}{dt}. \quad (4.46)$$

We assume, for simplicity, that structural growth in carbon terms is 100% efficient and there is no loss of material due to respiration or other processes (a loss would cause Y_X to be < 1). It has been proposed that growth efficiency increases during compensatory growth after starvation. An increased growth efficiency would provide another possible mechanism by which an organism could 'catch up' with missed growth.

Synthesis and breakdown of reserves

It is assumed that there are optimal levels of both substrate (metabolic) C and of reserve C which serve as targets; these are S_{opt} and R_{opt} (Eqn 4.40). The output flux from substrate (S) to reserves (R) is (kg C day^{-1}):

$$O_{S \to R} = \mu_{S \to R} W_X \left(\frac{S}{S_{opt}} \right)^{q_{S \to R}}.$$
$$\mu_{S \to R} = 0.5\,\text{day}^{-1}, S_{opt} = 0.02\,\text{kg substrate C (kg structural C)}^{-1},$$
$$q_{S \to R} = 2. \quad (4.47)$$

$\mu_{S \to R}$ is a rate constant. $q_{S \to R}$ is a dimensionless constant which defines the degree of control exercised over the level of S. A high value of $q_{S \to R}$ would cause Eqn 4.47 to behave like a step function at $S = S_{opt}$. Conversion of S into R is assumed to occur without loss.

Mobilization of reserves gives an output from the R pool into the S pool of:

$$\begin{aligned} O_{R\to S} &= \mu_{R\to S} W_R \left(\frac{S_{opt}}{S + K_{R\to S}} \right)^{q_{R\to S}}. \\ \mu_{R\to S} &= 0.004\ \text{day}^{-1},\ q_{R\to S} = 2, \\ K_{R\to S} &= 0.005\ \text{kg substrate C (kg structural C)}^{-1}. \end{aligned} \quad (4.48)$$

$\mu_{R\to S}$ is a rate constant and $q_{R\to S}$ is a dimensionless 'control' constant. The $K_{R\to S}$ term in the denominator is needed to prevent reserve mobilization from 'running away' when $S\to 0$. Output from the R pool is put into the S pool without loss.

Differential equations

Total inputs to and outputs from the metabolic S pool are:

$$\begin{aligned} I_S &= I_{i\to S} + O_{R\to S}. \\ O_S &= O_{S\to mai} + O_{S\to X} + O_{S\to R}. \end{aligned} \quad (4.49)$$

Inputs are from intake and breakdown of reserves (Eqns 4.40 and 4.48). Outputs are to maintenance, structural growth and reserves (Eqns 4.42, 4.45 and 4.47). The differential equation for the S pool is:

$$\frac{dW_S}{dt} = I_S - O_S. W_S(t = 0) = 0.02\ \text{kg substrate C.} \quad (4.50)$$

For the reserve R pool (with Eqns 4.47 and 4.48):

$$\frac{dW_R}{dt} = O_{S\to R} - O_{R\to S}. W_R(t = 0) = 1\ \text{kg reserve C.} \quad 4.51)$$

For the structural pool W_X and for the developmental variable y, Eqns 4.43 and 4.44 above are applied.

Simulations

Figure 4.9 illustrates the dynamics of *ad libitum* feeding compared with 50 days of starvation imposed from 100 to 150 days ($c_i = 0$ in Eqn 4.40). Whatever the feeding regime, then with the assumptions in Eqns 4.43 and 4.44 (namely that $K_{SX} = K_{Sy}$), the asymptote of structural dry weight M_X is always 100 times its $t = 0$ value. The reserve concentration (Eqn 4.39) increases (Fig. 4.9c) until intake, responding to the decreasing hunger factor of the organism (Fig. 4.9d), is exactly balanced by maintenance (Fig. 4.9b). However, not only are the weight asymptotes unchanged, but some catching up for the 50-day starvation occurs because maintenance is depressed and intake is increased post-starvation (Fig. 4.9b). Catching up can be enhanced if it is also assumed that growth is more efficient in a starving organism. Varying the feeding regimes can cause overshoot or undershoot (with higher or lower weight asymptotes), if it is assumed that developmental and structural growth Michaelis–Menten constants K_{SX} and K_{Sy}

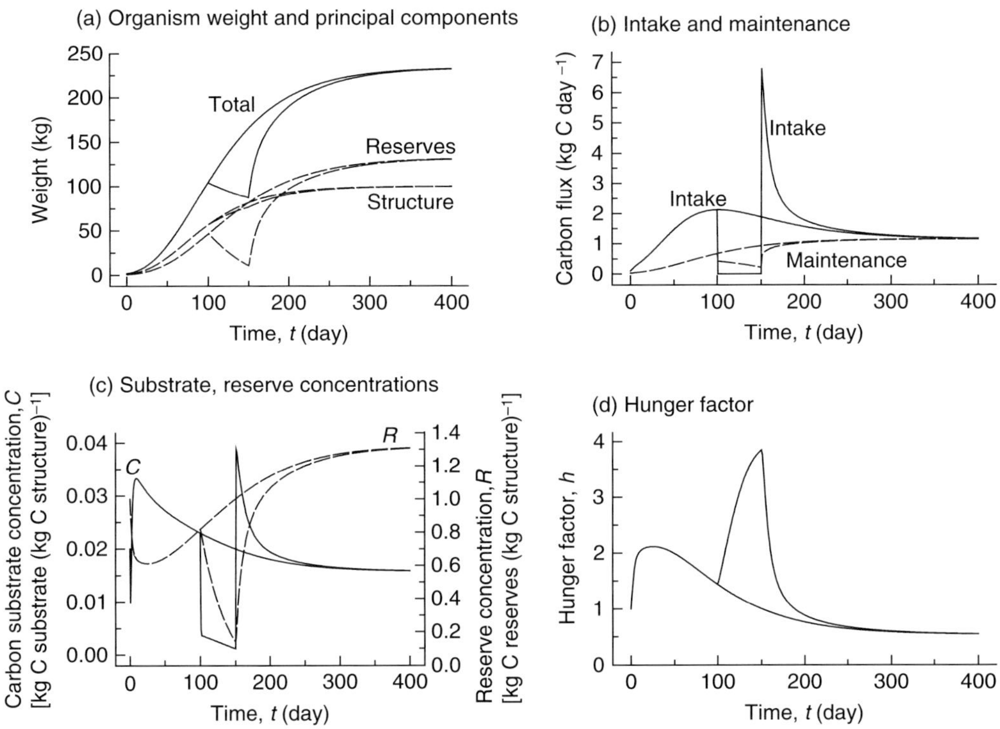

Fig. 4.9. Compensatory growth: starvation and recovery. In the first simulation, the organism is provided with *ad libitum* feed throughout. In the second simulation, food is removed entirely at 100 days and restored at 150 days. Otherwise, all parameters are as given.

of Eqns 4.43 and 4.44 are different so that the response to changing substrate concentration S is different.

The model as illustrated in Fig. 4.9 gives rise to the same final state. By changing a structural development parameter, K_{Sy} (Eqn 4.44), weight can overshoot or undershoot as a result of a period of starvation. This is illustrated in Fig. 4.10. In Fig. 4.10a, K_{Sy} is increased to 0.002 (from 0.001 in Fig. 4.9). This causes development rate to decrease more than growth rate when starvation occurs and substrate concentration S is decreased. The asymptote of the underlying Gompertz growth equation is increased with decreasing developmental rate (Thornley and France, 2007, Eqn 5.27). In Fig. 4.10b, K_{Sy} is assigned a very small value so that, essentially, developmental rate is not affected by substrate concentration or starvation. Because structural growth rate is less under starvation conditions, final asymptote is decreased.

There are many other ways in which compensating growth and overshoots/undershoots can be modelled. Broekhuizen *et al.* (1994) assume that there is hysteresis in the way in which the hunger factor operates. Effectively, increasing hunger acts more quickly than decreasing hunger so that, overall, intake is increased.

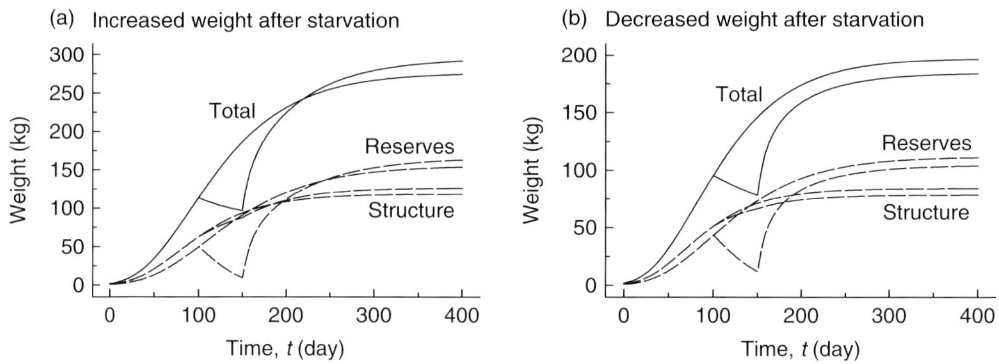

Fig. 4.10. Overshoot and undershoot in weight during compensatory growth with 50 days of starvation (100 to 150 days) (Fig. 4.9). (a) $K_{Sy} = 0.002$ kg substrate C (kg structural C)$^{-1}$ (Eqn 4.44). (b) $K_{Sy} = 0.1 \times 10^{-6}$ kg substrate C (kg structural C)$^{-1}$. Otherwise, all parameters are as given.

Modelling compensatory growth is a fascinating topic. It is a phenomenon which applies across biology (although most work has been done with animals) and at organ and organism levels. It is a problem which simple growth models (Thornley and France, 2007: Chapter 5) are unable to explain. The challenge is to find the minimal elaborations of the simple growth models which can describe the phenomenon and which may serve as useful management tools.

Allometry and Scaling

Allometry (= *allo* + *metry*) means growth of part of a body (W_1) at a different proportional rate from that of the whole body (W). Allometric mass growth can be expressed:

$$W_1 = aW^q, \tag{4.52}$$

where a is a normalization constant (units: mass^{1-q}) and q is a dimensionless allometric parameter. Taking logarithms gives a linear equation:

$$\ln W_1 = \ln a + q \ln W. \tag{4.53}$$

Differentiating with respect to time t, the proportional (or specific) rates of growth of the part and the whole are related by:

$$\frac{1}{W_1}\frac{dW_1}{dt} = q\frac{1}{W}\frac{dW}{dt}. \tag{4.54}$$

Note that the proportional rates of growth of part and whole are different if $q \neq 1$, so that the relative size, $W_1 W^{-1}$, changes as the organism grows.

The allometric relationship was first used by Huxley (1924) with reference to growth of animals and their parts. Equation 4.52 is now used quite generally for relating other attributes of organisms: lifespan, weight of limbs, basal metabolic rate, cross-sectional area of the aorta and heartbeat (Schmidt-Neilsen, 1984). Allometric relationships can be used within a species, to reflect the dynamics of growth, or between species, to reflect a possibly general relationship between body size and some attribute.

Organism size can vary over some 21 orders of magnitude and is an important determinant of processes and structures in the organism. There has long been a search for simple allometric 'laws' and much discussion over whether 3/4 or 2/3 is the most appropriate exponent for basal metabolic rate. While organism size and geometrical constraints are perhaps of foremost importance, evolutionary history, the environment and other conditions of growth may all contribute. Our position is that allometric equations can provide valuable general understanding, but they are inevitably approximate and do not substitute for a mechanistic view.

Arguably, the use of the allometric equation is declining. Although the method can be empirically convenient, it has little or no explanatory power and there is usually no reason for choosing the allometric equation over other empirical equations. Indeed, alternatives may be preferable. In animal models for agricultural use, it is often convenient to scale quantities like basal metabolic rate and maximum intake according to some measure of animal size (Eqns 4.41 and 4.40), and there are few mechanistic alternatives.

In the context of body parts, the non-additivity of allometric components is a serious limitation. That is, adding (or subtracting) two (or more) allometric equations does not yield an allometric equation. Consider an organism of weight W comprising two parts, with:

$$W = W_1 + W_2. \tag{4.55}$$

Writing:

$$W_1 = a_1 W^{q_1}, \tag{4.56}$$

substituting in Eqn 4.55 and solving for W_2 gives:

$$W_2 = W - a_1 W^{q_1}. \tag{4.57}$$

We would like to be able to write:

$$W_2 = a_2 W^{q_2}, \tag{4.58}$$

but this is simply not possible.

Application of simple geometrical factors

This section considers how geometry can be applied to some aspects of allometry.

If an organism is approximately spherical, then its surface area $\propto W^{2/3}$. Any deviation from spherical leads to an exponent $> 2/3$ (this is because a given volume has minimum surface area if it takes spherical shape). An area:weight exponent > 1 would hardly make biological sense (i.e. doubling organism weight more than doubles surface area). Assuming basal metabolic rate (*BMR*) is determined by the ability of the organism to lose heat through its surface, then we expect:

$$BMR \propto W^q, 2/3 \le q \le 1. \tag{4.59}$$

Evidence suggests that q is in the range 0.66 to 0.75 (Dodds *et al.*, 2001). Similarly, voluntary food intake $\propto W^{0.7}$ approximately.

A branching model for allometric scaling

Recently, a branching model has been proposed in relation to allometric scaling equations in biology (West *et al.*, 1997). This provides a valuable additional perspective on allometric scaling. Part of the model is outlined below in simplified form. Dodds *et al.* (2001) provide a valuable critique of the approach.

The main premise is that organisms are sustained by branching networks which supply all parts of the organism. Three assumptions are made. First, a space-filling branching network is required. Second, the final branch of the network (such as a capillary in a mammal) has a constant size. And, last, the energy required to distribute resources is minimum.

A scheme is drawn in Fig. 4.11 which could apply to blood flow in an animal. Branches are assumed to be cylindrical and are of order $i = 0, 1, 2, \ldots$. A branch of order i has length l_i, radius r_i and pressure drop of Δp_i across it. The flux through element i is $f_i = \pi r_i^2 \bar{u}_i$ where $\bar{u}_i$ is the average fluid velocity. There are $n_i = \beta^i$ branches of order i; β is the branching ratio, assumed independent of order i. Assume fluid is conserved across the system, then:

$$f_0 = n_i f_i = n_i \pi r_i^2 \bar{u}_i = n_m \pi r_m^2 \bar{u}_m. \tag{4.60}$$

The second assumption is that the terminal units ($i = m$) are invariant. Therefore, length l_m, radius r_m, pressure drop of Δp_m and $\bar{u}_m$ are independent of organism size. Because fluid flow supplies nutrients for metabolism, therefore basal metabolic rate, BMR, is given by:

$$\begin{aligned} BMR &\propto f_0 \propto n_m \propto \beta^m. \\ \therefore \ln(BMR) &= \text{constant} + m \ln \beta \end{aligned} \tag{4.61}$$

To minimize the energy dissipated in the system, it can be shown that branching is stationary or self-similar. This means that the branching ratio β is constant across orders (as assumed in Fig. 4.11), but also the radius (ρ) and length (λ) ratios:

$$\rho = \frac{r_{i+1}}{r_i}, \lambda = \frac{l_{i+1}}{l_i}, \tag{4.62}$$

do not change with order i. Therefore, expressing numbers (n_i), radius (r_i) and length (l_i) of order i in terms of those of the invariant terminal unit ($i = m$):

$$n_i = \beta^i = \frac{n_m}{\beta^{m-i}}, r_i = \frac{r_m}{\rho^{m-i}}, l_i = \frac{l_m}{\lambda^{m-i}}. \tag{4.63}$$

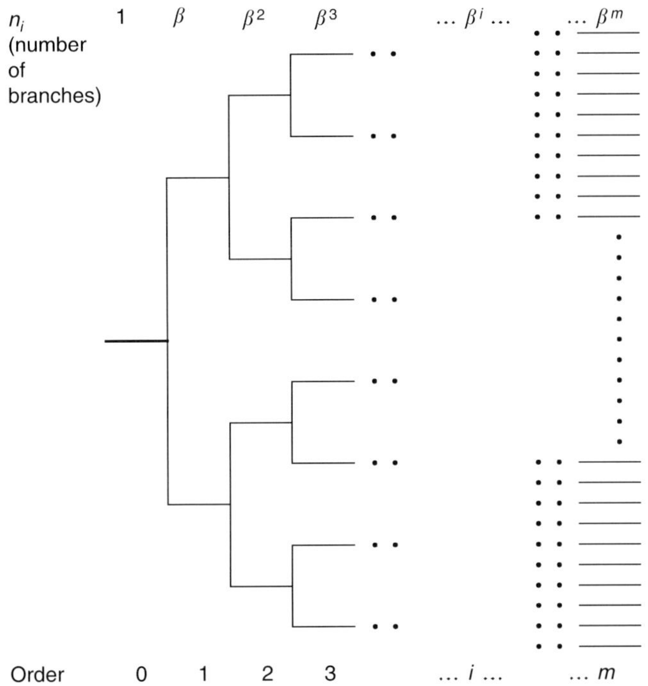

Fig. 4.11. Branching scheme for allometry. i is the branch order number. n_i is the number of branches of order i. m generations of branching events are shown. For simplicity, simple bifurcation (doubling) is illustrated. In general, branching ratio is β, relating number of branches or order i to number of order $i+1$ by factor β.

Total volume of fluid present, V, is (summing over numbers n_i and volume V_i of an ith-order element):

$$V = \sum_{i=0}^{m} n_i V_i = \sum_{i=0}^{m} \beta^i \pi r_i^2 l_i$$
$$= \left[\frac{(\beta\rho^2\lambda)^{-(m+1)} - 1}{(\beta\rho^2\lambda)^{-1} - 1} \right] \beta^m V_m; \tag{4.64}$$
$$V_m = \pi r_m^2 l_m.$$

Assuming that $\beta\rho^2\lambda < 1$ and $m \gg 1$, this can be approximated:

$$V = \frac{V_0}{1 - \beta\rho^2\lambda} = V_m = \frac{(\rho^2\lambda)^{-m}}{1 - \beta\rho^2\lambda}, \text{ where}$$
$$V_0 = \frac{V_m}{\rho^{2m}\lambda^m}. \tag{4.65}$$

Remembering that V_m is invariant and assuming that fluid volume $V \propto$ weight W, therefore:

$$W \propto (\rho^2\lambda)^{-m}, \tag{4.66}$$

$$\therefore \ln W = \text{constant} - m \ln(\rho^2\lambda).$$

Two further assumptions are needed. First, the branching network is 'space filling'. Arguably, this is the natural branching arrangement for ensuring that all parts of the organism structure are supplied with metabolites (Warner and Wilson, 1976, in a fine paper, discuss this point in relation to the human bronchial tree). Because $l_i \gg r_i$, the geometric volume (not the fluid volume) associated with the ith order can be approximated by (taking a spherical volume of diameter l_i for each ith order element):

$$n_i \frac{4\pi}{3}\left(\frac{l_i}{2}\right)^3. \tag{4.67}$$

Because this is constant by assumption (with respect to order number i), we can write:

$$\begin{aligned} n_i l_i^3 &= n_{i+1} l_{i+1}^3. \\ \therefore 1 &= \beta\lambda^3. \end{aligned} \tag{4.68}$$

Second, branching is area preserving. This is not a good assumption for animals, but is mostly a good assumption for plants where the vascular system comprises many small elements with continuity throughout the system (the 'pipe-model' theory: Shinozaki *et al.*, 1964). Area preservation across branching implies that:

$$\begin{aligned} n_i r_i^2 &= n_{i+1} r_{i+1}^2. \\ \therefore 1 &= \beta\rho^2. \end{aligned} \tag{4.69}$$

Using these last two equations, therefore:

$$\lambda = \frac{1}{\beta^{1/3}},\ \rho = \frac{1}{\beta^{1/2}},\ \rho^2\lambda = \frac{1}{\beta^{4/3}}. \tag{4.70}$$

Substituting into Eqn 4.66:

$$\ln W = \text{constant} + \frac{4m}{3}\ln\beta. \tag{4.71}$$

Combining this with Eqn 4.61 leads to:

$$\ln(BMR) = \frac{3}{4}\ln W + \text{constant}, \tag{4.72}$$

$$\therefore \text{BMR} \propto \text{W}^{3/4}.$$

We have shown that basal metabolic rate is $\propto$ body weight raised to the power of 0.75.

Other interesting allometric relations can be deduced. For the radius of the vascular system in the main stem (or that of the aorta), r_0 (using Eqns 4.63, 4.70 and 4.71):

$$\begin{aligned} r_0 &= \frac{r_m}{\rho_m} = r_m\beta^{m/2}, \\ \ln r_0 &= \text{constant} + \frac{m}{2}\ln\beta, \\ \ln r_0 &= \text{constant} + \frac{3}{8}\ln \text{W}, \\ r_0 &\propto \text{W}^{3/8}. \end{aligned} \tag{4.73}$$

Similarly, for the length of the stem, l_0,

$$l_0 \propto W^{1/4}. \tag{4.74}$$

These equations are a geometric consequence of the assumptions. Area-preserving branching is close to the norm for plant vascular systems but, in mammalian vascular systems, branching is not area preserving. Murray (1927) suggested that arterial branching is volume preserving ($1 = \beta\rho^3$; cf. Eqn 4.69; also called cubic-law branching) and that this tends to be true in small trees. Examination of Table 5 in Barker *et al.* (1973) suggests that a birch tree is area preserving; however, for an apple tree and the pulmonary artery, branching is somewhat area enhancing ($\beta\rho^2 = 1.2$), but far from volume preserving; for the bronchial tree (where the fluid is gas), branching is volume preserving.

West *et al.* (1997) continue to examine energy dissipation in relation to laminar flow and pulsed flow. The latter is relevant to birds and mammals. They showed that fluid pressure was independent of body size, but we were unable to understand their later analyses. The simplified analysis given above provides the flavour of their interesting but controversial approach (Dodds *et al.*, 2001).

Scaling in relation to maturity

Butterfield *et al.* (1983) suggested a method of scaling body components in relation to size at maturity, which may be of value for particular applications (Butterfield, 1988).

Consider an animal comprising weight components: bone (W_b), protein (W_p) and fat (W_f), and a residual, W_{res}, with total W given by:

$$W = W_b + W_p + W_f + W_{res}. \tag{4.75}$$

Assume it is possible to define a mature value for each variable: W_b^*, W_p^*, W_f^* and W^*. W^* might be viewed as the weight of an animal with a prescribed fraction of fat suitable for a particular market. The (dimensionless) progress towards maturity of each variable can be measured by variables ω with:

$$\omega_b = \frac{W_b}{W_b^*},\ \omega_p = \frac{W_p}{W_p^*},\ \omega_f = \frac{W_f}{W_f^*},\ \omega = \frac{W}{W^*}. \tag{4.76}$$

An empirical quadratic equation defines progress towards maturity of the *i*th component, ω_i, in terms of progress towards maturity of the whole, ω, with:

$$\omega_i = q_i\omega + (1 - q_i)\omega^2. \tag{4.77}$$

Parameter q_i (range: 0 to 2) specifies how quickly component *i* matures relative to the total weight. If $q = 1$, then $\omega_i = \omega$; component *i* matures at the same rate as the whole animal. If $q < 1$, this represents a late maturing tissue. If $q > 1$, this represents an early maturing tissue. Equation 4.77 is drawn in Fig. 4.12 for four values of q. It can be seen that, if $q > 2$ (e.g. $q = 3$), then the mature weight of the part is exceeded before the animal is mature; this is the reason why $q \le 2$.

Maturity parameters q are additive if a weighted value of the q-values of the parts is taken. For example, for a sheep weighing 100 kg at maturity, with q-values and mature weights for bone, protein and fat of $q_b = 1.4$, $W_b^* = 7.5$ kg,

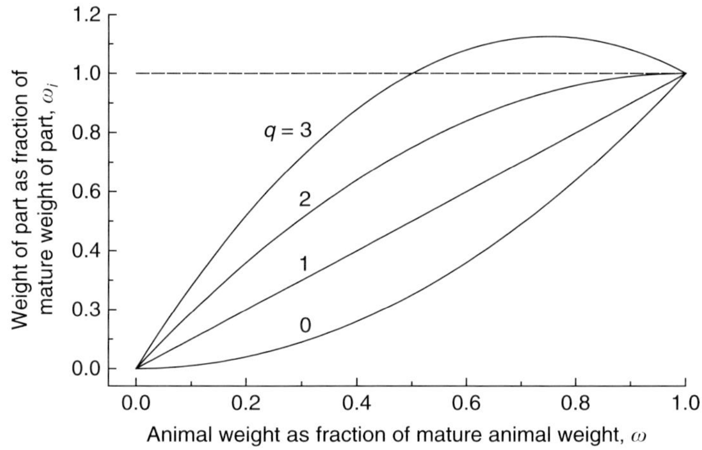

Fig. 4.12. Scaling of weight of part in relation to weight of whole, both being expressed as fractions of their mature weight. ω_i (Eqn 4.76) is the fractional weight of a part ($i = b$ (bone), p (protein), f (fat)); ω is the fractional weight of the whole. These are assumed to obey the empirical quadratic Eqn 4.77.

$q_p = 1.3$, $W_p^* = 25$ kg, $q_f = 0.1$, $W_f^* = 17.5$ kg, the q-value for the carcass (bone + protein + fat), q_{bpf} ($W_{bpf}^* = 50$ kg) is:

$$q_{bpf} = \left(1.4 \times \frac{7.5}{50}\right) + \left(1.3 \times \frac{25}{50}\right) + \left(0.1 \times \frac{17.5}{50}\right) = 0.9. \quad (4.78)$$

Biological Oscillators

Oscillations can occur in relatively simple inorganic chemical systems, such as the Belousov–Zhabotinski reaction (Field *et al.*, 1972), as well as in the hugely more complex biological arena. They can be important at many levels in biology, from the metabolic to the ecological, in both animals and plants, including bacteria. Oscillations are often concerned with circadian (daily) and annual rhythms. In such cases, a biological clock of approximately the desired frequency can be 'entrained' (or constrained) by environmental stimuli (Devlin, 2002). An internal oscillator may provide an organism with a method for anticipating and preparing for environmental events. The mathematics of oscillations is an enormous topic; few biological problems are amenable to mathematical analysis; the literature can be frustrating to those who look for a succinct concrete presentation, albeit based on highly simplifying assumptions. In this section, two simple examples are described to illustrate possibilities and principles. Oscillations may be related to possibilities for chaos.

Gene-metabolism oscillator

A scheme for a gene-metabolism oscillator is drawn in Fig. 4.13. There are three state variables, shown in the boxes. Messenger RNA (mRNA, m) is a gene product

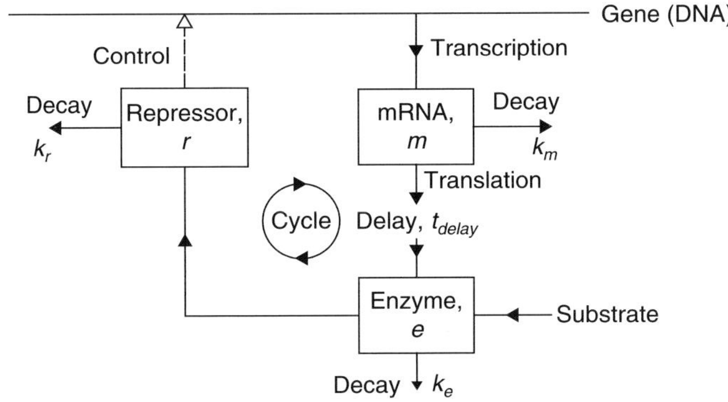

Fig. 4.13. Gene-metabolism oscillator model. Gene expression as messenger RNA (*m*) is controlled by a repressor (*r*), whose active form is a product of metabolism. *r* is generated by enzyme *e* from substrate. *e* is produced when *m* is translated in protein synthesis. t_{delay} represents the time taken for translation to take place. All three state variables (*m*, *e* and *r*) are subject to decay, with rate constants, k_m, k_e and k_r. The mathematical description is in Eqns 4.79.

generated by transcribing DNA. It decays (k_m) and, after a delay of time t_{delay}, is translated into enzyme *e*. *e* acts on a substrate to produce a repressor *r*. Also, *e* is subject to decay (k_e). Repressor *r* controls (by repression) the rate of expression of the gene, by means of a sigmoidal switch-off function (Thornley and France, 2007, Section 4.3.2; Eqn 4.61; Fig. 4.4.9). This is a simplified version of more complex ideas. Non-dimensionally, the mathematics takes the form:

$$\begin{aligned}
\frac{dm}{dt} &= \frac{1}{1+r^q} - k_m m,\\
\frac{de}{dt} &= m(t - t_{delay}) - k_e e,\\
\frac{dr}{dt} &= e - k_r r.\\
q = 4, k_m &= k_e = k_r = 0.5,\ t_{delay} = 2.\\
t = 0,\ e &= r = 1;\ t \le 0, m = 1.
\end{aligned} \tag{4.79}$$

The term $m(t - t_{delay})$ denotes the value of state variable *m* at a time t_{delay} before the present time *t*. t_{delay} is the time it takes for a given amount of mRNA to be expressed as protein (enzyme). The parameter values given here give rise to oscillations. There is always a steady-state solution, when:

$$\frac{1}{1+r^q} = k_m k_e k_r r, \tag{4.80}$$

but this may not be stable. Stability is decreased by increasing *q* (sigmoidicity), decreasing the *k* (decay constants) and increasing the delay (time to convert messenger RNA into protein). Increasing *q* increases the slope of the switch-off

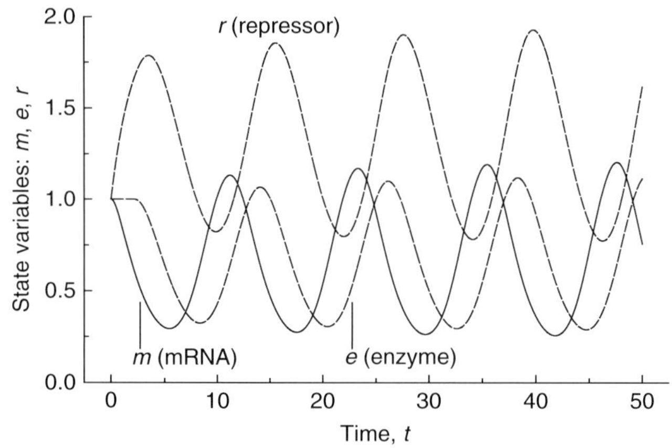

Fig. 4.14. Simulation of the scheme of Fig. 4.13 and Eqns 4.79.

response of mRNA synthesis to repressor r. However, a value of $q > 4$ is not biologically realistic. Decreasing the k simply reduces the damping losses in going round the cycle. Increasing the delay time 'decouples' the system in time: a small positive fluctuation in e (say) causes r to increase, mRNA synthesis to decrease and, after the delay, e to decrease. A small positive fluctuation in e would, without the cycle, be followed by a decrease, but, with the cycle, the decrease may be reinforced, giving oscillations. The problem is easily programmed and explored numerically, although mathematical analysis is possible and the problem has been much investigated (e.g. Murray, 1977: pp. 178–192).

Figure 4.14 illustrates a numerical solution of Eqns 4.79. It can be seen that r lags e by about 1 time unit and e lags m by about 3 time units ($1 + t_{delay}$). Because m synthesis is repressed by r, the trough in r is followed by a peak in m about 1 time unit later. The discrete delay t_{delay} could be approximately represented by a series of compartments.

Alternative-pathways oscillator

The scheme is based on a bi-stable system proposed by Thornley (1972) for application to the either/or problem of vegetative or reproductive growth at the plant apex. Such systems have been further considered by Thornley and Johnson (2000: pp. 151–158) and by Cherry and Adler (2000). An advantage of the scheme is that it demonstrates clearly how a bi-stable two-state variable scheme can be turned into an oscillator by making a parameter into a third state variable.

Figure 4.15 shows the basic scheme. There are two metabolites, x and y, each of whose synthesis is inhibited by the other metabolite. Both metabolites decay linearly. Non-dimensionally, the differential equations are:

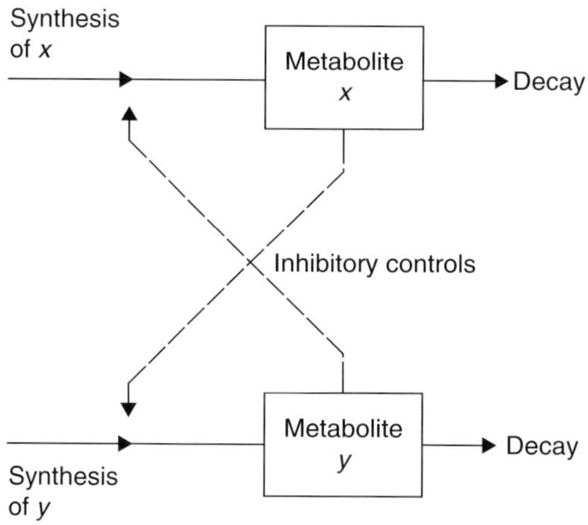

Fig. 4.15. Metabolic oscillator model involving two alternative pathways. *y* inhibits synthesis of *x* and *x* inhibits synthesis of *y*. Eqns 4.81 describe the scheme mathematically.

$$\begin{aligned} \frac{dx}{dt} &= \frac{1}{1+(y/h)^q} - x, \\ \frac{dh}{dg} &= \frac{1}{1+(y/h)^q} - y. \\ g &= h = 0.8,\ q = 4. \\ t &= 0: x = 0.5,\ y = 0.1. \end{aligned} \tag{4.81}$$

g, h and q are parameters.

First consider the steady-state solutions, given by equating Eqns 4.81 to zero. They are obtained by eliminating x (or y), or, more helpfully, by the intersection of the two equations:

$$\begin{aligned} y_1 &= \frac{1}{1+(x/g)^q}, \\ x = \frac{1}{1+(y_2/h)^q} &\text{ or } y_2 = h\sqrt[\frac{1}{q}]{\left(\frac{1-x}{x}\right)}. \end{aligned} \tag{4.82}$$

Equations 4.82 are drawn in Fig. 4.16 for various values of parameters g and h. With the default symmetrical parameters of Eqns 4.81, there is an unstable solution with $x = y$ at U, and two stable solutions at S_1 and S_2 (Fig. 4.16b). Dynamically, the system point moves to S_1 or S_2 depending on which side of the $y = x$ line the point is started from. If h is decreased to 0.6 (Fig. 4.16a), then solutions U and S_2 disappear and the system point moves to S_1. Conversely, if h is increased to 1 (Fig. 4.16c), then the system point always moves to S_2. Thus, if we contrive matters so that, if the system point is at S_2 in Fig. 4.16b and c, then h decreases and the system point must eventually move to S_1 in Fig. 4.16a. If we ensure also that, when the system point is at S_1 in Fig. 4.16a and b, h increases, then, in due course, the system point must move back to S_2 in Fig. 4.16c.

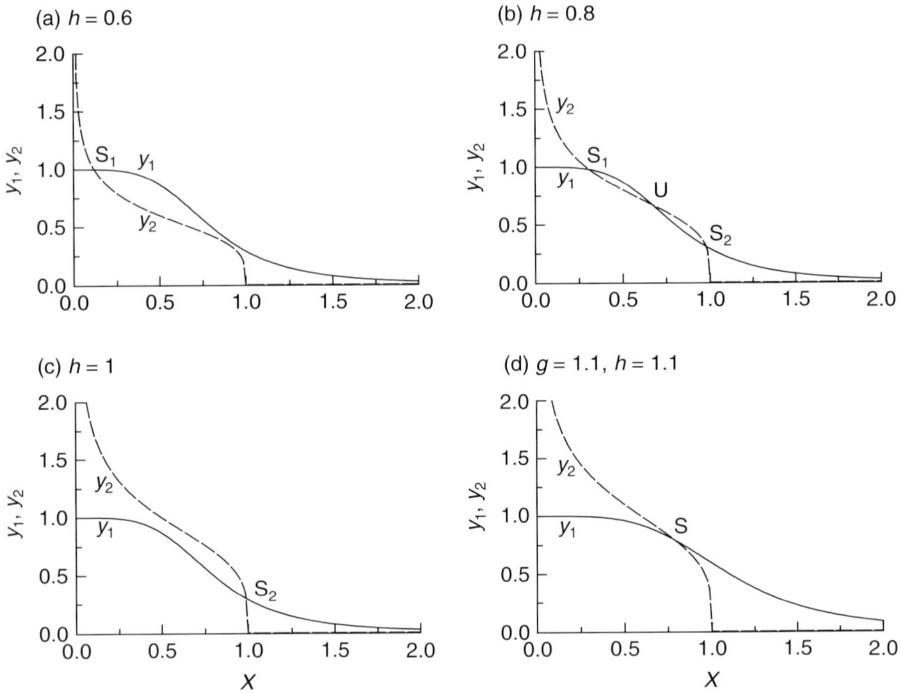

Fig. 4.16. Steady states of scheme of Fig. 4.15. Eqns 4.82 for y_1 and y_2 are plotted against x, the intersection points giving steady-state solutions for Eqns 4.81. S denotes a stable steady state and U an unstable steady state. $g = 0.8$ in (a), (b) and (c). h is as indicated.

Clearly, this provides the basis of an oscillator, in that the system flips between the two states S_1 and S_2 which, due to our assumption, are no longer stable. A system with (at least) two stable steady states can provide the basis of an oscillator or biological clock. Figure 4.16d illustrates a solution where there is only one stable steady state, which would not fulfil this requirement.

Equations 4.81 can be made to oscillate by making h a dynamic variable, with:

$$\frac{dh}{dt} = 0.1(x - 0.7). \tag{4.83}$$

$$t = 0; h = 0.8.$$

Simulations are shown in Fig. 4.17. x and y move in opposition (180° phase difference), as expected from Fig. 4.16, whereas h leads x by about 90°. The relative movements of x and h can be related to Fig. 4.16a, b and c.

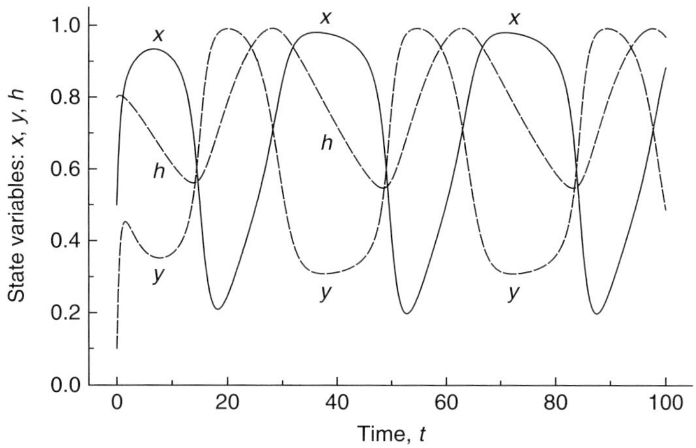

Fig. 4.17. Oscillations for the alternative-pathways scheme of Fig. 4.15, given by integrating Eqns 4.81 and 4.83 for the three state variables *x*, *y* and *h*.

References

Barker, S.B., Cumming, G. and Horsfield, K. (1973) Quantitative morphometry of the branching structure of trees. *Journal of Theoretical Biology* 40, 33–43.

Birch, C.P.D. (1999) A new generalized logistic sigmoid growth equation compared with the Richards growth equation. *Annals of Botany* 83, 713–723.

Bradley, M.C., Perrin, N. and Calow, P. (1991) Energy allocation in the cladoceran *Daphnia magna* Straus, under starvation and re-feeding. *Oecologia* 86, 414–418.

Broekhuizen, N., Gurney, W.S.C., Jones, A. and Bryant, A.D. (1994). Modelling compensatory growth. *Functional Ecology* 8, 770–782.

Butterfield, R.M. (1988) *New Concepts of Sheep Growth*. Griffin Press, Australia.

Butterfield, R.M., Griffiths, D.A., Thompson, J.M., Zamora, J. and James, A.M. (1983) Changes in body composition relative to weight and maturity in large and small strains of Australian merino rams. 1. Muscle, bone and fat. *Animal Production* 36, 29–37.

Cherry, J.L. and Adler, F.R. (2000) How to make a biological switch. *Journal of Theoretical Biology* 203, 117–133.

Devlin, P.F. (2002) Signs of the time: environmental input to the circadian clock. *Journal of Experimental Botany* 53, 1535–1550.

Dodds, P.S., Rothman, D.H. and Weitz, J.S. (2001) Re-examination of the '3/4-law' of metabolism. *Journal of Theoretical Biology* 209, 9–27.

Field, R.J., Körös, E. and Noyes, R.M. (1972) Oscillations in chemical systems II. Thorough analysis of temporal oscillations in the Bromate–Cerium–Malonic acid system. *Journal of the American Chemical Society* 94, 8649–8664.

Huxley, J.S. (1924) Constant differential growth ratios. *Nature, London* 114, 895–896.

Murray, C.D. (1927) The physiological principle of minimum work applied to the angle of branching of arteries. *Journal of General Physiology* 9, 835–841.

Murray, J.D. (1977) *Lectures on Nonlinear-differential-equation Models in Biology*. Clarendon Press, Oxford, UK.

Royal Society (1975) *Quantities, Units and Symbols*. Symbols Committee, Royal Society of London, London.

Schmidt-Neilsen, K. (1984) *Scaling: Why is Animal Size so Important?* University Press, Cambridge, UK.

Shinozaki, K., Yoda, K., Hozumi, K. and Kira, T. (1964) A quantitative analysis of plant form – the pipe model theory. *Japanese Journal of Ecology* 14, 97–105.

Thornley, J.H.M. (1972) A model of a biochemical switch and its application to flower initiation. *Annals of Botany* 36, 861–872.

Thornley, J.H.M. (1998) *Grassland Dynamics: An Ecoystem Simulation Model*. CAB International, Wallingford, UK.

Thornley, J.H.M. and France, J. (2005) An open-ended logistic-based growth function. *Ecological Modelling* 184, 257–261.

Thornley, J.H.M. and France, J. (2007) *Mathematical Models in Agriculture*, 2nd edn. CAB International, Wallingford, UK.

Thornley, J.H.M. and Johnson, I.R. (2000) *Plant and Crop Modelling,* Blackburn Press, Caldwell, New Jersey.

Thornley, J.H.M., Shepherd, J.J. and France, J. (2007) An open-ended logistic-based growth function: analytical solutions and the power-law model. *Ecological Modelling* 204, 531–534.

Warner, W.H. and Wilson, T.A. (1976) Distribution of end points of a branching network with decaying branch length. *Bulletin of Mathematical Biology* 38, 219–237.

West, G.B., Brown, J.H. and Enquist, B.J. (1997) A general model for the origin of allometric scaling laws in biology. *Science* 276, 122–126.

Wilson, P.N. and Osbourn, D.F. (1960) Compensatory growth after undernutrition in mammals and birds. *Biological Reviews of the Cambridge Philosophical Society* 37, 324–363.

5 The Dilemma in Models of Intake Regulation: Mechanistic or Empirical

D.P. POPPI

Schools of Animal Studies and Veterinary Science, The University of Queensland, Australia

Introduction

The regulation of intake has been studied for a long time because it plays such a central role in the performance of livestock. Variation in intake accounts for most of the difference in live weight gain or milk production in livestock. Knowledge of intake is also important to determine stocking rate or utilization rate of pasture in management models. It has long been known that intake by ruminants varies with different pasture types and their maturity, feed types and supplements (Blaxter *et al.*, 1956; Minson, 1971; Coleman *et al.*, 2004).

There have been many theories as to the control of intake and, within defined conditions, a number of physical and metabolic factors have been identified as closely controlling intake. However, the challenge has been to devise some all-encompassing model by which this large variety of factors may be taken into account. Baile and Forbes (1974) initially collated the large number of factors which control intake and Forbes (1980) produced a dynamic intake model which gave a reasonable representation of the daily pattern of intake. Since then, a large number of models have been produced, all with various aims, to try to predict intake from some characteristic of the feed (Thornton and Minson, 1972, 1973; Forbes, 1980; Poppi *et al.*, 1994; Weston, 1996; Ellis *et al.*, 1999; Pittroff and Kothmann, 1999) and Forbes (1995) has collated in his book most ideas pertaining to intake regulation. It is not the purpose of this review to investigate all these factors again, but rather to outline the role of models in examining this issue and to highlight the common difficulties in using mechanistic or empirical models in problem solving. The Weston model (Weston, 1996) appears to have great potential to examine a number of issues regarding intake regulation.

The Problem

There is much confusion in examining intake regulation through a modelling approach because the objectives of the models vary markedly. One major objective has been to predict intake from some characteristic of the diet so as to forecast animal performance and this is the basis of many current animal models used in the management of animals either at pasture or confined in some way (e.g. Grazfeed (Freer *et al.*, 1997) and Cornell CNCPS (Fox *et al.*, 2003)). Recently, McLennan (2005) has shown that the equations utilized to predict nutrient use, and hence live weight gain, in these models were reasonably accurate when actual intakes were used, but that the prediction of intake was widely variable, such that application of these models, especially with respect to tropical pastures, was not accurate enough to be useful. The relevant statistics for the regressions were:

CNCPS model:

$Y = 0.123 + 0.947\ X$, ($R^2 = 0.71$; $rsd = 0.159$; $sep = 0.185$; $bias = 17.3\%$),

where Y was the observed live weight gain and X was the predicted live weight gain.

SCA model:

$Y = -0.031 + 1.171\ X$ ($R^2 = 0.79$; $rsd = 0.141$; $sep = 0.153$; $bias = 9.6\%$),

where Y and X were as described above (McLennan, 2005).

Empirical approaches based on some regression approach, usually between intake and digestibility or some chemical description of the feed, have proved more useful, but are limited to the database used to derive the relationship and may also have great variability. For example, Minson (1990) showed an overall relationship between intake and digestibility but that there was large variation between cultivars and species. More recently, Lyons and Stuth (1992), Coates (2000, 2004) and Gibbs (2005) have shown reasonable relationships between the variables of intake, digestibility and crude protein (CP) content and faecal near-infrared spectrophotometry (NIRS), which should prove useful in field application.

Another application has been to predict intake from animal performance by back calculation through the nutrient use models (Baker, 2004; McLennan, 2005). This also has relevance in grazing studies where historical data for live weight gain from various pasture communities exist, so intake can be estimated and used in determining safe stocking rates or pasture utilization rates. This approach depends on the accuracy of the equations used to determine nutrient use, rather than an equation to predict intake per se.

Another quite distinct objective has been to derive mechanistic models by which to understand how intake is controlled. In this way, the means to manipulate intake become clearer and the sensitivity of intake to various factors and their interaction may be determined. This may lead to selection for certain parameters in plant breeding (e.g. leaf per cent, digestibility) or in management for certain characteristics (stage of maturity, soluble sugars). This approach has proved very useful in advancing our understanding of the control of intake (Ellis *et al*., 1999; Pittroff and Kothmann, 1999), but not very useful in having a simple, accurate method to predict intake. This is the dilemma facing scientists studying intake regulation, and the proponents of either approach are largely influenced by the questions they pose to themselves. To understand intake regulation, one must devise mechanistic models. To predict intake with sufficient accuracy to be useful and within a time frame by which appropriate management decisions can be instigated, the empirical approach appears most practical and, at present, faecal NIRS offers the most potential (Lyons and Stuth, 1992; Poppi, 1996; Coates, 2000, 2004).

In this review, a simple mechanistic model of forage intake (Weston, 1996), based on the interaction between physical and metabolic mechanisms of intake, will be examined as an example of how mechanistic approaches advance our understanding and help devise new means of manipulating intake. In contrast, the faecal NIRS approach will also be examined as an example of an empirical approach with wide application.

Brief History

Poppi *et al*. (1994) and Ellis *et al*. (1999) have outlined the physical and metabolic factors which affect intake of forages, and how they might interact, and have reviewed some of the models relating to this. Briefly, Blaxter *et al*. (1956, 1961) outlined a relationship between intake and digestibility and proposed a mechanism whereby rate of digestion and rate of passage allied to a constant rumen fill could explain the positive relationship between intake and digestibility. A vast body of work since then has examined many facets of this and has been most recently reviewed by Coleman *et al*. (2004). The most comprehensive analysis of this was by Minson (1990), who showed with tropical forages that, while there was a general relationship, there was large variation between cultivars and species. He also showed that the relationship was better for temperate forages, with less variation than tropical forages, and that leaf percentage accounted for much of the variation.

The physical mechanism proposed by Blaxter *et al*. (1956, 1961) relied on the concept of a constant level of rumen fill across forages, and the variation in rate of passage and digestion, as affected by chemical and physical characteristics of the forage, accounted for differences in rate of disappearance of feed from the rumen and, hence, intake. These pathways of disappearance of feed from the rumen could be combined into a single entity defined as retention time or the average time feed stays in the rumen. It followed mathematically that, if rumen fill was constant, then there would be a direct relationship between intake and retention time of the form:

$$I \text{ (g dry matter (DM) h}^{-1}) = \text{rumen fill (g DM)} \times 1/\text{retention time of DM (h)}.$$

Waldo *et al*. (1972) proposed a simple model (Fig. 5.1) which outlined how rate of digestion, rate of passage and potential digestibility interacted within this general concept of Blaxter's model.

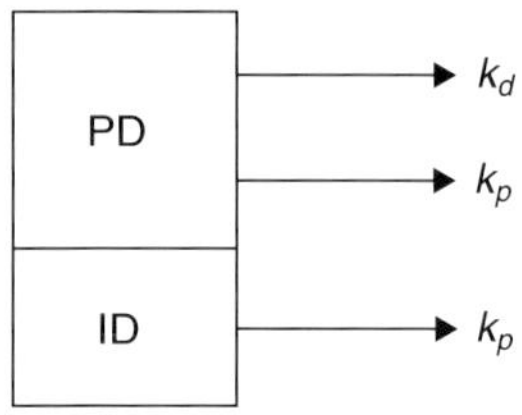

Fig. 5.1. The disappearance of potentially digestible (PD) and indigestible (ID) dry matter from the rumen by passage (fractional passage rate k_p) and digestion (fractional digestion rate k_d) (adapted from Waldo *et al.*, 1972).

Digestibility could be expressed as:

$$\text{Digestibility} = (k_d/(k_d + k_p))\ PD,$$

where k_d = fractional digestion rate (h^{-1}), k_p = fractional passage rate (h^{-1}), and PD = potential digestibility (of DM, organic matter (OM) or neutral detergent fibre (NDF), depending on the fraction of interest).

Thus, digestibility was not a causal factor of intake but the end result of the rate of digestion and rate of passage, the same factors which controlled intake. This mathematical model by Waldo *et al.* (1972) has withstood the test of time, albeit with some modifications, e.g. particle size (Poppi *et al.*, 1981b). Waldo's model introduced the concept of potential digestibility and the interaction of rate of passage and rate of digestion of the cellulose fraction. It follows that the cell wall fraction is the most important fraction for a physical model of intake regulation as it is not completely digestible (potential digestibility is < 100%, whereas cell contents are assumed to be 100% digestible), it occupies space and contributes to distension, and hence fill, and it has the slowest digestion and passage rates of any chemical entity of the plant. Thus, Thornton and Minson (1972, 1973) were able to show a good linear relationship between intake or digestible OM intake and retention time across temperate and tropical forages, as expected from a theoretical basis. Furthermore, Poppi *et al.* (1981a) showed the same highly correlated relationship across both sheep and cattle eating separated leaf and stem fractions. DM, OM and NDF relationships were demonstrated but, on theoretical grounds, one would expect a better relationship based on NDF, given that it has the longest retention in the rumen of all the chemical fractions of which a forage is composed. Thus, a concept of retention time allied to a mechanistic interaction of potential digestibility, rate of digestion and rate of passage appeared to explain the regulation of intake of forages, mathematically best captured by the model of Waldo *et al.* (1972).

However, as more work was done, some discrepancies emerged, particularly in relation to the concept of a constant rumen fill. Egan (1970) showed with low protein diets that the rumen was not full and varied with the addition of urea or casein. Thornton and Minson (1973) showed that the packing density of rumen contents was higher with legume diets, but that rumen digesta weight was lower and that there was, thus, a different linear relationship between intake and retention time because rumen fill differed between the two forage types. Gherardi and Black (1989) showed in a very elegant study that rumen fill declined as the level of post-ruminal metabolizable energy (ME) intake increased. Weston (1985, 1996) proposed a model by which rumen fill declined as ME intake or net energy (NE) intake increased, or as the NE deficit declined. Thus, there was an interaction between physical and metabolic mechanisms whereby rumen fill varied and so the direct relationship between intake and retention time could not be universal if rumen fill varied. Thus, there was a good relationship between intake and retention time when rumen fill was relatively constant (Thornton and Minson, 1972, 1973; Poppi *et al.*, 1981a) but a poor one when rumen fill varied (Thornton and Minson, 1973). In the early studies, the ME intake was still low in relation to potential ME (or NE) use and so rumen fill was at a maximum level and did not vary markedly across diets. In the later studies, where higher quality diets or supplements were used, this did not hold. Variation in rumen fill is thus the key to devising a robust model of intake regulation because rate of digestion and rate of passage are independent of intake and are characteristics set by the forage rather than the animal. Level of intake of a specific forage had little effect on retention time of OM in the rumen (Minson, 1966). Rate of digestion is a function of the inherent chemical composition and physical structure of the cell wall, and rate of passage is a function of particle disintegration and rumen digesta mat structure, both affecting dispersion within and escape of particles from the rumen. Understanding and being able to predict rumen fill and how it varies with forage quality would enable the models of Minson (1966) and Waldo *et al.* (1972) to have more universal application across a range of forage types. Weston (1996) has proposed a way in which this might be achieved.

The Weston Model

Three key papers outline the features of this model: Weston (1985, 1996) and Gherardi and Black (1989). The model relies on the observation that rumen fill or load is inversely proportional to NE intake when NE intake is varied across a wide range for lambs. Gherardi and Black (1989) showed that, with lambs, rumen OM load declined linearly as post-ruminal ME (or NE) infusion increased and that the regression was very similar to other independent data sets based on lambs consuming hays of different quality and intake. This has been presented in two ways in these papers, one based on ME (or NE) intake and the other based on NE deficit (or the difference between the maximum capacity to use NE and the supply of NE). These are illustrated in Fig. 5.2.

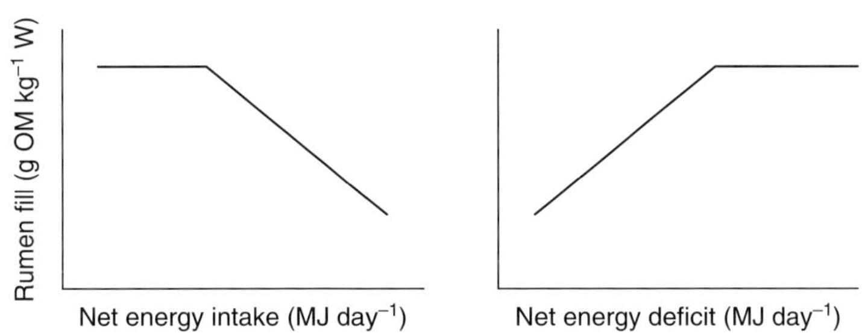

Fig. 5.2. The change in rumen fill of OM in response to net energy intake or the net energy deficit (adapted from Weston, 1996).

Weston (1996) has further outlined that, by using NE deficit, the application becomes more universal as it enables animals in different physiological states to be accommodated, in that those with a higher capacity to use NE (e.g. lactating animals, young male animals) will maintain the maximum rumen load limit up to a higher NE intake before declining at the same rate as NE intake increases. This explains why lactating animals have a higher rumen fill than dry animals (Hutton, 1963; Hutton *et al.*, 1964). The model is thus an elegant description about how rumen fill varies with NE intake or NE deficit. Retention time (or OM residence time, as used by Weston (1996)) accounted for the differences in NE intake. Thus, a simple physical model does not apply, as rumen fill should remain constant across the range of retention times until the NE deficit is met. It does this for low quality diets when the NE deficit is high, in line with the model outline (Fig. 5.2), but not as diet quality increases (or retention time decreases). Thus, as the deficit of NE declines, there is an interaction between physical (constant rumen fill) and some undefined metabolic factors (defined by Weston as the difference between the capacity to use energy and the supply of energy), such that the animal is not prepared to distend the rumen to the maximum constant extent. Hence, rumen fill declines as NE intake increases. Rumen fill may be defined in various ways. The simplest is total weight but, in computing intake and retention time, the weight of DM, OM or NDF is commonly used. NDF is probably a better term as NDF contributes space, and hence distension, and is the slowest disappearing fraction from the rumen. However, most data are presented as DM or OM, and OM will be used here to enable utilization of values from the above papers.

The Weston model provides an explanation for observations of rumen fill, intake and retention time. However, a problem is in its application. Forage can be defined in terms of digestibility and CP, and there may be historical data giving an approximate retention time of such material in the rumen. However, without some knowledge of intake, rumen fill cannot be computed. The question is: what is the likely intake of this forage? It becomes a circular argument trying to apply the Weston model to this because, in calculating intake, knowledge of rumen fill is required and, to estimate this, the NE intake or NE deficit needs to be known, which requires a knowledge of intake. The following section outlines a simple way in which the Weston model may be applied to this problem for forages varying in digestibility and to explain and calculate the substitution phenomena whereby intake of the basal forage diet declines as supplement intake increases. Forages deficient in CP are not considered because the rumen fill of sheep consuming these forages is less than maximum (Egan, 1970), although, if the capacity of sheep to use energy is set by absorbed amino acid supply, then Weston's model could also be used to examine this phenomenon.

Application of the Weston model to forages varying in retention time

The problem posed is how to estimate intake and rumen fill of forages varying in quality by application of the concepts of the Weston model. Quality may be defined by the intake and digestibility characteristics of the forage, which are related, as outlined earlier, to the retention time of forage within the rumen. Generally, all that is known about a forage is an estimate of its digestibility and limited data on chemical composition. Thornton and Minson (1972, 1973) showed a general relationship between digestibility or some chemical content (e.g. lignin) and retention time, and there are historical values for retention time of forages. The latter may not be accurate enough to examine small differences between forages, but are certainly adequate enough to define the range of forages from temperate to tropical forages (Thornton and Minson, 1973). Retention time is a characteristic of a forage, as it varies little with the level of feeding of a particular forage (Minson, 1966), with lactation (Hutton, 1963; Hutton *et al.*, 1964) and with the physiological age of the animal (Cruickshank *et al.*, 1990).

The following approach is constrained to OM because that is the form in which the available data are presented, but it would be better to follow the physical aspects by reference to NDF and the energy aspects by reference to OM. The process and equations have been simplified to illustrate how Weston's model may be applied and to demonstrate how mechanistic model application can help us understand the processes of intake regulation. Whether this is better than a simple empirical application is discussed in the final section.

The approach follows the steps:

1. Estimate retention time from digestibility, chemical composition or historical values for that forage.
2. Calculate rumen fill from Gherardi and Black's (1989) equation, an empirical approach.
3. Calculate intake from equation:

$$\text{Intake (g day}^{-1}) = \text{rumen fill OM (g)} \times 24/\text{retention time (h)}.$$

To be able to do this, rumen fill needs to be calculated. In this exercise, the data of Gherardi and Black (1989) were used. This approach uses a mix of empirical components (a linear regression to derive data) and mechanistic components (net energy deficit and associated metabolism). They presented a regression equation for rumen fill as:

$$\text{Rumen digesta OM (g kg}^{-1}\text{ RFFFLW)} = 50.65 - 28.6\text{ ME intake (MJ day}^{-1}\text{ kg}^{-1}\text{ MRFFFLW)},$$

where RFFFLW is rumen digesta-free, fleece-free live weight (kg) and MRFFFLW is metabolic rumen digesta-free, fleece-free live weight ($kg^{0.75}$). These are simplified to live weight (W) and metabolic live weight (MW), respectively.

This equation is of the form:

$$F = c - m\,MEIMW,$$

which may be converted to:

$$MEIMW = (c - F)m^{-1} \tag{5.1}$$

where F is rumen fill (g OM kg^{-1} W), c is the intercept, m is the slope and $MEIMW$ is ME intake per unit metabolic weight (MJ ME kg^{-1} MW day^{-1}).

Similarly, from the definition of retention time:

$$I = 24\,F\,T^{-1},$$

where I is intake of OM (g kg^{-1} W day^{-1}) and T is retention time of organic matter in the rumen (h). This can be converted to MEIW:

$$\text{MEIW (MJ ME kg}^{-1}\text{ W day}^{-1}) = (24\,F{*}D{*}15.83)/(1000\,T), \quad (5.2)$$

where MEIW is ME intake MJ ME kg^{-1} W day^{-1}, D is the OM digestibility and 15.83 is the MJ ME kg^{-1} digestible OM (AFRC, 1992).

Now, it follows that:

$$\text{Eqn 5.1}{*}MW = \text{Eqn 5.2}{*}W. \quad (5.3)$$

This may be solved to yield:

$$F = (c{*}T{*}MW)/(T{*}MW + 0.38\,D{*}W{*}m)$$

And from this:

$$\text{OM intake (g kg}^{-1}\text{ W day}^{-1}) = 24\,F\,T^{-1}.$$

Thus, from a knowledge of retention time and digestibility, rumen fill and intake may be calculated.

This equation was applied using the values from Gherardi and Black (1989) where: $m = 28.6$, $c = 50.65$, $W = 30$ kg for the purposes of this simulation, $MW = 12.82$ and using T and D values derived from the literature and personal data (Table 5.1). The actual values are not relevant for this simulation and could be derived by other means, e.g. the equation published by Thornton and Minson (1973).

Figure 5.3 outlines the changes in rumen fill and intake as retention time increases, the pattern of which agrees with expectation. Most tropical forages have retention times of 20–30 h and most temperate forages have retention times of 5–10 h.

Application of the Weston model to examining the response to a supplement

When animals are supplemented, substitution occurs. This is the substitution of a proportion of the basal forage diet for a given amount of supplement. The extent of substitution varies with the supplement and the basal diet and appears related more to the total digestible nutrients (TDNs) or the ME content of the supplement than the level of DM intake of the supplement (Moore *et al.*, 1999; Marsetyo, 2003; McLennan, 2004). Gherardi and Black (1989) clearly showed that

Table 5.1. The retention time (T) and OM digestibility (D) values used to simulate changes across a wide range of forages.

T (h)	5	10	15	20	30
D	0.85	0.8	0.7	0.6	0.5

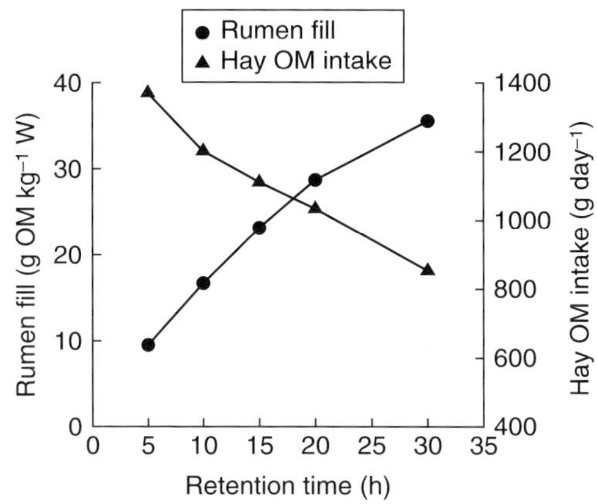

Fig. 5.3. The effect of retention time (T) of forage in the rumen on rumen fill of OM (•, g OM kg^{-1} W) and hay OM intake (▲, g OM day^{-1}) for a 30 kg lamb, as predicted by the Weston model and equations presented in the text.

post-ruminal infusion of ME resulted in a decline in rumen fill and a decline in intake of the basal forage diet. This would agree with Weston's model based on energy deficit and rumen fill. What exactly sets the level of fill with respect to the energy deficit is unknown, but the phenomena can be used in an empirical manner by assuming a relationship between fill and ME intake or NE deficit (Fig. 5.2 and equations given by Gherardi and Black, 1989). This is the same conceptual approach as used above to examine the response of intake and rumen fill to forages varying in retention time.

Situation 1: A supplement with no fibre (e.g. molasses) or a post-ruminal infused supplement

Equation 5.3 may be modified to accommodate the use of a supplement such that:

$$\text{Eqn } 5.1{*}MW = (\text{Eqn } 5.2{*}W) + (MEIS{*}W), \qquad (5.4)$$

where $MEIS$ = ME intake of the supplement (MJ ME kg^{-1} W day^{-1}).

This can be solved as:

$$F = ((c{*}MW{*}T) - (MEIS{*}W{*}m{*}T))/((0.38\ \mathrm{D}{*}W{*}m) + (MW{*}T)),$$

where F refers only to the rumen fill of hay assuming no fill from rapidly digested sugars or post-ruminal infusions.

The response of hay intake and rumen fill to increasing supplement intake for a 30 kg lamb consuming a low (D = 0.5, T = 30 h) or high quality (D = 0.8, T = 10 h) forage is shown in Fig. 5.4. These are once again in accord with the pattern observed in practice. There is a greater substitution effect with supplementation of the high quality forage compared with the low quality hay (53 g versus 38 g hay MJ^{-1} ME of supplement, respectively), an observed phenomenon in the literature (Marsetyo, 2003; McLennan, 2004). However, if

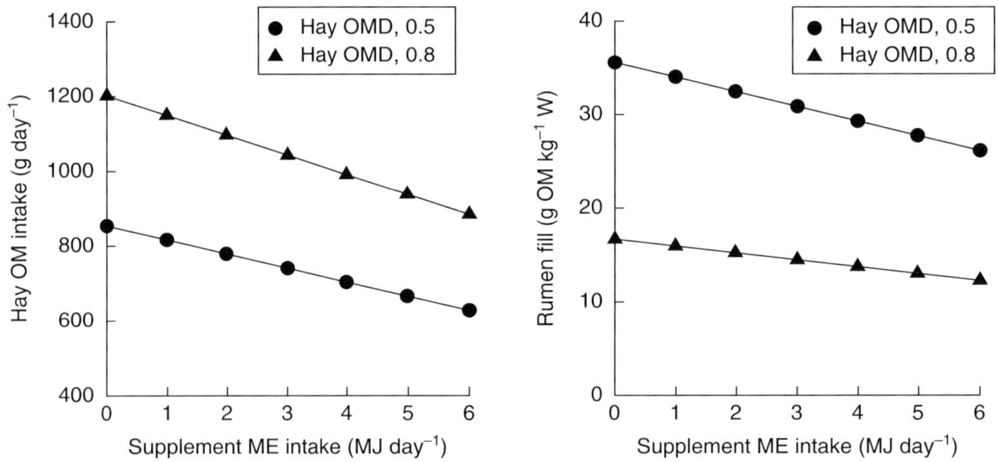

Fig. 5.4. The effect of supplement metabolizable energy (ME) intake (MJ day^{-1}) on rumen fill (g OM kg^{-1} W) and OM intake (g day^{-1}) of a hay diet with an OM digestibility of 0.5 (•) or 0.8 (▲) for a 30 kg lamb, as predicted by the Weston model and equations presented in the text.

intake is expressed as a proportion of the original hay intake (no supplement), then the proportional decline is identical for both forage types, which it must be if substitution occurs on an ME basis alone and rumen fill varies with ME intake, as assumed by applying the Weston model. There is supporting evidence for this from a wide collation of data by Moore *et al.* (1999), Dixon and Stockdale (1999), Marsetyo (2003) and McLennan (2004).

Situation 2: Supplements with fibre and variable retention time characteristics

Most supplements, whether they are protein meals, grains or legume forages, have significant amounts of fibre and other carbohydrate sources which contribute to retention time of the supplement in the rumen, and hence rumen fill. Situation 1 does not model these circumstances. By applying the same principles as above from Weston's model, the retention time characteristics and ME content (MJ ME kg^{-1} DM) of the supplement can be used to examine the intake and rumen fill from the hay diet as the level of supplement is increased.

Equation 5.4 needs to be modified to distinguish between rumen fill from the hay and rumen fill from the supplement.

$$FT = FH + FS,$$

where FT is total rumen fill or amount of OM in the rumen (g OM kg^{-1} W), FH is the amount of hay OM in the rumen (g OM kg^{1} W) and FS is the amount of supplement OM in the rumen (g OM kg^{-1} W).

Retention time for the hay and supplement needs to be defined as: TH = retention time of hay and TS = retention time of supplement.

This now takes the form:

$$(c - FT)*MW/m = ((0.38\ FH*D*W)/TH) + (MEIS*W). \qquad (5.5)$$

For a defined intake, retention time and ME content of the supplement, the rumen fill of the supplement can be calculated as:

$$FS = (TS*IS)/24,$$

where IS = intake of supplement g OM kg^{-1} W day^{-1}, and IS = (defined ME intake (MJ ME kg^{-1} W day^{-1}) × 1000)/ME content of supplement (MJ ME kg^{-1} OM).

Equation 5.5 can be solved as:

$$FH = ((c*MW*TH) - (FS*MW*TH) - (MEIS*W*m*TH))/((0.38\ D*W*m) + (MW*TH)).$$

From FH, intake of hay can be calculated by application of equation:

$$IH = 24FH/TH.$$

The results of the following simulations (Table 5.2) are seen in Table 5.3 and Figs 5.5 and 5.6.

These simulation results (Table 5.3 and Figs 5.5 and 5.6) highlight a number of conclusions:

- The higher the quality of the forage, the greater the substitution rate.
- The higher the ME content of the supplement, the greater the substitution rate when expressed as g hay g^{-1} supplement intake, but the lower the substitution rate when expressed as g hay MJ^{-1} ME supplement intake, which arises because the less rumen fill from the supplement, the higher the ME content of the supplement.
- The longer the retention time of the supplement in the rumen as a result of lower rates of digestion and/or passage of the supplement from the rumen, the greater the substitution rate expressed in either way.
- The ME content of the supplement and the retention time of the supplement explain the variability between supplement types in the substitution rate of supplement for hay, even when supplement intake is expressed on the basis of ME intake and intake is expressed as a percentage of the intake of the hay alone.
- When intake of hay by supplemented animals is expressed as a percentage of the hay intake of control or non-supplemented animals, then the decline

Table 5.2. Hay and supplement characteristics used in simulations.

Description	Low quality		High quality	
Forage				
OM digestibility	0.5		0.8	
Retention time of hay (h)	30		10	
Supplement				
ME content (MJ ME kg^{-1} OM)	10	10	13	13
Retention time of supplement (h)	10	15	10	15

Table 5.3. The rate of substitution (g hay MJ^{-1} ME supplement or g hay g^{-1} supplement) for supplements varying in ME content and retention time characteristics and hay quality defined in Table 5.2.

Forage	Low quality	Low quality	Low quality	Low quality
ME content of supplement (MJ ME kg^{-1} OM)	10	10	13	13
Retention time of supplement (h)	10	15	10	15
Substitution rate (g hay OM MJ^{-1} ME supplement)	61	73	56	65
Substitution rate (g hay OM g^{-1} supplement OM)	0.61	0.72	0.72	0.84
Forage	**High quality**	**High quality**	**High quality**	**High quality**
ME content of supplement (MJ ME kg^{-1} OM)	10	10	13	13
Retention time of supplement (h)	10	15	10	15
Substitution rate (g hay OM MJ^{-1} ME supplement)	86	102	78	91
Substitution rate (g hay OM g^{-1} supplement OM)	0.86	1.02	1.02	1.18

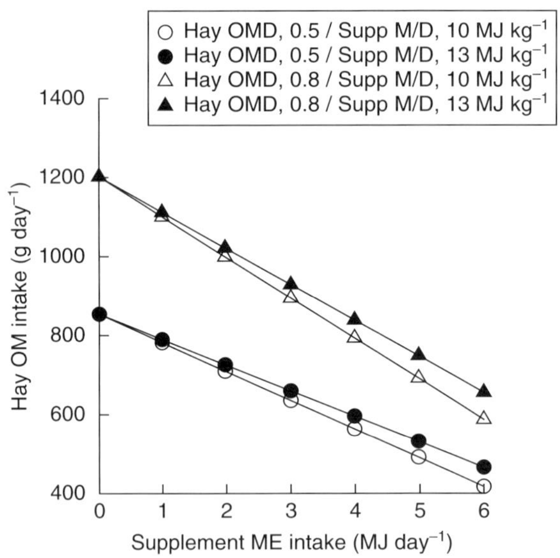

Fig. 5.5. The effect of a supplement varying in ME content (open symbols 10 MJ kg^{-1} DM, closed symbols 13 MJ kg^{-1} DM) and metabolizable energy (ME) intake (MJ day^{-1}) on OM intake (g day^{-1}) of a hay diet with an OM digestibility of 0.5 (circle symbols) or 0.8 (triangle symbols) for a 30 kg lamb, as predicted by the Weston model and equations presented in the text. The retention time of the supplement in the rumen was fixed at 15 h.

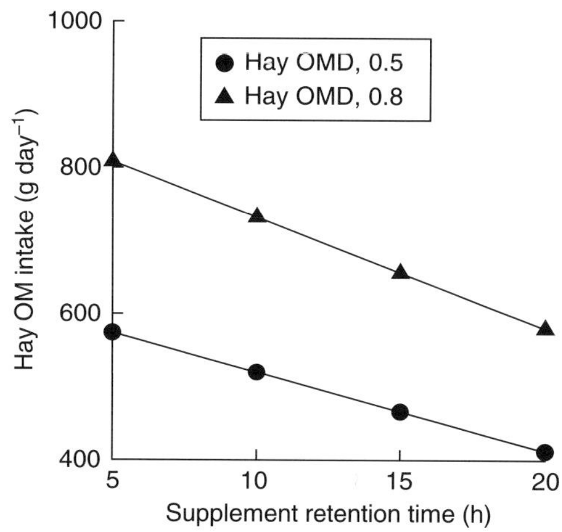

Fig. 5.6. The effect of retention time of a supplement with a metabolizable energy (ME) content of 13 MJ ME kg^{-1} DM and ME intake of 6 MJ day^{-1} on OM intake of a hay diet with an OM digestibility of 0.5 (•) or 0.8 (▲) for a 30 kg lamb, as predicted by the Weston model and equations presented in the text.

is identical for both low and high quality hay, as it must be if substitution is based on ME intake and rumen fill.

- Differences occur between supplements based on the above characteristics.

These conclusions agree closely with those derived by Marsetyo (2003) and McLennan (2004) in a series of experiments examining the response of cattle to supplements of varying composition and digestion characteristics (Fig. 5.7), and also with a review by Schiere and de Wit (1995), and is evidence that the Weston model provides a framework to understand the intake regulation of animals in a variety of circumstances. This is also an excellent example of how a mechanistic model has wide application to understand observations outside the immediate data set from which it was devised.

Way Forward

This application of Weston's model suggests that the basic hypothesis upon which it is based is robust. There are a number of suggestions to advance this model.

- The relationship between rumen fill and ME intake needs to be established for cattle, especially with respect to level of rumen OM and NDF fill.
- The calculations and relationships need to be defined in terms of the energy deficit rather than actual energy intake for a particular class of animal, as was done here. This should make the relationship more universal across physiological states and varying capacity to use energy, as suggested by Weston (1996).

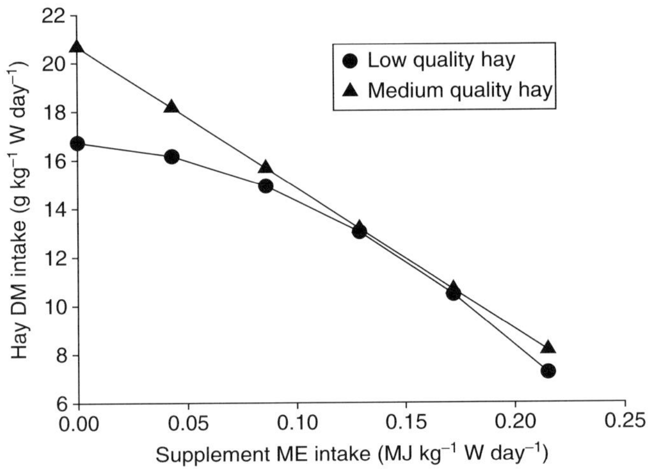

Fig. 5.7. The effect of metabolizable energy intake (ME) (MJ kg^{-1} W day^{-1}) of a barley grain supplement on the hay DM intake (g DM kg^{-1} W day^{-1}) of a low digestibility hay (•, OM digestibility 52.8%) or of a medium digestibility hay (▲, OM digestibility 62.4%).

- The retention time of supplements within rumens arising from different basal diets needs to be established. Vega and Poppi (1997) showed that the major influence on passage rate of particles was not the source of the particles but rather the rumen in which they were placed. This would suggest that retention time of supplement would vary markedly, depending on the basal diet and its retention time. However, rate of digestion of supplements is very high in comparison to rate of passage of the supplement particle and overall retention time may not be markedly affected, irrespective of the rumen in which it is placed.

Empirical Approaches

The choice of an empirical model over a mechanistic model is one of expediency. The desire to develop a purely mechanistic model is laudable and greatly aids our understanding of the control of intake, as outlined above. However, the output is more variable (Poppi *et al.*, 1994) and the inputs require more parameters of greater complexity, requiring significant time to derive. All these factors mean that mechanistic models at present are largely impractical for routine intake predictions, leading Poppi (1996) to conclude: 'The quick and dirty method of associative relationships, while lacking the elegance of mechanistic models, will always win out in the game of expedience.'

The most common empirical model is the regression relationship between intake and digestibility (or ME content) and this concept is used in various forms in most common animal models, in part or solely to predict intake, e.g. Grazfeed

(Freer *et al.*, 1997) and Cornell CNCPS (Fox *et al.*, 2003). Lippke (1980) (and also expanded upon in Ellis *et al.*, 1999) developed a set of multiple regression equations based on chemical composition to predict intake. These were:

$$\text{Digestible energy intake (kcal kg}^{-1}\text{ MW day}^{-1}) = 244.1 + 6.972\ \text{CP} - 3.49\ \text{ADF},$$

and

$$\text{Dry matter intake (g kg}^{-1}\text{ MW day}^{-1}) = 143.1 + 0.8699\ \text{CP} - 1.859\ \text{ADF}.$$

These empirical models do not advance our understanding of intake regulation but they do have the potential to identify important characteristics which have a major influence on intake regulation. They are generally useful only within the confines of the data set upon which they are based and, in any case, should be used only within the limits set by that database. The criteria upon which they should be judged are accuracy and ease of use. A prediction of intake to within 10% of the actual value is adequate for most aspects of ration formulation and management of pastures (feed budgets, etc.) and grazing animals. The intake–digestibility (or ME content), chemical composition (NDF, etc.) relationships meet these criteria within limited specific databases (e.g. Minson, 1990) but fail dismally across a wider range of forage types. Minson (1990) showed a wide variation in such relationships between cultivars and species. Also, the time required obtaining a digestibility estimate or a chemical composition is too long to be of routine use in management. Faecal NIRS offers the potential to overcome this for grazing animals.

Faecal NIRS is a method developed by Lyons and Stuth (1992), Stuth *et al.* (1999) and Coates (2004) to predict dietary DM digestibility and CP content by analysis of a faecal sample. It relies on an empirical approach of developing a regression relationship between the NIR spectrum of a faecal sample and the dietary DM digestibility or CP content. The field of NIRS has seen major advances in equipment and statistical procedures which have improved its reliability and acceptance within the scientific community. It is generally accepted that the spectrum reflects underlying chemical bonds and, as such, has a mechanistic relationship to chemical composition. In classical studies, the spectrum is regressed, after various statistical manipulations, against known levels of a compound determined by classical chemical analysis or bioassay. This is the basis upon which routine silage analysis and other feed types are analysed by direct NIRS. However, with grazing animals, especially on the rangelands, it is impossible to obtain representative samples of what the animal is eating upon which to do such analysis. A faecal sample represents an average sample of digested material that the animal has selected from a wide kaleidoscope of plant species and parts, especially in the heterogeneous pasture communities.

Faecal NIRS analyses a faecal sample which has undergone digestion and so it is the residue which is being analysed and, rather than a regression of the spectrum against the chemical content of the residue, the spectrum is regressed against the composition of the material originally ingested. It is for this reason that this approach has been criticized, even by proponents of NIRS methodology, as it goes against the basic principle upon which NIRS is based, i.e. the relationship between an NIR spectrum and a classically measured amount of a compound in the sample. However, in empirical terms, it seeks to determine if there is a statistical relationship between a faecal NIR spectrum and any aspect of diet quality. On that basis, it is no different conceptually from the early studies on faecal N and prediction of diet quality (Lancaster, 1949). Recently, Gibbs (2005) has outlined a mechanistic basis for why such a relationship might exist based on the concept that the NIR spectrum of the faecal residue reflects indigestible material having bonds which reflect the underlying structure and composition of the plant cell wall. From our understanding gained through mechanistic models of how plant cell wall structure and composition affects retention time and rates of passage and digestion (Coleman *et al*., 2004), there is a reasonable association, therefore, between the structure and composition of what cannot be digested to what was present in the original material. This is dependent on following strict NIRS protocols of sample numbers, sample variation in source and composition, and accepted chemical methods or bioassays in analysis of the original feed samples. So long as these accepted NIRS principles are followed, and so long as an acceptable relationship (based on R^2, standard error of calibration (SEC), etc.) is obtained between a faecal spectrum and the composition of interest in the feed sample, this approach is valid. Using this approach, Coates (2004) has obtained acceptable relationships with sufficient accuracy for determining DM digestibility, CP content and proportion of C3 and C4 plants in the diet of cattle. With grazing animals, this method surpasses any previous methods for its ease of use and accuracy for these parameters. Gibbs (2005) has further developed relationships for predicting the digestibility and CP content of both the supplemented diet and the underlying basal forage. This has extended the application of faecal NIRS to supplemented and unsupplemented diets, further increasing the usefulness of such an approach to grazing animals.

Given these features, the issue of interest here is the prediction of intake from a faecal NIRS. Once again, the approach is simple: look for an acceptable relationship with a wide database. One approach is to use the good prediction of DM digestibility from faecal NIRS and to use the published intake–digestibility relationships to predict intake. Given the large variation in such relationships, as outlined in the mechanistic section on intake regulation, this approach is not likely to provide a way forward. The alternative is to look for a direct relationship between faecal NIRS and intake. Coleman *et al*. (1989), Coates (2004) and Gibbs (2005) have all found such a relationship. The R^2 was similar to that derived by conventional chemical or *in vitro* analysis (Minson, 1990; Forbes, 1995), which ranged from 0.70 to 0.85 on wide data sets. So faecal NIRS was similar to, but not much better than, conventional analysis, but obviously more convenient. Coates (2004) found a better relationship (R^2 0.95 to 0.97 for digestible dry matter intake), which nutritionally is a more desirable parameter than just intake alone. Despite all this, the accuracy needs to be put into the context of alternative methods for measuring or predicting intake of grazing animals. In this context, faecal NIRS is superior on all aspects. The question is whether the accuracy is adequate for field application if one is to aspire to a measurement within 10% of the actual value. Currently, on Coates' data this is not the case, but the R^2 and CEV are reasonable and probably within acceptable limits to make appropriate management decisions with grazing animals. Coates (2004) showed that the SEC for prediction of intake (g DM kg^{-1} LW day^{-1}) by faecal NIRS ranged from 1.80 to 2.17 and that the R^2 ranged from 0.74 to 0.79. Comparable values for predicting digestible dry matter intake (g DDM kg^{-1} LW day^{-1}) by faecal NIRS were better, with SEC ranging from 1.16 to 1.42 and R^2 from 0.88 to 0.89. It would be interesting to see if a good relationship might be obtained between faecal NIRS and retention time because, if there were such a relationship, then Weston's model could be applied, using faecal NIRS data in the field.

Faecal NIRS may be used in two ways for predicting intake. First, as outlined above, a direct relationship may be obtained between faecal NIR spectrum and intake. However, intake needs to be measured accurately and this can only be done with pen-fed animals, as the errors in alternative methods in the field are too great. These relate to the use of oesophageal fistulated animals, measurement of digestibility by *in vitro* methods and estimation of faecal output by marker dilution methods. Thus, it becomes uncertain as to whether the error is due to the faecal NIRS method or the original measurement of intake. For these reasons, accurate pen-based measurements are the most appropriate method. Such studies have shown that intake can be predicted with acceptable accuracy, although probably not to within 10% (Coates, 2004). However, one issue arises about this relationship which needs to be carefully considered. These forage types will have variable leaf proportion and Laredo and Minson (1973) and Poppi *et al.* (1981b) have shown that leaf per cent markedly affects intake. In these studies, the digestibility of leaf and stem was the same, but intake and retention time differed markedly between leaf and stem of tropical forages.

Grazing animals select mainly leaf, so the leaf relationship may differ from a mixed leaf and stem relationship. Given that faecal NIRS appears to focus on the indigestible components of the cell wall fraction in estimating digestibility, it would appear better to establish a relationship between intake of grazing animals and faecal NIRS. This could be done by using faecal NIRS to measure DM digestibility in the grazing animal (which has been established above as an acceptable method) in combination with faecal output measurements by marker dilution from controlled release capsules. Intake can then be calculated from digestibility and faecal output. Such an approach would avoid the potential errors involved in pen-fed studies with variable leaf per cent. It would involve considerable effort in accessing a range of forages as part of the required NIRS protocol, but potentially would provide a valuable empirical approach for grazing animals.

The second way to use faecal NIRS to measure intake is to use it to predict DM digestibility and ME content. From a knowledge of live weight gain either measured directly or from historical data, nutrient use models can be used to back-calculate to derive the required intake to give that live weight gain from the estimated ME content (Baker, 2004). McLennan (2005) has examined the accuracy of this approach using an extensive database where intake, digestibility and live weight gain were measured with pen-fed animals. This approach uses the empirical equations for energy use, as outlined in various feeding standards and models, e.g. SCA (1990), AFRC (1993), Grazfeed (Freer *et al.*, 1997), Cornell CNCPS (Fox *et al.*, 2003). He found that these equations were robust and had high R^2 (from 0.91 to 0.95). Both approaches will have their uses but, in establishing an empirical approach to estimating intake of grazing animals, it would be worth investigating whether the marker dilution, faecal NIRS approach gives a good relationship for grazing animals. Such an outcome would have wide and useful application to grazing animals, especially those that graze in extensive conditions as occur within northern Australia.

Conclusions

The application of a mechanistic model (Weston, 1996), and the derivation of a method to estimate intake from such a model, has provided a means by which intake and its response to supplements of various types may be explained. This is an example of the usefulness of mechanistic models in understanding and examining novel situations. The role of an empirical approach based on faecal NIRS to estimate intake has been outlined and it is concluded that this approach offers the best way to estimate intake with grazing animals.

Acknowledgements

I acknowledge the many hours of convivial discussion and debate on this topic with D. Coates, W.C. Ellis, S.J. Gibbs, S.R. McLennan and R.H. Weston and I thank S.R. McLennan for assistance with the simulations and figures.

References

AFRC (1992) Nutritive requirements of ruminants: protein. *Nutrition Abstracts and Reviews* 62, 787–835.

AFRC (1993) *Energy and Protein Requirements of Ruminants*. CAB International, Wallingford, UK.

Baile, C.A. and Forbes, J.M. (1974) Control of feed intake and regulation of energy balance in ruminants. *Physiological Reviews* 54, 160–214.

Baker, R.D. (2004) Estimating herbage intake from animal performance. In: Penning, P.D. (ed.) *Herbage Intake Handbook*. The British Grassland Society, Hurley, UK, pp. 95–120.

Blaxter, K.L., Graham, N.Mc.C. and Wainman, F.W. (1956) Some observations on the digestibility of food by sheep, and on related problems. *British Journal of Nutrition* 10, 69–91.

Blaxter, K.L., Wainman, F.W. and Wilson, R.S. (1961) The regulation of food intake by sheep. *Animal Production* 3, 51–61.

Coates, D.B. (2000) Faecal NIRS – what does it offer today's grazier? *Tropical Grasslands* 34, 230–239.

Coates, D.B. (2004) Faecal NIRS – technology for improving nutritional management of grazing cattle. Final Report Project NAP3.121, Meat and Livestock Australia.

Coleman, S.W., Stuth, J.W. and Holloway, J.W. (1989) Monitoring the nutrition of grazing cattle with near-infrared analysis of feces. In: *Proceedings of the XVI International Grassland Congress*, Nice, France, pp. 881–882.

Coleman, S.W., Moore, J.E. and Wilson, J.R. (2004) Quality and utilisation. In: Moser, L.E., Burson, B.L. and Sollenberger, L.E. (eds) *Warm-Season (C4) Grasses*, Agronomy Monograph No. 45. American Society of Agronomy, Crop Science Society of America, Soil Science Society of America, Madison, WI 53711, pp. 267–308.

Cruickshank, G.J., Poppi, D.P., Sykes, A.R. and Familton, A.S. (1990) Effect of age, abomasal cannulation and rumen catheterisation on intake and site of digestion by early-weaned lambs. *Journal of Agricultural Science, Cambridge* 114, 49–54.

Dixon, R.M. and Stockdale, C.R. (1999) Associative effects between forages and grains: consequences for feed utilisation. *Australian Journal of Agricultural Research* 50, 757–773.

Egan, A.R. (1970) Nutritional status and intake regulation in sheep. VI. Evidence for variation in setting of an intake regulatory mechanism relating to the digesta content of the reticulo-rumen. *Australian Journal of Agricultural Research* 21, 735–746.

Ellis, W.C., Poppi, D.P., Matis, J.H., Lippke, H., Hill, T.M. and Rouquette, F.M. (1999) Dietary–digestive–metabolic interactions determining the nutritive potential of ruminant diets. In: Jung, H.-J.G. and Fahey, G.C. (eds) *Nutritional Ecology of Herbivores, Proceedings of the Vth International Symposium on the Nutrition of Herbivores*. American Society of Animal Science, Savoy, Illinois, pp. 423–481.

Forbes, J.M. (1980) A model of short-term control of feeding in the ruminant: effects of changing animal or feed characteristics. *Appetite* 1, 21–41.

Forbes, J.M. (1995) *Voluntary Food Intake and Diet Selection in Farm Animals*. CAB International, Wallingford, UK.

Fox, D.G., Tylutki, T.P., Tedeschi, L.O., Van Amburgh, M.E., Chase, L.E., Pell, A.N., Overton, T.R. and Russell, J.B. (2003) The net carbohydrate and protein system for evaluating herd nutrition and nutrient excretion, CNCPS version 5.0. Model documentation, Animal Science Mimeo 213, Department of Animal Science, Cornell University, Ithaca, New York.

Freer, M., Moore, A.D. and Donnelly, J.R. (1997) GRAZPLAN: decision support systems for Australian grazing enterprises – II. *Agricultural Systems* 54, 77–126.

Gherardi, S.G. and Black, J.L. (1989) Influence of post-rumen supply of nutrients on rumen digesta load and voluntary intake of a roughage by sheep. *British Journal of Nutrition* 62, 589–599.

Gibbs, S.J. (2005) Faecal near infrared reflectance spectroscopy to predict diet quality of cattle fed supplements. PhD thesis, The University of Queensland, Brisbane, Australia.

Hutton, J.B. (1963) The effect of lactation on intake in the dairy cow. *Proceedings of the New Zealand Society of Animal Production* 23, 39–52.

Hutton, J.B., Hughes, J.W., Newth, R.P. and Watanabe, K. (1964) The voluntary intake of the lactating dairy cow and its relation to digestion. *Proceedings of the New Zealand Society of Animal Production* 24, 29–42.

Lancaster, R.J. (1949) Estimation of digestibility of grazed pasture from faeces nitrogen. *Nature* 163, 330–331.

Laredo, M.A. and Minson, D.J. (1973) The voluntary intake, digestibility and retention time by sheep of leaf and stem fractions of five grasses. *Australian Journal of Agricultural Research* 24, 875–888.

Lippke, H. (1980) Forage characteristics related to intake, digestibility and gain by ruminants. *Journal of Animal Science* 50, 952–961.

Lyons, R.K. and Stuth, J.W. (1992) Faecal NIRS equations for predicting diet quality of free-ranging cattle. *Journal of Range Management* 45, 238–244.

McLennan, S.R. (2004) More effective supplements for the northern beef industry. Final Report NAP3.122, Meat and Livestock Australia.

McLennan, S.R. (2005) Improved prediction of the performance of cattle in the tropics. Final Report NBP.331, Meat and Livestock Australia

Marsetyo (2003) Feeding strategies to reduce intake substitution of forages by supplements in beef cattle. PhD thesis, The University of Queensland, Brisbane, Australia.

Minson, D.J. (1966) The apparent retention of food in the reticulo-rumen at two levels of feeding by means of an hourly feeding technique. *British Journal of Nutrition* 20, 765–773.

Minson, D.J. (1971) The digestibility and voluntary intake of six varieties of Panicum. *Australian Journal of Experimental Agriculture and Animal Husbandry* 11, 18–25.

Minson, D.J. (1990) *Forage in Ruminant Nutrition*. Academic Press, London.

Moore, J.E., Brant, M.H., Kunkle, W.E. and Hopkins, D.I. (1999) Effect of supplementation on voluntary forage intake, diet digestibility and animal performance. *Journal of Animal Science* 77, 122–135.

Pittroff, W. and Kothmann, M.M. (1999) Dietary–digestive–metabolic interactions determining the nutritive potential of ruminant diets. In: Jung, H.-J.G. and Fahey, G.C. (eds) *Nutritional Ecology of Herbivores, Proceedings of the Vth International Symposium on the Nutrition of Herbivores*. American Society of Animal Science, Savoy, Illinois, pp. 366–422.

Poppi, D.P. (1996) Predictions of feed intake in ruminants from analyses of food composition. *Australian Journal of Agricultural Research* 47, 489–504.

Poppi, D.P., Minson, D.J. and Ternouth, J.H. (1981a) Studies of cattle and sheep eating leaf and stem fractions of grasses. I. The voluntary intake, digestibility and retention time in the reticulo-rumen. *Australian Journal of Agricultural Research* 32, 99–108.

Poppi, D.P., Minson, D.J. and Ternouth, J.H. (1981b) Studies of cattle and sheep eating leaf and stem fractions of grasses. III. The retention time in the rumen of large feed particles. *Australian Journal of Agricultural Research* 32, 123–137.

Poppi, D.P., Gill, M. and France, J. (1994) Integrating theories of intake regulation in growing ruminants. *Journal of Theoretical Biology* 167, 129–145.

SCA (1990) *Feeding Standards for Australian Livestock, Ruminants*. Standing Committee on Agriculture, Ruminant Subcommittee, CSIRO, Melbourne, Australia.

Schiere, J.B. and Wit, J. de (1995) Feeding urea ammonia treated rice straw in the tropics. II. Assumptions on nutritive value and their validity for least cost ration formulation. *Animal Feed Science and Technology* 51, 45–63.

Stuth, J.H., Freer, M., Dove, H. and Lyons, R.K. (1999) Nutritional management for free-ranging livestock. In: Jung, H.-J.G. and Fahey, G.C. (eds) *Nutritional Ecology of Herbivores, Proceedings of the Vth International Symposium on the Nutrition of Herbivores*. American Society of Animal Science, Savoy, Illinois, pp. 696–751.

Thornton, R.F. and Minson, D.J. (1972) The relationship between voluntary intake and mean apparent retention time in the rumen. *Australian Journal of Agricultural Research* 23, 871–877.

Thornton, R.F. and Minson, D.J. (1973) The relationship between apparent retention time in the rumen, voluntary intake, and apparent digestibility of legume and grass diets in sheep. *Australian Journal of Agricultural Research* 24, 889–898.

Vega, A. De and Poppi, D.P. (1997) Extent of digestion and rumen condition as factors affecting passage of liquid and digesta particles in sheep. *Journal of Agricultural Science, Cambridge* 128, 207–215.

Waldo, D.R., Smith, L.W. and Cox, E.L. (1972) Model of cellulose disappearance from the rumen. *Journal of Dairy Science* 55, 125–129.

Weston, R.H. (1985) The regulation of feed intake in herbage-fed young sheep. *Proceedings of the Nutrition Society of Australia* 10, 55–62.
Weston, R.H. (1996) Some aspects of constraint to forage consumption by ruminants. *Australian Journal of Agricultural Research* 47, 175–197.

6 Models to Measure and Interpret Exchange of Metabolites Across the Capillary Bed of Intact Organs

J.P. Cant and F. Qiao

Centre for Nutrition Modelling, Department of Animal and Poultry Science, University of Guelph, Canada

Introduction

The exchange of metabolites between tissue and blood has captivated humans for centuries and, accordingly, has spawned a vast diaspora of experimental and theoretical wanderings. Interest has been logged in exchange of respiratory gases, energy metabolites like glucose, acetate and β-hydroxybutyrate, precursors for biosynthetic processes, secretory products, hormones, xenobiotics, the list goes on. Even in the modern age of genomics and complexity studies, the site of circulatory exchange retains a central role as the vital interface through which gene expression in individual tissues is communicated and responsive to events in the rest of the body.

A popular and useful technique to study mechanisms of exchange is to remove cells from the organ of interest and culture them *in vitro*, using various protocols to track molecular traffic from one side of the plasma membrane to another. Here, parameters are easily obtained to describe the concentration-dependence of transmembrane exchange, for example. However, if the goal is to use such parameters to explain phenomena in the whole animal, two major problems arise: (i) the *in vitro* rates of metabolism may be slower by half, or more, than *in vivo* due to loss of cell–cell contact and the appropriate extra-cellular milieu of hormones, growth factors, etc.; and (ii) the interplay between a stationary cell community and the circulatory system that replenishes and washes away extracellular solutes is unaccounted for. Parameterizing solute exchange *in vivo*, on the other hand, while yielding more relevant numbers, is plagued with technical difficulties arising from the influence of the body, i.e. not being able to manipulate solute concentrations over a sufficiently wide range or to obtain direct measurements of the exchange process. All is not lost, however, as these problems can be overcome with a mathematical model formulated to extract meaningful information from *in vivo* observations.

Despite, or perhaps as a consequence of, its long and varied history, there exists an entire catalogue of methods by which uptake and release of blood metabolites across an intact organ are routinely measured and interpreted. The factor that differentiates the various methods is the model that has been presumed to explain the observations and yield information of biological value. In this chapter, we attempt to set out, in a systematic manner, the main modelling methods available to the experimenter and their underpinnings so that the reader may select those best suited to his or her needs.

Steady-state Models

The primary basis for most *in vivo* exchange models is that, given the anatomy of blood circulation, one can measure the concentration of solutes in the entire arterial inflow and venous effluent from an organ. Arteries branch into arterioles that supply capillaries where exchange occurs and that drain into venules, which collect in larger veins that exit the organ (Fig. 6.1). The target system, then, whether it is the mammary gland, the liver, or the lungs, is simply treated as a black box with a single inlet and a single convective outlet (Fig. 6.2), both of which can be sampled to ascertain solute concentrations. In addition, there is a non-convective

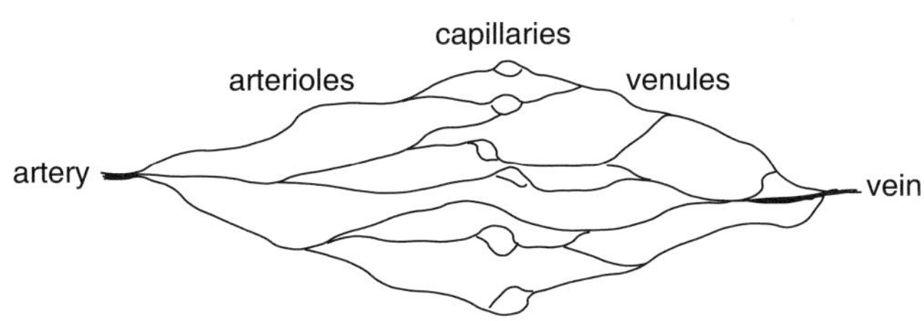

Fig. 6.1. A simple depiction of the capillary bed of a tissue (adapted from Meier and Zierler, 1954).

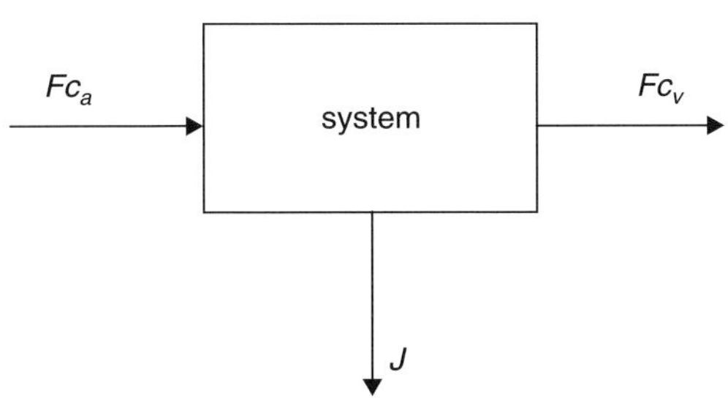

Fig. 6.2. Depiction of the organ as a black box where F represents blood flow (ml s^{-1}) through the system, c_a and c_v are arterial and venous concentrations (μmol ml^{-1}), respectively, of a solute, and J is a net non-convective outflux (μmol s^{-1}).

outlet from the black box to the surroundings, which cannot be directly sampled but is of prime interest in the experiment. At steady state, the net non-convective outflux J (μmol s^{-1}) of the nutrient, or uptake, equals the difference between convective influx and convective outflux through the system:

$$J = F(c_a - c_v), \tag{6.1}$$

where F is the blood flow rate (ml s^{-1}) and c_a and c_v represent the solute concentrations (μmol ml^{-1}) in arterial and venous samples, respectively; $c_a - c_v$ is the arteriovenous difference.

Arterial blood is considered sufficiently well mixed that metabolite concentrations in any one artery accurately represent concentrations in any other artery of interest, provided there are no exogenous arterial infusions ongoing. Thus, while the vein of interest must be sampled to measure c_v, any readily accessible artery such as a carotid or intracostal may be sampled to obtain c_a. Consideration must also be given to the circulatory anatomy unique to the organ under study. For example, the liver receives blood both from the hepatic portal vein that drains viscera and from the hepatic artery, and so c_a is obtained as essentially a blood flow-weighted average of the two concentrations. The inguinal mammary glands of a ruminant are drained by two large veins – the external pudic and the subcutaneous mammary abdominal – but only the subcutaneous mammary is typically sampled for calculation of net uptake J on the assumption that there is adequate mixing in venous anastomoses to equate solute concentrations between the two. A complication that arises in animals following successive lactations is that blood flow may be reversed in the external pudic so that blood draining non-mammary tissues will enter the mammary abdominal vein and contaminate the arteriovenous difference (Linzell, 1960; Thivierge *et al*., 2000). Furthermore, catheterization defines the organ as that system isolated by the artery and vein, which often represents a heterogeneous mix of cell types – e.g. muscle, bone, adipose and skin in the hind limb or stomach, small intestine, large intestine, pancreas and spleen in the portal-drained viscera – that are indistinguishable in the model of Fig. 6.2.

Solution of Eqn 6.1 requires an estimate of blood flow rate F. Several methods, beyond the scope of this chapter, exist for its estimation, but a simple approach involves rearrangement of Eqn 6.1 for a solute that is neither taken up nor released during transit through the system. The indicator solute is infused continuously into the target system, typically on the arterial side, although upstream venous infusion is an option as well (e.g. Linzell, 1966). Monitoring the indicator infusion rate gives the value of non-convective flux J, which can be used to calculate F from steady-state concentrations of the indicator, c_a and c_v. Commonly used indicators in the dye-dilution technique are indocyanine green and para-aminohippuric acid.

The net uptake J of a metabolite may be described as a clearance (ml s^{-1}):

$$Cl = \frac{J}{c_a} \tag{6.2}$$

which has the same units as a volume flow but is a non-convective flow, in contrast to convective blood flow.

An alternative expression is the net uptake as a proportion of arterial influx, or extraction percentage:

$$E = \frac{J}{Fc_a} = \frac{c_a - c_v}{c_a}, \tag{6.3}$$

which can be calculated without an estimate of blood flow. Extraction carries the attractive appearance of a parameter or slope not unlike a mass-action coefficient that describes affinity of a tissue for the circulating metabolite and could be used in predicting tissue responses to circulatory perturbations. Unfortunately, neither E nor Cl are constant across a range of blood flow rates (Cant *et al.*, 1993; Baron *et al.*, 1994; Dupuis *et al.*, 1996) and, where blood flow can change according to metabolic activity of the organ, make unsatisfactory parameters for robust prediction.

Hanigan *et al.* (1998) point out that if the black box in Fig. 6.2 is a well-mixed compartment of extracellular fluid, as would occur with rapid mixing in capillaries arranged in parallel in an organ, then the venous concentration of solute, c_v, is equal to the extracellular concentration. Accordingly, clearance should be calculated as a proportion of c_v. Hanigan *et al.* (1998) defined the venous clearance parameter (ml s^{-1}) as:

$$K = \frac{J}{c_v} \tag{6.4}$$

In this representation, the effect of a change in F is manifest in the extracellular solute concentration c_v in that a faster F, by replenishing supplies, will increase the concentration, and vice versa. The precise formulation is given by a re-arrangement of mass balance Eqn 6.1, substituting Eqn 6.4, as:

$$c_v = \frac{Fc_a}{F + K}. \tag{6.5}$$

With c_v carrying the F effect, K is taken to represent the exchange process over a range of blood flow values.

Cant and McBride (1995) took a slightly different tack to the problem of F interference in uptake parameterization. Following Renkin (1959) and Crone (1963), the capillary where exchange occurs is assumed to be a selectively permeable cylinder that exchanges with an extravascular space of constant radius along its length (Fig. 6.3). If net transport out of the capillary is a first-order process such that:

$$\frac{dc_{sc}(t)}{dt} = -kc_{sc}(t) \tag{6.6}$$

where $c_{sc}(t)$ is the solute concentration within the capillary at time t of transit from arterial to venous side and k is the rate constant (s^{-1}), then the venous concentration c_{sc_v} is the integral of Eqn 6.6:

$$c_{sc\_v} = c_a e^{-k\frac{V_{sc}}{F_{sc}}} \tag{6.7}$$

where the ratio of volume V_{sc} to volume flow F_{sc} in a single capillary is the capillary transit time. Equation 6.6 is considered a distributed-in-space model of

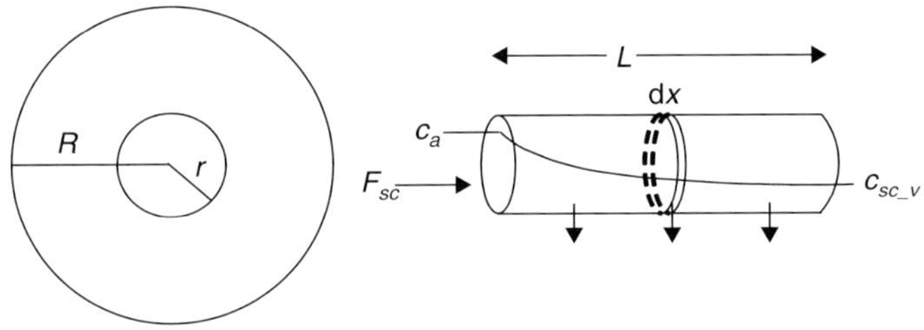

Fig. 6.3. Idealized cross-section of a capillary of radius *r* serving a cylinder of tissue of radius *R* and longitudinal view of that capillary where *L* is the length (cm), *dx* is a thin segment of that length (cm), F_{sc} is blood flow (ml s^{-1}) and c_a and c_{sc_v} are arterial and venous concentrations (μmol ml^{-1}), respectively, of a permeable solute. This is the representation assumed in Crone–Renkin models.

capillary exchange. Assuming a parallel arrangement of *n* identical capillaries into which *F* is distributed equally allows the whole-organ c_v to be calculated as:

$$c_v = c_a e^{-k\frac{V_{sc}n}{F}} \tag{6.8}$$

Estimation of *k* from steady-state arteriovenous difference data using Eqn 6.8 requires a measurement of the number of open capillaries *n*, which is, for most intents, not possible. Instead, the parameter product $kV_{sc}n$ may be calculated from the substitution of Eqn 6.8 into Eqn 6.3:

$$kV_{sc}n = -\ln(1-E)F. \tag{6.9}$$

Though unsatisfactory as a means to isolate the intrinsic parameters of solute exchange, Eqn 6.8 has been used in conjunction with a blood flow simulation model to predict the consequences of changes in *F* that may arise from capillary recruitment (i.e. a change in *n*), arteriolar resistance, or the arteriovenous pressure differential (Cant and McBride, 1995; Cant *et al.*, 2002, 2003).

So far, only net uptake or exchange has been discussed, but it is rare for a transporter to be able to move a solute in only one direction across the plasma membrane of a cell. As a general rule, if there is uptake, there is, simultaneously, release and the arteriovenous difference in steady state is the net result of both directions of transport. In some situations, and for some purposes, net uptake is a satisfactory measure of the utilization of a solute by an organ, but consider an organ that can both synthesize the solute of interest *de novo* and remove it from blood – net uptake could severely underestimate the true extent of utilization of this solute. Likewise, the gastrointestinal tract can extract nutrients from blood but also derive them by absorption from the lumen. To counter such problems, application of Eqns 6.1–6.9 to steady-state concentrations of a molecular tracer of the solute of interest has been used to yield information about unidirectional uptake (e.g. Kristensen *et al.*, 1996; Carter and Welbourne, 1997). The simplest approach is to assume that, once taken into the cells of an organ, the tracer is so diluted with intracellular tracee that the subsequent unidirectional release of tracer is negligible. Accordingly, *E* of tracer (Eqn 6.3), when multiplied by the arterial influx of tracee Fc_a, gives the unidirectional uptake of unlabelled solute. However, the simple approach still underestimates unidirectional uptake due to the tracer infusion time required to reach a steady state of solute labelling in blood, during which intracellular labelling, and therefore release of tracer, may increase beyond a negligible level. This recycling of tracer can be corrected with more complex models of the steady-state fluxes of tracer from arterial blood, between extra- and intracellular compartments and to venous blood, that have been developed particularly for solution of steady-state amino acid kinetics and that require measures of the extent of intracellular labelling from tissue biopsies or surrogate proteins in blood or milk (Cheng *et al.*, 1985; Biolo *et al.*, 1992; France *et al.*, 1995). These models and variants are discussed in detail in Chapter 12 of this volume.

Equation 6.1, upon which all the subsequent calculations and interpretations are based, is valid only for the steady-state condition during which flows and concentrations do not fluctuate. The main reason for this requirement was presented by Zierler (1961) as due to the time required for blood to move from the artery to the venous sampling site. If arterial concentration, even of a non-transportable substrate, increases abruptly, say, the venous concentration will not increase likewise until that pulse front reaches the sampling site after passing through the organ. Furthermore, there is no single transit time through the organ but a distribution of transit times along pathways of different lengths (Fig. 6.1), which convert the sharp pulse front into a broad wave of increasing concentrations in the vein. During this time, the arteriovenous difference $c_a - c_v$ will not represent net uptake but will be a consequence of the non-steady state. Likewise, a change in F will cause an artificial arteriovenous difference to arise.

The requirement for a steady state causes a few problems in the study of transport. First of all, the steady state is difficult to maintain, particularly in long-term experiments during which F may fluctuate considerably. Secondly, it may not be possible to explore a range of concentrations of the solute of interest without changing the physiological status of the animal. If one is attempting to parameterize the concentration-dependence of glucose transport by an organ, for example, infusion of glucose i.v. to obtain a steady state will cause insulin concentrations to rise and possibly change the concentration-dependence. Similarly, changes in concentrations of other metabolites in blood due to the glucose infusion could affect glucose utilization by the organ of interest. Fortunately, the theory of how the vascular system contributes to the delay between arterial and venous sampling sites can be used to correct the non-steady-state venous concentration profile following a controlled pulse dose of the solute of interest into the arterial influx and yield valuable information about transport. The bolus injection of nutrients can elicit a dynamic concentration profile over a wide range for a short period of time without influencing the physiological status of the animal. For this reason, non-steady-state techniques are considered superior to the constant infusion technique for estimating local kinetics of *in vivo* metabolism. Compared to the constant infusion, however, bolus injections are rarely utilized in practice to probe the nature of interactions between a circulating solute and an organ, apparently because of a perceived difficulty in the mathematics required to interpret observations. The computer essentially renders such opposition obsolete and we hope that, with the following review of classic and recent advances in non-steady-state modelling of capillary exchange, this powerful technique, which can yield information often considered accessible only *in vitro*, can be brought to bear on current problems of interest.

Non-steady-state Models

For non-steady-state modelling, an indicator solute that is not taken up into cells is rapidly injected as a bolus into the arterial inflow along with the transportable solute of interest, hereon called the 'nutrient' to differentiate it from the indicator, although the reader should bear in mind that the technique has much broader applicability and the word nutrient could be substituted by any solute of interest such as a waste product, intermediary metabolite, hormone, drug, etc. A series of venous blood samples is collected in rapid succession and the cross-organ time courses of simultaneous dilution of indicators and nutrients are obtained (Fig. 6.4). The non-transportable solute indicates what would happen to the nutrient if there were no uptake through the system. In terms of the black box depiction (Fig. 6.2), the difference between the nutrient and the indicator is that the indicator does not have access to the non-convective outflow. This is the same requirement as for steady-state measurement of F by dye dilution using Eqn 6.1, and the same compounds, e.g. indocyanine green and para-aminohippuric acid, may be used as indicators.

The space into which an indicator distributes is important to consider. There are vascular indicators such as ^{51}Cr-labelled erythrocytes, ^{131}I-labelled albumin, indocyanine green and Evans blue, extracellular indicators such as ^{14}C-labelled sucrose, inulin, mannitol and para-aminohippuric acid, and intracellular indicators such as ^{3}HHO and D_2O. In Fig. 6.4, one nutrient (hippurate) and four

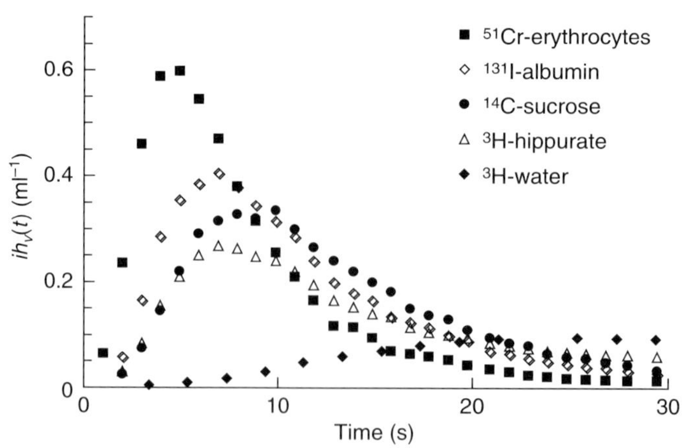

Fig. 6.4. Concentrations of multiple indicators and hippurate in the venous outflow of an organ following rapid injection of a bolus dose in the arterial supply (data from Schwab *et al.*, 2001).

indicator outflow curves are illustrated. For easy comparison of indicator and nutrient curves, venous concentration of each ($c_v(t)$) is normalized to:

$$h(t) = \frac{c_v(t)}{q_0} \text{ or } ih(t) = \frac{ic_v(t)}{iq_0}, \tag{6.10}$$

where q_0 is the dose (μmol) of indicator or nutrient injected (the leading '*i*' denotes a reference indicator as opposed to a test nutrient). Because there is no extraction from the system, the area under each normalized curve of indicator concentrations is identical. The area represents complete outflow of the entire dose injected. The peak of the vascular indicator (^{51}Cr-erythrocytes) curve is higher than that of the other three indicator curves because it does not distribute outside the vascular space. The curves of sucrose and albumin have a lower peak and a longer tail than the erythrocyte curve because they have larger volumes of extracellular distribution and, therefore, longer average residence times in the system. Although labelled albumin is often considered to be a vascular indicator, the difference between labelled erythrocyte and albumin curves shows that albumin distributes over a larger space and is, therefore, to some degree, extravascular. The water curve has the lowest peak and longest tail because it distributes in both extracellular and intracellular spaces and has the longest residence time in the system. The area under the hippurate curve is smaller than for either of the indicators because of uptake and sequestration in cells. In this way, the dilution curves contain information about physical characteristics of the system and fluxes through it. Coefficients that mathematically describe the curves can be used to investigate the kinetics of nutrient transport and sequestration in cells of the system.

Coefficients from indicator dilution curves

Blood flow rate

As with the constant infusion experiment, the faster the blood flows through the system, the more diluted the indicator concentration will be. In a bolus injection experiment, the venous concentration of indicator changes with sampling time so an average concentration is obtained as area under the curve. Thus, *F* is calculated as:

$$F = \frac{iq_0}{iA} = \frac{1}{ia}, \tag{6.11}$$

where iA (s μmol ml^{-1}) is the area under the concentration–time curve and ia (s ml^{-1}) is the area under the normalized concentration–time curve. *F* should be the same for each of the different indicators in a single injection because all of the areas ia under each indicator normalized outflow curve are identical. Note that *F* may represent plasma flow or blood flow depending on where the indicator is distributed and how it is analysed. If the indicator is distributed extracellularly and its concentration is measured in plasma, *F* will represent plasma flow and the blood flow can be calculated by dividing by (1.0 – packed cell volume). If labelled erythrocytes are the indicator and whole blood is directly counted,

F represents blood flow and plasma flow can be calculated by multiplying F by (1.0 – packed cell volume).

For F measurement, there must be 100% recovery of injected indicator from the venous outflow, which means there can be no remainder, origination, recirculation or loss in the system. The first three can be avoided by selection of the appropriate indicator compound for the tissue under study, but recirculation is unavoidable and usually occurs long before complete recovery of the dose has been achieved. If recirculation commences part-way along the downslope of the outflow curve, a monoexponential function from the upper part of the downslope is used to approximate how the lower part of the downslope would appear if recirculation were absent and there was none of the dose remaining in the system. This type of correction was introduced by Hamilton *et al.* (1928) and is called Hamilton's exponential extrapolation. A slope b (s^{-1}) is obtained by statistical fit of downslope observations before recirculation occurs (Fig. 6.5). The area under the normalized concentration curve, ia (s ml^{-1}), is then obtained in two parts. From time 0 until t_r just before recirculation appears, each normalized observation is multiplied by the time interval of sampling Δt and summed. The remaining area from t_r to infinity is obtained by integration of the monoexponential equation $ih(t) = ih(t_r)e^{-b(t-t_r)}$ as $ih(t_r)/b$. Thus:

$$ia = \int_0^{\infty} ih(t)\mathrm{d}t = \sum_{j=1}^{n} ih_j \Delta_t + ih(t_r)/b, \tag{6.12}$$

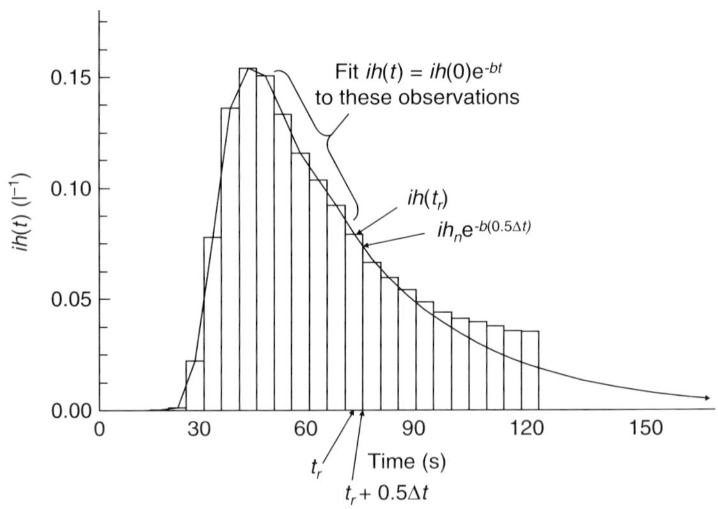

Fig. 6.5. Illustration of Hamilton's exponential extrapolation to correct normalized concentrations of para-aminohippuric acid, $ih(t)$ (l^{-1}), in the vein draining the mammary glands of a lactating cow for recirculation and incomplete recovery of the dose injected into the arterial supply. The slope b (s^{-1}) is obtained by statistical fit of downslope observations before recirculation appears in the sample after time t_r (s). This parameter is then used to extrapolate the remainder of the dilution curve to infinity from the estimated normalized concentration at the end of the nth sampling interval, $ih_n e^{-b(0.5\Delta t)}$ (l^{-1}), where n is the number of observations before time t_r.

where n is the number of observations before time t_r.

Caution must be exercised in using $ih(t_r)$. Because of continuous blood sampling, each observation of $h(t)$ is the average normalized concentration during the sampling time interval. The corresponding time for plotting concentrations is conventionally the midpoint of the sampling time interval but, in such cases, the term $\sum_{j=1}^{n} ih_j \Delta t$ is the area up to time $t_r + 0.5\Delta t$. The appropriate extrapolated area becomes:

$$ia = \int_0^\infty h(t)dt = \sum_{j=1}^{n} ih_j \Delta t + ih_n e^{-b(0.5\Delta t)} / b, \tag{6.13}$$

where $ih_n e^{-b(0.5\Delta t)}$ is the estimated normalized concentration at the end of the nth sampling interval.

Transit time

Transit time is an important concept in the interpretation of venous dilution curves. Indicator molecules will take different times to traverse the numerous parallel vascular pathways that exist from injection to sampling site (Fig. 6.1). Arteries and arterioles will cause a delay of the input into the capillaries; venules and veins will cause a delay of the output. The arterial and venous delays are in series and can be summed to one delay. Vascular indicators will follow the same pathways as blood in the vascular bed. However, extravascular indicators not only follow blood flow through the vascular bed but are further delayed in capillaries because of exchange with interstitial fluid. The diffusion delay is positively related with the volume into which the indicator is distributed and negatively related with the blood flow rate.

A typical venous dilution curve with recirculation is shown in Fig. 6.5, with vertical bars representing normalized venous concentrations of indicator $ih(t)$ from the beginning of injection into the arterial catheter. If each $ih(t)$ is divided by ia so that total area under the curve equals 1.0, then the area under each bar represents a fraction of the total dose injected. The corresponding time point represents the time needed for that fraction of dose to traverse the whole system, which includes the injection catheter, the sampling system, non-exchanging vessels and exchanging capillaries of the vascular system, and any extravascular space accessible to the indicator. An average of these transit times weighted according to the fraction of dose that appears at each time is then obtained as:

$$\bar{t}_{\text{total}} = \frac{\int_0^\infty t \cdot ih(t)dt}{ia}. \tag{6.14}$$

The delay in the arterial catheter is short because of the fast injection speed and the small volume of the catheter, so it is ignored in most indicator dilution studies. A sampling delay t_s (s) can be calculated from the volume of sampling tubing divided by the sampling flow rate. The t_s will shift the outflow curve to the right without changing its shape when dispersion is negligible in sampling tubing. A mean transit time $\bar{t}$ (s) is generally calculated, according to Eqn 6.14, as:

$$\bar{t} = \bar{t}_{\text{total}} - t_s = \frac{\sum_{j=1}^{n} (j\Delta t \cdot ih_j \, \Delta t) + ih_n e^{-b(0.5\Delta t)} / b^2}{ia} - t_s, \quad (6.15)$$

where *ia* is given by Eqn 6.13. As with the area calculation (Eqn 6.13), Hamilton's exponential extrapolation is used to correct for recirculation of indicator and incomplete recovery of the dose.

Similar to the mean transit time is a mean residence time t_b (s) based on the assumption that the system is a well-mixed compartment:

$$\bar{t}_b = \frac{1}{b}, \quad (6.16)$$

where b is the monoexponential downslope of the indicator dilution curve (Fig. 6.5). In contrast to a range of lengths of distinct pathways through the vascular and extravascular network of an organ, here, $\bar{t}_b$ represents the average of durations indicator is retained in the compartment due to a declining probability of exit as indicator concentration in the compartment falls. The compartment, representing extracellular and intracellular space, is of a size dependent on the type of indicator used and is fed by permeable capillaries. The fact that indicator curves end monoexponentially (Lassen and Perl, 1979) may indicate there is a well-mixed compartment within the system. Estimates of $\bar{t}_b$ are always smaller than the corresponding $\bar{t}$ from Eqn 6.15, even when corrected for the common large-vessel transit time that results in the delay between injection and first appearance of indicator at the venous sampling site (Goresky, 1963), because the latter term includes heterogeneous transit through non-exchanging vessels before and after the capillary.

Volume of distribution

There are two approaches to calculate distribution volume V (ml). The mean transit time method considers:

$$V_{\bar{t}} = F\bar{t}, \quad (6.17)$$

where $\bar{t}$ is calculated according to Eqn 6.15, and the compartmental assumption yields:

$$V_b = \frac{F}{b}. \quad (6.18)$$

$V_{\bar{t}}$ represents that part of the vascular bed included in the mean transit time (capillaries plus heterogeneous non-exchanging vessels) for vascular indicators, and the vascular bed plus extravascular space for extravascular indicators. Where b is obtained from the downslope of the indicator dilution curve and ignores the vascular time delay from artery to venous sampling site, V_b represents the volume of the extravascular system and is reliable only if that system behaves as a well-mixed compartment.

Multiple indicator/nutrient dilution models

The coefficients in the above section, calculated directly from indicator outflow curves, represent physiological properties of the system under study. However, one of the major purposes of the multiple indicator/nutrient dilution (MID) experiment, where more than one indicator plus a nutrient of interest may be injected simultaneously into the arterial inflow of an organ, is to measure rates of transport or sequestration of the nutrient. Physiological characteristics of the system leading to indicator dilution apply equally to the nutrient, so that the difference between nutrient and indicator dilution curves represents uptake. How, exactly, the uptake rates can be ascertained from this difference is the subject of several mathematical models. The single capillary where exchange of the nutrient occurs is the basic unit for most models. However, only whole system outflows are measured in the MID experiment. These whole system outflows reflect not only exchanges in capillaries but also dispersion along sampling tubes and non-exchanging blood vessels. Each model takes different account of the single capillary exchange and how the vasculature influences whole-organ outflow (Fig. 6.6).

Crone–Renkin model

Several investigators (Wählander *et al.*, 1993; Frisbee and Barclay, 1998; Farr *et al.*, 2000) have used the Crone–Renkin model (Renkin, 1959; Crone, 1963) of single capillary extraction to calculate the permeability of the target system to nutrients of interest. In these studies, a vascular indicator is injected simultaneously with an extracellular indicator that does not enter cells, such as ^{14}C-sucrose or ^{14}C-mannitol. The difference between the two indicator dilution curves (Fig. 6.4) is due to their different volumes of distribution and may contain information about the permeability of the capillary wall to the extracellular indicator. Concepts introduced in the derivation of the permeability model are useful for understanding other mathematical models developed for interpretation of MID data. Thus, they will be reviewed here in detail.

Figure 6.3 shows a single capillary as a Krogh cylinder of length 1.0. Consider, then, a thin disc within the cylinder of relative thickness dx. Mass balance of an extracellular indicator within this segment is as follows:

$$\text{in from arterial side} = \text{out to venous side} + \text{out through vessel wall}$$
$$F_{sc}h_{sc}(x) = F_{sc}h_{sc}(x+\mathrm{d}x) + PS_{sc}\mathrm{d}x \cdot h_{sc}(x), \tag{6.19}$$

where F_{sc} is the capillary blood flow (ml s^{-1}), $h_{sc}(x)$ is the normalized indicator concentration at point x in the capillary and PS_{sc} is the product of the permeability of the capillary wall to the extracellular indicator P (ml cm^{-2} s^{-1}) and the surface area of the wall S (cm^2). Thus, $PS_{sc}\mathrm{d}x$ is that fraction of the total permeability–surface area product that is available in dx. It is assumed that there is no flux of extracellular indicator back into the capillary once it has left. Also, it is assumed that there is no diffusion occurring along the length of the capillary. Given that the decline in nutrient concentration from one side of the

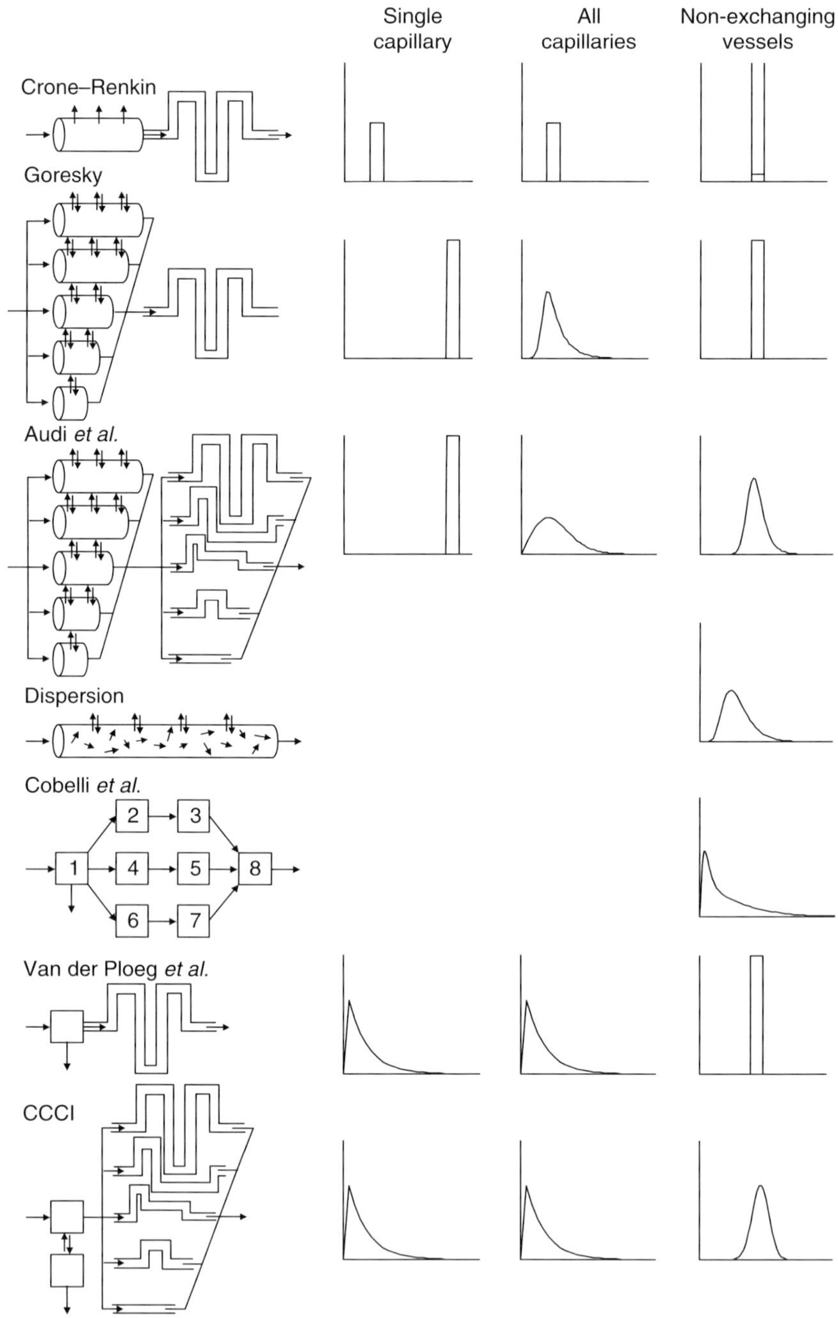

Fig. 6.6. Comparative illustration from Qiao *et al.* (2005a: used with permission) of alternative indicator dilution models showing simulated outflow of extracellular indicator from a single capillary, from all capillaries and from non-exchanging vessels of an organ after rectangular pulse input. Convolution of all capillaries with non-exchanging vessels generates the whole-organ outflow curve. CCCI, compartmental capillary, convolution integration.

disc to the other is $dh_{sc}(x) = h_{sc}(x + dx) - h_{sc}(x)$, Eqn 6.19 can be rearranged to:

$$\frac{dh_{sc}(x)}{dx} = -\frac{PS_{sc}}{F_{sc}} h_{sc}(x). \tag{6.20}$$

Equation 6.20 has the same theoretical origins as Eqn 6.6 for the steady-state, distributed-in-space model of nutrient extraction (Cant and McBride, 1995), except that disappearance through the capillary is described with a permeability coefficient instead of a first-order rate constant and the integrand is presented as a function of distance instead of time. Integrating in terms of x over the entire length of the capillary yields the normalized venous concentration:

$$h_{sc\_v} = h_a e^{-\frac{PS_{sc}}{F_{sc}}}. \tag{6.21}$$

On a timescale, one must consider the single capillary transit time t_{sc} (s) as a delay between entrance of the disc into the capillary and exit on the venous side to obtain:

$$h_{sc\_v}(t) = h_a(t - t_{sc})e^{-\frac{PS_{sc}}{F_{sc}}}. \tag{6.22}$$

For vascular indicators, $PS_{sc} = 0$ by definition, so $ih_{sc\_v}(t) = ih_a(t - t_{sc})$. Because both indicators start out at the same normalized concentration ($h_a = ih_a$), the venous concentration of the test extracellular indicator $h_{sc\_v}(t)$ is the proportion $e^{-PS_{sc}/F_{sc}}$ of the arterial input concentration of the reference vascular indicator $ih_a(t - t_{sc})$ or its associated venous concentration $ih_{sc\_v}(t)$, as illustrated in Fig. 6.7. In other words, the venous concentration of the vascular indicator is equal to what the extracellular indicator concentration was when it entered the capillary. Extraction in a single capillary, as introduced in Eqn 6.3, can thus be obtained from concentrations of the two indicators on the venous side of the capillary as:

$$E_{sc}(t) = \frac{ih_{sc\_v}(t) - h_{sc\_v}(t)}{ih_{sc\_v}(t)}, \tag{6.23}$$

which, according to Eqn 6.21, is also equal to:

$$E_{sc}(t) = 1.0 - e^{-\frac{PS_{sc}}{F_{sc}}}. \tag{6.24}$$

Thus, not unlike Eqn 6.9 for the steady-state model of Cant and McBride (1995), capillary permeability can be parameterized from an extraction measurement in the single capillary as:

$$PS_{sc} = -\ln(1 - E_{sc})F_{sc}, \tag{6.25}$$

where E_{sc} is written instead of $E_{sc}(t)$ because the proportion PS_{sc}/F_{sc} in Eqn 6.24 is constant for the duration of the experiment.

Obviously, E_{sc} and PS_{sc} cannot be calculated directly from indicator dilution curves (Fig. 6.4) because the concentrations in outflow from a single capillary, $ih_{sc\_v}(t)$ and $h_{sc\_v}(t)$, are unknown; only whole system outflows $h_v(t)$ and $ih_v(t)$ following a pulse dose are measured. Assuming all capillaries are identical, PS

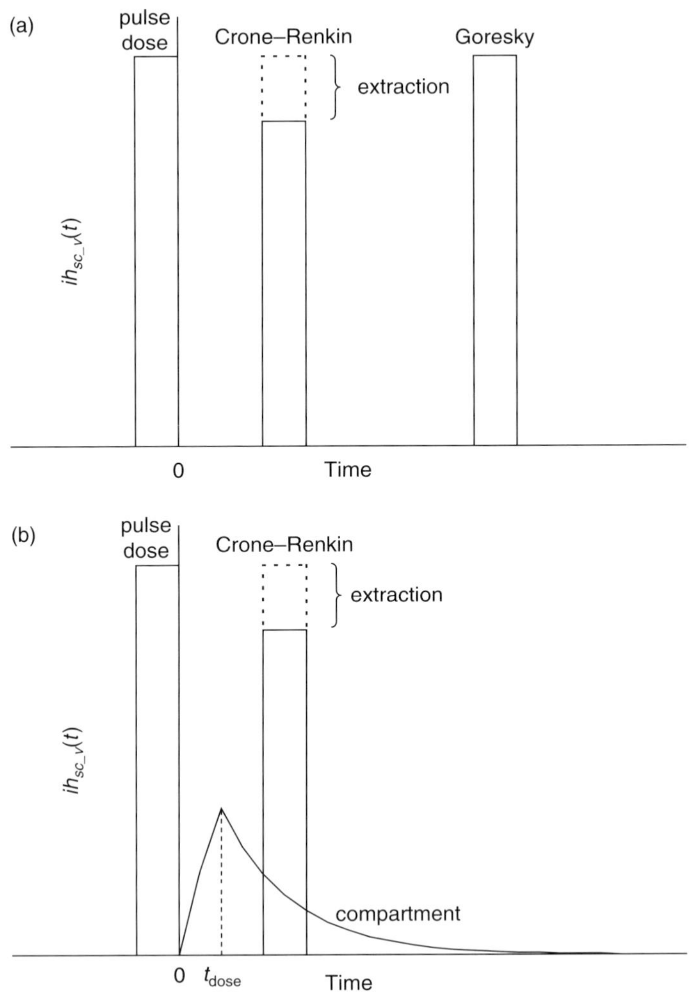

Fig. 6.7. Profile of extracellular indicator concentrations, $ih_{sc\_v}(t)$, in the outflow from a single capillary following rectangular pulse input of duration t_{dose} (s) according to the Crone–Renkin and Goresky models (a) or the Crone–Renkin and compartmental capillary models (b), from Qiao *et al.* (2005a: used with permission).

for the whole system is derived by multiplying both sides of Eqn 6.25 by the number of open capillaries in the system, so that:

$$PS = -\ln(1 - E_{sc})F, \tag{6.26}$$

where F is whole-organ blood flow rate. To use Eqn 6.26 to calculate PS, the E_{sc} term is approximated from observed vascular and extracellular indicator outflows from the entire system as:

$$E(t) = \frac{ih_v(t) - h_v(t)}{ih_v(t)}. \tag{6.27}$$

The assumption here is that both indicators exit from the single capillary at the same time, the extracellular one at a lower concentration due to extraction and, to produce the characteristic whole-tissue outflow curve over time, this venous labelled blood mixes with a proportion of unlabelled blood from capillaries that the pulse dose has not yet reached or has already passed. This proportion changes with time, eventually to the point that all venous blood is unlabelled. As long as both indicators are mixing with the same volumes of unlabelled blood, $E(t) = E_{sc}$.

Unfortunately, the $E(t)$ calculated from real ID curves is not constant across all time points and declines rapidly to below zero (Crone and Levitt, 1984). In practice, PS is calculated from E obtained as the mean of $E(t)$ only during the upslope of dilution curves, within the first few seconds of indicator appearance. The equality between $E(t)$ and E_{sc} is abrogated by washout of the extracellular indicator from the system. After the pulse dose of indicators has passed through the capillary, extracellular fluid is loaded with indicator molecules that will wash back into the venous outflow, which contains no reference vascular indicator, and thereby artificially reduces $E(t)$. In fact, washout does not wait for the dose to finish traversing the capillary, but will commence immediately on appearance of test indicator in the extracellular space. Thus, though the first few $E(t)$ values of paired indicator dilution curves may be constant, they underestimate unidirectional extraction due to indicator washout. The mass balance in the capillary (Eqn 6.19) ignores the concentration of indicator in the surrounding interstitium.

Maximum extraction (E_{max}) model

Yudilevich and colleagues adapted the Crone–Renkin model to estimate rates of unidirectional nutrient uptake by organs (Yudilevich *et al.*, 1979; Yudilevich and Mann, 1982). The difference between the Yudilevich and Crone–Renkin approaches is in the indicators. The reference is an extracellular indicator, such as ^{14}C-mannitol or ^{14}C-sucrose, instead of a vascular indicator. In addition, the nutrients of interest differ from the reference indicator in that they are sequestered by cells through metabolism, binding, storage or secretion. An equivalent of the PS product, calculated from the maximum extraction (E_{max}) of the injected nutrient relative to the extracellular indicator (Eqn 6.27), is used as a clearance parameter to estimate unidirectional uptake of nutrient as:

$$J = -\ln(1 - E_{\max})Fc_a(0), \qquad (6.28)$$

where $c_a(0)$ is the background arterial concentration of the target nutrient. This paired indicator/nutrient model suffers the same drawback as the Crone–Renkin model in that only a portion of the dilution curve is explained. The $E(t)$ of nutrient relative to extracellular indicator starts low, increases to a peak value and then decreases, and even becomes negative at the tail (Linehan and Dawson, 1979; Yudilevich and Mann, 1982; Calvert and Shennan, 1996). The $E(t)$ is influenced by factors such as heterogeneity of transit times and efflux from the intracellular space, in addition to the exchange rate of interest, so it is essentially arbitrary that E_{max} is assigned to represent unidirectional uptake. The E_{max} might be better considered an index of uptake that has been useful in identifying saturation kinetics from dilution curves obtained at different nutrient perfusion rates or evaluating inhibition and activation of transport (Yudilevich and Mann, 1982; Calvert and Shennan, 1996).

Goresky models

The Crone–Renkin models do not explain how an input curve of a few seconds or less is transformed to a whole-organ outflow dispersed over many seconds. Goresky (1963) introduced two elements into the modelling that allowed entire dilution curves to be described. The first was a consideration of extravascular spaces of the capillary supply zone and the second was a distribution of capillary transit times (Fig. 6.6).

The single capillary of Goresky (1963) is similar to that of the Crone–Renkin model, except that time and distance are considered simultaneously (Fig. 6.8), and both a vascular space A and an extravascular space B into which solutes can distribute are considered in order to predict indicator concentration at the venous end of a capillary of length L. Mass balance in the disc of thickness dx within vascular space A, assuming negligible longitudinal diffusion, is:

net added to A = in from arterial side – out to venous side – net out to B

$$V_{sc\_A}\frac{h_{sc\_A}(x,t+\mathrm{d}t)-h_{sc\_A}(x,t)}{\mathrm{d}t}=F_{sc}h_{sc\_A}(x-\mathrm{d}x,t)-F_{sc}h_{sc\_A}(x,t)-V_{sc\_B}\frac{h_{sc\_B}(x,t+\mathrm{d}t)-h_{sc\_B}(x,t)}{\mathrm{d}t} \tag{6.29}$$

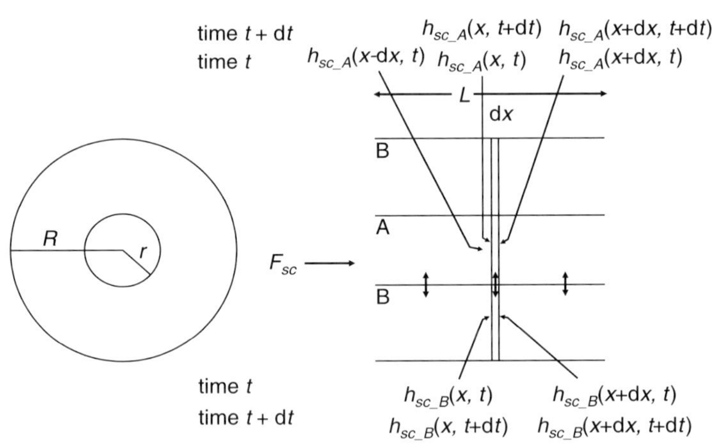

Fig. 6.8. Idealized cross-section of a capillary of radius r (space A) serving a cylinder of tissue of radius R (space B) and longitudinal section of that capillary where L is the length (cm), dx is a thin segment of that length (cm), F_{sc} is blood flow (ml s^{-1}), $h_{sc\_A}(x,t)$ represents the normalized indicator/nutrient concentration (μmol ml^{-1}) in space A at some point along the length x at time t and $h_{sc\_B}(x,t)$ represents the normalized concentration in space B at some point along the length x at time t (adapted from Goresky, 1963). This is the representation assumed in Goresky models.

where V_{sc_A} and V_{sc_B} represent the volumes (ml) of spaces A and B, respectively, $h_{sc\_A}(x,t)$ represents the normalized indicator/nutrient concentration (μmol ml^{-1}) in space A at some point along the length x at time t, $h_{sc\_B}(x,t)$ represents the normalized concentration in space B at some point along the length x at time t, and F_{sc} is capillary blood flow. Given $F_{sc} = V_{sc\_A}v_F/\mathrm{d}x$, where v_F is the velocity of blood flow in the capillary (cm s^{-1}), Eqn 6.30 becomes:

$$V_{sc\_A}\frac{h_{sc\_A}(x,t+\mathrm{d}t)-h_{sc\_A}(x,t)}{\mathrm{d}t} = -V_{sc\_A}v_F\frac{h_{sc\_A}(x,t)-h_{sc\_A}(x-\mathrm{d}x,t)}{\mathrm{d}x} - V_{sc\_B}\frac{h_{sc\_B}(x,t+\mathrm{d}t)-h_{sc\_B}(x,t)}{\mathrm{d}t} \quad (6.30)$$

Setting $\gamma = V_{sc\_B}/V_{sc\_A}$ yields the following partial differentials:

$$v_F\frac{\partial h_{sc\_A}(x,t)}{\partial x}+\frac{\partial h_{sc\_A}(x,t)}{\partial t}+\gamma\frac{\partial h_{sc\_B}(x,t)}{\partial t}=0 \quad (6.31)$$

Finally, assuming that lateral diffusion between vascular and extracellular spaces at any point along the capillary is instantaneous yields the following partial differentials for mass balance in a pulsed dose:

$$v_F\frac{\partial h_{sc\_A}(x,t)}{\partial x}+(1+\gamma)\frac{\partial h_{sc\_A}(x,t)}{\partial t}=0 \quad (6.32)$$

Goresky (1963) obtained the analytical solution to Eqn 6.32 for a capillary of length L (cm):

$$h_{sc\_v}(t) = h_a(t-[1+\gamma]L/v_F). \quad (6.33)$$

where $[1 + \gamma]L/v_F$ is the capillary transit time. For vascular indicators, $\gamma = 0$ and Eqn 6.33 becomes identical to Eqn 6.22 of the Crone–Renkin model, where $PS_{sc} = 0$ and $t_{sc} = L/v_F$. In contrast to the Crone–Renkin model, though, Eqn 6.33 indicates that extravascular indicators traverse the capillary with $1/(1 + \gamma)$ of the blood velocity v_F. Appearance at the venous end is delayed because of mixing between a non-convective extravascular space and a convective vascular space, but the shape and size of the outflow curve is unchanged from the input function because this mixing is instantaneous. The arterial input function $h_a(t)$ of injected dose can be assumed to be a rectangular pulse function of duration t_{dose} (s):

$$h_a(t) = \frac{1}{F\cdot t_{\mathrm{dose}}}p(t), \quad (6.34)$$

where:

$$p(t) = \begin{cases}1 & 0 < t \le t_{\mathrm{dose}}\\ 0 & \text{otherwise}\end{cases}. \quad (6.35)$$

Substituting Eqn 6.34 into Eqn 6.33 yields a capillary venous outflow:

$$h_{sc\_v}(x,t) = \frac{1}{F\cdot t_{\mathrm{dose}}}p(t-[1+\gamma]L/v_F) \quad (6.36)$$

which is depicted in Fig. 6.7. For vascular indicators, both the Goresky model and the Crone–Renkin model are the same in that the input function $ih_a(t)$ traverses a single capillary cylinder without changing its shape. In the Crone–Renkin model, the extracellular indicator exits the capillary at the same time as the vascular indicator, but at a reduced concentration due to extraction. In contrast, in the Goresky model, the concentration of the extracellular indicator in the outflow $h_{sc\_v}(t)$ is the same as in the input, but is delayed over the vascular indicator by a factor of $1 + \gamma$. This delay without changing shape is analogous to ideal flow of a retained solute through a chromatography column.

The dispersion of an arterial pulse dose of indicators into its venous concentration profile is a matter of transit time heterogeneity (Meier and Zierler, 1954). Goresky (1963) proposed that the heterogeneity of vascular indicator transit times was due to different lengths of capillaries (L) to yield a transit time distribution function $f(\tau)$ where $\tau = L/v_F$ (Fig. 6.6). The values of v_F, F_{sc} and γ were assumed to be identical for all capillaries. According to this formulation, when blood is sampled from the venous outflow of the organ, it contains a mixture of fractions originating from the venous outflows of capillaries of different lengths. Mathematically, the normalized indicator concentration flowing out of the whole organ is a convolution of the concentrations flowing out of each capillary (Eqn 6.36) and their respective transit times:

$$ih(t) = \int_0^t \frac{1}{F \cdot t_{\mathrm{dose}}} p(t - [1+\gamma]\tau) f(\tau) \mathrm{d}\tau, \tag{6.37}$$

where the term $f(\tau)d\tau$ represents the fraction of all single capillary transit times with values between τ and $\tau + \mathrm{d}\tau$.

A vascular indicator, for which $\gamma = 0$, provides the capillary transit time distribution function:

$$f(t) = F \cdot ih_{vas}(t + t_0) \tag{6.38}$$

where $ih_{vas}(t)$ is the normalized vascular indicator outflow profile and t_0 (s) is the large vessel transit time common to all pathways through the organ. With Eqn 6.38 and assuming an instantaneous t_{dose}, Goresky (1963) solved Eqn 6.37 to yield the final equation relating extravascular indicator concentrations to those of the vascular indicator:

$$ih(t) = \frac{1}{1+\gamma} ih_{vas}\left(\frac{t - t_0}{1+\gamma} + t_0\right). \tag{6.39}$$

Equation 6.39 predicts that the outflow profile of the extravascular indicator ($ih(t)$) superimposes on to that of the vascular indicator ($ih_{vas}(t)$) after multiplying concentration by $1 + \gamma$ and time of appearance by $1/(1 + \gamma)$. Superimposition is the basis of extracellular volume estimation (i.e. γ) from MID curves with the Goresky model.

The utility of the distributed-in-space model, first introduced by Goresky (1963), lies in its role in identifying the basic physiology of the interaction of an organ with its intravascular phase. For nutrients, more complicated mechanisms of transport and metabolism are involved beyond simple diffusion into extravascular space. An irreversible cellular uptake model (Goresky, 1964) and a barrier-limited transport model (Goresky *et al.*, 1973) were constructed by simply adding additional terms to the right side of Eqn 6.32. The transport and net removal of D-galactose by intact dog liver were investigated by rapid injection of ^{51}Cr-labelled erythrocytes, ^{14}C-labelled sucrose and ^{3}H-D-galactose simultaneously into the portal vein and, from rapidly sampled hepatic venous blood, normalized outflow-time patterns were obtained (Goresky *et al.*, 1973). Similar to the product of P and S that cannot be separated into its individual parameters in the Crone–Renkin model, four parameter products were estimated by fits of a barrier-limited transport model to the curves: an extracellular space ratio $p\gamma$, a cellular influx rate constant multiplied by the ratio of the cellular space to the total vascular + extracellular space outside cells $k_1\theta/(1 + p\gamma)$, a cellular efflux rate constant divided by the partition coefficient for galactose in cells k_2/f_u, and a sequestration constant divided by the partition coefficient for galactose in cells k_3/f_u. The capacity for galactose entry into cells was found to be 40 times that for sequestration by phosphorylation and, whereas the K_m for sequestration was less than 0.8 μmol ml^{-1}, that for entry was approximately 30 μmol ml^{-1}.

Alternative representations of the distribution of indicator transit times through the whole organ have been incorporated into the Krogh cylinder models. Goresky (1963) assigned all of the heterogeneity of transit times to characteristics of capillaries but later work (Goresky *et al.*, 1970; Rose and Goresky, 1976; Rose *et al.*, 1977) explored the consequences of assuming heterogeneity in non-exchanging vessels. In the extreme case of assigning all heterogeneity to the non-exchanging vessels, in which capillary transit time is a single value, the concentration profile of extracellular indicators in organ outflow was predicted to exhibit an identical shape to the vascular indicator profile (see Fig. 6.4) and be delayed in time only (Goresky *et al.*, 1970). Because such differences between extracellular and vascular indicators have not been observed, the hypothesis that non-exchanging vessels account for all of the heterogeneity in transit through an organ was rejected. However, indicator dilution curves across the heart were best fit with a distribution of non-exchanging vessel transit times, setting pathway length as a function of capillary transit time (Rose and Goresky, 1976). The majority of the heterogeneity, though, was again attributed to capillaries. It is important to note that both these conclusions about the magnitude of non-exchanging vessel heterogeneity were derived from the Krogh cylinder model, which has indicators exiting individual capillaries as pulse functions undispersed from those that enter (Fig. 6.7). Audi *et al.* (1994) described the distribution of capillary and non-exchanging vessel transit times as two separate curves, the convolution of which yields the whole-organ outflow (Fig. 6.6). Estimation of mean transit time, variance σ^2 and a third central moment or skewness m^3 for each curve, not unlike the lagged normal density function used by Bassingthwaighte *et al.* (1966), indicated that non-exchanging vessels accounted for approximately 27% of the dispersion of pulse-dosed extracellular indicators in isolated, perfused rabbit lung (Audi *et al.*, 1995).

Dispersion models

An alternative distributed-in-space model that has been used in studies of drug elimination in the liver is the dispersion model of Roberts and Rowland (1986). It is based on the hypothesis that a pulse dose of an extracellular indicator injected into the arterial supply of an organ will disperse, due to the heterogeneity of blood flow, into an inverse Gaussian distribution of concentrations in the collecting vein (Fig. 6.2). The single capillary is not explicitly represented. Exchange of injected nutrients between extracellular and intracellular spaces is represented with first-order rate constants to yield the following analytic solution in the Laplace domain for the profile of nutrient concentrations in the organ outflow (Yano *et al.*, 1989):

$$h_v(s) = \frac{q_0}{F}\exp\left[\frac{FV_e}{2D_c}\left\{1 - \sqrt{1 + \frac{4D_c}{F^2}\left(s + k_1 + k_3 - \frac{k_1 k_2}{s + k_2}\right)}\right\}\right], \tag{6.40}$$

where s is the Laplace operator, q_0 is the dose injected (μmol), V_e is the whole system extracellular volume (ml), D_c is the dispersion coefficient corrected for F and V_e, and k_1, k_2 and k_3 are rate constants (s^{-1}) for nutrient influx, efflux and sequestration, respectively. The five unknown parameters are estimated by non-linear fits of Eqn 6.40 to a single nutrient dilution curve without the use of any indicators (Yano *et al.*, 1989).

Tirona *et al.* (1998) fitted Eqn 6.40 to nutrient dilution curves across the rat liver and compared parameter estimates with those obtained from fits of the Goresky barrier-limited transport model to the same curves. Vascular and extracellular indicators had also been injected to obtain the volumes of distribution necessary for solution of the Goresky equations. Estimates of V_e and k_1 agreed well between the two models, but efflux and sequestration rate constants k_2 and k_3 differed considerably. The venous extracellular indicator profile predicted by the dispersion model deviated from the tail of the observed sucrose curve, indicating that the inverse Gaussian function was not an appropriate transit time distribution. The differences in tail fits between the two models were probably responsible for the differences in k_2 and k_3 estimates.

Compartmental capillary models

Cobelli *et al.* (1989) proposed a network of well-mixed compartments (Fig. 6.6) to account for the heterogeneity of transit times through an organ. Three parallel pairs of identical compartments between injection and sampling compartments were found to be adequate to fit the downslope of extracellular indicator and transportable substrate concentrations in the venous drainage of the human forearm. Each pathway from compartment 1 to 8 is essentially a series of first-order delays as pulse-dosed indicator molecules mix with unlabelled blood and washout, mix with the next compartment and washout, and so on. Uptake of nutrient is considered possible from the intermediate compartments only. The parallel pathways are a representation of the different routes indicator molecules may take as they proceed through an organ, but the compartments in series have no direct physiological corollary. The single capillary and non-exchanging vessels are not represented explicitly.

Van der Ploeg *et al.* (1995) used a single well-mixed compartment in series with a venous transit time delay (Fig. 6.6) to estimate O_2 distribution volumes in goat hearts from a step change in blood flow. Assuming multiple identical compartments in series to approximate Krogh cylinder behaviour, as in the Crone–Renkin model, yielded gross overestimates of coronary volume (Van der Ploeg *et al.*, 1995). It was concluded that the Krogh cylinder was an inappropriate model of coronary O_2 exchange. Distributing flow heterogeneously to nine parallel pathways, each consisting of a well-mixed compartment and transit time delay in series, yielded volume estimates that differed only 8–15% from those of the single pathway model.

Recently, we developed a compartmental capillary, convolution integration (CCCI) approach to model paired indicator/nutrient dilution curves (Qiao *et al.*, 2005a) by adapting ideas from previous models of nutrient exchange across organs. The indicator is extracellular, as in the Yudilevich *et al.* (1979) adaptation of the Crone–Renkin model, but a split of the heterogeneity of transit times between exchanging and non-exchanging vessels, as implemented by Audi *et al.* (1995), is assumed. However, instead of interpreting the capillary transit function from a distributed-in-space model of the single capillary, the well-mixed compartment of Van der Ploeg *et al.* (1995) is used. Audi *et al.* (1995) indicated that capillary dispersion modelled by a single exponential decay, which is characteristic of the well-mixed compartment, was consistent with observations of the capillary transit time function in isolated rabbit lungs. Capillaries in many tissues form close-knit networks (Prosser *et al.*, 1996), which cause extensive mixing of the fluid elements and where multiple capillaries may be draining a common extracellular space (Wang and Bassingthwaighte, 2001). The steady-state model of Hanigan *et al.* (1998; Fig. 6.2) considered the capillary and its surrounding fluid as a well-mixed compartment and the same simplification was appropriate for non-steady-state modelling of O_2 exchange in goat hearts (Van der Ploeg *et al.*, 1995). With the capillary transit function simulated by washout from a compartmental model, the remaining transit time heterogeneity is assigned to non-exchanging vessels before and after the capillary. A convolution integral is implemented to integrate from identical single capillary outflow profiles to the whole system outflow according to this heterogeneity of transit times in non-exchanging vessels.

In the CCCI model, it is assumed that, upon reaching the capillary, indicators and nutrients instantaneously mix with the extracellular space it serves. Nutrient is transported across a barrier into the intracellular space from which it can also exit. The extracellular space and intracellular space are treated as two well-mixed compartments (Fig. 6.9). Because the model was designed for numerical solution, assumptions to simplify analytical solution were not required, such as an instantaneous dose or normalized concentrations. Thus, the model can be applied to a nutrient that already exists in circulation and there is no need for a labelled solute. The mechanisms of indicator or nutrient movement within the single capillary can be expressed in ordinary differential equations. A general description of the single compartmental capillary model is:

$$\frac{dc_{sc\_v}(t)}{dt} = [(c_a(t) - c_{sc\_v}(t))F - j_1(t) + j_2(t)]\frac{1}{V_e}, \tag{6.41}$$

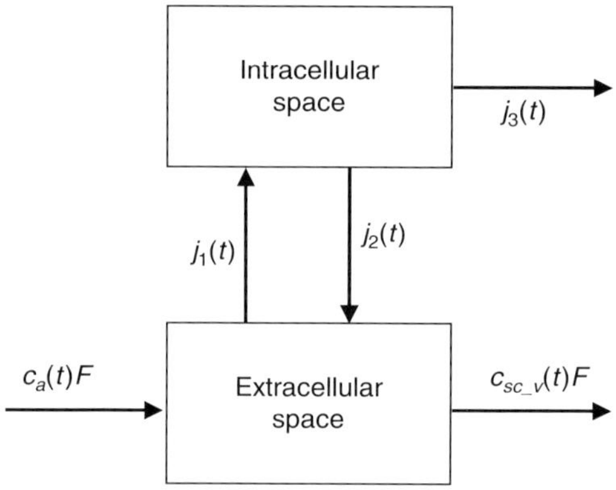

Fig. 6.9. Diagrammatic representation of the single capillary submodel of the compartmental capillary, convolution integration (CCCI) model where F represents blood flow (ml s^{-1}) through the system, c_a (Eqn 6.43) and c_{sc_v} are arterial and venous concentrations (μmol ml^{-1}), respectively, of a solute and j_1, j_2 and j_3 represent the influx, efflux and metabolism rates (μmol s^{-1}), respectively.

and:

$$\frac{dc_{sc\_c}(t)}{dt} = [j_1(t) - j_2(t) - j_3(t)]\frac{1}{V_c}, \tag{6.42}$$

where V_e is the extracellular volume (ml) of the organ, V_c is the intracellular volume (ml), c_{sc_c} is the intracellular concentration (μmol ml^{-1}), and j_1, j_2 and j_3 represent the influx, efflux and metabolism rates (μmol s^{-1}), respectively.

The input arterial function, $c_a(t)$, is based on a rectangular pulse dose (Eqn 6.35):

$$c_a(t) = \frac{q_0}{Ft_{dose}}p(t) + c_a(0), \tag{6.43}$$

where q_0 is the dose injected, and $c_a(0)$ is the background arterial concentration. If only the extracellular indicator is of interest, $j_1 = j_2 = j_3 = 0$, so that Eqn 6.42 is ignored and Eqn 6.41 has the analytical solution:

$$c_{sc\_v}(t) = \begin{cases} \dfrac{q_0}{F \cdot t_{dose}}(1 - e^{-\frac{F}{V_e}t}) & 0 < t \le t_{dose} \\ \dfrac{q_0}{F \cdot t_{dose}}(1 - e^{-\frac{F}{V_e}t_{dose}})e^{-\frac{F}{V_e}(t - t_{dose})} & \text{otherwise} \end{cases}. \tag{6.44}$$

Figure 6.7 compares indicator venous outflows from a single capillary simulated by the Crone–Renkin model and the well-mixed compartmental model. The indicator reaches peak concentration at t_{dose}. How fast it is washed out of the capillary distribution space is positively related with F and negatively related with V_e (Eqn 6.44).

The Gaussian, or normal distribution, function is used to describe the density distribution of vascular transit times as:

$$f(t) = \frac{1}{\sqrt{2\pi}\sigma}e^{-\frac{(t - \bar{t}_\mu)^2}{2\sigma^2}}, \tag{6.45}$$

where $\bar{t}_\mu$ represents the mean of transit times ascribed to the non-exchanging blood vessels before and after the capillary, which includes a common large vessel transit time, and σ represents standard deviation of the mean. Both indicator and nutrient share the same non-exchanging vessel pathways, described by $f(t)$. The entire system outflow profile is the convolutionary accumulation of each single capillary outflow in these different delays as:

$$c_v(t) = \int_0^t c_{sc\_v}(t-\tau)f(\tau)\mathrm{d}\tau. \tag{6.46}$$

To fit experimental data from paired indicator/nutrient dilution curves, the parameters F and V_e can be calculated directly from the indicator curve according to Eqns 6.11 and 6.18, respectively. Then, to estimate t_μ and σ of the non-exchanging vessel transit time function, Eqns 6.41, 6.45 and 6.46 can be simulated numerically with an iterative algorithm (e.g. Levenberg–Marquardt) for narrowing in on the lowest residual sum of squares between predicted and observed indicator concentrations $ic_v(t)$. To solve Eqn 6.46, at each increment of simulated time, c_{sc_v} and the area under the $f(t)$ function $\int f(n)$, can be placed in respective arrays and multiplied:

$$c_v(t) = \begin{bmatrix} c_{sc\_v}(1) & 0 & . & . & . & . & 0 \\ c_{sc\_v}(2) & c_{sc\_v}(1) & 0 & . & . & . & 0 \\ c_{sc\_v}(3) & c_{sc\_v}(2) & c_{sc\_v}(1) & 0 & . & . & 0 \\ . & . & . & . & . & . & 0 \\ . & . & . & . & . & . & 0 \\ . & . & . & . & . & . & 0 \\ c_{sc\_v}(n) & c_{sc\_v}(n-1) & c_{sc\_v}(n-2) & . & . & . & c_{sc\_v}(1) \end{bmatrix} \begin{bmatrix} \int_0^1 f(1) \\ \int_1^2 f(2) \\ \int_2^3 f(3) \\ . \\ . \\ . \\ \int_{n-1}^n f(n) \end{bmatrix}, \tag{6.47}$$

where n is the number of integration intervals. To estimate parameters of the j_1, j_2 and j_3 nutrient fluxes, Eqns 6.41, 6.42, 6.45 and 6.46 are simulated, using F, V_e, t_μ and σ from fits to the associated extracellular indicator curve, to find the lowest residual sum of squares between predicted and observed nutrient concentrations $c_v(t)$.

Because the single capillary model is compartmental and distinct from the transit time function, it can be easily modified to include or exclude various hypothetical compartments and exchange or transformation routes. Four candidate submodels of glucose exchange within the single capillary of the mammary glands of lactating cows were evaluated for their ability to describe venous glucose dilution curves following rapid injection of para-aminohippuric acid plus glucose into the external iliac artery (Qiao *et al.*, 2005b). The submodels differed in how fluxes j_1, j_2 and j_3 were described, e.g. with zero-, first-order or Michaelis–Menten equations. Combining extracellular and intracellular space into one compartment was superior to considering an exchange parameter between the two spaces in its goodness-of-fit to glucose dilution curves and identifiability of parameters. The rapidity of exchange relative to sequestration is similar to the findings, previously discussed, of Goresky *et al.* (1973) for galactose dilution across the liver of dogs. Michaelis–Menten parameters of mammary glucose sequestration were not identifiable (Qiao *et al.*, 2005b). Glucose sequestration followed first-order kinetics between 0 and 7 μmol ml^{-1} extracellular glucose with an average rate constant of 0.006 s^{-1} or a clearance of 44 ml s^{-1}. The ratio of intracellular glucose distribution space to extracellular indicator distribution space was 0.34, which was considerably lower than the expected intracellular volume and suggested, in agreement with the *in vitro* results of Xiao *et al.* (2004), the existence of an intracellular occlusion compartment with which extracellular glucose rapidly exchanges. This example highlights how the modelling can illuminate mechanisms that might conventionally only be probed *in vitro*, yet the parameters describing the processes are relevant to the intact organ in the live animal and, therefore, possess greater utility for understanding whole-animal function.

Conclusion

Steady-state models of nutrient exchange across organs that are major nutrient users and transformers, such as the gut, liver, muscle and mammary glands, yield equations that are simple to apply in order to generate useful biological information from data. However, the steady-state paradigm itself is limited in scope and is not easily harnessed to the parameterization of kinetics of nutrient transport and metabolism. More complex models have been developed to interpret the non-steady states of nutrient dilution across an organ using one or more indicators to assist in the parameterization. The MID experiment is easy to perform if the arterial supply of the organ can be catheterized. However, the challenge is in the mathematical modelling of the data afterwards. Past practice in MID modelling has been to find analytical solutions to the models, which has tended to blanket them in obscurity to the experimenter and may be one reason why the technique, though powerful in its ability to yield parameters relevant to metabolism *in vivo*, has been little used in the nutritional sciences. We have described here a new CCCI model that may be solved numerically using readily available simulation software and which treats the site of nutrient exchange in an organ as a compartmental submodel that may be easily customized to the idiosyncratic flows of the nutrient under study according to the familiar rate:state formalism. This model is also complete in that it considers the heterogeneity of transit times through the organ so that the entire venous dilution curve is accounted for. Simulation of the non-steady state of nutrient exchange appears to be a fruitful field for the modeller, as well as for the experimenter interested in the behaviour of intact organs within animals.

Considerations when selecting a model for use include its tractability to the user, whether underlying assumptions hold (e.g. that indicator washout from the extracellular space is negligible for the Crone–Renkin models, t_{dose} is instantaneous for the Goresky models, or the extracellular space is a well-mixed compartment for the CCCI model), the utility of resulting parameters to the research problem and how well predictions fit with observations. This review of the underpinnings of several alternative models of MID provides the reader with a starting point to explore the models further.

References

Audi, S.H., Krenz, G.S., Linehan, J.H., Rickaby, D.A. and Dawson, C.A. (1994) Pulmonary capillary transport function from flow-limited indicators. *Journal of Applied Physiology* 77, 332–351.

Audi, S.H., Linehan, J.H., Krenz, G.S., Dawson, C.A., Ahlf, S.B. and Roerig, D.L. (1995) Estimation of the pulmonary capillary transport function in isolated rabbit lungs. *Journal of Applied Physiology* 78, 1004–1014.

Baron, A.D., Steinberg, H., Brechtel, G. and Johnson, A. (1994) Skeletal muscle blood flow independently modulates insulin-mediated glucose uptake. *American Journal of Physiology* 266, E248–E253.

Bassingthwaighte, J.B., Ackerman, F.H. and Wood, E.H. (1966) Application of the lagged normal density curve as a model for arterial dilution curves. *Circulation Research* 18, 398–415.

Biolo, G., Chinkes, D., Zhang, X.-J. and Wolfe, R.R. (1992) A new model to determine *in vivo* the relationship between amino acid transmembrane transport and protein kinetics in muscle. *Journal of Parenteral and Enteral Nutrition* 16, 305–315.

Calvert, D.T. and Shennan, D.B. (1996) Evidence for an interaction between cationic and neutral amino acids at the blood-facing aspect of the lactating mammary epithelium. *Journal of Dairy Research* 63, 25–33.

Cant, J.P. and McBride, B.W. (1995) Mathematical analysis of the relationship between blood flow and uptake of nutrients in the mammary glands of a lactating cow. *Journal of Dairy Research* 62, 405–422.

Cant, J.P., DePeters, E.J. and Baldwin, R.L. (1993) Mammary amino acid utilization in dairy cows fed fat and its relationship to milk protein depression. *Journal of Dairy Science* 76, 762–774.

Cant, J.P., Trout, D.R., Qiao, F. and Purdie, N.G. (2002) Milk synthetic response of the bovine mammary gland to an increase in the local concentration of arterial glucose. *Journal of Dairy Science* 85, 494–503.

Cant, J.P., Berthiaume, R., Lapierre, H., Luimes, P.H., McBride, B.W. and Pacheco, D. (2003) Responses of the bovine mammary glands to absorptive supply of single amino acids. *Canadian Journal of Animal Science* 83, 341–355.

Carter, P. and Welbourne, T. (1997) Glutamate transport regulation of renal glutaminase flux *in vivo*. *American Journal of Physiology* 273, E521–E527.

Cheng, K.N., Dworzak, F., Ford, G.C., Rennie, M.J. and Halliday, D. (1985) Direct determination of leucine metabolism and protein breakdown in humans using L-[1-13C, 15N]-leucine and the forearm model. *European Journal of Clinical Investigation* 15, 349–354.

Cobelli, C., Saccomani, M.P., Ferrannini, E., Defronzo, R.A., Gelfand, R. and Bonadonna, R. (1989) A compartmental model to quantitate *in vivo* glucose transport in the human forearm. *American Journal of Physiology* 257, E943–E958.

Crone, C. (1963) The permeability of capillary in various organs as determined by use of the 'indicator diffusion' method. *Acta Physiologica Scandinavica* 58, 292–305.

Crone, C. and Levitt, D.G. (1984) Capillary permeability to small solutes. In: Renkin, E.M. and Michel, C.C. (eds) *Handbook of Physiology, Section 2, The Cardiovascular System*. American Physiological Society, Bethesda, Maryland, pp. 411–466.

Dupuis, J., Goresky, C.A., Rouleau, J.L., Bach, G.G., Simard, A. and Schwab, A.J. (1996) Kinetics of pulmonary uptake of serotonin during exercise in dogs. *Journal of Applied Physiology* 80, 30–46.

Farr, V.C., Prosser, C.G. and Davis, S.R. (2000) Effects of mammary engorgement and feed withdrawal on microvascular function in lactating goat mammary glands. *American Journal of Physiology* 279, H1813–H1818.

France, J., Bequette, B.J., Lobley, G.E., Metcalf, J.A., Wray-Cahen, D., Dhanoa, M.S., Backwell, F.R.C., Hanigan, M.D., MacRae, J.C. and Beever, D.E. (1995) An isotope dilution model for partitioning leucine uptake by the bovine mammary gland. *Journal of Theoretical Biology* 172, 369–377.

Frisbee, J.C. and Barclay, J.K. (1998) Microvascular hematocrit and permeability – surface area product in contracting canine skeletal muscle *in situ*. *Microvascular Research* 55, 153–164.

Goresky, C.A. (1963) A linear method for determining liver sinusoidal and extravascular volumes. *American Journal of Physiology* 204, 626–640.

Goresky, C.A. (1964) Initial distribution and rate of uptake of sulfobromophthalein in the liver. *American Journal of Physiology* 207, 13–26.

Goresky, C.A., Ziegler, W.H. and Bach, G.G. (1970) Capillary exchange modelling. Barrier-limited and flow-limited distribution. *Circulation Research* 27, 739–764.

Goresky, C.A., Bach, G.G. and Nadeau, B.E. (1973) On the uptake of materials by the intact liver. The transport and net removal of galactose. *Journal of Clinical Investigations* 52, 991–1009.

Hamilton, W., Moore, J., Kinsman, J. and Spurling. R. (1928) Simultaneous determination of the pulmonary and systemic circulation times in man and of a figure related to cardiac output. *American Journal of Physiology* 84, 338–344.

Hanigan, M.D., France, J., Wray-Cahen, D., Beever, D.E., Lobley, G.E., Reutzel, L. and Smith, N.E. (1998) Alternative models for analyses of liver and mammary transorgan metabolite extraction data. *British Journal of Nutrition* 79, 63–78.

Kristensen, N.B., Danfær, A., Tetens, V, and Agergaard. N. (1996) Portal recovery of intraruminally infused short-chain fatty acids in sheep. *Acta Agricultura Scandinavica* 46A, 26–38.

Lassen, N. and Perl, W. (1979) *Tracer Kinetic Methods in Medical Physiology*. Raven Press, New York.

Linehan, J.H. and Dawson, C.A. (1979) A kinetic model of prostaglandin metabolism in the lung. *Journal of Applied Physiology* 47, 404–411.

Linzell, J.L. (1960) Valvular incompetence in the venous drainage of the udder. *Journal of Physiology* 153, 481–491.

Linzell, J.L. (1966) Measurement of venous flow by continuous thermodilution and its application to measurement of mammary blood flow in the goat. *Circulation Research* 18, 745–754.

Meier, P. and Zierler, K.L. (1954) On the theory of the indicator–dilution method for measurement of blood flow and volume. *Journal of Applied Physiology* 6, 731–744.

Prosser, C.G., Davis, S.R., Farr, V.C. and Lacasse, P. (1996) Regulation of blood flow in the mammary microvasculature. *Journal of Dairy Science* 79, 1184–1197.

Qiao, F., Trout, D.R., Quinton, V.M. and Cant, J.P. (2005a) A compartmental capillary, convolution integration model to investigate nutrient transport and metabolism *in vivo* from paired indicator/nutrient dilution curves. *Journal of Applied Physiology* 99, 788–798.

Qiao, F., Trout, D.R., Xiao, C. and Cant, J.P. (2005b) Kinetics of glucose transport and sequestration in lactating bovine mammary glands measured *in vivo* with a paired indicator/nutrient dilution technique. *Journal of Applied Physiology* 99, 799–806.

Renkin, E.M. (1959) Transport of potassium-42 from blood to tissue in isolated mammalian skeletal muscles. *American Journal of Physiology* 197, 1205–1210.

Roberts, M.S. and Rowland, M. (1986) A dispersion model of hepatic elimination: 1. Formulation of the model and bolus considerations. *Journal of Pharmacokinetics and Biopharmaceutics* 14, 227–260.

Rose, C.P. and Goresky, C.A. (1976) Vasomotor control of capillary transit time heterogeneity in the canine coronary circulation. *Circulation Research* 39, 541–554.

Rose, C.P., Goresky, C.A. and Bach, G.G. (1977) The capillary and sarcolemmal barriers in the heart. An exploration of labeled water permeability. *Circulation Research* 41, 515–533.

Schwab, A.J., Tao, L., Yoshimura, T., Simard, A., Barker, F. and Pang, K.S. (2001) Hepatic uptake and metabolism of benzoate: a multiple indicator dilution, perfused rat liver study. *American Journal of Physiology* 280, G1124–G1136.

Thivierge, M.C., Petitclerc, D., Bernier, J.F., Couture, Y. and Lapierre, H. (2000) External pudic venous reflux into the mammary vein in lactating dairy cows. *Journal of Dairy Science* 83, 2230–2238.

Tirona, R.G., Schwab, A.J., Geng, W. and Pang, K.S. (1998) Comparison of the dispersion and Goresky models in outflow profiles from multiple indicator dilution rat liver studies. *Drug Metabolism and Disposition* 26, 465–475.

Van der Ploeg, C.P.B., Dankelman, J., Stassen, H.G. and Spaan, J.A.E. (1995) Comparison of different oxygen exchange models. *Medical and Biological Engineering and Computing* 33, 661–668.

Wählander, H., Friberg, P. and Haraldsson, B. (1993) Capillary diffusion capacity for Cr-EDTA and cyanocobalamine in spontaneously beating rat hearts. *Acta Physiologica Scandinavica* 147, 37–47.

Wang, C.Y. and Bassingthwaighte, J.B. (2001) Capillary supply regions. *Mathematical Biosciences* 173, 103–114.

Xiao, C., Quinton, V.M. and Cant, J.P. (2004) Description of glucose transport in isolated bovine mammary epithelial cells by a three-compartment model. *American Journal of Physiology* 286, C792–C797.

Yano, Y., Yamaoka, K., Aoyama, Y. and Tanaka, H. (1989) Two-compartment dispersion model for analysis of organ perfusion system of drugs by fast inverse Laplace transform (FILT). *Journal of Pharmacokinetics and Biopharmaceutics* 17, 179–202.

Yudilevich, D.L. and Mann, G.E. (1982) Unidirectional uptake of substrates at the blood side of secretory epithelia: stomach, salivary gland, pancreas. *Federation Proceedings* 41, 3045–3053.

Yudilevich, D.L., Eaton, B.M., Short, A.H. and Leichtweiss, H.P. (1979) Glucose carriers at maternal and fetal sides of the trophoblast in guinea pig placenta. *American Journal of Physiology* 237, C205–C212.

Zierler, K.L. (1961) Theory of the use of arteriovenous differences for measuring metabolism in steady and non-steady states. *Journal of Clinical Investigations* 40, 2111–2125.

7 Modelling Protozoal Metabolism and Volatile Fatty Acid Production in the Rumen

J. Dijkstra,[1] E. Kebreab,[2,3] J. France[3] and A. Bannink[4]

[1]Animal Nutrition Group, Wageningen Institute of Animal Sciences, Wageningen University, The Netherlands; [2]National Centre for Livestock and Environment, Department of Animal Science, University of Manitoba, Canada; [3]Centre for Nutrition Modelling, Department of Animal and Poultry Science, University of Guelph, Canada; [4]Division Nutrition and Food, Animal Sciences Group, Wageningen University Research Centre, The Netherlands

Introduction

The reticulo-rumen (hereafter, rumen) of ruminants harbours microorganisms that are capable of digesting fibrous materials and are not susceptible to attack by ruminant enzymes. This allows ruminants to partly digest plants, such as grass, which have a high fibre content and low nutritional value for simple-stomached animals. Rumen microorganisms ferment a portion of the ingested material, while the other portion of the ingested material is passed on to the omasum and, subsequently, abomasum. Most of the rumen microbes, predominantly bacteria (10^9–10^{11} ml^{-1}), protozoa (10^4–10^6 ml^{-1}) and fungi (fungal zoospores density 10^3–10^5 ml^{-1}), are obligate anaerobes. Species diversity and activity of the microbial population varies according to changing dietary conditions, and numerous interactions between microbes exist (Dehority, 2003). The products of microbial activities in the rumen constitute the principal food of the host. These products are the fermentation acids (volatile fatty acids, VFA) absorbed mainly from the rumen and the microbial cells (particularly protein, but also polysaccharides and lipids) passing from the rumen and digested in the intestine.

As qualitative knowledge of rumen fermentation processes increased, it became possible to develop quantitative approaches to increase our understanding further (Dijkstra *et al.*, 2005a). To date, several models of whole rumen function have been developed which integrate knowledge on various aspects of the processes in the rumen. These models do not necessarily share common objectives (for a history of rumen models, see Dijkstra and Bannink, 2000). The evaluation of models generally depends on an appraisal of the total effort in relation to the objectives of the modelling exercise (Thornley and France, 2007). This chapter does not intend to compare several rumen models because other papers have already described comparative aspects on, for example, whole rumen function (Offner and Sauvant, 2004), diet-specific input parameters (Bannink *et al.*, 1997b) and microbial protein synthesis (Dijkstra *et al.*, 1998a). The aim of this chapter is to describe two key aspects in the supply of absorbed nutrients: (i) the quantitative representation of protozoal metabolism; and (ii) the quantitative representation of VFA production in the rumen.

Rumen Protozoa

The role of rumen protozoa in the rumen fermentation processes has been the subject of much debate, and our knowledge of rumen protozoa and their function is limited compared with that of rumen bacteria. The contribution of protozoa to total rumen microbial biomass may equal that of bacteria, suggesting that there may be an important role of protozoa in ruminal fermentation processes. Yet, in numerous defaunation experiments, their presence has been demonstrated to be non-essential for the ruminant (Williams and Coleman, 1997). Most protozoa feed predominantly on smaller microorganisms, particularly bacteria. Bacterial protein breakdown in the rumen is significantly reduced upon removal of protozoa (Sharp *et al.*, 1994). The modifications brought about as a result of defaunation are generally large, but not systematic (review Eugène *et al.*, 2004). Although there is considerable basic knowledge of protozoal metabolism, *in vivo* data on the roles of protozoa within the rumen and on dietary factors affecting protozoal metabolism are scarce. The limited knowledge about protozoal metabolism is mostly because of their dependence on live bacteria, which confounds their *in vitro* culture results (Dehority, 2003). A requirement for live bacteria appears to be manifested in particular in culture periods longer than 2–4 days. The protozoal dependency on live bacteria may be partly, but not completely, related to a nutritive bacterial contribution to protozoal metabolism (Fondevila and Dehority, 2001). Results of biochemical, cultural and microscopic studies indicate that the overall contribution of protozoa to rumen fermentation processes depends on the complex interactions between protozoa, bacteria and dietary characteristics (Jouany, 1989). Thus, attempts to explain the non-systematic modifications resulting from removal of protozoa should include these relationships. An increased understanding of interactions between several components of a biological system needs an integrative approach. Such an integrative approach, with the aim to increase understanding of interactions between several components of a biological system, is possible through mathematical representation of the processes involved as a series of non-linear differential equations. However, the explicit representation of protozoal metabolism within mathematical models of rumen fermentation has received only limited attention (Dijkstra *et al.*, 1998a).

Protozoal metabolism model

Dijkstra (1994) developed a mechanistic rumen model that incorporated specific aspects of rumen protozoa, including predation of microorganisms and autolysis of protozoa. A full description of the model and derivation of parameter values has been given previously (Dijkstra *et al.*, 1992; Dijkstra, 1994). A simplified diagram of the model and the fluxes representing recycling of microbial N due to protozoal metabolism is given in Fig. 7.1. The model comprises 19 state variables. These state variables relate to the carbohydrate entities (rumen degradable and undegradable fibre, starch and mono- or disaccharides derived from hydrolysis of fibre, starch and sugars), nitrogen-containing entities (rumen degradable and undegradable protein and ammonia), fatty acid-containing entities (lipid and VFA) and microbial entities (amylolytic bacteria, fibrolytic bacteria and protozoa). General protozoal characteristics, which differ from bacterial characteristics and have been represented in the model, include: engulfment of starch to form storage polysaccharides; no utilization of ammonia to synthesize amino acids *de novo*; preference for insoluble over soluble protein as an N source; engulfment and digestion of bacteria and protozoa; relatively low maximum growth rates; selective retention within the rumen; and death and subsequent lysis related to nutrient availability. The majority of the transaction kinetics are described using standard expressions from enzyme kinetics (Michaelis–Menten equations). The model is driven by continuous inputs of nutrients (calculated from the amount of feed fed and the chemical composition of the diet, including estimates of solubility, degradability and digestion turnover times of feed components) and by fractional outflow rates of fluid and solid phases from the rumen, as well as rumen

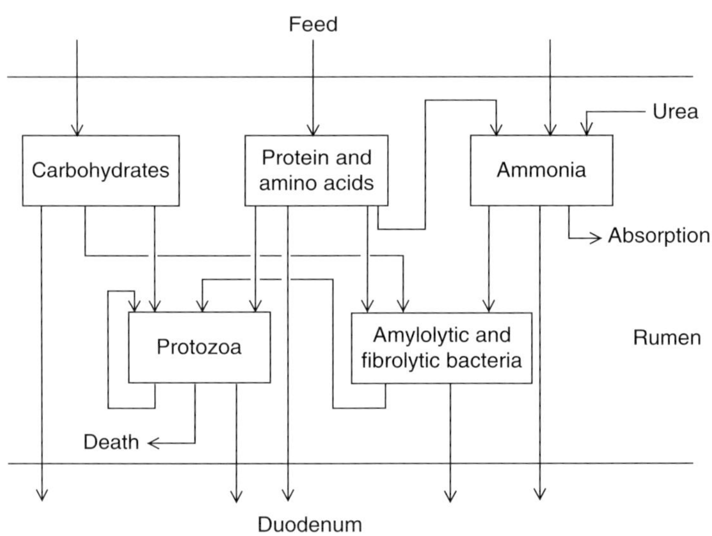

Fig. 7.1. Simplified diagrammatic representation of the rumen protozoa model (adapted from Dijkstra *et al.*, 1998b). Boxes enclosed by solid lines indicate aggregated state variables and arrows indicate fluxes.

fluid pH. The computer program was written in the simulation language ACSL and the model was solved by integration of 19 state variables with a fourth-order Runge–Kutta method.

The uptake of bacteria and protozoa by other protozoa and the death and subsequent lysis of protozoa related to nutrient availability are key elements in the structural stability of the model and will therefore be described in more detail. A general condition for stable coexistence is that the number of nutrients, having rate-limiting effects on the competitors, equals or exceeds the number of populations in the system (De Freitas and Fredrickson, 1978). For the present model, in most dietary situations, energy substrates would limit growth, while N substrates would affect microbial growth at relatively low N availability only. Since two major pools of energy substrates (amylolytic and fibrolytic hexose) are included in the present model, only two microbial groups are expected to coexist. Therefore, in the present model: (i) uptake of microorganisms by protozoa; and (ii) protozoal death rate related to build-up of fermentation end products within protozoa, were included to obtain biologically realistic coexistence of the populations. Analogous to the stabilizing effect of production of specific autoinhibitors on the coexistence of populations (De Freitas and Fredrickson, 1978), this representation of protozoal metabolism and interactions with bacteria allowed stable coexistence under a wide range of dietary inputs. Similarly, a chemostat model of four substrates and three functional classes of microbes in the rumen (amylolytic and fibrolytic bacteria and protozoa), in which a number of parameter values described by Dijkstra (1994) were adopted, showed a wide range of dietary situations for which all three populations coexisted (Witten and Richardson, 2003). Uptake of prey by predators (here, bacteria and protozoa, respectively) has often been described by Lotka–Volterra equations. However, the application of these equations to predator–prey systems has been questioned because of the biologically unrealistic results (Bazin, 1981) and the structural instability of the model (Brown and Rothery, 1993). In the present model, uptake of bacteria and protozoa is represented by Michaelis–Menten equations similar to the rectangular hyperbola proposed by Holling (1959) to represent predation rate, with parameters described previously (Dijkstra *et al.*, 1992):

$$U_{Mi,MiPo} = v_{MiPo}\, Q_{Po} \,/\, (1 + M_{Mi,MiPo}/C_{Mi}), \tag{7.1}$$

where $U_{Mi,MiPo}$ (g day^{-1}) is the engulfment of microorganisms (Mi; includes amylolytic and fibrolytic bacteria and protozoa), v_{MiPo} (g Mi g^{-1} Po day^{-1}) is the velocity of uptake of Mi by protozoa (Po), Q_{Po} (g) is the amount of protozoa, $M_{Mi,MiPo}$ (g l^{-1}) is the affinity constant for engulfment of Mi, and C_{Mi} (g l^{-1}) is the concentration of Mi in rumen contents.

The representation in Eqn 7.1 assumes that, at low concentrations of microbes, protozoa would search thoroughly to secure an adequate uptake of microbial matter, whereas, at high microbial concentrations, protozoa would reduce their search efforts because of satiation. On a wide range of predator species, the rectangular hyperbola has been found to provide a good fit to experimental data (Brown and Rothery, 1993). Amylolytic and fibrolytic bacteria were considered to be engulfed in the proportion in which they were present. This is based on experimental observations which indicate that, although selective engulfment of bacteria by some protozoal species might occur, no consistent pattern between protozoal species could be found (review Coleman, 1989). The ability of rumen protozoa to engulf and digest attached bacteria as compared with bacteria free in rumen fluid is a matter of conjecture. The engulfment of solid feed particles by protozoa is well known and this is also expected to result in engulfment of bacteria attached to these particles. On the other hand, the hypothesis of protection from engulfment by means of attachment has been supported by observations that, upon defaunation, the fluid-phase, non-fibrolytic bacteria increased to a far higher extent than did attached bacteria (Weimer, 1992). It should be noted, though, that the preference of protozoa for starch and sugars rather than fibre will result in a relatively higher availability of starch and sugars compared with fibre upon defaunation, and hence a smaller expected increase in attached, fibrolytic bacteria compared to non-attached bacteria. Interestingly, Rasmussen *et al.* (2005) reported that some bacterial pathogens, like *Salmonella*, appear to be resistant to degradation in vacuoles of mixed rumen protozoa. Survival of several types of *Salmonella* in protozoal vacuoles, in particular multi-resistant types, results in higher intestinal cell invasion capacity. On the other hand, toxin-producing *Escherichia coli* were not engulfed by or attached to mixed ciliate protozoa (Burow *et al.*, 2005). Representation of uptake and digestion of bacteria by protozoa is further complicated because of adaptive mechanisms that bacteria develop to survive protozoal predation. Adaptive mechanisms to increase the survival of bacteria under predation pressure include changing cell surface properties, secretion of bioactive metabolites, modification of swimming speed, or formation of micro-colonies (Matz and Kjelleberg, 2005). Thus, it appears that the mathematical representation of selective engulfment and digestion of bacteria by protozoa may well be further improved.

In the protozoa model, uptake of microorganisms was assumed to be reduced due to the presence of starch within the protozoa (Coleman, 1992). This was represented by a sigmoidal function (Eqn 7.2) based on observations that bacterial uptake rate was not limited when protozoa were filled with relatively small amounts of starch, whereas engulfment of bacteria was never completely inhibited, even if protozoa appeared to be completely filled with starch, in which ν_{MiPo} is represented as:

$$\nu_{MiPo} = \nu^*_{MiPo} / [1 + (Q_{Sp} / (Q_{Po} + Q_{Sp}) / J_{Sp,MiPo})^{\theta_{Sp,MiPo}}], \quad (7.2)$$

where ν^*_{MiPo} (g Mi g^{-1} Po day^{-1}) is the maximum velocity of uptake of Mi by protozoa, Q_{Sp} (g) is the amount of storage polysaccharides in protozoa (Sp), $J_{Sp,MiPo}$ (g g^{-1}) is the inhibition constant of Sp in Mi uptake and $\theta_{Sp,MiPo}$ is the steepness parameter for this uptake. Sensitivity analyses indicated that the recycling of microbial biomass was rather sensitive to variations in $J_{Sp,MiPo}$ (Dijkstra, 1994) and more data to estimate the value of $J_{Sp,MiPo}$ were needed.

Particularly on diets rich in easily degradable carbohydrates, protozoa have been observed to degenerate and burst (Williams and Coleman, 1997). The cause of protozoal lysis is probably the inability of protozoa to control soluble substrate entry and the subsequent intracellular build-up of acidic fermentation products. Thus, in the model, the amount of VFA produced from fermentation of substrate per unit of time and protozoal biomass will determine the death rate of protozoa. A sigmoidal response is assumed to obtain low death rates at low nutrient availabilities, with a rapid increase when hexose entities fermented to VFA are increased:

$$U_{Po,PoDe} = v^*_{PoDe}\, Q_{Po} \,/\, [1 + (M_{VFA,PoDe} \,/\, P_{VFA,HxVFA} \,/\, Q_{Po})^{\theta_{VFA,PoDe}}], \quad (7.3)$$

where $U_{Po,PoDe}$ (g day^{-1}) is protozoal death rate, v^*_{PoDe} (day^{-1}) is the maximum fractional death rate, $M_{VFA,PoDe}$ (mol day^{-1}) is the affinity constant related to VFA production within protozoa, $P_{VFA,HxVFA}$ (mol g^{-1} day^{-1}) is the VFA production within protozoa and $\theta_{VFA,PoDe}$ is steepness parameter related to this protozoal VFA production.

The model provides a framework in which knowledge on protozoal–bacterial interrelationships is integrated and hypotheses formulated to represent key aspects of protozoal and bacterial metabolism. Comparisons between model predictions and experimental observations, using the ^{14}C dilution technique in cattle and sheep, indicated reasonable agreement for protozoal biomass in the rumen (Dijkstra, 1994). At present, a widely accepted marker to measure the protozoal fraction of microbial protein (separate from the bacterial fraction) is lacking and this limits comparison of observed and simulated values. New molecular techniques such as real-time polymerase chain reaction (PCR), targeting the gene encoding 18S rDNA to quantify the amount of protozoal biomass (Sylvester *et al*., 2004), may be promising tools to obtain more quantitative data.

Model application

Engulfment and lysis of bacteria and protozoa contribute significantly to recycling of microbial material within the rumen, thus potentially reducing the flow of microbial protein to the duodenum. The protozoa model was applied to quantify recycling in various dietary situations (Dijkstra *et al*., 1998b). In steady state, the turnover of microbial N in the rumen (g day^{-1}) is calculated from uptake of bacteria and protozoa (Eqns 7.1 and 7.2) and protozoal death (Eqn 7.3) as:

$$\text{turnover} = f_{N,Po}\,(U_{Mi,MiPo} + U_{Po,PoDe}), \quad (7.4)$$

where $f_{N,Po}$ is the fraction of N in the polysaccharide free microbial DM (0.118 g N g^{-1} DM). Division of the calculated turnover (Eqn 7.4) by Q_{Mi} gives the fractional turnover rate (day^{-1}). The ruminal recycling of microbial N (%) in steady state represents the proportion of microbial N synthesized but not washed out of the rumen and is given by:

$$\text{recycling} = \text{turnover} \,/\, [\text{turnover} + f_{N,Po}\, U_{Mi,MiEx}] \times 100\%, \quad (7.5)$$

where $U_{Mi,MiEx}$ (g day^{-1}) is the outflow of bacterial and protozoal DM to the duodenum.

Predicted microbial N recycling according to Eqn 7.5 varies with level of intake and diet composition. This is illustrated by simulations of all-hay (diet H), all-maize silage (diet M) and mixed (diet B; 333 g kg^{-1} DM each of hay, barley and mixed concentrate) diets at low (9.2 kg day^{-1}) and high (17.1 kg day^{-1})

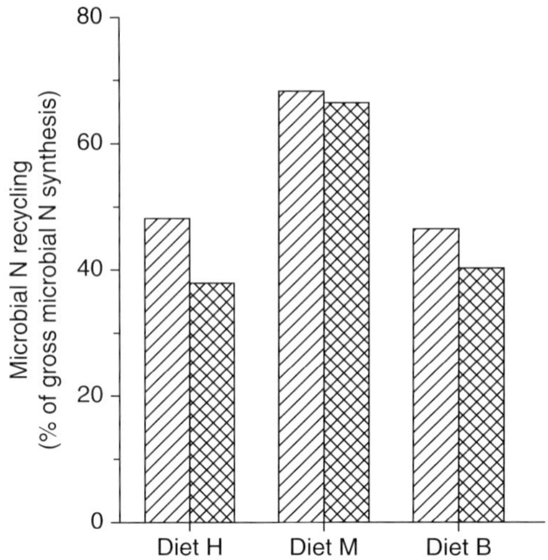

Fig. 7.2. Microbial N recycling (per cent of gross microbial N synthesis) in the rumen of cattle predicted using the model of Dijkstra (1994). Diets were all-hay (diet H), all-maize silage (diet M) and mixed (diet B; 333 g kg^{-1} DM each of hay, barley and mixed concentrate) diets at low (9.2 kg day^{-1}) (striped bars) and high (17.1 kg day^{-1}) (crossed bars) daily DMI.

daily dry matter intake (DMI) (Fig. 7.2). The gross microbial N synthesis at low and high DMI is 213 and 393 g N day^{-1} (diet H), 179 and 352 g N day^{-1} (diet M), and 240 and 430 g N day^{-1} (diet B), respectively. Predicted recycling varies between 37.9 and 68.3% of gross microbial N synthesis. Simulated microbial recycling is extensive, in particular for diets containing high (but not unlimited) amounts of starch, because starch promotes protozoal proliferation. However, when starch is in excess of a certain level (this level being dependent upon other diet characteristics), protozoal lysis becomes more pronounced and protozoal biomass and activity may decrease. In line with such simulations, Firkins *et al.* (1992) reported high recycling of microbial N (76–90% of gross microbial N synthesis) on diets high in starch (85% maize silage diets) compared with diets high in lucerne chaff or wheat straw. Similarly, diets low in protein will stimulate the development of protozoa relative to that of bacteria, since protozoa usually do not encounter protein deficiencies as they engulf large amounts of bacterial protein. An increased DMI is expected to reduce recycling because of increased fractional rates of passage. However, this intake effect is most pronounced with diet H and least with diet M. Thus, the model contributes to understanding of the response of microbial protein synthesis to changes in diet composition.

Overall, recycling of microbial protein wastes energy, although the VFA production may well be increased due to recycling. The released amino acids may be deaminated and this gives rise to further wastage of N as urea in urine. Direct quantifications of microbial N recycling have been obtained using isotope tracer methods (see Dijkstra *et al.*, 1998b), but the number of studies are few. The approach in the present study was to quantify variation in microbial N recycling, due to protozoal activities, by representing the underlying processes in an integrated model of rumen fermentation. Hence, the estimated microbial turnover and recycling relate solely to protozoal activities. This is in line with experimental data on protozoal turnover *in vivo* and on the impact of protozoa on bacterial turnover *in vitro* presented before. However, in the absence of protozoa, other mechanisms that determine bacterial recycling may become significant. For example, bacterial N recycling decreased from 49% in faunated sheep to 33% in defaunated animals (Koenig *et al.*, 2001). Thus, in the absence of protozoa, there is still considerable recycling of bacterial N. This is not included in the present model. Preliminary simulations with the model in which the protozoal pool was set to zero to simulate defaunated animals overpredicted substrate degradation within the rumen and bacterial N flow to the duodenum (Dijkstra, unpublished results). Application of the model to compare faunated and defaunated animals thus requires a representation of the factors responsible for bacterial N recycling not related to protozoal activities.

The simulated variation in predicted recycling will have a large impact on the efficiency of microbial protein synthesis. The effect of recycling and of availability of amino acids versus ammonia as a source of N on bacterial protein efficiency is shown graphically in Fig. 7.3. In these calculations, 20% of bacterial DM is assumed to be storage polysaccharides and the crude protein content is assumed to be 60%. Synthesis of 1 g of bacterial protein (i.e. 1.7 g of bacterial DM) based on ammonia or on preformed amino acids is assumed to require 3.1 and 2.6 g OM, respectively (Dijkstra *et al.*, 1992). Calculations are shown in which the contribution of ammonia-N to total bacterial-N varies between 20 and 100%. The effect of recycling on net microbial protein requirement is much larger than the effect of N precursor (ammonia versus preformed amino acids). For example, at 30% recycling, 3.9 to 4.4 g OM is required g^{-1} net bacterial protein synthesized, whereas, at 60% recycling, 6.8 to 7.8 g OM is required g^{-1} net bacterial protein synthesized. Thus, the large variation in microbial protein yield generally observed in experiments with different diets may be partly explained by variation in microbial recycling. Given the large impact of microbial turnover

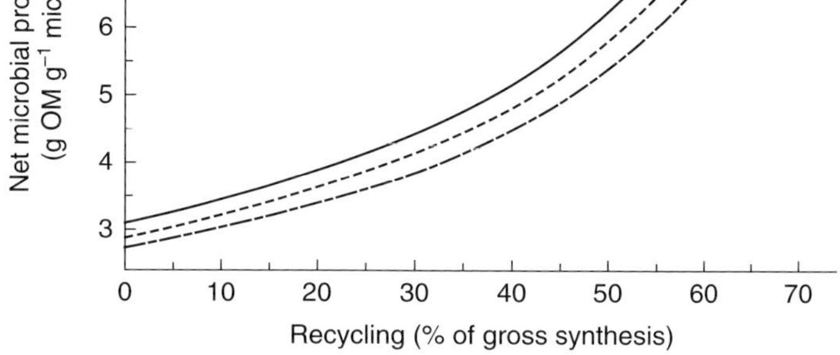

Fig. 7.3. Effect of microbial N recycling and of ratio of ammonia to amino acids on net microbial protein requirement. See text for explanation of derivation of values.

on microbial efficiency, the small amount of experimental research on turnover as compared with large research efforts on substrate degradation is striking (Dijkstra *et al.*, 2005b), and much more research should focus on this item. Quantification of microbial recycling will help to establish more accurate estimates of microbial protein yield factors to be applied in protein evaluation systems.

VFA Production

Ruminal VFAs are produced as end products of microbial fermentation. VFAs represent the major source of absorbed energy and, with most diets, account for approximately 80% of the energy disappearing in the rumen. The need to maintain redox balance through reduction and reoxidation of pyridine nucleotides (NAD) controls fermentation reactions. Excess reducing power generated during the conversion of hexose to acetate or butyrate is utilized in part during the formation of propionate, but mainly by conversion to methane. Thus, adequate knowledge of the types of VFA formed contributes to the proper prediction of methane formation in the rumen (Mills *et al.*, 2001). Carbohydrates are by far the major source of VFAs in the rumen. Dietary proteins also may be a significant source with diets characterized by a high ratio of rumen degradable protein to rumen degradable carbohydrates. The majority of the VFAs produced in the rumen are lost by absorption across the rumen wall. At low pH values, VFAs with a higher carbon chain have a higher fractional absorption rate due to their greater lipid solubility (Lopez *et al.*, 2003). During passage across the rumen wall, the VFAs are metabolized to varying extents so that the amounts entering the bloodstream are generally found to be less than the quantities absorbed from the rumen (review Brockman, 2005).

The concentration of VFA in the rumen at any given time reflects the balance between the rate of production and rate of loss. Immediately after feeding, production usually exceeds loss and the concentration increases but, subsequently, the situation is reversed and the concentration falls. The relative concentrations of the individual acids, commonly referred to as the fermentation pattern, are a reliable index of the relative production rates of the acids when forage diets are given, but would appear less reliable with concentrate diets (review France and Dijkstra, 2005). The fermentation pattern is determined by the composition of the microbial population, which, in turn, is largely determined by the basal diet, particularly the type of dietary carbohydrate, and by the rate of depolymerization of available substrates (review Dijkstra, 1994). For example, high-fibre forage diets encourage the growth of acetate-producing bacterial species and the acetate:propionate:butyrate molar proportions would typically be in the 70:20:10 region. On the other hand, starch-rich concentrate diets favour the development of propionate-producing bacterial species and are associated with an increase in the proportion of propionate at the expense of acetate (Bannink *et al.*, 2006). As described previously, certain diets encourage the development of a large protozoal population and this is accompanied by an increase in butyrate rather than propionate production (Williams and Coleman, 1997). If levels of substrate available for fermentation are high, either from increased intake or increased rates of depolymerization, a shift in fermentation pattern from acetic acid to propionic acid occurs to dispose of excess reducing power (Dijkstra, 1994). In addition to the type of dietary carbohydrate, many other factors, including the physical form of the diet, level of intake, frequency of feeding and the use of chemical additives, may also affect the fermentation pattern.

After absorption, acetate and butyrate are used primarily as energy sources through oxidation via the citric acid cycle. Acetate is also the principal substrate for lipogenesis, whilst propionate is used largely for gluconeogenesis and, with most diets, is the major source of glucose (Brockman, 2005). The balance between the supply of the glucogenic propionate relative to that of the non-glucogenic acetate and butyrate influences the efficiency with which the VFAs are used for productive purposes (Sutton, 1985). Thus, not only the total supply of VFA but also the molar proportions are main determinants of feed utilization by ruminants. Moreover, the proportions of VFA are important in determining the composition of milk produced by dairy cattle (Sutton, 1985). A number of methods have been used to estimate the rates of individual and total VFA production in the rumen. These methods may be conveniently divided into two groups: methods not employing isotopic tracers and those employing tracers based on the application of compartmental analysis to interpret isotope dilution data (see review France and Dijkstra, 2005). Since the most accurate method (employing isotopes) is difficult and expensive, only VFA concentrations are measured routinely in rumen fermentation trials. Hence, efforts were made to predict the stoichiometry of rumen fermentation using various modelling approaches, and these will be discussed further.

VFA stoichiometry method, Koong *et al.* (1975) and Murphy *et al.* (1982)

Koong *et al.* (1975) were among the first to propose a method to obtain estimates of stoichiometric coefficients for fermentation of various dietary components. In this approach, each carbohydrate utilized in the rumen was considered to be partly fermented and partly incorporated into microbial biomass, whereas amino acids derived from protein degradation were assumed to be completely fermented. Stoichiometric coefficients were then applied that define the proportion of the substrate (carbohydrates and protein) fermented to acetate, propionate, butyrate and valerate. These coefficients were varied in sequential runs and model predictions compared to experimental estimates for various diets.

A major limitation in this approach was the requirement for experimental estimates of VFA production rather than commonly measured VFA concentrations. Murphy *et al.* (1982) changed the model of Koong *et al.* (1975) so that VFA molar proportions could be used in comparisons of experimental and predicted values. Murphy *et al.* (1982) obtained a data set mainly with beef cattle and sheep and divided the data set into a roughage group (more than 50% roughage in diet DM) and a concentrate group. Substrates were divided into soluble carbohydrates, starch, cellulose, hemicellulose and pectin. Based on preliminary

Table 7.1. Stoichiometric yield parameters (mol VFA mol^{-1} fermented substrate) for production of acetic acid (Ac), propionic acid (Pr), butyric acid (Bu) and branched chain plus valeric acid (Vl) from fermentation of substrates on roughage (R) and concentrate (C) diets (Murphy *et al.*, 1982).

	Ac		Pr		Bu		Vl	
Substrate	R	C	R	C	R	C	R	C
Soluble sugars	1.38	0.90	0.41	0.42	0.10	0.30	0.00	0.04
Starch	1.19	0.80	0.28	0.60	0.20	0.20	0.06	0.10
Cellulose	1.32	1.58	0.17	0.12	0.23	0.06	0.03	0.09
Hemicellulose	1.13	1.12	0.36	0.51	0.21	0.11	0.05	0.07
Protein	0.40	0.36	0.13	0.16	0.08	0.08	0.33	0.33

analyses of their model which indicated similar VFA molar proportions for pectin, organic acids and sugars, these three substrates were included in the soluble carbohydrates fraction. The estimated stoichiometric coefficients are presented in Table 7.1.

Soluble carbohydrate and starch stoichiometric parameters were quite different between the roughage and concentrate groups. Also, fermentation parameters of hemicellulose and cellulose differed significantly, probably related to those microbial species capable of utilizing hemicellulose but not cellulose (Baldwin, 1995). The Murphy coefficients were subsequently applied in mechanistic models of whole rumen function in dairy cattle (Baldwin *et al.*, 1987; Dijkstra *et al.*, 1992). Subsequently, Argyle and Baldwin (1988) adapted the values of the stoichiometric coefficients related to starch and soluble carbohydrates to account for the effect of rumen pH as established *in vitro*. However, based on dairy cattle data, the extensive evaluations of Bannink *et al.* (1997a,c) indicated that predictions of VFA molar proportions based on Murphy coefficients were not adequate.

VFA stoichiometry method, Pitt *et al.* (1996)

Like Argyle and Baldwin (1988), Pitt *et al.* (1996) recognized that the type of VFA produced is closely related to the pH of rumen fluid. They derived VFA relationships based on the Cornell Net Carbohydrate and Protein System. In this system, three carbohydrate fractions are distinguished: structural carbohydrates, starch and pectin and soluble sugars. The amount of fermented substrate was divided into production of acetate, propionate and butyrate, as well as lactic acid, all according to the pH of rumen fluid. Only structural carbohydrates were assumed not to produce lactic acid. Lactic acid, in turn, is fermented to acetate, propionate and butyrate according to the pH of rumen fluid. Stoichiometric parameters were derived from one principal source of *in vitro* data on fermentation of starch, sucrose, pectin, xylans and cellobiose at initial pH values of 6.0 or 6.7.

The application of a pH-dependent relationship between substrate fermentation and the type of VFA formed helps to overcome the rather arbitrary division into roughage and concentrate diets applied by Murphy *et al.* (1982). However, the principal sources of information on the division of fermentation end products are rather limited and based entirely on *in vitro* data. The direct application of *in vivo* situations is questionable. From a limited evaluation against *in vivo* data, Pitt *et al.* (1996) showed that predicted individual molar proportions of VFA were poorly correlated with observed values and that they were insensitive to variations in the evaluation studies. When Pitt *et al.* (1996) applied the Murphy *et al.* (1982) coefficients, the overall goodness-of-fit was lower, but the variation in predicted VFA molar proportions was more in line with observed variation. Moreover, from inspection of the graphical information Pitt *et al.* (1996) provided, it appears that the goodness-of-fit for each individual acid was better when the Murphy equations were applied than when the Pitt equations were used. Hence, the Pitt *et al.* (1996) coefficients are not sufficient for feed evaluation purposes.

VFA stoichiometry method, Friggens *et al.* (1998)

Rather than being based on substrate degradation in the rumen, in the Friggens *et al.* (1998) method, the VFA molar proportions are predicted from feed chemical entities. Friggens *et al.* (1998) tested 16 feeds at three inclusion rates in grass silage-based rations fed to sheep. Principal components regression was used to relate the observed proportions of VFA to the chemical composition of the total feed. Significant terms in the regressions were crude protein, starch, sugars and (by difference) cellulose. The regression equations are shown in Table 7.2.

No independent evaluation of the predictions was provided by Friggens *et al.* (1998). Friggens used the data set to evaluate the Murphy coefficients and discerned much less variation in predicted molar proportions of the major VFA than in observed values. It should be noted that substrate degradabilities were estimated from the disappearance of substrate from nylon bags incubated for 24 h in dairy cattle. The direct application of 24-h nylon bag results in cattle to

Table 7.2. Regression coefficients for the relationship between various dietary chemical entities (in per cent of diet DM) and molar proportions (in per cent of total) of acetic acid (Ac), propionic acid (Pr) and butyric acid (Bu), where valeric acid is calculated as 100% minus the other three VFA molar proportions (Friggens *et al.*, 1998).

		Regression coefficients			
	Intercept	Protein	Starch	Soluble sugars	Cellulose
Ac	56.46	–0.086	0.056	0.104	0.373
Pr	36.96	–0.117	–0.223	–0.299	–0.394
Bu	5.15	0.110	0.128	0.234	–0.023

in vivo sheep rumen degradability is highly questionable, however, as it does not take into account the effect of differences in retention times or rumen fluid characteristics. For example, the applied values of 100% degradability of cellulose in wheat, 98% cellulose degradability in sugarbeet pulp, or 2% cellulose degradability in field beans are unlikely to occur *in vivo*. Finally, such an approach is unable to predict differences in VFA molar proportions from various ingredient sources that have the same amount of a particular substrate. For example, since maize starch is more resistant to ruminal degradation than barley starch, an increased molar proportion of propionic acid occurs with barley (Sutton, 1985), whereas the Friggens *et al.* (1998) coefficients would not lead to differences in predicted VFA molar proportions. Also, technological treatment to change rumen degradabilities will give rise to changes in observed VFA molar proportions, but predicted molar proportions remain unchanged in the Friggens *et al.* (1998) approach.

VFA stoichiometry method, Kohn and Boston (2000)

According to Kohn and Boston (2000), attempts to predict the type of VFA produced in the rumen should be based on mechanisms, rather than on empirical relationships between type of substrate and type of VFA. They argued that thermodynamic control would occur when the reactants were sufficiently limited relative to products for the reactions not to proceed, according to the second law of thermodynamics. Therefore, Kohn and Boston (2000) developed a model of glucose fermentation in which thermodynamic limits to VFA and gas production were incorporated, by including fractional rate constants for reverse reactions. Simulations indicated that high rates of substrate fermentation induced a shift in fermentation pathway from the production of acetic acid to the production of propionic acid, which is thermodynamically more feasible under those conditions. The attractiveness of this approach is its mechanistic basis. However, only glucose is considered as a substrate and the type of microorganism involved in the fermentation reactions is not represented. Some information on model behaviour was presented, but evaluation of the model against actual data was not included. Thus, the thermodynamic approach, though promising from a mechanistic point of view, will have to be developed further before it can be applied in whole rumen models.

VFA stoichiometry method, Nagorcka *et al.* (2000)

Nagorcka *et al.* (2000) hypothesized that previously derived stoichiometric coefficients were related to substrate only and that distinct fermentation pathways that characterize different microbial groups should also be included. Hence, Nagorcka *et al.* (2000) developed fermentation coefficients that depended both on the substrate and on the type of microbial group fermenting the substrate. Three microbial groups were considered: amylolytic bacteria (fermenting sugars and starch, hemicellulose and protein), fibrolytic bacteria (fermenting hemicellulose,

Table 7.3. Stoichiometric yield parameters (mol VFA mol^{-1} fermented substrate) for production of acetic acid (Ac), propionic acid (Pr), butyric acid (Bu) and branched chain plus valeric acid (Vl) from fermentation of starch and soluble sugars (SS), cellulose (CE), hemicellulose (HC) and protein (PT) by amylolytic bacteria (Ba), fibrolytic bacteria (Bf) and protozoa (Po) (Nagorcka *et al.*, 2000).

	Ac			Pr			Bu			Vl		
	Ba	Bf	Po	Ba	Bf	Po	Ba	Bf	Po	Ba	Bf	Po
SS	0.90	NF	0.99	0.85	NF	0.02	0.10	NF	0.49	0.02	NF	0.00
CE	NF	1.30	0.99	NF	0.53	0.22	NF	0.09	0.49	NF	0.00	0.00
HC	1.00	1.00	1.00	0.36	0.34	0.00	0.23	0.25	0.50	0.00	0.00	0.00
PT	0.50	0.50	0.50	0.15	0.15	0.15	0.13	0.13	0.13	0.24	0.24	0.24

cellulose and protein) and protozoa (fermenting sugars and starch, hemicellulose, cellulose and protein). The rumen protozoa model of Dijkstra (1994) described in a previous section was applied to predict the activities of the three microbial groups. The stoichiometric coefficients derived are presented in Table 7.3.

Upon comparison with independent data used by Dijkstra *et al.* (1992) to evaluate the Murphy coefficients, an improvement in prediction accuracy was obtained. Thus, the separation of various microbial groups that may ferment the same substrate may be attractive to incorporate higher variation in predicted molar proportions of VFA. In particular, protozoa are known to produce relatively large amounts of butyric acid (Williams and Coleman, 1997) and fermentation of starch and sugars by protozoa should give rise to higher levels of butyric acid than fermentation by bacteria. However, the aggregation of sugars and starch into one entity for VFA formation hampers necessary distinction in the type of VFA produced between starch and sugars. Also, the assumption of hemicellulose degradation by amylolytic bacteria that is assumed to pass from the rumen with the liquid phase, in the model, is not an attractive representation, from the biological perspective, as bacteria have to attach to particles in order to degrade hemicellulose.

VFA stoichiometry method, Sveinbjörnsson *et al.* (2006)

Sveinbjörnsson *et al.* (2006) developed a submodel for rumen VFA production to be used in the Nordic dairy-cow model Karoline. Before they developed this submodel, they evaluated the adequacy of the Murphy *et al.* (1982) coefficients and of the concentrate coefficients of Bannink *et al.* (2006) (see next section). On the range of diets of interest, VFA molar proportions were poorly predicted by these coefficients. The extremely low R^2 values for acetate and propionate (ranging between 0.001 to 0.010), however, cast some doubt on the accuracy of the evaluation, since these low values are far below any other independent evaluation of the Murphy coefficients. Subsequently, Sveinbjörnsson *et al.* (2006)

Table 7.4. Stoichiometric yield parameters (mol mol^{-1} total VFA) for production of acetic acid (Ac), propionic acid (Pr), butyric acid (Bu) and valeric acid (Vl) and regression coefficients for DMI level (kg DM kg^{-1} live weight day^{-1}) and concentrate ether extract (g kg^{-1} DM) from fermentation of substrates (Sveinbjörnsson *et al.*, 2006). Branched chain fatty acid molar proportion is 0.33 with protein and 0 with other substrates.

	VFA molar proportions						Regression coefficients	
	Protein	Lactic acid	Forage NDF	Concentrate NDF	Starch	Rest OM fraction	DMI level	Concentrate ether extract
Ac	0.402	0.255	0.815	0.792	0.669	0.585	−0.508	−0.333
Pr	0.172	0.514	0.080	0.125	0.180	0.227	0.665	0.442
Bu	0.080	0.231	0.105	0.083	0.151	0.188	−0.250	−0.099

derived stoichiometric coefficients using, in principle, the approach of Murphy *et al.* (1982) for acetate, propionate and butyrate. The substrates with significant effects were forage NDF, concentrate NDF, starch, crude protein, lactic acid and a rest fraction of OM. Furthermore, feeding level and concentrate ether extract in the diet explained a significant part of the variation in VFA pattern and were added to the coefficients. The stoichiometric coefficients derived are presented in Table 7.4.

Sveinbjörnsson *et al.* (2006) used a particular data set with diets from Nordic countries characterized by high levels of grass silage and concentrates based largely on barley and rapeseed meal to derive the coefficients. They acknowledged that the coefficients derived would not necessarily be applicable to dairy cattle diets used in other countries. In the Sveinbjörnsson *et al.* (2006) coefficients, as compared with the Murphy *et al.* (1982) and Bannink *et al.* (2006) coefficients, starch appears to have a smaller effect on the molar proportion of propionate. Higher feed intake levels reduced acetate and butyrate molar proportions in favour of propionate molar proportions. Since higher feed intake levels are associated with reduced pH levels of rumen fluids, the previous attempts of Argyle and Baldwin (1988) and Pitt *et al.* (1996) to include a pH dependency yielded a qualitatively similar effect. An independent evaluation was not performed by Sveinbjörnsson *et al.* (2006). Evaluation of the coefficients on a subset of the data set used to derive the coefficients again indicated a much smaller variation in predicted than in observed VFA molar proportions.

VFA stoichiometry method, Bannink *et al.* (2006)

Bannink *et al.* (2006) adapted the model of Murphy *et al.* (1982), assuming a fixed incorporation of each substrate into microbial biomass. This model was fitted to data from experiments with dairy cattle obtained from literature in which truly degraded substrate and VFA molar proportions were presented. The stoichiometric coefficients are presented in Table 7.5.

As in previous attempts, Bannink *et al.* (2006) observed that the variation in predicted molar proportions was smaller than that in observed molar proportions.

Table 7.5. Stoichiometric yield parameters (mol VFA mol^{-1} fermented substrate) for production of acetic acid (Ac), propionic acid (Pr), butyric acid (Bu) and branched chain plus valeric acid (Vl) from fermentation of substrates on roughage (R) and concentrate (C) diets (Bannink *et al.*, 2006).

	Ac		Pr		Bu		Vl	
Substrate	R	C	R	C	R	C	R	C
Soluble sugars	1.29	1.06	0.16	0.31	0.24	0.26	0.04	0.06
Starch	0.98	0.97	0.43	0.62	0.21	0.15	0.08	0.05
Cellulose	1.12	1.37	0.41	0.23	0.17	0.20	0.07	0.00
Hemicellulose	0.88	1.02	0.35	0.24	0.32	0.32	0.06	0.05
Protein	0.62	0.49	0.32	0.20	0.09	0.19	0.07	0.23

They established a simulated data set to investigate this problem further and demonstrated that the statistical method applied, combined with the necessity of molar proportions to add up to unity, invariably led to a low variation in predicted molar proportions. Even so, the coefficients thus established were not different from the true coefficients applied in the simulation study. Although these coefficients seem to be applicable for a wide range of diets, the empirical nature of the approach is still a point of interest. Of major concern is the assumption that a change in fractional rate of substrate fermentation will shift fermentation pathways away from the production of acetate to the production of (in particular) propionate, because of the thermodynamic principles described before (Kohn and Boston, 2000). Inclusion of pH as a factor may assist in this respect, since increased rates of fermentation are generally associated with decreased pH values. At present, this set of coefficient estimates may significantly improve the prediction of VFA production by extant models of whole rumen function because of the extensive and wide database used to derive the coefficients.

Conclusions

Protozoal metabolism and VFA production in the rumen are key aspects in predicting the supply of absorbed nutrients in ruminants. Protozoa play a major role in nutrient recycling within the rumen and in efficiency of microbial protein synthesis. Surprisingly few efforts have been made to quantify the mechanisms responsible for recycling. The development of a model of protozoal metabolism has helped to understand the contribution that protozoa make to nutrient supply from the rumen in various dietary situations. The simulations indicate areas for further improvement of quantitative understanding. In contrast to protozoal metabolism, many approaches to predict the profile of VFAs absorbed have been presented. Most of these are rather empirical in nature and relate the type of VFA produced to the type of substrate fermented. Evaluation of various approaches indicates that the prediction of the type of VFA produced is still unsatisfactory and further developments, preferably based on mechanisms, are necessary.

References

Argyle, J.L. and Baldwin, R.L. (1988) Modeling of rumen water kinetics and effects of rumen pH changes. *Journal of Dairy Science* 71, 1178–1188.

Baldwin, R.L. (1995) *Modeling Ruminant Digestion and Metabolism.* Chapman and Hall, London.

Baldwin, R.L., Thornley, J.H.M. and Beever, D.E. (1987) Metabolism of the lactating dairy cow. II. Digestive elements of a mechanistic model. *Journal of Dairy Research* 54, 107–131.

Bannink, A., De Visser, H. and Van Vuuren, A.M. (1997a) Comparison and evaluation of mechanistic rumen models. *British Journal of Nutrition* 78, 563–581.

Bannink, A., De Visser, H., Dijkstra, J. and France, J. (1997b) Impact of diet-specific input parameters on simulated rumen function. *Journal of Theoretical Biology* 184, 371–384.

Bannink, A., De Visser, H., Klop, A., Dijkstra, J. and France, J. (1997c) Causes of inaccurate prediction of volatile fatty acids by simulation models of rumen function in lactating cows. *Journal of Theoretical Biology* 189, 353–366.

Bannink, A., Kogut, J., Dijkstra, J., France, J., Kebreab, E., Van Vuuren, A.M. and Tamminga, S. (2006) Estimation of the stoichiometry of volatile fatty acid production in the rumen of lactating cows. *Journal of Theoretical Biology* 238, 36–51.

Bazin, M.J. (1981) Mixed culture kinetics. In: Bushell, M.E. and Slater, J.H. (eds) *Mixed Culture Fermentations*. Academic Press, London, pp. 25–51.

Brockman, R.P. (2005) Glucose and short-chain fatty acid metabolism. In: Dijkstra, J., Forbes, J.M. and France, J. (eds) *Quantitative Aspects of Ruminant Digestion and Metabolism*, 2nd edn. CAB International, Wallingford, UK, pp. 291–310.

Brown, D. and Rothery, P. (1993) *Models in Biology: Mathematics, Statistics and Computing*. John Wiley and Sons Ltd, Chichester, UK.

Burow, L.C., Gobius, K.C., Vanselow, B.A. and Klieve, A.V. (2005) A lack of predatory interaction between rumen ciliate protozoa and Shiga-toxin producing *Escherichia coli*. *Letters in Applied Microbiology* 40, 117–122.

Coleman, G.S. (1989) Protozoal–bacterial interactions in the rumen. In: Nolan, J.V., Leng, R.A. and Demeyer, D.I. (eds) *The Roles of Protozoa and Fungi in Ruminant Digestion*. Penambul Books, Armidale, Australia, pp. 13–27.

Coleman, G.S. (1992) The rate of uptake and metabolism of starch grains and cellulose particles by *Entodinium* species, *Eudiplodinium maggii*, some other entodiniomorphid protozoa and natural protozoal populations taken from the ovine rumen. *Journal of Applied Bacteriology* 73, 507–513.

Dehority, B.A. (2003) *Rumen Microbiology*. Nottingham University Press, Nottingham, UK.

Dijkstra, J. (1994) Simulation of the dynamics of protozoa in the rumen. *British Journal of Nutrition* 72, 679–699.

Dijkstra, J. and Bannink, A. (2000) Analyses of modelling whole rumen function. In: Theodorou, M.K. and France, J. (eds) *Feeding Systems and Feed Evaluation Models*. CAB International, Wallingford, UK, pp. 299–322.

Dijkstra, J., Neal, H.D.St.C., Beever, D.E. and France, J. (1992) Simulation of nutrient digestion, absorption and outflow in the rumen: model description. *Journal of Nutrition* 122, 2239–2256.

Dijkstra, J., France, J. and Davies, D.R. (1998a) Different mathematical approaches to estimating microbial protein supply in ruminants. *Journal of Dairy Science* 81, 3370–3384.

Dijkstra, J., France, J. and Tamminga, S. (1998b) Quantification of the recycling of microbial nitrogen in the rumen using a mechanistic model of rumen fermentation processes. *Journal of Agricultural Science, Cambridge* 130, 81–94.

Dijkstra, J., Forbes, J.M. and France, J. (2005a) *Quantitative Aspects of Ruminant Digestion and Metabolism*, 2nd edn. CAB International, Wallingford, UK.

Dijkstra, J., Kebreab, E., Bannink, A., France, J. and Lopez, S. (2005b) Application of the gas production technique in feed evaluation systems for ruminants. *Animal Feed Science and Technology* 123–124, 561–578.

Eugène, M., Archimède, H. and Sauvant, D. (2004) Quantitative meta-analysis on the effects of defaunation of the rumen on growth, intake and digestion in ruminants. *Livestock Production Science* 85, 81–97.

Firkins, J.L., Weiss, W.P. and Piwonka, E.J. (1992) Quantification of intraruminal recycling of microbial nitrogen using nitrogen-15. *Journal of Animal Science* 70, 3223–3233.

Fondevila, M. and Dehority, B.A. (2001) Preliminary study on the requirements of *Entodinium exiguum* and *E. caudatum* for live or dead bacteria when cultured *in vitro*. *Reproduction Nutrition Development* 41, 41–46.

France, J. and Dijkstra, J. (2005) Volatile fatty acid production. In: Dijkstra, J., Forbes, J.M. and France, J. (eds) *Quantitative Aspects of Ruminant Digestion and Metabolism*, 2nd edn. CAB International, Wallingford, UK, pp. 157–175.

Freitas, M.J. De and Fredrickson, A.G. (1978) Inhibition as a factor in the maintenance of the diversity of microbial ecosystems. *Journal of General Microbiology* 106, 307–320.

Friggens, N.C., Oldham, J.D., Dewhurst, R.J. and Horgan, G. (1998) Proportions of volatile fatty acids in relation to the chemical composition of feeds based on grass silage. *Journal of Dairy Science* 81, 1331–1344.

Holling, C.S. (1959) Some characteristics of simple types of predation and parasitism. *Canadian Entomologist* 91, 385–398.

Jouany, J.P. (1989) Effects of diet on populations of rumen protozoa in relation to fibre digestion. In: Nolan, J.V., Leng, R.A. and Demeyer, D.I. (eds) *The Roles of Protozoa and Fungi in Ruminant Digestion*. Penambul Books, Armidale, Australia, pp. 59–74.

Koenig, K.M., Newbold, C.J., McIntosh, F.M. and Rode, L.M. (2001) Effects of protozoa on bacterial nitrogen recycling in the rumen. *Journal of Animal Science* 78, 2431–2445.

Kohn, R.A. and Boston, R.C. (2000) The role of thermodynamics in controlling rumen metabolism. In: McNamara, J.P., France, J. and Beever, D.E. (eds) *Modeling Nutrient Utilization in Farm Animals*. CAB International, Wallingford, UK, pp. 11–24.

Koong, L.J., Baldwin, R.L., Ulyatt, M.J. and Charlesworth, T.J. (1975) Iterative computation of metabolic flux and stoichiometric parameters for alternate pathways in rumen fermentation. *Computer Programs in Biomedicine* 4, 209–213.

Lopez, S., Hovell, F.D.D., Dijkstra, J. and France, J. (2003) Effects of volatile fatty acids supply on their absorption and on water kinetics in the rumen of sheep sustained by intragastric infusions. *Journal of Animal Science* 81, 2609–2616.

Matz, C. and Kjelleberg, S. (2005) Off the hook – how bacteria survive protozoan grazing. *Trends in Microbiology* 13, 302–307.

Mills, J.A.N., Dijkstra, J., Bannink, A., Cammell, S.B., Kebreab, E. and France, J. (2001) A mechanistic model of whole-tract digestion and methanogenesis in the lactating dairy cow: model development, evaluation and application. *Journal of Animal Science* 79, 1584–1597.

Murphy, M.R., Baldwin, R.L. and Koong, L.J. (1982) Estimation of stoichiometric parameters for rumen fermentation of roughage and concentrate diets. *Journal of Animal Science* 55, 411–421.

Nagorcka, B.N., Gordon, G.L.R. and Dynes, R.A. (2000) Towards a more accurate representation of fermentation in mathematical models of the rumen. In: McNamara, J.P., France, J. and Beever, D.E. (eds) *Modeling Nutrient Utilization in Farm Animals*. CAB International, Wallingford, UK, pp. 37–48.

Offner, A. and Sauvant, D. (2004) Comparative evaluation of the Molly, CNCPS, and LES rumen models. *Animal Feed Science and Technology* 112, 107–130.

Pitt, R.E., Van Kessel, J.S., Fox, D.G., Pell, A.N., Barry, M.C. and Van Soest, P.J. (1996) Prediction of ruminal volatile fatty acids and pH within the net carbohydrate and protein system. *Journal of Animal Science* 74, 226–244.

Rasmussen, M.A., Carlson, S.A., Franklin, S.K., McCuddin, Z.P., Wu, M.T. and Sharma, V.K. (2005) Exposure to rumen protozoa leads to enhancement of pathogenicity of and invasion by multiple-antibiotic-resistant *Salmonella enterica* bearing SGI1. *Infection and Immunity* 73, 4668–4675.

Sharp, R., Hazlewood, G.P., Gilbert, H.J. and O'Donnell, A.G. (1994) Unmodified and recombinant strains of *Lactobacillus plantarum* are rapidly lost from the rumen by protozoal predation. *Journal of Applied Bacteriology* 76, 110–117.

Sutton, J.D. (1985) Digestion and absorption of energy substrates in the lactating cow. *Journal of Dairy Science* 68, 3376–3393.

Sveinbjörnsson, J., Huhtanen, P. and Udén, P. (2006) The Nordic dairy cow model Karoline – development of VFA sub-model. In: Kebreab, E., Dijkstra, J., Bannink, A., Gerrits, W.J.J. and France, J. (eds) *Nutrient Digestion and Utilization in Farm Animals: Modelling Approaches*. CAB International, Wallingford, UK, pp. 1–14.

Sylvester, J.T., Karnati, S.K.R., Yu, Z., Morrison, M. and Firkins, J.L. (2004) Development of an assay to quantify rumen ciliate protozoal biomass in cows using real-time PCR. *Journal of Nutrition* 134, 3378–3384.

Thornley, J.H.M. and France, J. (2007) *Mathematical Models in Agriculture*, 2nd edn. CAB International, Wallingford, UK.

Weimer, P.J. (1992) Cellulose degradation by ruminal microorganisms. *Critical Reviews in Biotechnology* 12, 189–223.

Williams, A.G. and Coleman, G.S. (1997) The rumen protozoa. In: Hobson, P.N. and Stewart, C.S. (eds) *The Rumen Microbial Ecosystem*. Blackie Academic and Professional, London, pp. 73–139.

Witten, G.Q. and Richardson, F.D. (2003) Competition of three aggregated microbial species for four substrates in the rumen. *Ecological Modelling* 164, 121–135.

8 Modelling Methane Emissions from Farm Livestock

J.A.N. Mills

School of Agriculture, Policy and Development, University of Reading, UK

Introduction

This chapter reviews how models have been developed to predict methane production from individuals, groups of animals and, more broadly, from farming systems. The aim of this chapter is to discuss the techniques used for model development and to summarize the progress made to date. The chapter also discusses aspects of methanogenesis that have yet to be addressed adequately if the aim of offering a robust quantitative description of the biology is to be met. However, it is not the purpose of this chapter to describe the experimental techniques used for the direct measurement of methane arising from animal production. The reader should consider the range of these techniques available (Lockyer and Jarvis, 1995; Leuning *et al.*, 1999; Boadi *et al.*, 2002; Laubach and Kelliher, 2005) and their likely strengths and limitations when used to generate data for modelling studies.

Until recently, gaseous emissions from ruminants had received little attention from scientists intent on improving animal productivity. However, with rising interest in the effects of global warming and its implications for climate change, the last 15 years have seen a large increase in research directed at quantifying and ultimately reducing emissions of greenhouse gases from ruminants. Methane, resulting from enteric fermentation, is the principal greenhouse gas from ruminant (and, to a lesser extent, non-ruminant) agriculture. According to the Intergovernmental Panel on Climate Change (IPCC) (2001), methane levels in the atmosphere have doubled over the last 200 years and, with the gas displaying a relatively short life in the atmosphere (10–12 years), methane mitigation strategies offer an effective route to combating global warming. At present, in the USA, methane from enteric fermentation comprises the third largest contribution to total emissions behind landfill sites and natural gas systems (Environmental Protection Agency, 2005). The environmental consequences aside, methane emissions represent an energetic inefficiency that impacts on profitability of livestock production through reduced feed conversion efficiency. Therefore, the rationale of the producers and the policy makers may be different, but the goal of reduced emissions is universal.

Emissions from the Animal

Globally, about 95% of enteric methane is from ruminants, a consequence of their large populations, body size and appetites, combined with the extensive degree of anaerobic microbial fermentation occurring in their gut. Only 10% of ruminant methane is a product of fermentation during manure storage and handling. However, for non-ruminants, the situation is reversed, although few quantitative accounts of methane emissions from non-ruminants exist. Where they do exist, they tend to be for the purposes of regional inventories and, hence, differences due to nutrition or management are not considered in detail. Kirchgessner *et al.* (1991) recorded a mean production of 1.75 kg methane $year^{-1}$ for pigs fed a typical diet in respiration chambers, which was in broad agreement with Crutzen *et al.* (1986), who estimated that individual pigs produced approximately 1.5 kg methane $year^{-1}$. This compares with their estimates of 8 kg $year^{-1}$ for sheep and upwards of 55 kg for dairy cattle. Therefore, perhaps unsurprisingly, little research has been directed at modelling emissions from enteric fermentation in non-ruminants and the following section will concentrate on models concerning ruminants.

Crucial to the evaluation of the many potential emission reduction strategies is an understanding of the underlying biological mechanisms. The most appropriate mitigation strategy for any given scenario depends on the farming system, itself the result of many complex interrelationships. This complexity and the desire to achieve significant reductions in emissions have led to several attempts to model methanogenesis from ruminant livestock. Mathematical models offer the potential to evaluate intervention strategies for any given situation, thereby providing a low cost and quick estimate of best practice. Models of methanogenesis can be classified within two main groups. First, there are the statistical models that relate directly the nutrient intake with methane output. Secondly, there are the dynamic mechanistic models that attempt to simulate methane emissions based on a mathematical description of ruminal fermentation biochemistry.

Statistical models

Statistical modelling has been used as a tool to describe empirical relationships between the animal and enteric methane production over many years (Kriss, 1930; Bratzler and Forbes, 1940; Blaxter and Clapperton, 1965). The statistical models tend to be well suited to practical application for rapid diet evaluation or larger-scale inventory purposes. Several statistical models constructed to predict methane emissions from cattle were summarized by Wilkerson *et al.* (1995).

Based on a comparative evaluation against independent data, Wilkerson *et al.* (1995) recommended adoption of the Moe and Tyrrell (1979) linear equation for predicting emissions from dairy cows (Eqn 8.1). Unfortunately for those seeking to assess global emissions from dairy cows, this model, along with many others, was developed solely on the basis of North American data. Of practical importance is that it requires cellulose and hemicellulose to be known and such detailed data are unavailable on many farms. The relationship is summarized as:

$$CH_4\,(\text{MJ day}^{-1}) = 3.38 + 0.51\text{NFC} + 2.14\text{HC} + 2.65\text{C}, \tag{8.1}$$

where NFC is non-fibre carbohydrate, HC is hemicellulose and C is cellulose (all in kg day^{-1}). The limitation of these statistical models lies with their tendency to be unreliable predictors of emissions when applied outside the production systems upon which they were developed. Factors including species, physiological age or condition, nutrition and management all contribute to variable emissions, thereby tying statistical models to the factors and range of data that were used in their construction. An example of this situation is shown in Fig. 8.1, where the relationship between dry matter intake (DMI) and methane output described by Axelsson (1949) is plotted. Given the prevalence of more recent models to rely on a linear form to describe what is clearly a curvilinear relationship, Axelsson's model showed considerable logic and foresight. However, Fig. 8.1 shows clearly that a simple quadratic relationship cannot be used to predict emissions beyond the range of intakes upon which the model was developed (3 to 12 kg DM day^{-1}), with negative methane emissions predicted above 24 kg DMI. It is the restrictions of the statistical modelling approach that give rise to their ever increasing number, with each practical situation demanding a specially derived relationship. As we have seen from Fig. 8.1, there is a problem where published models are used outside their intended data range and, therefore, model comparisons are in danger of portraying a contradictory picture of model performance, depending on the data set used for their evaluation. A better approach

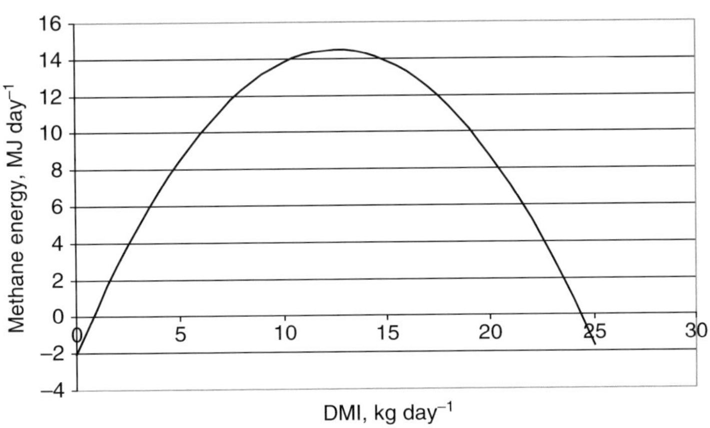

Fig. 8.1. Methane emissions from dry matter intake as predicted by Axelsson (1949).

may be to constrain evaluations of such models to the confines of the system for which they were developed and, as far as application is concerned, to think instead of selecting appropriate statistical models on a case-by-case basis.

Another danger of the empirical approach seen with many statistical models is that they imply cause and effect where none actually exists, especially when the aim of a study is to produce the strongest possible correlation for a given set of data. For example, the following model was proposed as one of five by Holter and Young (1992) with the objective to predict methane production from dairy cows:

$$\begin{aligned} CH_4(\%GE) = {} & 2.898 - 0.0631M + 0.297MF - 1.587MP + 0.0891CP \\ & + 0.101FADF + 0.102DMI - 0.131EE + 0.116DMD \\ & - 0.0737CPD, \end{aligned} \qquad (8.2)$$

where M is milk yield (kg day^{-1}), MF is milk fat (%), MP is milk protein (%), CP is crude protein, FADF is forage ADF (%DMI), EE is dietary fat (%), DMD is dry matter digestibility (%) and CPD is crude protein digestibility. This model implies a significant effect of milk yield and constituents on methane output. Milk yield and constituent concentrations are themselves the function of the animal's nutrition and other factors, as pointed out by the authors. However, this relationship already accounts for the effect of major nutrients and DMI and, for those applying the model as a predictive tool, the implications could be misleading.

In an attempt to improve on existing statistical models for UK-based dairy cow diets, Mills *et al.* (2003) tried to harness the advantages of speed and simplicity associated with the statistical approach, while introducing a degree of mechanism to include known nutritional effects on methane output as follows:

$$CH_4(\text{MJ day}^{-1}) = a - (a+b)e^{-cx}, \qquad (8.3)$$

where a and b are the upper and lower bounds of methane production, respectively, and c is a shape parameter determining the rate of change of methane production with increasing metabolizable energy (ME) intake, as defined by x. c is calculated as follows:

$$c = -0.0011\left[\frac{St}{ADF}\right] + 0.0045, \qquad (8.4)$$

where St is the starch concentration in the diet (g kg^{-1} DM) and ADF is the acid detergent fibre concentration (g kg^{-1} DM). Through application of a non-linear approach, this model displays the typical diminishing returns response observed with increasing intake, as described by Axelsson (1949), but absent from many later models. However, as shown in Fig. 8.2, the relationship based on the Mitscherlich equation is refined by altering the slope of the curve according to the form of dietary carbohydrate. This model tries to strike a balance between ease of use and additional complexity and, therefore, wider application. However, it is known that many other nutritional factors absent from this model can impact significantly on methane output and, as such, this model is still restricted in its application. When used to estimate the likely influence of the trend towards increased levels of starch in the diet at the expense of fibrous carbohydrate, as seen in many European farming systems, this model provides a quick solution.

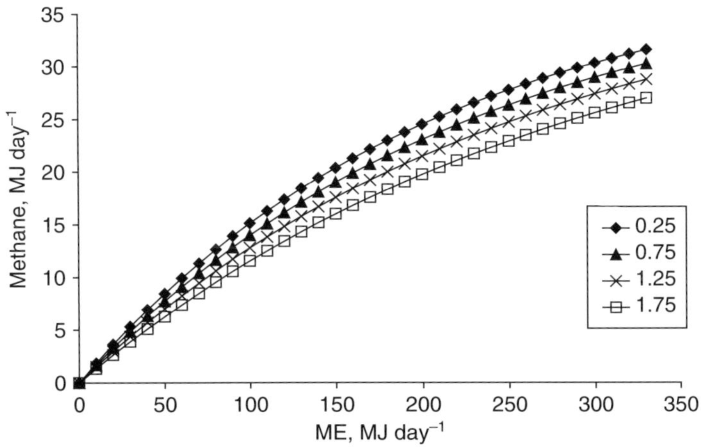

Fig. 8.2. A statistical model of methane emissions from dairy cows defining the response to energy intake as affected by starch to ADF ratio (g kg^{-1} DM) (Mills *et al.*, 2003).

Dynamic mechanistic models

Unlike their statistical counterparts, dynamic models include time as a variable and they tend to be more mechanistic in their construction. This type of model has been applied successfully on several occasions to predict methane emissions from ruminants (Mills *et al.*, 2003). However, they too are not without their limitations and they may not deliver quick solutions based on very limited dietary information. By definition, mechanistic models describe in more detail the fermentation processes occurring in the gut that result ultimately in the formation of methane as a sink for excess hydrogen. Within a model of rumen digestion, Baldwin *et al.* (1987) described a scheme for calculating the sources and sinks of this reducing power during fermentation (Fig. 8.3). Ulyatt *et al.* (1991) evaluated this model using independent data for New Zealand livestock and compared predictions with those from the models of Blaxter and Clapperton (1965) and Moe and Tyrrell (1979). Ulyatt *et al.* (1991) reported improved predictions when using the mechanistic model; however, the predictions were not without bias. The same scheme was subsequently incorporated into the whole rumen model of Dijkstra *et al.* (1992), first by Benchaar *et al.* (1998) and then with revisions by Mills *et al.* (2001), and used to evaluate the potential impact of various mitigation options.

When integrated with a larger model of rumen digestion and metabolism, schemes such as that displayed in Fig. 8.3 have the advantage that any model input can be assessed as to its effect on methane production, assuming that the underlying biology is represented sufficiently. Indeed, this model has been applied to suggest the most effective nutritional strategies for limiting emissions while maintaining an adequate nutrient supply to the host animal (Mills *et al.*, 2003) and also in the broader context of limiting emissions of both methane and

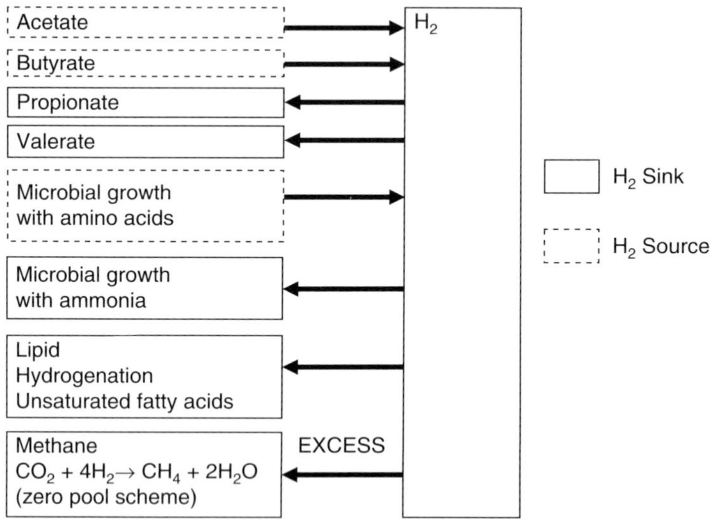

Fig. 8.3. A mechanistic scheme for methane production in the rumen (Baldwin *et al.*, 1987; Mills *et al.*, 2001).

nitrogen pollutants from dairy production (Kebreab *et al.*, 2006). While practical experimentation can demonstrate the effect of individual treatments for a given animal type and environment, mechanistic models are able to extend the value of these results by providing indications of response outside the bounds of the experimental treatments. Mills *et al.* (2001) demonstrated the potential to reduce environmental pollution and to improve production efficiency in dairy cows through increasing intake, increasing supplementation and changing the non-structural carbohydrate source. Such a tool can, therefore, form part of an integrated system to help producers and policy makers manage the threat of climate change with respect to livestock production.

Despite recent efforts to model the nutritional influence on ruminant methane emissions, there exist several nutritional and non-nutritional factors that have yet to be given adequate consideration within models of rumen function. The tendency for existing mechanistic schemes to underestimate higher-level emissions from dairy cows (Mills *et al.*, 2001) may demonstrate the need to expand the models to account for some of these effects. For example, the description of microbial metabolism within extant mechanistic models is restricted in part by their limited characterization of different microbial groups, with even the more complex models relying on one (Baldwin *et al.*, 1987) or two (Dijkstra *et al.*, 1992) distinct subdivisions of the microbial population. Further developments in this area have been constrained by the availability of suitable quantitative data and the problems associated with modelling the interrelationships observed between multiple microbial groups competing for the same substrates (Baldwin, 1995). Recent indications of the dynamic metabolic behaviour observed with different levels of substrate availability for individual microbial species (Soto-Cruz *et al.*, 2002) suggest that additional complexity will need to be integrated within mechanistic models if we are to refine further our estimates of methane output.

A significant barrier to applying any model that attempts to relate available nutrition to methane emissions has been the poor description of intake. Many statistical models of intake in ruminants are available but, by their nature, they are tied to the specific environment in which they were created. Therefore, both mechanistic and statistical models of methane output have tended to require intake to be defined as an input to the model. This is not a problem where intake has been measured directly for a given diet, as is often the case in studies directed at model evaluation, but it does create substantial problems where models are required to predict future emissions with no estimates of likely intake, such as is the case for inventory purposes.

It has been shown that as the rate of fermentation increases due to the feeding of increased readily fermentable carbohydrate, the rate of methane emission declines per unit of feed degraded (Pelchen and Peters, 1998). This fits neatly with observations of reduced methanogenic activity as rumen pH declines. However, Mills *et al.* (2001) do not account directly for this effect, with only a crude effect of pH on cellulolytic activity as a whole being present in the original model (Dijkstra *et al.*, 1992). Simulating the effects of rumen pH on the diverse microbial groups present in the rumen remains a challenge, but perhaps an even greater task is to model adequately the diurnal fluctuations in pH itself.

Figure 8.3 shows the concept of sources and sinks for excess hydrogen produced during the anaerobic fermentation process, with conversion to methane acting as the final sink following all other transactions. Our knowledge of fermentation biology is more advanced than this scheme would suggest, with several other sources and sinks likely to play a role in the overall process. Compounds such as nitrates and sulphates act as sinks and are unaccounted for in the present model. Oxygen transfer at the rumen epithelium may be significant, but experimental estimates are lacking. Apparently minor microbial species may also play a role in controlling emissions. Czerkawski (1986) suggests that, in some animals, acetotrophic methanogens could convert acetate directly to methane, while, conversely, acetogens could lead to lower methane emissions in other animals (Joblin, 1999). Dynamic models have yet to include these effects and progress is likely to remain limited in these areas without additional quantitative observations.

Non-nutritional factors, including the effects of direct pharmacological interventions such as rumen modifiers (e.g. ionophores) and selective vaccination, have yet to be incorporated into mechanistic models. Yet again, the lack of subdivisions between distinct microbial groups in existing models has thwarted what could have been a relatively straightforward application of these simulation models whereby one or another group is selectively limited or destroyed. Based on genetic sequencing observations, Whitford *et al.* (1997) suggest that only a small fraction of rumen microbes have, in fact, been cultured, with quantitative metabolic data on known species appearing infrequently. At the same time, we can assume that methane control agents such as vaccines are likely to display high host specificity. Models that fail to account for these targeted responses will be of limited use in assessing their likely impact on animal production systems.

The task of incorporating additional microbial groups is not a simple one given the numerous metabolic relationships present with other groups or species. For example, Dijkstra (1994) describes the integration of an explicit protozoal pool within the model of rumen function. At first glance, this should create the potential to account for the variable effects of defaunation on methane production (Hegarty, 1999). However, to be properly representative for a broad range of diets, such an exercise would require additional elements describing specific microbial species and their ability to live in or on specific species of protozoa (Finlay *et al.*, 1994).

Another, less obvious problem occurs when one tries to model the long-term consequences of such interventions. Extant models of rumen function have been developed to describe the steady-state biology as characterized by an animal well adapted to its diet and environment. In practice, intervention studies rarely consider treatments in these terms, leading to questions about the longer-term efficacy of these methods. Indeed, Johnson *et al.* (1994) indicated that the effect of monensin and lasalocid was not sustained beyond 16 days of treatment. This is most likely the result of adaptation by the rumen microorganisms, given their short generation time and genetic diversity. If enough data were available to describe the long-term effects of pharmacological treatments, there would still exist an opportunity to model the adaptation to these treatments. This applies equally to the potential to model the transitional response following a conventional nutritional change.

Existing modelling research has focused on animals adapted to their diet for good reason, namely because this is quantitatively more important as far as emission inventories and animal production are concerned. However, the process of adaptation from one diet to the next is of significant biomathematical interest. A quantitative description of the transitional phase would further our understanding of gastric fermentation, possibly identifying key control mechanisms in the shift from one type of fermentation to another. Any attempts to model this phase would almost certainly require a more reductionist approach than has been published previously for models of whole rumen function. Microbial competition for nutrients will impact fermentation end products, with the relative proportions of different microbial groups dependent on their abilities to metabolize dietary nutrients, intermediate compounds from other groups and even other microbes themselves, such as in the case of protozoa and their predatory behaviour. A model capable of accurately simulating transient changes in emissions through dietary manipulation will have to account for these intermicrobial relationships.

A longer-term view is also important when considering how to account for changes in methane emissions with the inevitable progression from one physiological state to another. As time advances, animals grow and develop as they move from juveniles to adults. Subsequently, they will also experience physiological changes as they progress through pregnancy and lactation. Homeorhetic control throughout this development is brought about through the endocrine system, itself a function of an individual's genes. Extant models assume these factors will ultimately manifest themselves as effects of intake and nutrition. However, it is conceivable that other modes of action to affect methane emissions are possible. For instance, it is known that intestinal morphology can change substantially following parturition, with Gibb *et al.* (1992) demonstrating a 15% increase in small intestinal length between calving and mid-lactation in Holstein dairy cows. The same study showed that a similar increase in mass was observed for rumen tissues and rumen contents. These changes will affect the extent of degradation in the rumen and also the quantity of nutrients available for fermentation in the hindgut. Unfortunately, the invasive and expensive nature of the experimentation required to provide further quantitative estimates of such physiological changes will limit the available data for model construction and evaluation.

Inter-animal variation

Several studies have observed that there can be significant variation in emissions between apparently similar individual ruminants subjected to the same experimental treatments. Such effects are most apparent when expressed as methane yield as a percentage of gross energy intake. Blaxter and Clapperton (1965) were first to demonstrate this phenomenon in sheep and cattle housed in open-circuit calorimeters. Subsequent work with sheep by Pinares-Patino *et al.* (2003) has indicated that this variation is a real long-term phenomenon, even in more natural grazing conditions, although the results of an earlier study were less conclusive (Pinares-Patino, 2000). Unfortunately for those wishing to model this variance, the underlying causes are not clear. It could be that nutritional factors such as differences in diet selection are partly responsible, in which case the challenge to the modeller is limited to defining differences in nutrient intake, as discussed previously. However, the studies described have attempted a reasonable control of nutritional composition. This raises the possibility of individuals displaying inherent differences in digestive efficiency, at least with regard to methane emissions and the recovery of dietary energy in animal product. These differences could result from variation in digestive morphology and the associated changes in digesta passage. There could also be significant differences in the composition of the microbial population, leading ultimately to variation in the balance of fermentation from one animal to another. The potential for improved prediction in existing models through further reductionism has already been highlighted as far as accounting for differences in nutrient intake. Clearly, where substantial inter-animal variation in the microbial population exists, the only determinate models suited to simulation of these effects will be those that provide the required minimum level of biological detail to describe such shifts in microbial metabolism. The description of digesta passage in mechanistic models of digestion is relatively undeveloped due to our poor quantitative knowledge of the relevant biology. Under experimental conditions, where an animal's rate of passage for certain digesta fractions can be measured, model parameters could already be adjusted accordingly in order to see if this mechanism explains the observed effect on emissions. It should be noted that the presence of significant animal-to-animal variation has important consequences for experimental design and selection of measurement technique. For example, Boadi *et al.* (2002) suggest that experiments designed to detect methane using the SF_6 tracer gas technique should use sufficient animals in order to ensure detection of genuine treatment differences.

Interspecies variation

As with animal-to-animal variance, differences between methane emissions for individuals of different ruminant species exposed to the same nutrition could be a function of digestive morphology or rumen microbial composition. The difference between sheep and cattle can be pronounced, with sheep tending to display lower emissions when expressed as a percentage of gross energy intake (Ulyatt *et al.*, 2002). It is likely that most of this difference can be explained through intake selection in a grazing environment, with sheep choosing a more digestible diet. As stated previously, statistical models tend to be blind to many factors that have the potential to alter emissions and the effect of species is no exception. However, it is possible that dynamic mechanistic models, such as those described herein, could be parameterized to enable application, despite the seemingly large jump from one ruminant species to another. Input parameters describing differences in digesta passage and nutrient intake should allow wider use of these models, emphasizing the advantage of an approach based on the fundamental biology. With regard to models of rumen function, the gap between sheep and cattle should not be considered large. Despite much focus on their subsequent application to dairy cows for socioeconomic reasons, extant dynamic models have several direct links to smaller ruminants, with many parameters and concepts used in their original development coming from research into species such as sheep.

Emissions from the Herd and Farm

Attempts to relate mechanistic model predictions of emissions to their consequences on a larger scale have been very limited and it has remained an area where static emission factors or simple statistical models have predominated. A herd of cows or flock of sheep comprises animals at different physiological states and on different nutrition. These factors, which are essentially functions of management, need to be considered when collating individual estimates of methane production in order to examine the effect of mitigation strategies on a larger scale. Of particular importance with dairy cows is the need to account for the change of herd structure over time. Modern dairy farming systems in the developed world do not conform to the standard model with mature animals calving once a year. Calving intervals for many animals are extended well beyond 400 days and age at first calving varies greatly, depending on the management system and effects of breed. Garnsworthy (2004) describes a dairy herd model that integrated and updated work from previous studies (Grossman *et al.*, 1999;

Stott *et al.*, 1999; Yates *et al.*, 2000) in an attempt to consider the effects of changes in herd management on methane and ammonia emissions. A particular focus of this work was to evaluate the effect of herd replacements on overall emissions. In principle, higher individual milk yields facilitate a smaller overall herd size and, hence, fewer replacements and a reduced yield of methane l^{-1} milk produced. However, high-producing herds are also associated with declining fertility levels and associated extended calving intervals and increased culling, which may negate at least part of this effect. Garnsworthy (2004) showed that the individual effects of milk yield and fertility, respectively, were of greater significance than changes to forage quality when it came to influencing total methane emissions. As stated previously, the effects of milk yield and fertility are certainly not independent of each other, especially when one considers the case for shorter calving intervals that increase the proportion of time an animal spends producing milk during early lactation. Garnsworthy (2004) demonstrated that improvements to herd fertility (conception rate) and the associated management (oestrus detection) produced significant benefits, regardless of level of intensity or the presence of production quotas. However, the effect of improving fertility from current UK levels (50% oestrus detection and 37% conception rate) to 'ideal' levels (70% oestrus detection and 60% conception rate) depended on the presence of quota restrictions and average milk yield per cow. With a 6000 l herd average and no quota, improving fertility by the stated amount indicated a 10% reduction in total herd emissions. For a 9000 l herd with a milk quota of 1 Ml year^{-1}, the associated reduction in methane was almost 25%. Garnsworthy (2004) thereby indicated the dangers of focusing too heavily on modelling single mitigation issues such as nutrition in an attempt to limit overall emissions.

Whilst Garnsworthy (2004) has helped to broaden the scope and application of models to predict methane emissions, there remain elements of the production system that have tended to be considered in isolation. At least for the sake of completeness, a farm model of emissions should include an estimate of production from manure storage and distribution. However, just as animal type, nutrition and management affect methane production from individual animals, there are a variety of factors that influence emissions during collection, storage and distribution of manure. This diversity introduces complexity to the task of simulating emissions and, together with their relative insignificance in relation to enteric emissions, these factors have contrived to limit modelling efforts to relatively crude inventories, the most well known of which is that used by the IPCC.

Regional Inventories

Inventories provide a mechanism to relate the modelling of emissions at the animal and farm level to higher levels of organization. Environmental policy is generally founded on the basis of regions, be they political or geographical, which span areas containing many different farms and farming systems. Therefore, inventories are required to demonstrate estimates of current emissions and to highlight historical trends in the light of existing national and international targets.

The IPCC publishes methodology for the construction of such large-scale inventories and describes a three-step process for estimating emissions for the purpose of regional or national inventories. Initially, the population is divided into subgroups corresponding to those classes of livestock for which separate emission factors can be estimated in the second step of the process. Separate emission factors are derived for enteric fermentation and manure storage. The final stage involves multiplying the emission factors by the subgroup populations and then combining to deliver an estimate of total emissions. On the face of it, this is a very straightforward process worthy of no further description. However, it should be noted that, while the official IPCC guidelines involve utilization of their recommended methodology to produce the individual emission factors using either a simplified (Tier 1) or more detailed (Tier 2) approach, it could be possible to substitute other models described above to arrive at the required factors. Having said this, care should be taken to avoid introducing unnecessary complexity into a system that is, by its very nature, full of broad assumptions about animal numbers and type.

Modelling to Evaluate Mitigation Strategies

Mitigation strategies at the level of the individual animal can be characterized broadly between two types: namely, pharmacological intervention and nutritional intervention. For ruminants in particular, the objective of many modelling exercises is to provide additional information on the efficacy of the range of potential mitigation strategies, or to define the environmental impact of other management changes that do not include effects on emissions as part of their primary objective. The snapshots represented by results from practical experimentation can be extended through the use of modelling techniques as described above. Dynamic simulation models are able to define the basis for any given effect and, therefore, not only are they able to describe quantitatively an effect on overall emissions, but they can help to understand causation.

Several papers have been published that show model predictions for various methane reduction strategies, many of which are summarized by Kebreab *et al.* (2006) and it is not intended to repeat their findings here. However, it is worth noting that there has tended to be a distinct division between analysis of effects on outputs from individual animals and the broader study of effects at the farm, regional or national scale.

Given that there is an 'overhead' of methane emissions associated with an animal's basal metabolism, results of modelling strategies to limit emissions from groups of animals over a sustained period of time have highlighted the major influence of changing animal numbers. For certain systems such as milk production, it is quite possible to produce a similar output of animal product (milk) from widely varying cow numbers, depending on the system adopted. Compared to intensive dairy regimes, extensive systems using long grazing seasons and minimal nutritional supplementation require a greater number of cows to achieve the same output of milk for any given time period. Such extensive methods can be popular for a variety of reasons focused on consumer choice and the resources available. However, Mills *et al.* (2001) and others have showed that, when concerned with methane emissions, the increased number of animals involved in the extensive system outweighs the greater individual feed intakes required under intensive management. In a logical extension to this type of analysis, it has been demonstrated that reproductive performance of a group of animals is a crucial factor in reducing unnecessary wastage from the system (cull animals) and ultimately limiting methane emissions through reduced rolling herd numbers (Garnsworthy, 2004). For pasture-based systems where the influence of supplemental nutrition is minimal, reproductive management may be the most effective tool in bringing about an overall abatement strategy.

Summary

This chapter suggests that further advances in modelling methane emissions will probably result from a deepening of the mechanistic description of the underlying fermentation biology in the gastrointestinal tract of farm livestock. At the animal level, statistical approaches will continue to be relevant where a specific solution is required and data to parameterize more complex mechanistic models are unavailable. Statistical models will continue to provide a useful input into inventory calculations for broader-scale modelling of emissions from groups of animals or regions. At this level, their straightforward operation and lack of unnecessary detail are an advantage. However, as the need for more accurate and meaningful inventories grows, it is likely that a more robust link between mechanistic, dynamic models and emission inventories will be formed. Ultimately, inventories built on such foundations will be better able to describe the potential consequences of changes in agricultural practice brought about by a changing physical and political environment.

For the time being, there remain significant gaps in our understanding of methane production from farm livestock, despite the recent efforts of many scientists to introduce a quantitative framework to studies on emissions. Models can play a major role not only in identifying these poorly understood areas, but also in helping to give direction to further experimental programmes as we try to resolve outstanding issues. The lack of consideration given to non-ruminant species, while understandable, is a cause for concern and those involved with producing national inventories of emissions would benefit from improved estimates for this class of livestock.

References

Axelsson, J. (1949) The amount of produced methane energy in the European metabolic experiments with adult cattle. *Annals of the Royal Agricultural College of Sweden* 16, 404–419.

Baldwin, R.L. (1995) *Modeling Ruminant Digestion and Metabolism*. Chapman and Hall, London.

Baldwin, R.L., Thornley, J.H.M. and Beever, D.E. (1987) Metabolism of the lactating cow. II. Digestive elements of a mechanistic model. *Journal of Dairy Research* 54, 107–131.

Benchaar, C., Rivest, J., Pomar, C. and Chiquette, J. (1998) Prediction of methane production from dairy cows using existing mechanistic models and regression equations. *Journal of Animal Science* 76, 617–627.

Blaxter, K.L. and Clapperton, J.L. (1965) Prediction of the amount of methane produced by ruminants. *British Journal of Nutrition* 19, 511–522.

Boadi, D.A., Wittenberg, K.M. and Kennedy, A.D. (2002) Validation of the sulphur hexafluoride (SF_6) tracer gas technique for measurement of methane and carbon dioxide production by cattle. *Canadian Journal of Animal Science* 82, 125–131.

Bratzler, J.W. and Forbes, E.B. (1940) The estimation of methane production by cattle. *Journal of Nutrition* 19, 611–613.

Crutzen, P.J., Aselmann, I. and Seiler, W. (1986) Methane production by domestic animals, wild ruminants, other herbivorous fauna, and humans. *Tellus* 38B, 271–284.

Czerkawski, J.W. (1986) *An Introduction to Rumen Studies*. Pergamon Press, Oxford, UK.

Dijkstra, J. (1994) Simulation of the dynamics of protozoa in the rumen. *British Journal of Nutrition* 72, 679–699.

Dijkstra, J., Neal, H.D.St.C., Beever, D.E. and France, J. (1992) Simulation of nutrient digestion, absorption and outflow in the rumen: model description. *Journal of Nutrition* 122, 2239–2256.

Environmental Protection Agency (2005) *US Emissions Inventory 2005: Inventory of US Greenhouse Gas Emissions and Sinks: 1990–2003*. US Environmental Protection Agency, Washington, DC.

Finlay, B.J., Esteban, G., Clarke, K.G., Williams, A.G., Embley, T.M. and Hirt, R.P. (1994) Some rumen ciliates have endo-symbiotic methanogens. *FEMS Microbiology Letters* 117, 157–162.

Garnsworthy, P.C. (2004) The environmental impact of fertility in dairy cows: a modeling approach to predict methane and ammonia emissions. *Animal Feed Science and Technology* 112, 211–223.

Gibb, M.J., Ivings, W.E., Dhanoa, M.S. and Sutton, J.D. (1992) Changes in body components of autumn-calving Holstein-Friesian cows over the first 29 weeks of lactation. *Animal Production* 55, 339–360.

Grossman, M., Hartz, S.M. and Koops, W.J. (1999) Persistency of lactation yield: a novel approach. *Journal of Dairy Science* 82, 2192–2197.

Hegarty, R.S. (1999) Reducing rumen methane emissions through elimination of rumen protozoa. *Australian Journal of Agricultural Research* 50, 1321–1327.

Holter, J.B. and Young, A.J. (1992) Methane prediction in dry and lactating Holstein cows. *Journal of Dairy Science* 75, 2165–2175.

Intergovernmental Panel on Climate Change (2001) *Climate Change 2001: The Scientific Basis*. Cambridge University Press, Cambridge, UK.

Joblin, K.N. (1999) Ruminal acetogens and their potential to lower ruminant methane emissions. *Australian Journal of Agricultural Research* 50, 1307–1313.

Johnson, D.E., Abo-Omar, J.S., Saa, C.F. and Carmean, B.R. (1994) Persistence of methane suppression by propionate enhancers in cattle diets. In: Aquilera, J.F. (ed.) *Energy Metabolism of Farm Animals*. EAAP Publication No. 76. CSIC Publishing Service, Mojacar, Spain.

Kebreab, E., Clark, K., Wagner-Riddle, C. and France, J. (2006) Methane and nitrous oxide emissions from Canadian animal agriculture: a review. *Canadian Journal of Animal Science* 86, 135–158.

Kirchgessner, M., Kreuzer, M., Muller, H.L. and Windisch, W. (1991) Release of methane and carbon dioxide by the pig. *Agribiological Research* 44, 103–113.

Kriss, M. (1930) Quantitative relations of dry matter of the food consumed, the heat production, the gaseous outgo and the insensible loss in body weight of cattle. *Journal of Agricultural Research* 40, 283–295.

Laubauch, J. and Kelliher, F.M. (2005) Measuring methane emission rates of a dairy cow herd (II): results from a backward-Lagrangian stochastic model. *Agricultural and Forest Meteorology* 129, 137–150.

Leuning, R., Baker, S.K., Jamie, I.M., Hsu, C.H., Klein, L., Denmead, O.T. and Griffith, D.W.T. (1999) Methane emission from free-ranging sheep: a comparison of two measurement methods. *Atmospheric Environment* 33, 1357–1365.

Lockyer, D.R. and Jarvis, S.C. (1995) The measurement of methane losses from grazing animals. *Environmental Pollution* 90, 383–390.

Mills, J.A.N., Dijkstra, J., Bannink, A., Cammell, S.B., Kebreab, E. and France, J. (2001) A mechanistic model of whole-tract digestion and methanogenesis in the lactating dairy cow: model development, evaluation, and application. *Journal of Animal Science* 79, 1584–1597.

Mills, J.A.N., Kebreab, E., Yates, C.M., Crompton, L.A., Cammell, S.B., Dhanoa, M.S., Agnew, R.E. and France, J. (2003) Alternative approaches to predicting methane emissions from dairy cows. *Journal of Animal Science* 81, 3141–3150.

Moe, P.W. and Tyrrell, H.F. (1979) Methane production in dairy cows. *Journal of Dairy Science* 62, 1583–1586.

Pelchen, A. and Peters, K.J. (1998) Methane emissions from sheep. *Small Ruminant Research* 27, 137–150.

Pinares-Patino, C.S. (2000) Methane emission from forage-fed sheep, a study of variation between animals. PhD thesis, Massey University, Palmerston North, New Zealand.

Pinares-Patino, C.S., Ulyatt, M.J., Lassey, K.R., Barry, T.N. and Homes, C.W. (2003) Persistence of difference between sheep in methane emission under generous grazing conditions. *Journal of Agricultural Science* 140, 227–233.

Soto-Cruz, O., Favela-Torres, E. and Saucedo-Castaneda, G. (2002) Modeling of growth, lactate consumption, and volatile fatty acid production by *Megasphaera elsdenii* cultivated in minimal and complex media. *Biotechnology Progress* 18, 193–200.

Stott, A.W., Veerkamp, R.F. and Wassell, T.R. (1999) The economics of fertility in the dairy herd. *Animal Science* 68, 49–57.

Ulyatt, M.J., Betteridge, K., Costall, D., Knapp, J. and Baldwin, R.L. (1991) *Methane Production by New Zealand Ruminants*. Report prepared for the New Zealand Ministry for the Environment. New Zealand Ministry for the Environment, Wellington.

Ulyatt, M.J., Lassey, K.R., Shelton, I.D. and Walker, C.F. (2002) Methane emission from dairy cows and wether sheep fed subtropical grass-dominant pastures in midsummer in New Zealand. *New Zealand Journal of Agricultural Research* 45, 227–234.

Whitford, M.E., Forster, R.J., Beard, C.E., Gong, J. and Teather, R.M. (1997) Phylogenetic analysis of rumen bacteria by comparative sequence analysis of cloned 16 S-rRNA genes. *Anaerobe* 4, 153–163.

Wilkerson, V.A., Casper, D.P. and Mertens, D.R. (1995) The prediction of methane production of Holstein cows by several equations. *Journal of Dairy Science* 78, 2402–2414.

Yates, C.M., Cammell, S.B., France, J. and Beever, D.E. (2000) Prediction of methane emissions from dairy cows using multiple regression analysis. *Proceedings of the British Society of Animal Science* 2000, 94.

9 Supporting Measurements Required for Evaluation of Greenhouse Gas Emission Models for Enteric Fermentation and Stored Animal Manure

C. WAGNER-RIDDLE,[1] E. KEBREAB,[2,3] J. FRANCE[3] AND J. RAPAI[1]

[1]Department of Land Resource Science, University of Guelph, Canada; [2]National Centre for Livestock and Environment, Department of Animal Science, University of Manitoba, Canada; [3]Centre for Nutrition Modelling, Department of Animal and Poultry Science, University of Guelph, Canada

Introduction

The potential environmental impact of animal production is wide-ranging, comprising aspects of human health, water, soil and air quality. Recently, concerns with increased atmospheric concentration of gases such as carbon dioxide (CO_2), methane (CH_4) and nitrous oxide (N_2O), and the related enhancement of the greenhouse effect, have prompted calls for quantification and better understanding of greenhouse gas (GHG) emissions related to animal production. These emissions occur in the form of CH_4 and N_2O at several stages of the animal–manure–soil–crop (AMSC) continuum and are a function of the carbon and nitrogen transfer between compartments, starting with animal feed intake and ending with nutrient uptake by crops (Fig. 9.1).

Limited data on GHG emissions associated with animal production are available worldwide (NRC, 2003). Efforts to address this research gap have focused on individual components of the AMSC continuum but, clearly, effective management of GHG emissions requires an understanding of the whole nutrient cycle. Most animal nutrition and enteric fermentation studies have not been concerned with GHG emissions 'downstream' from the 'animal' compartment (Fig. 9.1). Likewise, studies on GHG emissions during storage or treatment of manure and after manure application are often carried out outside an animal

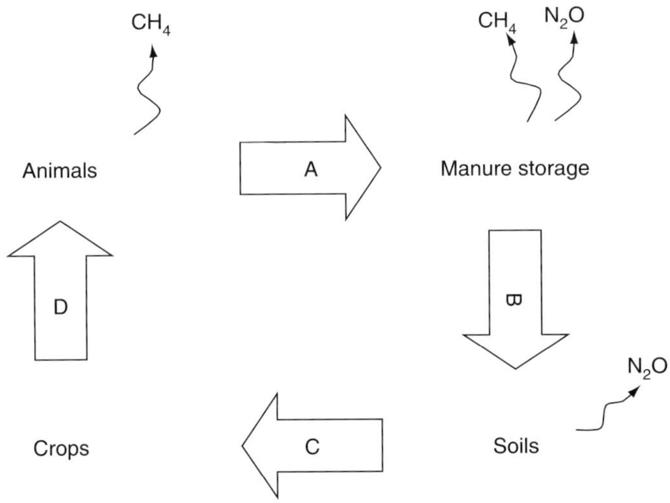

Fig. 9.1. Transfer of nitrogen and carbon in animal production systems from animals to manure storage in the form of faeces and urine (A), from manure storage to soils through field application of manure (B), from soils to crops through plant uptake (C) and from crops or pasture to animals through feed intake (D). Potential emissions of greenhouse gases, methane and nitrous oxide, are shown for each compartment of the cycle.

nutrition context. Hence, the usefulness of emission data obtained is compromised, in particular, for future efforts on modelling of GHG for the AMSC continuum.

The objectives of this chapter are to: (i) briefly review processes and controlling factors involved in GHG production and emission associated with animal production; (ii) review currently used models that describe GHG emissions from animal production; and (iii) identify supporting measurements and reporting standards for GHG emission studies to improve the usefulness of obtained data. In our discussion, we will first address these objectives for CH_4 emissions from enteric fermentation and then for CH_4 and N_2O emissions from manure storage.

Methane Emissions from Enteric Fermentation

Processes and controlling factors

Enteric CH_4 production arises principally from microbial fermentation of hydrolysed dietary carbohydrates such as cellulose, hemicellulose, pectin and starch. The primary substrates for ruminal methanogenesis are hydrogen (H_2) and CO_2. Most of the H_2 produced during fermentation of hydrolysed dietary carbohydrates, much of which is generated during the conversion of hexose to acetate or butyrate via pyruvate, ends up in CH_4. Significant quantities of ruminal CH_4, particularly with high-protein diets, can also arise from microbial fermentation of amino acids, the end products of which are ammonia, volatile fatty acids (VFAs), CO_2 and CH_4 (Mills *et al.*, 2001). The environmental consequences aside, CH_4 emissions represent an energetic inefficiency that impacts on profitability of livestock production through reduced feed conversion efficiency. Therefore, the rationale of the producers and the policy makers may be different, but the goal of reduced emissions is universal.

The amount of CH_4 produced by an animal is influenced by many factors. These include dietary factors such as type of carbohydrate in the diet, level of feed intake, level of production (e.g. annual milk production in dairy), digesta passage rate, presence of ionophores, degree of saturation of lipids in the diet, environmental factors such as temperature and genetic factors such as efficiency of feed conversion (Kebreab *et al.*, 2006a).

Modelling methanogenesis

Crucial to the evaluation of the many potential emission reduction strategies is an understanding of the underlying biological mechanisms. The most appropriate mitigation strategy for any given scenario depends on the farming system, itself the result of many complex interrelationships. This complexity and the desire to achieve significant reductions in emissions have led to several attempts to model methanogenesis from ruminant livestock. Mathematical models offer the potential to evaluate intervention strategies for any given situation, thereby providing a low cost and quick estimate of best practice. Models of methanogenesis can be classified within two main groups. First, there are the statistical models that directly relate the nutrient intake with methane output, which includes emission factors provided by the Intergovernmental Panel on Climate Change, IPCC (2000) (Table 9.1). Secondly, there are the dynamic mechanistic models that attempt to simulate methane emissions based on a mathematical description of ruminal fermentation biochemistry.

Statistical models

Statistical modelling has been used as a tool to describe empirical relationships between the animal and enteric CH_4 production over many years (e.g. Blaxter and Clapperton, 1965). The statistical models tend to be well suited to practical application for rapid diet evaluation or larger-scale inventory purposes. The IPCC publishes methodology for the construction of large-scale inventories and describes a three-step process for estimating emissions for the purpose of regional or national inventories. Initially, the population is divided into subgroups corresponding to those classes of livestock for which separate emission factors can be estimated in the second step of the process. Separate emission factors are derived for enteric fermentation and manure storage. The final stage involves multiplying the emission factors by the subgroup populations and then combining to deliver an estimate of total emissions (Table 9.1). On the face of it, this is a very straightforward process worthy of no further description. However, it should be noted that, while the official IPCC guidelines involve utilization of their recommended

Table 9.1. Comparison of model inputs required for emission factor and process-based models of greenhouse gas emission from animals and manure storage.

Type of model	Parameter modelled	Units	Inputs	Source
Emission factor	CH_4 (enteric fermentation)	kg CH_4 per head $year^{-1}$	– number of animals – type of animals (species, lactating) – emission factor (EF) for each type of animal	IPCC (2000)
	CH_4 (enteric fermentation)	MJ CH_4 day^{-1}	– metabolizable energy intake – starch and acid detergent fibre intake	Mills *et al.* (2003)
	CH_4 (manure storage)	kg CH_4 per head $year^{-1}$	– number of animals using manure storage – type of manure storage – volatile solids excreted per animal (VS) – methane conversion factor (MCF) – ultimate methane yield (B_o)	IPCC (2000)
	N_2O (manure storage)	kg N_2O-N (kg $N_{excreted}$)$^{-1}$	– type of manure storage – N content of manure – number of animals using storage	IPCC (2000)
	CH_4 (manure storage)	kg CH_4 per head $year^{-1}$	– animal production stage/class – animal age and body weight – amount of meat/ milk produced – feed type – feed intake – manure management	Phetteplace *et al.* (2001)
Process-based	CH_4 (enteric fermentation)	kg CH_4 day^{-1} MJ CH_4 day^{-1} moles CH_4 day^{-1}	– dry matter intake – volatile fatty acids (and lactic acid) in diet – NDF, degradable NDF, total starch, degradable starch, soluble sugars – N content, ammonia N in diet, undigestible protein – rate of degradation of starch and protein	Kebreab *et al.* (2004)

(*Continued*)

Table 9.1 *Continued.*

Type of model	Parameter modelled	Units	Inputs	Source
	CH_4 (manure storage)	g CH_4 day^{-1}	– proportion of degradable and non-degradable VS in manure – daily VS loading rate in-house and outside store – emptying frequency – potential and actual methane yield – manure in-house residence time – housing air temperature – monthly mean air temperature (assumed equal to slurry temperature)	Sommer *et al.* (2004)
	CH_4 (manure digestion)	l CH_4 day^{-1}	– initial volume – daily VS loading rate or input rate – volatile fatty acids (C_2 – C_5) – total nitrogen, NH_4 – temperature	Hill (1982), Hill *et al.* (1983), Hill and Cobb (1996)

methodology to produce the individual emission factors using either a simplified (Tier 1) or more detailed (Tier 2) approach, it could be possible to substitute other models to arrive at the required factors. Having said this, care should be taken to avoid introducing unnecessary complexity into a system that is, by its very nature, full of broad assumptions about animal numbers and type.

Extant statistical models that estimate methane emissions have been reviewed by Kebreab *et al.* (2006a). Similar to the emission factors, the statistical models will provide a useful input into inventory calculations for broader-scale modelling of emissions from groups of animals or regions; however, one should be aware of their inadequacies. The limitation of these statistical models lies with their tendency to be unreliable predictors of emissions when applied outside the production systems upon which they were developed. Factors including species, physiological age or condition, nutrition and management all contribute to variable emissions, thereby tying statistical models to the factors and range of data that were used in their construction.

Process-based models

Unlike their statistical counterparts, dynamic models include time as a variable and they tend to be more mechanistic in their construction. This type of model has been applied successfully on several occasions to predict methane emissions from ruminants (Mills *et al.*, 2003). However, they too are not without their limitations and they may not deliver quick solutions based on very limited dietary information. By definition, mechanistic models describe in more detail the fermentation processes occurring in the gut that result ultimately in the formation of CH_4 as a sink for excess H_2. Baldwin *et al.* (1987) described a scheme for calculating the sources and sinks of this reducing power during fermentation. Ulyatt *et al.* (1991) evaluated this model using independent data for New Zealand livestock and compared predictions with those from the models of Blaxter and Clapperton (1965) and Moe and Tyrrell (1979). They highlighted the improved prediction seen when using the mechanistic model, although they noted that the predictions were not without bias. The same scheme was subsequently incorporated into the whole rumen model of Dijkstra *et al.* (1992) by Mills *et al.* (2001) and used to evaluate the potential impact of various mitigation options. Indeed, this model has been applied to suggest the most effective nutritional strategies for limiting emissions while maintaining an adequate nutrient supply to the host animal (Mills *et al.*, 2003), and also in the broader context of limiting emissions of both CH_4 and nitrogen pollutants from dairy production (Kebreab *et al.*, 2006b). The model requires detailed information on diet such as dry matter intake, types of carbohydrates and their degradabilities, protein concentration and degradability and amount of lipid in the diet.

Future developments in modelling and data requirements

There have been numerous studies conducted since the mid-1960s which have the potential to be used as a source for development/refinement of models to predict CH_4 emissions from enteric fermentation accurately (Table 9.2).

Table 9.2. Selected results from the literature examining CH_4 and N_2O emissions from animal and manure storage.

Source	Type of animal/manure	System	Recorded value	Measurement method/period
Belyea *et al.* (1985)	Dairy	Enteric fermentation	8.9 MJ day^{-1}	Respiration mask
Boadi and Wittenberg (2002)	Dairy	Enteric fermentation	9.5 MJ day^{-1}	Tracer gas (SF_6)
Boadi and Wittenberg (2002)	Beef	Enteric fermentation	9.5 MJ day^{-1}	Tracer gas (SF_6)
Boadi *et al.* (2002)	Steers	Enteric fermentation	11.4 MJ day^{-1}	Tracer gas (SF_6)
Johnson *et al.* (2002)	Dairy	Enteric fermentation	21.4 MJ day^{-1}	Tracer gas (SF_6)
Kinsman *et al.* (1995)	Dairy	Enteric fermentation	20.3 MJ day^{-1}	Infrared gas analyser from barn
McCaughey *et al.* (1999)	Beef	Enteric fermentation	13.7 MJ day^{-1}	Tracer gas (SF_6)
McCaughey *et al.* (1997)	Steers	Enteric fermentation	8.9–11.3 MJ day^{-1}	Tracer gas (SF_6)
Sauer *et al.* (1998)	Dairy	Enteric fermentation	20.7 MJ day^{-1}	Infrared gas analyser from barn
McGinn *et al.* (2004)	Beef	Enteric fermentation	9.1 MJ day^{-1}	Chamber
Husted (1994)	Swine Dairy	Liquid manure storage	0.4–35.8 g CH_4 m^{-3} day^{-1} 0.0–34.5 g CH_4 m^{-3} day^{-1}	Periodically from 1 October 1991 to 31 September 1992
Khan *et al.* (1997)	Dairy	Liquid manure storage	2–100 kg CH_4 ha^{-1} day^{-1}	4 days in May 1995, and 2 days in August 1995
Kaharabata *et al.* (1998)	Swine Dairy	Liquid manure storage	74 kg CH_4 m^{-2} $year^{-1}$ 56.5 kg CH_4 m^{-2} $year^{-1}$	12 June to 20 November 1995
Sharpe and Harper (1999)	Swine	Liquid manure storage	52.3 kg CH_4 ha^{-1} day^{-1}	Periodically over the entire year of 1996

Harper *et al.* (2000)	Swine	Liquid manure storage	0–3.6 kg N_2O ha^{-1} day^{-1}	Summer 1994 to summer 1996
Sommer *et al.* (2000)	Dairy	Liquid manure storage	<0.01–1.4 g CH_4 m^{-3} h^{-1}	Autumn 1996, summer 1997
Sharpe *et al.* (2002)	Swine	Liquid manure storage	5.3–115.3 kg CH_4 ha^{-1} day^{-1}	Periodically from May 1997 to February 1998
Massé *et al.* (2003)	Dairy	Liquid manure storage	Short storage: 1.46–2.17 l CH_4 m^{-3} day^{-1} Long storage: 1.06–14.83 l CH_4 m^{-3} day^{-1}	Laboratory, 180 days or 272 days storage periods, total solids (5%, 10%), and temperature (10°C, 15°C) varied
	Swine		Short storage: 5.36–30.00 l CH_4 m^{-3} day^{-1} Long storage: 4.97–28.08 l CH_4 m^{-3} day^{-1}	
Külling *et al.* (2003)	Dairy	Liquid manure storage	13.6–16.1 µg CH_4 m^{-2} s^{-1} 0.20–0.40 µg N_2O-N m^{-2} s^{-1}	Laboratory, 5–7 weeks storage, comparing diets
Wolter *et al.* (2004)	Swine	Solid manure storage	6–63 mg CH_4-C kg^{-1}(DM) day^{-1} 6–28 mg N_2O-N kg^{-1}(DM) day^{-1}	Periodically over 113 days
Laguë *et al.* (2005)	Swine	Liquid manure storage	3.75 g CO_2 eq kg^{-1} day^{-1}	Periodically from 2001 to 2003
DeSutter and Ham (2005)	Swine	Liquid manure storage	60–210 g CH_4 m^{-2} day^{-1}	Daily over 1 year (2001)
Pattey *et al.* (2005)	Dairy	Liquid, solid manure storage	1.52–15.96 g CH_4 kg^{-1}(DM) (3 month)$^{-1}$ 0.101–0.582 g N_2O kg^{-1}(DM) (3 month)$^{-1}$	Twice weekly over 14 weeks
Pattey *et al.* (2005)	Beef	Liquid, solid manure storage	0.14–9.76 g CH_4 kg^{-1}(DM) (3 month)$^{-1}$ 0.017–0.162 g N_2O kg^{-1}(DM) (3 month)$^{-1}$	Twice weekly over 11 weeks
Park *et al.* (2006)	Swine	Liquid manure storage	4.6×10^{-3}–1.05 mg CH_4 m^{-2} s^{-1} 101.8–337.6 ng N_2O m^{-2} s^{-1}	Half-hourly over 15 months, July 2000 to May 2002

As described above, methanogenesis is affected by various factors and those studies report a select set of conditions, which limit their usability in integrating the studies. At the minimum, every study needs to report feed intake (amount and description) and methane output. Even at this basic level, a significant barrier to applying any model that attempts to relate available nutrition to CH_4 emissions has been the poor description of intake. It has been shown that, as the rate of fermentation increases due to the feeding of increased readily fermentable carbohydrate, the rate of CH_4 emission declines per unit of feed degraded (Pelchen and Peters, 1998). This fits neatly with observations of reduced methanogenic activity as rumen pH declines. Therefore, intake data should include amount and types of carbohydrate consumed. The data would be useful for modelling if the feed components (in kg day^{-1}), such as starch, non-digestible fibres (NDF), simple sugars, protein and lipids with associated degradabilities of carbohydrates and protein, were given (Table 9.3). A longer-term view is also important when considering how to account for changes in CH_4 emissions with the inevitable progression from one physiological state to another. As time advances, animals grow and develop and they move from juveniles to adults. Subsequently, they will also experience physiological changes as they progress through pregnancy and lactation. Therefore, the physiological state of the animal (e.g. non-lactating, if lactating then days in milk, parity, etc.) would give strength to the data. Animal weight should be reported in case there is a need for scaling by some of the models. Unlike other models that predict nutrient balances (and therefore require measurement of various outputs), CH_4 models are input-driven; therefore, the better the quality of input in terms of dietary description, the more freedom in selecting or developing a model. With advances in measurement techniques, it is assumed that CH_4 output is accurately measured in a controlled environment.

Several studies have observed that there can be significant variation in emissions between apparently similar individual ruminants subjected to the same experimental treatments. Such effects are most apparent when expressed as methane yield as a percentage of gross energy intake. Blaxter and Clapperton (1965) were first to demonstrate this phenomenon in sheep and cattle housed in open-circuit calorimeters. Subsequent work by Pinares-Patino *et al.* (2003) has indicated that this is a real long-term effect, even in more natural grazing conditions, although the results of an earlier study were less conclusive (Pinares-Patino, 2000). Unfortunately for those wishing to model this variance, the underlying causes are not clear. It could be that nutritional factors such as differences in diet selection are partly responsible, in which case the challenge to the modeller is limited to defining differences in nutrient intake.

Greenhouse Gas Emissions from Manure Storage

Globally, approximately 0.2–2.5 Tg N_2O-N and 34 Tg CH_4 are produced annually from manure storage (Berges and Crutzen, 1996). Manure is stored in liquid or solid form or, alternatively, in cases where animals are left in pasture, no

Table 9.3. Supporting measurements related to animal populations required in greenhouse gas emissions studies. Data should be collected by animal class. Frequency of measurements recommended is weekly, bi-weekly or as changes occur.

Parameter	Units (SI units)	Essential?
Species	–	Yes
Number of animals	–	Yes
Age	(day, month, year, as appropriate)	Yes
Weight (start)	kg	Yes
Weight gain	kg day^{-1}	Yes
Physiological state	–	Yes
Daily feed intake (weight as consumed)	kg day^{-1}	Yes
Feed intake management	–	
Diet composition:		
dry matter content	%	Yes
forage:concentrate ratio	–	Yes
non-digestible fibres	%	Yes
ash	%	Yes
crude protein	%	Yes
lipids	%	
total N	%	
total C	%	
total P	%	
total S	%	
Additives	g kg^{-1} DM	
Excreted total nitrogen	kg per head	Yes
Excreted forms of nitrogen:		
NH_4^+	% (or kg per head)	
urine N	kg per head	Yes
faecal N	kg per head	
Excreted volatile solids	kg per head	
Rumen pH	–	
Rumen microbes	g l^{-1}	
Alternate H_2 sinks (e.g. ionophores)	g kg^{-1} DM	
Management	–	
Genetic selection (breed)	–	

storage is used. Faeces and urine excreted by animals, plus bedding and/or water used in barns, are flushed or removed into storage until field application is carried out. The IPCC (2000) provides a description of the main types of storage systems, as popular use of these systems varies worldwide. Typically, storage systems are grouped according to the total solids (TS) content of the manure, with solid, semi-solid and liquid systems referring to >20, 10–20 and <10% TS, respectively. Liquid manure systems are considered important sources of

CH_4, whereas solid storage is estimated to be a significant source of both CH_4 and N_2O (Janzen *et al.*, 1998).

Availability of organic matter and anaerobic conditions in manures favour the production of CH_4 by methanogens, with some consumption of CH_4 occurring in the portion of the manure with high O_2 content, such as in crusts (Petersen *et al.*, 2005). Presence of ammonium and some O_2 in solid or aerated liquid manures may lead to N_2O production through nitrification; however, this process usually results in relatively low N_2O emissions. Denitrification is considered the main microbial process resulting in N_2O emissions from manure and this process is dependent on nitrate production through nitrification and requires low O_2 availability. Ultimately, modelling of GHG emissions from stored manure requires an in-depth understanding of the microbial processes producing and consuming these gases, as well as their controlling factors. Truly mechanistic, dynamic, process-based models attempt to describe these processes at the biological level, with state variables (e.g. acetic acid concentration, nitrate concentration) changing according to the rate of microbial consumption or production (e.g. methanogenesis, methanotrophy, nitrification, denitrification), as affected by controlling factors (e.g. O_2 for denitrification) or inhibition factors (e.g. NH_3 for methanogenesis). Empirically based models use macroscale variables (e.g. water content) as surrogates and often combine several fundamental concepts into one factor that is applicable for a certain set of conditions. The 'emission factor' approach (IPPC, 2000) is an example of the latter and is discussed in detail in the following section. A discussion on process-based models follows.

Emission factor approach

Modelling GHG emissions from manure storage has largely been carried out using the emission factor (EF) approach, as detailed by IPCC methodology (IPCC, 2000, 2006). In this approach, emissions of CH_4 are obtained by multiplying the population of animals in each livestock category by an EF (kg CH_4 per head year^{-1}) specific for the given category and country or region. The approach for N_2O is similar, with EF expressed in kg N_2O-N (kg N)$^{-1}$ excreted. For CH_4, a refinement of this approach has been proposed, where EF is a function of maximum methane production potential for a given manure type, volatile solid (VS) content of manure, as estimated from animal diet (dry matter intake, energy digestibility and ash content), and a CH_4 conversion factor (MCF) that takes climate and type of manure storage into account (Tier 2).

The EF approach is well suited for national GHG inventories, as it requires activity data that can be obtained relatively easily, such as number of animals. The disadvantage of this approach is that mitigation practices often cannot be evaluated, as many important processes for GHG emission are not captured in the EF equations. For example, in the case of Tier 2 EF (IPCC, 2000), changes in animal diet other than VS content would not affect predicted CH_4 emissions, while there is experimental evidence that low protein diets can result in lower CH_4 emissions (Velthof *et al.*, 2005). Further refinement of the EF approach to capture animal and manure management practices would require an extensive data set of emission measurements. It is important to ensure that current and future efforts in GHG flux measurements collect supporting data that would allow for derivation of emission factors as a function of various animal and manure management indicators.

In a recent study, Park *et al.* (2006) measured half-hourly CH_4 fluxes from liquid swine manure stored in concrete tanks, which were averaged to obtain monthly flux means and then converted to a monthly emission per animal, using the storage tanks' surface area and the number of animals at each farm. Data obtained for the three measurement sites were then pooled and an annual CH_4 emission factor was obtained by summing monthly emissions and interpolating for 2 months with missing data (September and December). Similarly, DeSutter and Ham (2005) obtained an EF for anaerobic lagoons through measurement of biogas fluxes over 1 year. In both studies, comparison with IPCC EF was possible since CH_4 fluxes were measured over the course of a year. Interestingly, the IPCC-derived EF overestimated measured EF in both studies. DeSutter and Ham (2005) speculated that CH_4 losses from barn storage pits could potentially account for the observed difference, as IPCC EF attempt to quantify CH_4 emissions from all manure generated per animal over 1 year. In the IPCC EF, this effect is quantified through the VS production per animal year^{-1}, which provides the substrate for CH_4 production. Not all VS produced ends up in outdoor storage, potentially explaining the observed discrepancy between measured and derived EF.

An independent measurement of fraction of excreted VS that reaches anaerobic lagoon storage would allow for a direct comparison of measured and IPCC-derived EF. This is also applicable to Park *et al.*'s (2006) study, which aimed at comparing US Environmental Protection Agency (USEPA)- and IPCC-derived MCF with a measured MCF for manure stored in tanks. While the measured MCF compared favourably with USEPA-derived values based on manure temperature (0.22–0.25), measurements of excreted VS and VS in manure would have allowed for further testing of the IPCC Tier 2 EF approach. Due to the inverse relationship between VS and MCF derived from EF, an uncertainty of ±30% in average estimated VS in manure would have resulted in changes in estimated MCF between 42 and –23%.

Process-based models

Few models describing the process that leads to GHG emissions from stored manure under ambient conditions currently exist. Husted (1994) measured CH_4 and CO_2 emission from pig and dairy manure stored in tanks (liquid) and in piles (solid) and proposed regression equations to predict CH_4 emission as a function of manure temperature. He also included regression equations for emissions from liquid manure with a crust on the surface.

Due to the controlled nature of the anaerobic digestion process, there are several models (Hill, 1982; Hill and Cobb, 1996; Keshtkar *et al.*, 2003;

Escudié *et al.*, 2005; and cited references therein) that describe methane production of digesters, bioreactors and lagoons. These models are based on the kinetics of fundamental processes (hydrolysis, acetogenesis, methanogenesis), their stoichiometric equations, the kinetics of bacterial growth, with described processes linked by mass-balance equations. The kinetics of bacterial growth is highly related to temperature. These models could form the basis for development of a process-based model of GHG emissions from liquid stored manure, but clearly such a model would need to include the complexity of O_2 diffusion into the liquid surface layer, CH_4 diffusion and ebullition to manure surface, manure temperature variations according to weather conditions, and other factors. For manure stored in solid piles, modelling of processes leading to GHG emissions is more complex, as conditions in the surface layer are mostly aerobic but in the centre of the pile anaerobic conditions are prevalent.

Models describing processes that lead to N_2O emissions from soils have been developed (Li *et al.*, 1992) and, in principle, these algorithms could be applied to emissions from solid manure storage. However, the spatial variability of air temperature, substrate concentration and airflow through manure piles (Wolter *et al.*, 2004) add additional complexities to the modelling effort.

Integrated models

Ideally, models dealing with the GHG from manure management should be integrated with models which describe processes that extend beyond the storage tank, that is, through the AMSC continuum. Understandably, such efforts do not use process-based approaches for the modelling of GHG emissions from each 'pool', but rather an emission factor approach, or simplified model for each pool, and focus on the flows of nutrients between different pools.

Schils *et al.* (2005) suggest a framework for full GHG accounting, where both direct and indirect emissions (e.g. from tractor usage) are estimated from the entire farm system, rather than from one component alone. The model divides a farm into five submodels, or pools, one of which is manure storage. Inputs to the manure pool are, in part, derived from outputs of the animal and enteric fermentation pool and, similarly, outputs from the manure pool are inputs for modelling emissions from manure-applied soils. IPCC emission factors are used in the model when data are not available. Specific inputs required to estimate CH_4 and N_2O using the Schils *et al.* (2005) model are listed in Table 9.1.

Sommer *et al.* (2004) proposed algorithms for a model that quantifies CH_4 emissions from liquid manure during storage and N_2O emissions from soils after field application of slurry (Table 9.1). Methane emission during storage is modelled as a function of degradable and non-degradable VS and indoor or outdoor air temperature (assumed equal to slurry temperature). Volatile solid accumulation between storage emptying is considered, although it is not clear if VS consumed during methanogenesis is subtracted from VS in storage. Nitrous oxide emission from soils is modelled as a function of VS, slurry N and soil water potential, and using emissions factors for denitrification and nitrification that occur in 'clumps' of added slurry and for nitrification that occurs in soils. Although this approach has the merit of linking CH_4 and N_2O fluxes through the carbon and nitrogen cycle, some of the empirical equations used are probably only valid for the specific slurries studied by Sommer *et al.* (2004). Also, these authors cite a lack of GHG emission data for manure storage available for testing of their model.

Phetteplace *et al.* (2001) used IPCC emission factors and equations in a farm-scale model of N_2O and CH_4. The model included factors such as milk or meat production, diet characteristics and manure management, which are more accurate when taken on a farm-by-farm basis rather than from a national average. Another farm-scale study used more recent figures for manure storage and N-excretion rates to prepare an improved IPCC model, which resulted in significantly higher estimates (Brown *et al.*, 2001).

A committee of researchers examining air emissions from animal feeding operations found a whole farm approach was needed for dealing with gaseous losses (NRC, 2003). Mitigation of GHG from farming operations is important, but should be viewed within the context of other pollution issues. It is important to be aware of the impact that mitigation measures may have on other pollution problems. Altering one aspect of a nutrient cycle can drastically affect other components within that cycle. For instance, management practices which result in reducing N_2O loss, yet cause an increase in NH_3 volatilization or mineral-N leaching to groundwater, should not be used for GHG mitigation, as the problem has just been altered to another form.

Supporting measurements required for modelling of greenhouse gas emissions from animal manure

The development of models to predict GHG emissions from manure storage requires the measurement and reporting of additional variables that are often missing in published studies. As discussed above, manure composition and characteristics such as pH, BVS, VFA (acetate, propionate, butyrate, valerate), temperature and O_2 concentration are very important for the understanding of processes leading to GHG production, and these variables should be quantified over the course of experiments designed to measure GHG fluxes (Table 9.4). The manure management practices of the studied farm should be described so that the measured gas fluxes can be interpreted accordingly. In particular, dynamic variables such as loading rate or input over time would allow for a link between manure tank and animals generating the manure. For outdoor storage, the environmental conditions (e.g. air temperature, rainfall) which will determine manure temperature are important, as these would be inputs for models aiming at describing gas fluxes from manure. These data are often available from local weather stations but, if unavailable from these sources, variables should be monitored by researchers during the study period. Finally, a complete description of the animal production operation, with emphasis on the barn units using the monitored storage tank, is fundamental (Table 9.4). This would ensure that, in the future, modelling of manure processes could be linked to animal nutrition modelling efforts.

Table 9.4. Supporting measurements related to animal manure required in greenhouse gas emissions studies. Frequency of measurements recommended is weekly, bi-weekly, or as changes occur, except for environmental variables, which should be measured daily or at hourly intervals.

Parameter	Units	Essential?
Type of storage	–	Yes
Surface area of storage (tank, windrow)	m^2	Yes
Width and length of storage (tank, windrow)	m	Yes
Volume of storage (tank, windrow)	m^3	
Depth or height of storage (tank, windrow)	m	Yes
Bedding materials:		
description	–	Yes
dry matter content	%	
timing of addition	Date, time	
amount added	Total (kg) and kg m^{-3} manure	
Manure removal:		
description (mechanical cleaning, flushing from barn to tank)	–	Yes
timing	Date, time	Yes
amount	m^3	Yes
duration	h	Yes
Manure handling:		
description (agitation, turning)	–	Yes
location (holding tank, lagoon)		
timing	Date, time	
duration	h	
Manure in storage (tank, windrow):		
total depth	m	Yes
depth of sludge (tank)	m	
description (presence of crust, etc.)	–	
temperature profile (3 depths)	°C	
timing of emptying/spreading	Date, time	
volume left (tank)	m^3	
Manure composition:		
dry matter content	%	Yes
volatile solids	%	
total C	%	Yes
total N	%	
ash	%	
NO_3^-	mg l^{-1}	
NH_4^+	mg l^{-1}	
sulfur	mg l^{-1}	
phosphorus	mg l^{-1}	
pH	–	

(Continued)

Table 9.4. *Continued.*

Parameter	Units	Essential?
Environment:		
air temperature	°C	Yes
wind speed	$m\ s^{-1}$	
wind direction	degrees	
precipitation	mm	
air humidity	%	
solar radiation	$W\ m^{-2}$	

Standards for reporting of greenhouse gas fluxes from manure

As discussed in Kebreab *et al.* (2006a), methods for quantification of gaseous fluxes from stored manure are based on methods developed for measurement of gaseous emissions from soils and can be classified into chamber or micro-meteorological methods. These methods yield a flux (in strict terms, a flux density), i.e. mass of gas per area per time, averaged over the measurement period (typically > 30 min). When chamber methods are deployed in a laboratory setting, a known volume or mass of manure is used, so that fluxes are often reported in units of mass of gas per volume (or mass) of manure per time (Massé *et al.*, 2003). In the case of continuous flow anaerobic digesters, treatment design takes into account VS loading rates, and methane production is often expressed as volume or mass of gas per mass of added VS per time (Umetsu *et al.*, 2005). Gas emissions from solid manure piles have been expressed on a manure dry matter basis, which requires careful monitoring of manure dry matter content, as decomposition significantly decreases this value over time (Wolter *et al.*, 2004; Pattey *et al.*, 2005). As detailed above, EF consists of expressing flux as mass of gas per head $year^{-1}$ for a given animal category. In order to account for differences in animal size, some authors have expressed fluxes as mass of gas kg^{-1} live animal weight per time (Laguë *et al.*, 2005). There is evidently a multitude of ways in which gas flux can be expressed; clearly making the task of comparing results from different studies very difficult (Table 9.2). Agreement on a reporting standard may be difficult due to the diverse disciplines involved in the study of processes and gas emissions from manure. However, we suggest that fluxes be reported 'as measured', which, for most field experiments, consists of a flux density, and that detailed description and measurements of the emitting substrate be reported simultaneously. For CH_4, which is produced from decomposition of VS, a measure of total amount of VS (degradable and non-degradable) in the manure tank, including daily/weekly loading rates or input, is recommended. For N_2O, total nitrogen in the manure, including the partitioning into organic and mineral (NH_4^+, NO_3^-) forms, needs to be quantified.

This raises issues related to manure sampling procedures due to the non-homogeneous nature of manure, particularly the stratification that occurs in liquid manures (Ndegwa and Zhu, 2003; DeSutter and Ham, 2005). In solid manure piles, stratification of mineral N forms can also occur, with NO_3^- usually only present in the drier surface layer, where, apparently, nitrification can take place (Brown *et al.*, 2001). Advances in infrared spectroscopy for real-time analysis of dry matter and organic matter in liquid manure samples may provide the option for frequent measurement of manure composition (Saeys *et al.*, 2005).

Finally, the detailed characterization of emitting substrate (i.e. manure composition over time) needs to be accompanied by a description of the animals generating the manure, their diet and the manure management used at the facility.

In summary, for GHG emissions from manure storage, studies that seek to measure gas fluxes or treatment impacts for mitigation are encouraged to include the following measurements:

1. *Emission rate expressed as mass CH_4 or N_2O per area and per time (e.g. mg m^{-2} s^{-1})*

CH_4 and N_2O flux must be reported as a function of time as recorded and not as long-time averages. Daily means are acceptable averages.

2. *Dimensions of manure storage and manure volume stored*

Dimensions are required in order to calculate volume and surface area of the emitting storage unit. The change in level of liquid manure in tank over time or the volume/mass input and output rate are also useful in order to associate emissions with a known manure volume/mass. For solid manure piles, monitoring of the volume and bulk density are required.

3. *Composition of manure (total solids, volatile solids, biodegradable volatile solids, volatile fatty acids, total nitrogen, ammonium)*

This information, combined with manure volume, would give a measure of substrate amount for total GHG emissions.

4. *Length of manure storage time*

Methane production has been shown to be related to the length of storage time for liquid dairy manure, but not for liquid swine manure (Massé *et al.*, 2003). Moreover, measured mean gas fluxes need to be integrated over the storage period in order to calculate annual emissions. Frequency of agitation or emptying of manure storages should be recorded and included in reporting.

5. *Animals using storage system*

IPCC emission factors are on a per head basis, thus comparison with these factors requires inclusion of the number of animals contributing to the emissions. Uniformity in reporting is desirable, as some studies report on the basis of animal units, by animal weight (e.g. kg CH_4 (1000 kg body weight)$^{-1}$), or by product weight (e.g. kg CH_4 (kg milk)$^{-1}$). Ideally, reporting should include number of animals per standard weight category and productivity level (weight gain, milk production, etc.), as well as animal diet and feed intake characterization.

Supporting measurements required for modelling of greenhouse gas emissions from animal manure

The development of models to predict GHG emissions from manure storage requires the measurement and reporting of additional variables that are often missing in published studies. As discussed above, manure composition and characteristics such as pH, BVS, VFA (acetate, propionate, butyrate, valerate), temperature and O_2 concentration are very important for the understanding of processes leading to GHG production, and these variables should be quantified over the course of experiments designed to measure GHG fluxes (Table 9.4). The manure management practices of the studied farm should be described so that the measured gas fluxes can be interpreted accordingly. In particular, dynamic variables such as loading rate or input over time would allow for a link between manure tank and animals generating the manure. For outdoor storage, the environmental conditions (e.g. air temperature, rainfall) which will determine manure temperature are important, as these would be inputs for models aimed at describing gas fluxes from manure. These data are often available from local weather stations, but if unavailable from these sources, variables should be monitored by researchers during the study period. Finally, a complete description of the animal production operation, with emphasis on the barn units using the monitored storage tank, is fundamental (Table 9.4). This would ensure that in the future, modelling of manure processes can be linked to animal nutrition modelling efforts.

Conclusions

Modelling has been used to summarize and give an added value to research conducted in relation to GHGs. Although there are a number of models developed thus far, further advances in modelling GHG emissions will probably result from a strengthening of the mechanistic description of the underlying microbial processes in the gastrointestinal tract of farm livestock, in stored manure and in soils. Statistical approaches will continue to be relevant where a specific solution is required and data to parameterize more complex mechanistic models are unavailable. Future research should report a detailed description of diet, such as type of energy, protein and their degradabilities, and amount of lipid; animals, such as weight, age and physiological state; manure, such as type and size of storage, composition, and environmental conditions.

References

Baldwin, R.L., Thornley, J.H.M. and Beever, D.E. (1987) Metabolism of the lactating cow. II. Digestive elements of a mechanistic model. *Journal of Dairy Science* 54, 107–131.

Belyea, R.L., Marin, P.J. and Sedgwick, H.T. (1985) Utilization of chopped and long alfalfa by dairy heifers. *Journal of Dairy Science* 68, 1297–1301.

Berges, M.G.M. and Crutzen, P.J. (1996) Estimates of global N_2O emissions from cattle, pig and chicken manure, including a discussion of CH_4 emissions. *Journal of Atmospheric Chemistry* 24, 241–269.

Blaxter, K.L. and Clapperton, J.L. (1965) Prediction of the amount of methane produced by ruminants. *British Journal of Nutrition* 19, 511–522.

Boadi, D.A. and Wittenberg, K.M. (2002) Methane production from dairy and beef heifers fed forages differing in nutrient density using the sulphur hexafluoride (SF_6) tracer gas technique. *Canadian Journal of Animal Science* 82, 201–206.

Boadi, D.A., Wittenberg, K.M. and McCaughey, W.P. (2002) Effects of grain supplementation on methane production of grazing steers using the sulphur hexafluoride (SF_6) tracer gas technique. *Canadian Journal of Animal Science* 82, 151–157.

Brown, L., Jarvis, S.C. and Headon, D. (2001) A farm-scale basis for predicting nitrous oxide emissions from dairy farms. *Nutrient Cycling in Agroecosystem* 60, 149–158.

DeSutter, T.M. and Ham, J.M. (2005) Lagoon-biogas emissions and carbon balance estimates of swine production facility. *Journal of Environmental Quality* 34, 198–206.

Dijkstra, J., Neal, H.D.St.C., Beever, D.E. and France, J. (1992) Simulation of nutrient digestion, absorption and outflow in the rumen: model description. *Journal of Nutrition* 122, 2239–2256.

Escudié, R., Conte, T., Steyer, J.P. and Delgenès, J.P. (2005) Hydrodynamic and biokinetic models of an anaerobic fixed-bed reactor. *Process Biochemistry* 40, 2311–2323.

Harper, L.A., Sharpe, R.R. and Parkin, T.B. (2000) Gaseous nitrogen emissions from anaerobic swine lagoons: ammonia, nitrous oxide, and dinitrogen gas. *Journal of Environmental Quality* 29, 1356–1365.

Hill, D.T. (1982) A comprehensive dynamic model for animal waste methanogenesis. *Transactions of the ASAE* 25, 1374–1380.

Hill, D.T. and Cobb, S.A. (1996) Simulation of process steady-state in livestock waste methanogenesis. *Transactions of the ASAE* 39, 565–573.

Hill, D.T., Tollner, E.W. and Holmberg, R.D. (1983) The kinetics of inhibition in methane fermentation of swine manure. *Agricultural Waste* 5, 105–123.

Husted, S. (1994) Seasonal variation in methane emission from stored slurry and solid manures. *Journal of Environmental Quality* 23, 585–592.

Intergovernmental Panel on Climate Change (IPCC) (2000) *Good Practice Guidance and Uncertainty Management in National Greenhouse Gas Inventories.* Cambridge University Press, Cambridge, UK.

Intergovernmental Panel on Climate Change (IPCC) (2006) IPCC Guidelines for National Greenhouse Gas Inventories, 2006. In: Eggleston, H.S., Buendia, L., Miwa, K., Ngara, T. and Tanabe, K. (eds) *National Greenhouse Gas Inventories Programme.* IGES, Japan. Available at: http://www.ipcc-nggip.iges.or.jp/public/2006gl/vol4.htm

Janzen, H.H., Desjardins, R.L., Asselin, J.M.R. and Grace, B. (1998) *The Health of Our Air: Toward Sustainable Agriculture in Canada.* Research Branch, Agriculture and Agri-Food Canada, Ottawa.

Johnson, K.A., Kincaid, R.L., Westberg, H.H., Gaskins, C.T., Lamb, B.K. and Cronrath, J.D. (2002) The effect of oilseeds in diets of lactating cows on milk production and methane emissions. *Journal of Dairy Science* 85, 1509–1515.

Kaharabata, S.K., Schuepp, P.H. and Desjardins, R.L. (1998) Methane emissions from above ground open manure slurry tanks. *Global Biogeochemical Cycles* 12, 545–554.

Kebreab, E., Mills, J.A.N., Crompton, L.A., Bannink, A., Dijkstra, J., Gerrits, W.J.J. and France, J. (2004) An integrated mathematical model to evaluate nutrient partition in dairy cattle between animal and environment. *Animal Feed Science and Technology* 112, 131–154.

Kebreab, E., Clark, K., Wagner-Riddle, C. and France, J. (2006a) Methane and nitrous oxide emissions from Canadian animal agriculture: a review. *Canadian Journal of Animal Science* 86, 135–158.

Kebreab, E., France, J., McBride, B.W., Odongo, N., Bannink, A., Mills, J.A.N. and Dijkstra, J. (2006b) Evaluation of models to predict methane emissions from enteric fermentation in North American dairy cattle. In: Kebreab, E., Dijkstra, J., Gerrits, W.J.J., Bannink, A. and France, J. (eds) *Nutrient Utilization in Farm Animals: Modelling Approach.* CAB International, Wallingford, UK, pp. 219–313.

Keshtkar, A., Mayssami, B., Abolhamd, G., Ghaforian, H. and Asadi, M.K. (2003) Mathematical modeling of non-ideal mixing continuous flow reactors for anaerobic digestion of cattle manure. *Bioresource Technology* 87, 113–124.

Khan, R.Z., Muller, C. and Sommer, S.G. (1997) Micrometeorological mass balance technique for measuring CH_4 emission from stored cattle slurry. *Biology and Fertility of Soils* 24, 442–444.

Kinsman, R., Sauer, F.D., Jackson, H.A. and Wolynetz, M.S. (1995) Methane and carbon dioxide emissions from dairy cows in full lactation monitored over a six-month period. *Journal of Dairy Science* 78, 2760–2766.

Külling, D.R., Menzi, H., Sutter, F., Lischer, P. and Kreuzer, M. (2003) Ammonia, nitrous oxide and methane emissions from differently stored dairy manure derived from grass- and hay-based rations. *Nutrient Cycling Agroecosystems* 65, 13–22.

Laguë, C., Gaudet, É., Agnew, J. and Fonstad, T.A. (2005) Greenhouse gas emissions from liquid swine manure storage facilities in Saskatchewan. *Transactions of the ASAE* 48, 2289–2296.

Li, C.S., Frolking, S. and Frolking, T.A. (1992) A model of nitrous-oxide evolution from soil driven by rainfall events. 1. Model structure and sensitivity. *Journal of Geophysical Research – Atmospheres* 97, 9759–9776.

McCaughey, W.P., Wittenberg, K. and Corrigan, D. (1997) Methane production by steers on pasture. *Canadian Journal of Animal Science* 77, 519–524.

McCaughey, W.P., Wittenberg, K. and Corrigan, D. (1999) Impact of pasture type on methane production by lactating beef cows. *Canadian Journal of Animal Science* 79, 221–226.

McGinn, S.M., Beauchemin, K.A., Coates, T. and Colombatto, D. (2004) Methane emissions from beef cattle: effects of monensin, sunflower oil, enzymes, yeast, and fumaric acid. *Journal of Animal Science* 82, 3346–3356.

Massé, D.I., Croteau, F., Patni, N.K. and Masse, L. (2003) Methane emissions from dairy cow and swine manure slurries stored at 10°C and 15°C. *Canadian Biosystems Engineering* 45, 6.1–6.6.

Mills, J.A.N., Dijkstra, J., Bannink, A., Cammell, S.B., Kebreab, E. and France, J. (2001) A mechanistic model of whole tract digestion and methanogenesis in the lactating dairy cow: model development, evaluation and application. *Journal of Animal Science* 79, 1584–1597.

Mills, J.A.N., Kebreab, E., Yates, C.M., Crompton, L.A., Cammell, S.B., Dhanoa, M.S., Agnew, R.E. and France, J. (2003) Alternative approaches to predicting methane emissions from dairy cows. *Journal of Animal Science* 81, 3141–3150.

Moe, P.W. and Tyrrell, H.F. (1979) Methane production in dairy cows. *Journal of Dairy Science* 62, 1583–1586.

National Research Council (NRC) (2003) *Air Emissions from Animal Feeding Operations.* National Academy Press, Washington, DC, 263 pp.

Ndegwa, P.M. and Zhu, J. (2003) Sampling procedures for piggery slurry in deep pits for estimation of nutrient content. *Biosystems Engineering* 85, 239–248.

Park, K.-H., Thompson, A.G., Marinier, M., Clark, K. and Wagner-Riddle, C. (2006) Greenhouse gases from stored liquid swine manure in a cold climate. *Atmospheric Environment* 40, 618–627.

Pattey, E., Trzcinski, M.K. and Desjardins, R.L. (2005) Quantifying the reduction of greenhouse gas emissions as a result of composting dairy and beef cattle manure. *Nutrient Cycling in Agroecosystems* 72, 173–187.

Pelchen, A. and Peters, K.J. (1998) Methane emissions from sheep. *Small Ruminant Research* 27, 137–150.

Petersen, S.O., Amon, B. and Gattinger, A. (2005) Methane oxidation in slurry storage crusts. *Journal of Environmental Quality* 34, 455–461.

Phetteplace, H.W., Johnson, D.E. and Seidl, A.F. (2001) Greenhouse gas emissions from simulated beef and dairy livestock systems in the United States. *Nutrient Cycling in Agroecosystems* 60, 99–102.

Pinares-Patino, C.S. (2000) Methane emission from forage-fed sheep, a study of variation between animals. PhD thesis, Massey University, Palmerston North, New Zealand.

Pinares-Patino, C.S., Ulyatt, M.J., Lassey, K.R., Barry, T.N. and Homes, C.W. (2003) Persistence of difference between sheep in methane emission under generous grazing conditions. *Journal of Agricultural Science* 140, 227–233.

Saeys, W., Mouazen, A.M. and Ramon, H. (2005) Potential for onsite and online analysis of pig manure using visible and near infrared reflectance spectroscopy. *Biosystems Engineering* 91, 393–402.

Sauer, F.D., Fellner, V., Kinsman, R., Kramer, J.K.G., Jackson, H.A., Lee, A.J. and Chen, S. (1998) Methane output and lactation response in Holstein cattle with monensin or unsaturated fat added to the diet. *Journal of Animal Science* 76, 906–914.

Schils, R.L.M., Verhagen, A., Aarts, H.F.M. and Sebek, L.B.J. (2005) A farm level approach to define successful mitigation strategies for GHG emissions from ruminant livestock systems. *Nutrient Cycling in Agroecosystems* 71, 163–175.

Sharpe, R.R. and Harper, L.A. (1999) Methane emissions from an anaerobic swine lagoon. *Atmospheric Environment* 33, 3627–3633.

Sharpe, R.R., Harper, L.A. and Byers, F.M. (2002) Methane emissions from swine lagoons in southeastern US. *Agriculture, Ecosystems and Environment* 90, 17–24.

Sommer, S.G., Petersen, S.O. and Søgaard, H.T. (2000) Atmospheric pollutants and trace gases: greenhouse gas emission from stored livestock slurry. *Journal of Environmental Quality* 29, 744–751.

Sommer, S.G., Petersen, S.O. and Møller, H.B. (2004) Algorithms for calculating methane and nitrous oxide emissions from manure management. *Nutrient Cycling in Agroecosystems* 69, 143–154.

Ulyatt, M.J., Betteridge, K., Costall, D., Knapp, J. and Baldwin, R.L. (1991) *Methane Production by New Zealand Ruminants.* Report prepared for the Ministry for the Environment, DSIR Grasslands, Palmerston North, New Zealand.

Umetsu, K., Kimura, Y., Takahashi, J., Kishimoto, T., Kojima, T. and Young, B. (2005) Methane emission from stored dairy manure slurry and slurry after digestion by methane digester. *Animal Science Journal* 76, 73–79.

Velthof, G.L., Nelemans, J.A., Oenema, O. and Kuikman, P.J. (2005) Gaseous nitrogen and carbon losses from pig manure derived from different diets. *Journal of Environmental Quality* 34, 698–706.

Wolter, M., Prayitno, S. and Schuchardt, F. (2004) Greenhouse gas emission during storage of pig manure on pilot scale. *Bioresource Technology* 95, 235–244.

10 Data Capture: Development of a Mobile Open-circuit Ventilated Hood System for Measuring Real-time Gaseous Emissions in Cattle

N.E. ODONGO,[1] O. ALZAHAL,[1] J.E. LAS,[1] A. KRAMER,[2] B. KERRIGAN,[3] E. KEBREAB,[1,4] J. FRANCE[1] AND B.W. MCBRIDE[1]

[1]Centre for Nutrition Modelling, Department of Animal and Poultry Science, University of Guelph, Canada; [2]Department of Animal Sciences, Wageningen University, The Netherlands; [3]54–2979 River Road, RR3 Chemainus, Canada; [4]National Centre for Livestock and Environment, Department of Animal Science, University of Manitoba, Canada

Introduction

Climate change refers to long-term changes in weather patterns caused by natural phenomena and human activities that alter the chemical composition of the atmosphere, resulting in the build-up of greenhouse gases (GHGs; Environment Canada, 2005). The main naturally occurring GHGs are water vapour, carbon dioxide (CO_2), ozone (O_3), methane (CH_4) and nitrous oxide (N_2O). One-third of the energy radiated to the earth by the sun is reflected back to space by the stratospheric ozone layer, clouds, deserts and snow cover. At normal atmospheric concentrations of GHGs, there is a balance between the energy retained and the energy lost, thus keeping the earth's temperature at approximately 15°C. Greenhouse gases reduce the net loss of infrared heat to space, while having little impact on the absorption of solar radiation, thereby causing the surface temperature to be warmer than it otherwise would be and producing the so-called greenhouse effect (Intergovernmental Panel on Climate Change (IPCC), 1997). Human activities are altering the concentration of GHGs and aerosols, both of which influence, and are influenced by, climate (IPCC, 1997). In general, temperatures and sea levels are expected to rise and the frequency of extreme weather events is expected to increase.

In 2002, Canada emitted about 731 megatonnes of CO_2 equivalent (Mt CO_2 eq) of GHGs to the atmosphere (Environment Canada, 2005). Approximately 81%

of the total GHG emissions were from the energy sector, while agriculture accounted for 8.1% (or 59 Mt), mainly from enteric fermentation (CH_4) and manure management (N_2O and CH_4; 49%) and soil management and cropping practices, e.g. fertilizer application (N_2O; 51%; Environment Canada, 2005). Enteric CH_4 is produced as an unavoidable by-product of organic matter fermentation in the rumen and it represents a loss of dietary energy of up to 12%. The amount of CH_4 produced by an animal is influenced by many factors, including type of carbohydrate in the diet, level of feed intake, level of production (e.g. annual milk production in dairy), digesta passage rate, presence of ionophores, degree of saturation of lipids in the diet, environmental factors such as temperature (McAllister *et al.*, 1996) and genetic factors such as feed conversion efficiency (Nkrumah *et al.*, 2006). In recent years, focus on the environmental impact agriculture has on GHGs has been intensifying and there is a need for an accurate inventory of GHGs in order to identify potential sources that can be mitigated. The IPCC publishes guidelines for national GHG inventories, which are used for official estimates of CH_4 emissions (e.g. IPCC, 1997). These guidelines might not be sufficiently sensitive or accurate given the types of animals currently kept or the diets fed today.

Several methods have been used to measure CH_4 emissions from ruminants. These range from whole-animal respiration calorimetry chambers with various types of gas analysers, to tracer techniques and whole-barn mass-balance techniques (Young *et al.*, 1975; McLean and Tobin, 1987; Johnson and Johnson, 1995). Whole-animal respiration chambers are the gold standard (Young *et al.*, 1975; McLean and Tobin, 1987; Johnson and Johnson, 1995). The principle behind open-circuit indirect calorimetry technique is that outside air is circulated around the animal's head, mouth and nose and expired air collected (McLean and Tobin, 1987). Gaseous exchange is then determined by measuring the total airflow through the system and the difference in concentration between inspired and expired air. However, although whole-animal open-circuit indirect respiration chamber systems have been used extensively in the literature (McLean and Tobin, 1987), they are expensive to construct and maintain.

Ventilated head-hoods or head-boxes, which are less expensive, can also be used to quantify gaseous exchange using the same principle. Various types of head-hood systems have been used with degrees of success in a number of nutritional and physiological studies (Bergman, 1964; Young *et al.*, 1975; McLean and Tobin, 1987; Ku-Vera *et al.*, 1990; Takahashi and Young, 1991, 1994; Kelly *et al.*, 1994; Nicholson *et al.*, 1996). The advantages and disadvantages of each method have been reviewed by Johnson and Johnson (1995). This technique involves the use of an airtight box that encloses the animal's head. The box is big enough to allow the animal to move its head in an unrestricted manner and allows access to feed and water. A sleeve or drape is placed around the animal's neck to minimize air leakage (Kelly *et al.*, 1994). Outside air is then circulated around the animal's head, mouth and nose through the sleeve and expired air collected (McLean and Tobin, 1987) and gaseous exchange quantified. The objective of this chapter is to update, describe and test a mobile, open-circuit ventilated hood system for measuring real-time gaseous exchange in large ruminants at the farm level.

Materials and Methods

System design

Ventilated hood

The head-hood was custom-made to enclose a large animal's head and was made from white polypropylene sheeting material (6 mm thickness; Johnston Industrial Plastics, Toronto, Ontario, Canada) mounted on steel frames (179 cm high by 74 cm deep by 105 cm wide). In the front end of the hood was an opening through which the animal's head was placed. A tightly woven tarp material (sleeve) was attached to the opening in the hood and secured around the animal's neck using a nylon drawstring, such that the animal could stand or lie down in the stanchions with its head in the hood (Figs 10.1 and 10.2). Air was drawn through the system using two pumps at the posterior end of the system, which created a slight negative pressure throughout the system, thus eliminating any leakage of expired air to the atmosphere. The air entered the system through the gaps between the animal and the sleeve around the animal's neck. The rear panel of the hood was lined with insulating foam along the metal frame to prevent air leakage when the panel door was closed. The panel was hinged on one side and fitted with two 5 cm butterfly clips on the other end to facilitate feeding and watering of the animal. On both sides and at the rear end of the hood were transparent acrylic windows to enable the animal to see its surroundings and allow visual inspection of the animal without disturbing the collection environment.

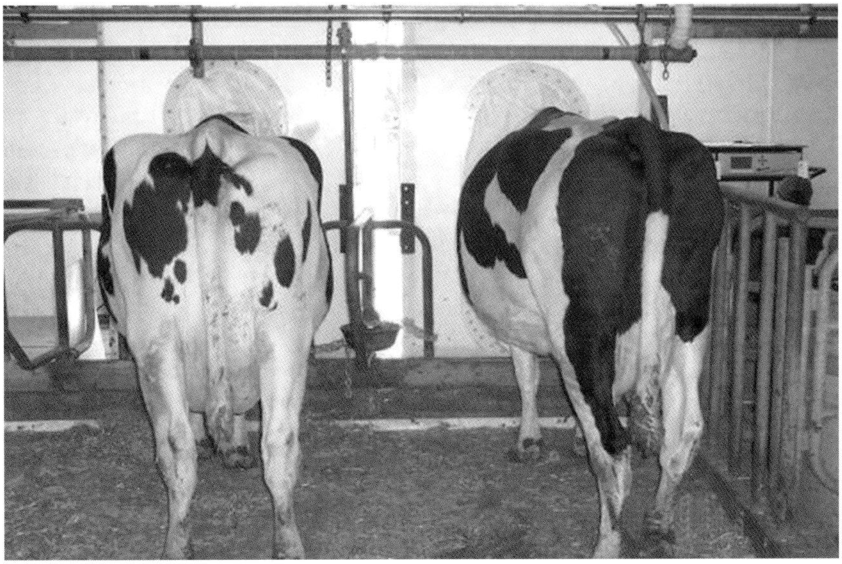

Fig. 10.1. Cows in the ventilated head-hoods during measurement of gaseous exchange (standing).

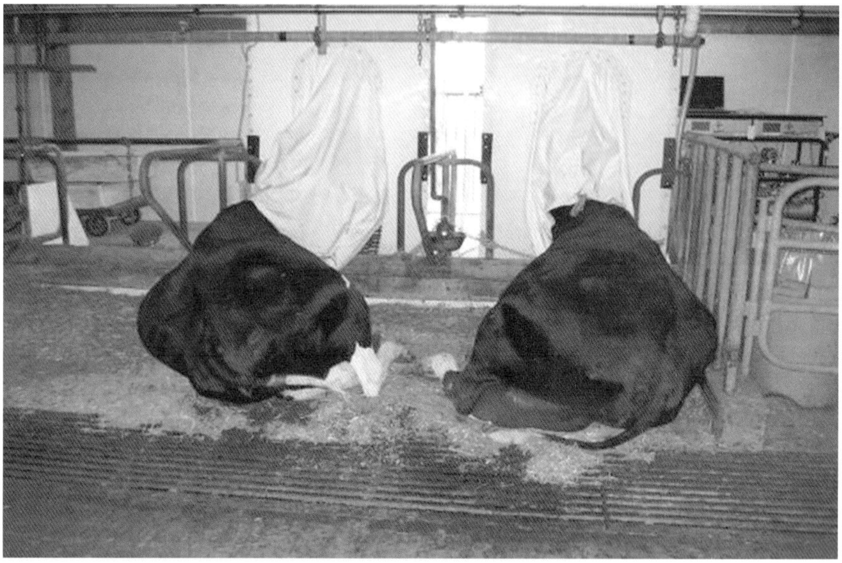

Fig. 10.2. Cows in the ventilated head-hoods during measurement of gaseous exchange (lying down).

Gas sampling

The calorimetry unit was based on two separate but linked sampling lines, each associated with one of the two hoods (Fig. 10.3) mounted on a cart on wheels (104 cm long by 89 cm high by 61 cm wide; Fig. 10.4). The main line (25.4 mm i.d.; reinforced polyethylene tubing; Kuri Tec Corporation, Cambridge, Ontario, Canada) moved the gases from the ventilated hoods to an oil-less vacuum pump system (model 3040 in series with model 1023-101Q; Gast Manufacturing, Inc., Benton Harbor, Michigan) and exhausting the gases to the outside. The two pumps were held in series to ensure airflow through the system was maintained at least at 600 l min^{-1} to ventilate the animals adequately. The lines were also fitted with bypass control valves (F, Fig. 10.3). Mounted in-line were: (i) an absolute pressure transmitter (model IAP10; Invensys Process Systems, Foxboro, Massachusetts) to measure absolute pressure; (ii) temperature and relative humidity sensors with built-in display (model HX93DA; Omega Engineering, Inc., Stamford, Connecticut) to measure and display temperature and relative humidity; and (iii) a differential pressure transmitter fitted with an integral flow orifice assembly (model IDP10; Invensys Process Systems, Foxboro, Massachusetts) to measure air flow.

A side arm (9.5 mm i.d.; reinforced polyethylene tubing; Kuri Tec Corporation, Cambridge, Ontario, Canada) withdraws a sample of the gases from the main line using a second airtight oil-less vacuum pump (model 1531-107B; Gast Manufacturing, Inc., Benton Harbor, Michigan) with a flow rate of approximately 30 l min^{-1}. The subsampling system was connected to four two-way solenoid operated valves (Omega Engineering, Inc., Laval, Quebec, Canada), which directed air from each hood in sequence to the analysers. The gases were passed through an acrylic drying column (anhydrous calcium sulphate; W.A. Hammond

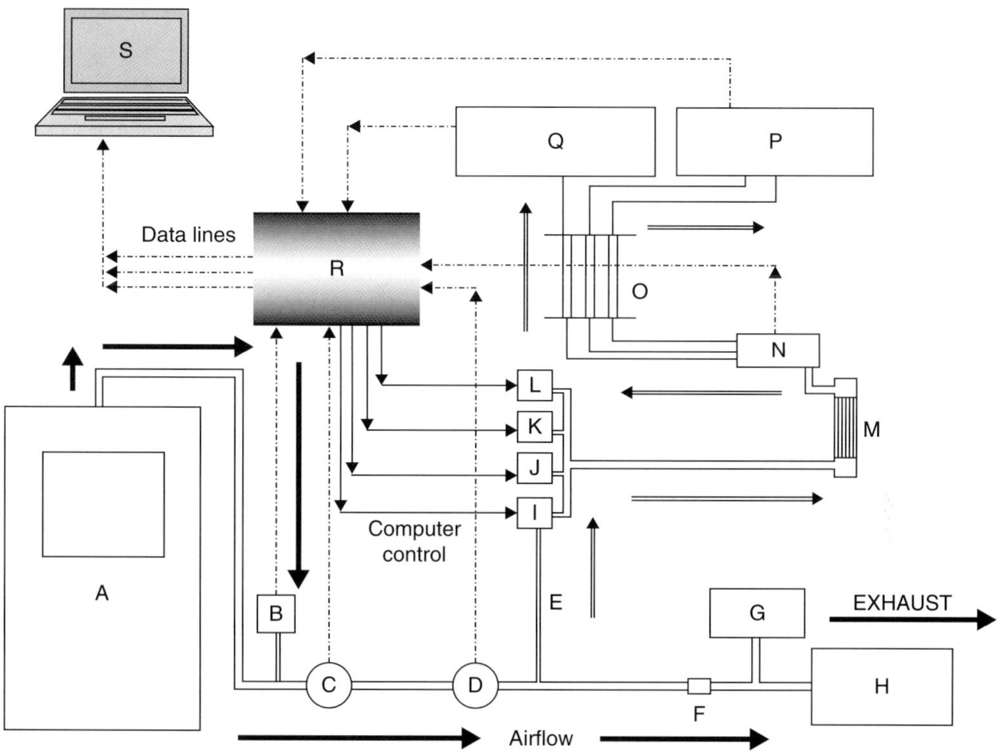

Fig. 10.3. Schematic of the calorimetry system attached to one hood (not to scale; see also picture of cart in Fig. 10.4). A, ventilated hood; B, temperature and relative humidity sensor; C, absolute pressure transmitter; D, differential pressure transmitter; E, subsampling side arm; F, bypass control valve; G, vacuum pump (Gast model 1023-101Q); H, vacuum pump (Gast model 3040, G and H are in series); a second line from the second hood (A2; not shown) was connected to the subsampling line E using a T-junction; I, J, K, L computer controlled two-way solenoid operated valves (hood air A1, hood air A2, room air, calibration gases, respectively); M, Drierite drying column; N, sampling pump (Gast model 1531-107B); O, instantaneous variable-area flow meters; P, oxygen analyser; Q, methane and carbon dioxide analyser; R, black box (system control and data acquisition panel); S, laptop computer. Airflow in the main line (thick solid arrow), airflow in the subsampling line (double-lined arrow), data lines to the black box (broken-lined arrow).

Drierite Co., Xenia, Ohio) to remove water vapour before being passed through three (one each for O_2, CO_2 and CH_4) variable-area flow meters (instantaneously visual flow monitor; ABB, Inc., Burlington, Ontario, Canada) and supplied at positive pressure to the analysers. All equipment, except the variable-area flow meters, was controlled by a computer attached to a data acquisition system capable of acquiring real-time data at intervals of 1 s.

Analytical apparatus

Gaseous emissions from the animals were removed from the hood through reinforced polyethylene tubing attached to the top of the hood using the vacuum

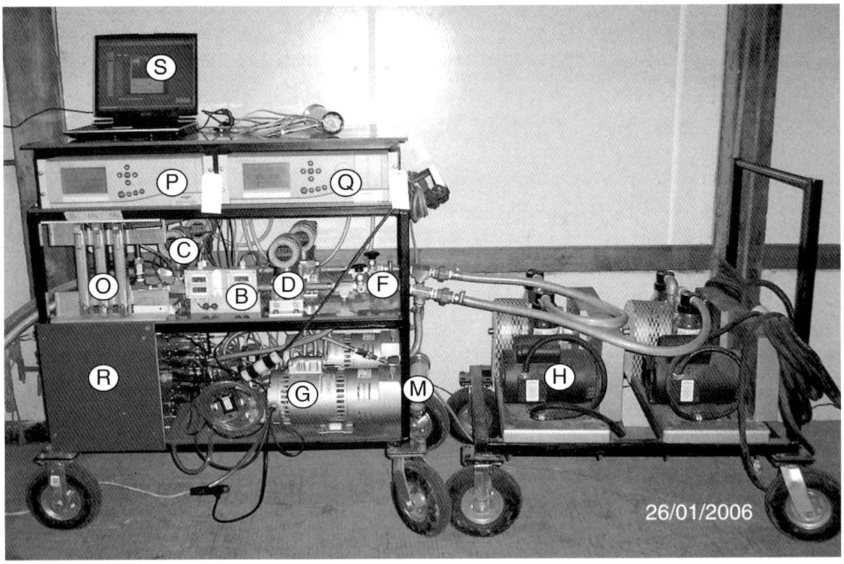

Fig. 10.4. Mobile open-circuit calorimetry equipment cart (B, temperature and relative humidity sensor; C, absolute pressure transmitter; D, differential pressure transmitter; F, bypass control valve; G, vacuum pump (Gast model 1023-101Q); H, vacuum pump (Gast model 3040, G and H are in series); M, Drierite drying column; O, instantaneous variable-area flow meters; P, oxygen analyser; R, methane and carbon dioxide analyser; R, black box (system control and data acquisition panel); S, laptop computer).

pumps on the cart. Methane and CO_2 concentrations in samples of inspired and expired air were measured using a non-dispersive infrared CH_4 and CO_2 analyser, while the concentration of O_2 was measured using a paramagnetic O_2 analyser (Servomex Xentra 4100 Gas Purity Analyser; Servomex Group Ltd, Crowborough, East Sussex, UK) with a response time of <12 s for the O_2 analyser and <20 s for the CH_4 and CO_2 analyser, respectively. The analysers were calibrated weekly, as described by McLean and Tobin (1987). Atmospheric air was sampled from a separate line located outside the building to calibrate the O_2 analyser (O_2 calibration range, 16.0–20.96%). Oxygen recovery was calibrated by the N_2 injection technique (by releasing a weighed amount of N_2 gas into the system), as described by Young *et al.* (1984). Zero and span calibration and linearity detection of the analysers was performed using zero grade N_2, 2.5% CO_2 and 1500 ppm CH_4 (BOC Gases Canada Ltd, Guelph, Ontario, Canada).

System control and data acquisition

System control and data acquisition were handled on a laptop computer, which was connected to three measurement-computing modules through universal serial bus (USB) connectors. One of the modules provided 24 high-drive digital input/output lines. Six of these lines were used to control solid-state relays, which in turn controlled four two-way solenoid operated valves (Omega Engineering,

Inc., Laval, Quebec, Canada) and switched the sampling pump on and off. The remaining two measurement-computing modules provided 16 input lines of single-ended voltage analogue-to-digital conversion, which were connected to the temperature and relative humidity sensor, an absolute pressure transducer and a differential pressure (flow) transducer for hood A and B, respectively, and the O_2, CH_4 and CO_2 analysers. The remaining seven input lines were not assigned but potentially could be used, for example, for rumen pH electrodes to monitor rumen pH in ruminally fistulated cows. All the transducer and sensor output signals were standard 4–20 milliamp currents, which were converted to voltage using simple resistors. A single fixed-voltage open-frame power supply was used to power the transducers that did not have their own power supply. Although the analogue-to-digital conversion modules had digital input/output lines, separate modules that drove the solid-state relays directly were used to avoid the need for additional drive circuitry. The software developed to operate this system was created using National Instruments Lab View 7.1 (National Instruments, Austin, Texas) running under Microsoft Windows XP. Real-time data at intervals of 1 s were automatically collected and downloaded into a computer. Monitoring the absolute pressure and wet and dry bulb temperature and relative humidity allowed correction of gas volumes to dry 0°C at 1 atmosphere (STPD – standard temperature (0°C), standard pressure (760 mm Hg absolute), dry) conditions.

System testing

Three experiments were conducted to test the calorimetry system. In Experiment 1, we compared the addition of fatty acids to the diet of dairy cows on enteric CH_4 emissions. A control versus a myristic acid (MA; 50 g kg^{-1} DM) treated total mixed ration (TMR) was compared using 12 mature Holstein dairy cows (710 ± 17.3 kg body weight) housed in a tie-stall facility at the Elora Dairy Research Centre (University of Guelph, Guelph, Ontario, Canada). The animals were offered *ad libitum* access to a TMR (% DM; maize silage, 33.2%; haylage, 22.1%; hay, 5.5%; high-moisture maize, 20.2%; and custom supplement, 18.9%) formulated to meet NRC (2001) requirements for a lactating dairy cow. In Experiment 2, we compared the effects of grain processing in the TMR on enteric CH_4 emissions using 12 Holstein dairy cows. The TMR was formulated as above, but the maize portion of the TMR was provided as either steam-flake (SF; density 479–509 g l^{-1}) or cracked maize (CC; density 719–749 g l^{-1}). Ingredients and chemical composition of the dietary treatments used in Experiments 1 and 2 are provided in Table 10.1. The experiments consisted of a 7-day pre-trial period when cows were fed the regular Elora Dairy Research Centre TMR to obtain baseline CH_4 emission, a 10-day adaptation period and a 1-day, 8-h collection period. The animals were fed and milked twice daily (feeding, 0800 and 1300; milking, 0500 and 1500). Feed intake and milk yields were recorded in both experiments and water was available at all times. In Experiment 3, we repeated Experiment 2 (steam-flake versus cracked maize) on a commercial dairy farm using eight mature component-fed (as-fed, kg per cow day^{-1}, maize silage, 12.6; balage, 9.5; mixed hay, 2.5; maize,

Table 10.1. Ingredients and chemical composition (DM basis) of the dietary treatments used in Experiments 1 and 2 provided as total mixed rations (TMR).

	Experiment 1		Experiment 2	
Parameter	Myristic acid	Control	Cracked maize[a]	Steam-flaked maize[b]
	% DM			
Ingredient composition:				
Hay	5.2	5.5	5.5	5.5
Haylage	21.1	22.1	22.1	22.1
Maize silage	31.7	33.2	33.2	33.2
Maize, steam-flaked	–	–	–	20.2
Maize, cracked	–	–	20.2	–
Maize, high moisture	19.3	20.2	–	–
Custom TMR dairy supplement[c,d]	22.8	18.9	18.9	18.9
Chemical composition:				
Dry matter, %	99.5	99.5	97.7	97.3
Crude protein, % (N × 6.25)	16.9	17.0	18.6	18.0
Soluble protein, %	3.74	4.49	4.78	7.67
Acid detergent fibre, %	19.9	24.5	22.6	24.5
Neutral detergent fibre, %	36.2	40.5	35.8	40.9
Lignin, % NDF	9.94	9.93	8.97	6.7
Calcium, %	1.09	1.00	0.81	0.90
Phosphorus, %	0.46	0.5	0.46	0.48
Potassium, %	1.31	1.54	1.37	1.48
Magnesium, %	0.24	0.27	0.25	0.25
Sodium, %	0.39	0.45	0.49	0.47
Net energy (lac), Mcal kg^{-1}	1.57	1.49	1.52	1.49
Fat, %	9.84	4.23	3.36	3.15
Ash, %	7.2	7.36	6.99	7.68

[a]Density 719–749 g l^{-1} (Floradale Feed Mill Limited, Guelph, Ontario, Canada).
[b]Density 479–509 g l^{-1} (Floradale Feed Mill Limited, Guelph, Ontario, Canada).
[c]Provided as a mash supplement (g kg^{-1}): maize gluten meal, 210; soybean meal, 250; beet pulp, 50; herring meal, 50; canola meal, 100; roasted soybeans, 100; soybean hulls, 41; custom vitamin/mineral mix (white salt, 23; dicalcium phosphate, 29; limestone, 45; bicarbonate, 35; magox-56%, 5; fibrozyme, 3; organic dairy micro premix, 5; sulfur 99.5%, 2.1; yea-sacc 1026, 2; rovimix H_2, 0.1; DCAD+, 9), 159; golden flake, 20; molasses, 20.
[d]Provided as a mash supplement (g kg^{-1}): myristic acid, 194; maize gluten meal, 170; soybean meal, 202; beet pulp, 50; herring meal, 40; canola meal, 86; roasted soybeans, 86; soybean hulls, 15; custom vitamin/mineral mix (white salt, 18; dicalcium phosphate, 23; limestone, 36; bicarbonate, 28; magox-56%, 4; fibrozyme, 2.4; organic dairy micro premix, 4.7; sulfur 99.5%, 1.9; yea-sacc 1026, 1.6; rovimix H_2, 0.1; DCAD+, 7.3), 127; golden flake, 15; molasses, 15.

5.5; and custom supplement, 5.0) Holstein dairy cows. The experiment consisted of a 14-day adaptation period and two 8-h enteric CH_4 emission measurements repeated after 6 consecutive days. Animals were allocated randomly to the calorimetry hoods. All experimental procedures were done with the approval of the University of Guelph Animal Care Committee in accordance with the guidelines of the Canadian Council on Animal Care.

Chemical analysis

Feed and orts samples were collected three times during each experiment and stored at –20°C for later analysis. Composited feed and orts samples were analysed for DM by oven drying at 60°C for 48 h (AOAC 16th edition, 3.002), ADF and NDF using Ankom2000 Fibre Analyser (Forage Analysis Procedures, National Forage Testing Association, AOAC 16th edition, 4.6.03) and CP using LECO FP 428 Nitrogen Analyser (AOAC 16th edition, 4.2.08). Ingredients and chemical composition of the diets used in Experiment 3 are presented in Table 10.2. Milk samples were also collected three times during the trials from

Table 10.2. Ingredients and chemical composition (DM basis) of component feeds used in Experiment 3 on the commercial dairy farm.

Parameter	Mixed balage	Mixed hay	Maize silage	Cracked maize[a]	Steam-flaked maize[b]	Custom supplement[c]
				%, DM basis		
Dry matter, %	51.1	84.5	40.1	86.0	85.6	88.3
Crude protein, % (N × 6.25)	18.9	18.9	8.3	8.5	9.1	29.9
Soluble protein, %	11.7	7.4	3.1	1.6	0.5	5.2
Acid detergent fibre, %	26.9	32.8	18.6	3.9	4.7	9.8
Neutral detergent fibre, %	38.0	41.9	40.1	11.1	11.2	32.7
Lignin, % NDF	18.5	19.0	4.8	1.8	2.7	4.6
Calcium, %	1.22	1.20	0.14	0.01	0.01	2.18
Phosphorus %	0.28	0.23	0.21	0.29	0.30	1.02
Potassium, %	2.78	3.20	0.91	0.40	0.40	1.02
Magnesium, %	0.29	0.22	0.17	0.12	0.12	0.59
Sodium, %	0.05	0.03	0.02	0.02	0.03	0.75
Net energy (lac), Mcal kg^{-1}	1.48	1.42	1.63	1.84	1.83	1.74
Fat, %	2.1	2.1	3.6	4.4	4.7	5.9
Ash, %	9.2	9.1	3.3	1.5	1.5	11.3

[a]Density 719–749 g l^{-1} (Floradale Feed Mill Limited, Guelph, Ontario, Canada).
[b]Density 479–509 g l^{-1} (Floradale Feed Mill Limited, Guelph, Ontario, Canada).
[c]Provided as a pellet (g kg^{-1}): mixed grain, rolled, 409.5; maize gluten meal, 50; soybean meal, 200; herring meal, 50; canola meal, 100; roasted soybeans, 100; custom vitamin/mineral mix (white salt, 20.4; dicalcium phosphate, 20; limestone, 39; magox-56%, 5.5; organic dairy micro premix, 3.6; sulfur, 99.5%, 2.0).

AM and PM milkings and preserved with 2-bromo-2nitropropane-1-2-diol. Milk samples were pooled daily (60:40, AM:PM) based on milk yield, and the pooled samples analysed for protein, fat and lactose using a near-infrared analyser (Foss System 4000, Foss Electric, Hillerd, Denmark) according to AOAC (1990) (Laboratory Services, University of Guelph, Guelph, Ontario, Canada).

Statistical analysis

The repeated measurements of the enteric CH_4 emissions were analysed as paired comparisons using PROC MIXED of SAS (v. 9.1; SAS Inst., Inc., Cary, North Carolina) using the model, $Y_{ij} = \mu + a_i + \beta_j + \varepsilon_i$, where Y_i = the dependent variable, m = overall mean, a_i = effect of treatment (i = 1, 2), β_j = effect of pair (j = 1, 2, ..., 6), and ε_i = random residual error. Baseline CH_4 emissions were used as covariate, and treatment means were compared using Tukey's multiple comparison procedures in SAS. Effects were considered significant at a probability $P < 0.05$.

Results and Discussion

Dry matter intake (DMI), milk yield, milk components and CH_4 production in Experiments 1, 2 and 3 are presented in Tables 10.3 and 10.4. All animals adapted easily to confinement in the hoods during CH_4 measurement and there were no indications of discomfort or stress in the animals. A typical real-time enteric CH_4 emission from lactating dairy cows is presented in Fig. 10.5. Addition of myristic acid in the diet reduced ($P < 0.05$) CH_4 output by 33% (613.6 versus 409.5 l day^{-1}, control versus myristic acid treated TMR), reduced DMI (16.0 versus 13.8, control versus myristic acid treated TMR) and increased ($P < 0.05$) fat test (4.0 versus 4.5, control versus myristic acid treated TMR; Table 10.3). Dohme *et al.* (2000) observed from *in vitro* studies that, with the addition of 53 g kg^{-1} DM of palm kernel oil, CH_4 production rates were reduced

Table 10.3. Effects of a control versus myristic acid treated total mixed ration on dry matter intake, milk yield, milk composition and enteric methane emissions in lactating dairy cows (n = 6).

Parameter	Control	Myristic acid	SE
Dry matter intake, kg day^{-1}	16.0^a	13.8^b	1.55
Milk yield, kg day^{-1}	14.9	13.3	1.59
Protein, %	3.6	3.6	0.09
Fat, %	4.0^a	4.5^b	0.16
Lactose, %	4.2	4.0	0.08
CH_4 output, l day^{-1}	613.6^a	409.5^b	80.98
CH_4 output, MJ day^{-1}	23.2^a	15.5^b	3.06

[a,b]Means within a row with different superscripts differ ($P < 0.05$).
Adapted from Odongo *et al.* (2007).

Table 10.4. Effects of grain processing (steam-flake versus cracked maize) on dry matter intake, milk yield, milk composition and enteric methane emissions in lactating dairy cows.

Parameter	Cracked maize	Steam-flake maize	SE
Experiment 2 ($n = 6$)			
Dry matter intake, kg day^{-1}	20.0	19.3	0.49
Milk yield, kg day^{-1}	23.7	24.3	0.88
Protein, %	3.5	3.6	0.14
Fat, %	3.8	3.8	0.25
Lactose, %	8.1	8.1	0.11
CH_4 output, l day^{-1}	525.4	577.7	41.16
CH_4 output, MJ day^{-1}	19.9	21.8	1.55
Experiment 3 ($n = 5$)			
Dry matter intake, kg day^{-1}	20.0	20.4	0.33
Milk yield, kg day^{-1}	27.8	28.6	1.02
Protein, %	3.3	3.4	0.05
Fat, %	4.6	4.9	0.20
Lactose, %	4.5	4.5	0.05
CH_4 output, l day^{-1}	615.7[a]	704.2[b]	24.2
CH_4 output, MJ day^{-1}	21.3[a]	24.3[b]	0.78

[a,b]Means within a row with different superscripts differ ($P < 0.05$).

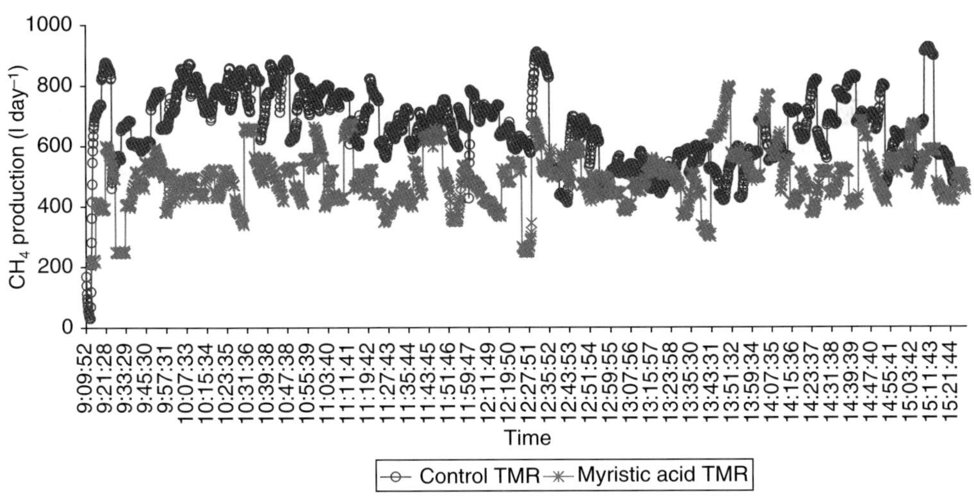

Fig. 10.5. Enteric methane production (l day^{-1}) in lactating dairy cows fed a control versus myristic acid treated total mixed ration.

by 34%. When coconut oil was fed to sheep at inclusion rates of 3.5 and 7%, daily CH_4 production was reduced by 28 and 73%, respectively (Machmuller and Kreuzer, 1999). However, a major problem associated with addition of excessive amounts of fat in the ration (>5 to 6%) is that it depresses fibre

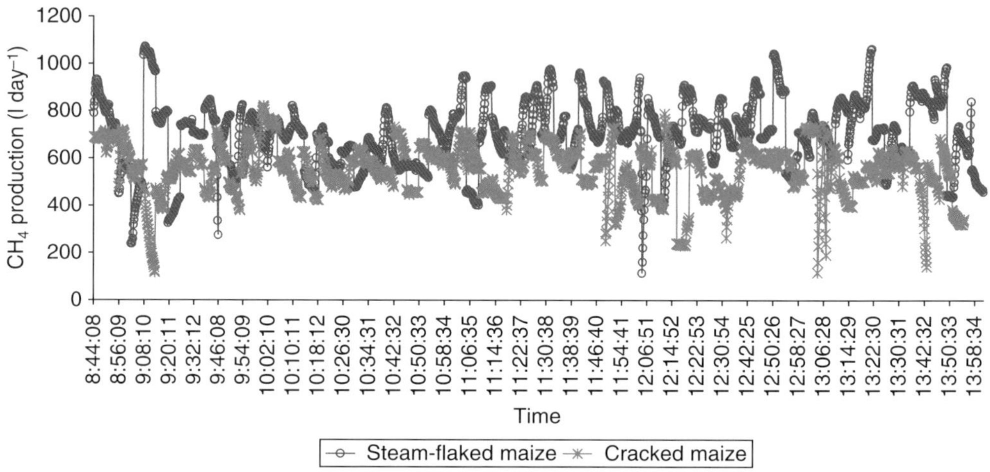

Fig. 10.6. Enteric methane production in lactating dairy cows component fed (as-fed, kg per cow day^{-1}, maize silage, 12.6; balage, 9.5; mixed hay, 2.5; maize, 5.5; and custom supplement, 5.0) steam-flaked maize versus cracked maize rations on a commercial dairy farm.

degradation in the rumen (Dong *et al.*, 1997; Mathison *et al.*, 1998) and reduces acetate production and milk fat content (Jenkins *et al.*, 1996; Ashes *et al.*, 1997).

In both Experiments 2 and 3, steam-flake (SF) and cracked maize (CC) in a TMR or as a component feed had no effect ($P > 0.05$) on DMI, milk yield and milk composition (Table 10.4). In Experiment 2, CC in the TMR numerically reduced enteric CH_4 emissions (Table 10.4). The average CH_4 emissions in this experiment ranged from 392.6 l day^{-1} for cows on the CC diet to 741.0 l day^{-1} for cows on the SF diet. In Experiment 3, CC ration reduced CH_4 emissions by 14% (615.7 versus 704.2, CC versus SF, respectively, $P < 0.05$). A typical real-time profile of CH_4 production in Experiment 3 is presented in Fig. 10.6. There were no differences ($P > 0.05$) in DMI, milk yield and milk composition (Table 10.4). Previous studies comparing the performance of cows fed SF versus CC have shown that milk yield of cows fed SF maize was superior to that of cows fed CC in high silage diets (Dann *et al.*, 1999) and cows fed coarsely ground maize in lucerne-based diets (Yu *et al.*, 1998). In Experiment 2, the milk yields of SF cows were not different from those of CC cows. In lactating cows, steam flaking increased the estimated net energy for lactation (NEL) of maize by 33% (Plascencia and Zinn, 1996), whereas, in feedlot cattle, steam flaking increased the net energy for maintenance (NEM) of maize by 13 to 16% (Lee *et al.*, 1982; Ramirez *et al.*, 1985; Zinn, 1987). Improvement in performance by feeding SF maize has been attributed to shifts in the proportion of starch digestion in the rumen versus the intestines of dairy cows (Theurer *et al.*, 1999). The amount of high quality protein presented to the small intestine is also increased by feeding SF grains. In three digestibility trials (Plascencia and Zinn, 1996; Joy *et al.*, 1997; Crocker *et al.*, 1998), lactating dairy cows fed SF maize digested 50% more starch in the rumen (52 versus 35%), increased post-ruminal digestibility of starch by 50% (93 versus 61%) and increased total tract digestibility by 25% (97 versus 78%; Theurer *et al.*, 1999) compared to CC maize. The microbial protein flow to the duodenum averaged 18% greater for cows fed SF compared to CC (1.23 versus 1.04 kg day^{-1}).

In the absence of country-specific emission factors, the IPCC published guidelines for national GHG inventories (IPPC, 1997) that are used for official estimates of CH_4 emissions. In Tier 1, IPCC (1997) assumed an average milk production of 6700 kg per head $year^{-1}$ and recommended that a default value of 118 kg CH_4 $year^{-1}$ (475 l day^{-1}) be used for highly productive, commercial North American dairy cows. The mean CH_4 production for the control treatment in the current study was, on average, 14% higher than the IPCC (1997) predictions. A recent study by Kebreab *et al.* (2006a) has also shown that the Tier I model underpredicts mean CH_4 emission in dairy cattle. As CH_4 is considered to have a global warming potential (GWP) 21 times that of CO_2 (IPCC, 1997), 118 kg of CH_4 is equivalent to 2.478 t of CO_2 in inventories of GHG production. The concept of GWP was developed to allow scientists and policy makers to compare the ability of each GHG to trap heat in the atmosphere relative to other gases. A GWP is defined as the time-integrated change in radiative forcing due to the instantaneous release of 1 kg of the gas expressed relative to the radiative forcing from the release of 1 kg of CO_2 (Environment Canada, 2005). For example, CH_4 emitted from the livestock sector accounts for 38% of all agricultural GHG emissions in Canada (Environment Canada, 2005). Understanding the relationship between diet and enteric CH_4 production is essential to reduce uncertainty in GHG emission inventories and to identify viable GHG reduction strategies. Canada's commitment under the Kyoto Protocol is to reduce net GHG emissions to 6% below 1990 levels between 2008 and 2012.

Mathematical models offer the potential to evaluate intervention strategies for any given situation, thereby providing a low cost and quick estimate of best practice. Models of methanogenesis can be classified within two main groups. First, there are the statistical models that directly relate the nutrient intake with CH_4 production. Secondly, there are the dynamic mechanistic models that attempt to simulate CH_4 emissions based on a mathematical description of ruminal fermentation biochemistry. The statistical models tend to be well suited to practical application for rapid diet evaluation or larger-scale inventory purposes. Several statistical models constructed to predict CH_4 emissions from cattle were summarized by Kebreab *et al.* (2006b). Unlike their statistical counterparts, dynamic models include time as a variable and they tend to be more mechanistic in their construction. This type of model has been applied successfully on several occasions to predict CH_4 emissions from ruminants (e.g. Mills *et al.*, 2003). However, they too are not without their limitations and they may not deliver quick solutions based on very limited dietary information. By definition, mechanistic models describe in more detail the fermentation processes occurring in the gut that result ultimately in the formation of CH_4 as a sink for excess hydrogen. The experimental results reported herein can be used to evaluate extant models and, if necessary, modify some elements of the model to make it more relevant to the North American type of management. Typically, CH_4 emissions from enteric fermentation represent about 6% of dietary gross energy loss, but this varies with diet from about 2% in feedlot cattle to 12% for animals on very poor quality forage (Johnson and Johnson, 1995). Mitigation strategies to reduce enteric CH_4 emissions from dairy cows have been reviewed by Boadi *et al.* (2004) and updated by Kebreab *et al.* (2006b).

Conclusion

The system described in this chapter is advantageous because it is simple, accurate and mobile. Although the principles behind the determination of gaseous exchange are the same as those of previously published reports (e.g. Young *et al.*, 1975; Kelly *et al.*, 1994), this system uses improvements in technology for the determination of O_2, CO_2 and CH_4 contents, measurements of airflow, absolute pressure, temperature and relative humidity, system control and data acquisition. All animals adapted easily to confinement in the hoods and there were no indications of discomfort or stress in the animals. This mobile ventilated head-hood system therefore provides an accurate and reliable means of measuring real-time gaseous exchange in ruminants at the farm level.

Acknowledgements

The authors would like to thank Mayhaven Farms for collaborating in this research, the staff of the Elora Dairy Research Centre, University of Guelph for their technical assistance and Elanco Animal Health, Division Eli Lilly Canada, Inc. and Dairy Farmers of Canada (Greenhouse Gas Mitigation Program for Canadian Agriculture) for financial support. We would also like to acknowledge the continued support received from the Ontario Ministry of Agriculture, Food and Rural Affairs and the Natural Sciences and Engineering Council of Canada (BWM).

References

Ashes, J.R., Gulati, S.K. and Scott, T.W. (1997) New approaches to changing milk composition: potential to alter the content and composition of milk fat through nutrition. *Journal of Dairy Science* 80, 2204–2212.

Association of Official Analytical Chemists (1990) *Official Methods of Analysis*, 15th edn. AOAC, Arlington, Virginia.

Bergman, E.N. (1964) A simple apparatus for long-term respiratory carbon-14 studies in ruminants. *American Journal of Veterinary Research* 25, 848–851.

Boadi, D., Benchaar, C., Chiquette, J. and Massé, D. (2004) Mitigation strategies to reduce enteric methane emissions from dairy cows: update review. *Canadian Journal of Animal Science* 84, 319–335.

Crocker, L.M., DePeters, E.J., Fadel, J.G., Perez-Monti, H., Taylor, S.J., Wyckoff, J.A. and Zinn, R.A. (1998) Influence of processed corn grain in diets of dairy cows on digestion of nutrients and milk composition. *Journal of Dairy Science* 81, 2394–2407.

Dann, H.M., Varga, G.A. and Putnam, D.E. (1999) Improving energy supply to late gestation and early postpartum dairy cows. *Journal of Dairy Science* 82, 1274–1281.

Dohme, F., Machmuller, A., Wasserfallen, A. and Kreuzer, M. (2000) Comparative efficiency of various fats rich in medium chain fatty acids to suppress ruminal methanogenesis as measured with RUSITEC. *Canadian Journal of Animal Science* 80, 473–482.

Dong, Y., Bae, H.D., McAllister, T.A., Mathison, G.W. and Cheng, K.J. (1997) Lipid-induced depression of methane production and digestibility in the artificial rumen system (RUSITEC). *Canadian Journal of Animal Science* 77, 269–278.

Environment Canada (2005) *Canada's Greenhouse Gas Inventory: 1990–2003*. Greenhouse Gas Division, Environment Canada, April 2005, Ottawa. Available at: http://www.ec.gc.ca/pdb/ghg/inventory_report/2003_report/2003_report_e.pdf

Intergovernmental Panel on Climate Change (1997) *Revised 1996 IPCC Guidelines for National Greenhouse Gas Inventories: Reference Manual. Vol. 3. Agriculture*. Intergovernmental Panel on Climate Change, Geneva, Switzerland.

Jenkins, T.C., Bateman, H.G. and Block, S.M. (1996) Butylsoyamide increases unsaturation of fatty acids in plasma and milk of lactating dairy cows. *Journal of Dairy Science* 79, 585–590.

Johnson, K.A. and Johnson, D.E. (1995) Methane emissions from cattle. *Journal of Animal Science* 73, 2483–2492.

Joy, M.T., DePeters, E.J., Fadel, J.G. and Zinn, R.A. (1997) Effects of corn processing on the site and extent of digestion in lactating cows. *Journal of Dairy Science* 80, 2087–2097.

Kebreab, E., France, J., McBride, B.W., Odongo, N., Bannink, A., Mills, J.A.N. and Dijkstra J. (2006a) Evaluation of models to predict methane emissions from enteric fermentation in North American dairy cattle. In: Kebreab, E., Dijkstra, J., Gerrits, W.J.J., Bannink, A. and France, J. (eds) *Nutrient Digestion and Utilization in Farm Animals: Modelling Approaches*. CAB International, Wallingford, UK.

Kebreab, E., Clarke, K., Wagner-Riddle, C. and France, J. (2006b) Methane and nitrous oxide emissions from Canadian animal agriculture – a review. *Canadian Journal of Animal Science* 86, 135–158.

Kelly, J.M., Kerrigan, B., Milligan, L.P. and McBride, B.W. (1994) Development of a mobile, open-circuit indirect calorimetry system. *Canadian Journal of Animal Science* 74, 65–71.

Ku-Vera, J.K., Macleod, N.A. and Orskov, E.R. (1990) Construction and operation of an open-circuit ventilated hood system for cattle nourished wholly by intragastric infusion of nutrients. *Animal Feed Science and Technology* 28, 109–114.

Lee, R.W., Galyean, M.L. and Lofgreen, G.P. (1982) Effects of mixing whole shelled and steam flaked corn in finishing diets on feedlot performance and site and extent of digestion in beef steers. *Journal of Animal Science* 55, 475–483.

McAllister, T.A., Okine, E.K., Mathison, G.W. and Cheng, K.J. (1996) Dietary, environmental and microbiological aspects of methane production in ruminants. *Canadian Journal of Animal Science* 76, 231–243.

Machmuller, A. and Kreuzer, M. (1999) Methane suppression by coconut oil and associated effects on nutrient and energy balance in sheep. *Canadian Journal of Animal Science* 79, 65–72.

McLean, J.A. and Tobin, G. (1987) *Animal and Human Calorimetry*. Cambridge University Press, New York.

Mathison, G.W., Okine, E.K., McAllister, T.A., Dong, Y., Galbraith, J. and Dmytruk, O.I.N. (1998) Reducing methane emissions from ruminant animals. *Journal of Applied Animal Research* 14, 1–28.

Mills, J.A.N., Kebreab, E., Yates, C.M., Crompton, L.A., Cammell, S.B., Dhanoa, M.S., Agnew, R.E. and France, J. (2003) Alternative approaches to predicting methane emissions from dairy cows. *Journal of Animal Science* 81, 3141–3150.

National Research Council (2001) *Nutrient Requirements of Dairy Cattle*, 7th rev edn. National Academy Press, Washington, DC.

Nicholson, M.J., Holton, J., Bradley, A.P. and Beatty, P.C.W. (1996) The performance of a variable-flow indirect calorimeter. *Physiological Measurement* 17, 43–55.

Nkrumah, J.D., Okine, E.K., Mathison, G.W., Schmid, K., Li, C., Basarab, J.A., Price, M.A., Wang, Z. and Moore, S.S. (2006) Relationships of feedlot feed efficiency, performance, and feeding behavior with metabolic rate, methane production, and energy partitioning in beef cattle. *Journal of Animal Science* 84, 145–153.

Odongo, N.E., Or-Rashid, M.M., Kebreab, E., France, J. and McBride, B.W. (2007) Effect of supplementing myristic acid in dairy cow rations on ruminal methanogenesis and fatty acid profile in milk. *Journal of Dairy Science* 90, 1851–1858.

Plascencia, A. and Zinn, R.A. (1996) Influence of flake density on the feeding value of steam-processed corn in diets for lactating cows. *Journal of Animal Science* 74, 310–316.

Ramirez, R.G., Kiesling, H.E., Galyean, M.L., Lofgreen, G.P. and Elliott, J.K. (1985) Influence of steam-flaked, steamed-whole or whole shelled corn on performance and digestion in beef steers. *Journal of Animal Science* 61, 1–8.

Takahashi, J. and Young, B.A. (1991) Prophylactic effect of L-cysteine on nitrate-induced alterations in respiratory exchange and metabolic rate in sheep. *Animal Feed Science and Technology* 35, 105–113.

Takahashi, J. and Young, B.A. (1994) The regulation of energy metabolism in sheep by nitrate and L-cysteine. *Proceedings of 13th Symposium on Energy Metabolism of Farm Animals*, Mojacar, Spain. EAAP Publication No. 76, Consejo Superior de Investigaciones Cientificas, p. 81.

Theurer, C.B., Huber, J.T., Delgado-Elorduy, A. and Wanderley, R. (1999) Invited review: summary of steam-flaking corn or sorghum grain for lactating dairy cows. *Journal of Dairy Science* 82, 1950–1959.

Young, B.A., Kerrigan, B. and Christopherson, R.J. (1975) A versatile respiratory pattern analyzer for studies of energy metabolism of livestock. *Canadian Journal of Animal Science* 55, 17–22.

Young, B.A., Fenton T.W. and McLean J.A. (1984) Calibration methods in respiratory calorimetry. *Journal of Applied Physiology* 56, 1120–1125.

Yu, P., Huber, J.T., Santos, F.A.P., Simas, J.M. and Theurer, C.B. (1998) Effects of ground, steam-flaked, and steam-rolled corn grains on performance of lactating cows. *Journal of Dairy Science* 81, 777–783.

Zinn, R.A. (1987) Influence of lasalocid and monensin plus tylosin on comparative feeding value of steam-flaked versus cracked corn in diets for feedlot cattle. *Journal of Animal Science* 65, 256–266.

11 Efficiency of Amino Acid Utilization in Simple-stomached Animals and Humans – a Modelling Approach

P.J. MOUGHAN

Riddet Centre, Massey University, New Zealand

Introduction

The simulation of mammalian growth processes allows investigators to formulate and test complex hypotheses concerning numerous interacting factors. When a model or model component fails ongoing testing, via the process of refutation, then a new hypothesis better fitting the experimental facts needs to be developed. Mathematical modelling has proven to be a powerful tool in increasing our understanding of the behaviour of complexly interactive and dynamic systems.

The objective of this contribution is to describe how early attempts by our group to model dietary nitrogen and amino acid metabolism in simple-stomached animals from a causal perspective led to a systematic approach to our own and others' protein metabolism research: a blueprint that has served well for over two decades. On the one hand, models reduce complex systems down into identifiable parts and allow the relative quantitative importance of these subunits to be compared but, on the other hand, they allow the behaviour of the whole system, involving multiple interactions among the parts, to be analysed and appreciated as one.

Scientists seldom work in isolation but, rather, their ideas are influenced by the thinking of others. In our case, the published works of Miller and Payne (1963) and Whittemore and Fawcett (1976) were particularly influential. The first biological model that we developed (Moughan, 1981; Moughan and Smith, 1984) had as its objective the prediction of dietary protein utilization in the pig for the purposes of describing dietary protein quality. The model was successful in accurately predicting urinary and faecal nitrogen excretions, and thus body nitrogen retention, and in ranking diverse diets in terms of their dietary protein quality. Such a model, by necessity, included a description of both amino acid and dietary energy metabolism and the inevitable interaction between the two.

It was thus possible, with relatively minor modification, to extend the protein quality model into a deterministic biological growth model (Moughan *et al.*, 1987). The latter model was extended (Moughan, 1989), verified and validated and was used commercially worldwide (under exclusive licence to Ralston Purina International) to predict biological and economic consequences of changes (nutritional, genetic, etc.) in pork production systems. In turn, the model became the base for the development of more sophisticated models, both in the Netherlands (the TMV modelling group) and in Canada (the Guelph University/Massey University modelling group led by Dr Kees de Lange).

These dietary protein quality and growth models not only allowed us to logicize our thinking into an overall coherent and testable framework but also, and very importantly, allowed us to examine the relative importance of variables influencing the growth processes and that of the model parameters themselves. The models highlighted the disproportionate effect of the simulated supply of amino acids available for body protein synthesis on the accuracy of prediction of body growth, given the postulate that rates of body water and ash retention are related to body protein retention. Moreover, simulation of body protein metabolism underscored the relatively low efficiency of utilization of dietary protein by pigs growing under practical conditions, with concomitant high rates of nitrogenous excretion (Moughan, 1991). Predicted (model) values for the efficiency of utilization of dietary crude protein are presented in Table 11.1 and are all well below 50%.

Table 11.1. Efficiency of utilization[a] of dietary crude protein (CP) and lysine in six commercial pig grower diets given at two feeding levels to 50 kg live weight gilts.

	Diet					
	1	2	3	4	5	6
Feeding level = 1710 g meal day^{-1}:						
Digestible CP intake (g day^{-1})	175	281	235	232	182	215
Protein deposited (g day^{-1})	48.9	110.0	73.5	106.9	74.3	115.0
PE (%)[b]	20.4	30.0	23.1	33.8	32.3	42.1
LE (%)[c]	37.2	38.3	38.5	43.5	54.0	59.0
Feeding level = 2270 g meal day^{-1}:						
Digestible CP intake (g day^{-1})	232	374	312	309	242	285
Protein deposited (g day^{-1})	71.4	115.0	104.1	115.0	105.2	115.0
PE (%)[b]	22.4	23.7	24.6	27.4	34.4	31.7
LE (%)[c]	40.9	30.2	41.1	35.3	59.0	45.0

[a]Predicted values from a pig growth simulation model. Assumes healthy animals growing in a thermoneutral environment.

[b]$PE = \frac{\text{Body protein deposited}}{\text{Diet crude protein intake}} \times \frac{100}{1}$

[c]$LE = \frac{\text{Body lysine deposited}}{\text{Diet total lysine intake}} \times \frac{100}{1}$

Adapted from Moughan (1991).

The predicted efficiency of utilization of dietary crude protein intake (PE) ranged from 20 to 42% at a low level of meal intake and from 22 to 34% at a higher level. On average, the ingested dietary protein was utilized with an efficiency close to 30%. The equivalent of around 70% of the ingested nitrogen was excreted from the pig's body. Part of this inefficiency can be explained by dietary amino acid imbalance, which may be purposeful and economically justifiable. Lysine was the first limiting amino acid in each of the six diets, so it is pertinent to examine the predicted efficiency of utilization of ingested lysine (LE), whereby the effect of amino acid imbalance is removed. As expected, the simulated values for LE (Table 11.1) were higher than the comparable values for PE. On average, the ingested lysine was utilized with an efficiency of close to 44%, but still over half the dietary lysine was not used for the net deposition of lean tissue. Simulation data such as those presented in Table 11.1 highlight the importance of understanding the physiological processes that lead to losses of amino acids from the body, and thus explain inefficiency of utilization of the dietary first-limiting amino acid for growth.

The absorption and metabolism of amino acids in animals is complex and highly integrated with continuous flux within and between body cells. It is useful, however, and inherently necessary when constructing a model of metabolism, to view amino acid metabolism as discrete physiological processes (Table 11.2).

Some understanding of the relative quantitative importance of these processes is afforded by the simulation data shown in Tables 11.3 and 11.4. The predicted data for lysine and protein flows relate to 50 kg live weight pigs differing in genetic potential for body protein retention, receiving a commercial barley-based diet at three levels of feed intake. The information given in Table 11.3 demonstrates that, particularly at higher food intakes, the process of inevitable catabolism may have an important effect on the utilization of the first limiting amino acid. Absorption and endogenous gut loss are also of importance, with body protein turnover being of lesser significance and cutaneous loss of only minor importance. Preferential catabolism may contribute relatively significantly

Table 11.2. Processes involved in the utilization of dietary amino acids by the growing pig.

Pre-uptake:
Ingestion of dietary amino acids
Absorption of amino acids from unprocessed feedstuffs
Absorption of amino acids from processed feedstuffs
Post-absorptive metabolism:
Use of amino acids for body protein maintenance
Use of amino acids for synthesis of non-protein nitrogen compounds
Transamination
Inevitable amino acid catabolism
Preferential catabolism of amino acids for energy supply
Amino acid imbalance
Catabolism of amino acids supplied above the amount required to meet the maximum rate of body protein retention

Table 11.3. Predicted (simulation model) utilization of dietary lysine by the 50 kg live weight growing pig, at three feeding levels[a] and three maximal rates of body protein deposition (Pdmax).

Feeding level ($g\ day^{-1}$)	Diet intake ($g\ day^{-1}$)			Losses ($g\ day^{-1}$)										Deposition ($g\ day^{-1}$)		
					Urine											
	Pdmax	Total lysine	Available lysine	Unabsorbed available lysine	Protein turnover	Inevitable catabolism	Imbalance	Excess supply	Preferential catabolism	Total	Cutaneous	Gut endogenous		Total lysine	Protein	Lipid
1505	100	13.8	13.1	1.8	0.7	3.2	0	0	1.0	4.9	0.08	1.6		4.78	72	72
	130	13.8	13.1	1.8	0.8	2.5	0.2	0	1.4	4.9	0.08	1.6		4.83	73	73
	160	13.8	13.1	1.8	0.8	2.1	0	0	1.8	4.7	0.08	1.6		4.91	74	74
2069	100	18.9	17.9	2.3	0.7	4.7	0	1.6	0	7.0	0.08	1.9		6.63	100	162
	130	18.9	17.9	2.3	0.8	4.7	0	0	0	5.5	0.08	1.9		8.20	124	145
	160	18.9	17.9	2.3	0.8	3.9	0.1	0	0	4.8	0.08	1.9		8.84	133	138
2633	100	24.1	22.9	3.1	0.7	6.0	0	4.4	0	11.1	0.08	2.1		6.63	100	277
	130	2.41	22.9	3.1	0.8	6.0	0	2.3	0	9.1	0.08	2.1		8.62	130	255
	160	24.1	22.9	3.1	0.8	6.0	0	0.3	0	7.1	0.08	2.1		10.61	160	233

[a]Correspond to 8, 11 and 14% metabolic live weight, $kg^{0.75}$.

Adapted from Moughan (1994).

Table 11.4. Predicted (simulation model) utilization of dietary crude protein by the 50 kg live weight growing pig, at three feeding levels and three maximal rates of body protein deposition (Pdmax).

	Feeding level (g day^{-1})[a]								
	1505			2069			2633		
Pdmax =	100	130	160	100	130	160	100	130	160
Available protein intake (g day^{-1})	268	268	268	368	368	368	468	468	468
Absorbed available protein intake (g day^{-1})	229	229	229	315	315	315	401	401	401
Body protein synthesis (g day^{-1})	516	566	616	516	566	616	516	566	616
Nitrogenous losses (g protein day^{-1})									
Cutaneous loss	1.8	1.8	1.8	1.8	1.8	1.8	1.8	1.8	1.8
Urine loss at maintenance	21	23	25	21	23	25	21	23	25
Gut loss at maintenance	34	34	34	47	47	47	59	59	59
Inevitable catabolism	69	66	56	95	95	95	121	121	121
Urine loss (imbalance)	17	11	12	26	25	16	31	30	30
Urine loss (excess supply)	0	0	0	25	0	0	66	35	4
Urine loss (preferential catabolism)	15	21	28	0	0	0	0	0	0
Protein deposition (g day^{-1})	72	73	74	100	124	133	100	130	160

[a]Levels correspond to 8, 11 and 14% of metabolic live weight, kg $^{0.75}$.

Adapted from Moughan (1994).

to amino acid loss in situations where metabolizable energy intake limits protein deposition. Similarly, excess amino acid supply can make a major contribution to inefficiency. The relative importance of dietary amino acid imbalance to protein utilization by the pig is shown more clearly in Table 11.4. For well-formulated commercial diets, the loss of amino acids due to imbalance is of lesser significance. It is clear from these data and from formalized sensitivity analyses (Moughan, 1985) that biological processes such as protein deposition (influenced by the upper limit to protein retention, Pdmax and dietary amino acid imbalance), protein digestion, inevitable amino acid catabolism, preferential amino acid catabolism and the combined maintenance processes are quantitatively significant processes in overall body protein metabolism. In adult humans, inevitable amino acid catabolism and the various component processes contributing to the maintenance requirement assume prominence (Moughan, 2005a).

The remainder of this chapter will address four of the more quantitatively important metabolic processes listed in Table 11.2 in the context of animal growth models and the model parameters used to describe them. This will serve to illustrate how modelling ideas have developed over the past two decades.

Key Processes Controlling Growth – Recent Advances in Modelling

Protein deposition

When diets are formulated, some amino acids will be supplied in excess of requirement, leading to dietary amino acid imbalance. Amino acid imbalance can be predicted based on the concepts of ideal amino acid balance (Cole, 1980) and body protein synthesis being an 'all or nothing' type phenomenon. In our early work (Moughan and Smith, 1984), the degree of dietary amino acid imbalance was calculated by reference to an ideal amino acid pattern using the Simplex linear programming algorithm, which had the advantage of allowing for amino acid transamination to yield dietary non-essential amino acids (NEAA) if the sum of NEAA was less than ideal.

The ideal pattern of amino acids for growth in rapidly growing animals has often been based on the amino acid composition of whole-body protein. An improvement on this is to simulate muscle protein deposition separately from splanchnic protein deposition, which has a different amino acid composition (P.J. Moughan, unpublished data), and to derive an ideal amino acid balance based on the different compositions weighted for differences in rates of deposition.

There is a cellular limit to the amount of daily protein synthesis, which appears to engage, at least in some species and strains of animal, within the constraints of appetite. It is thus necessary to set constraints within models for the rate of whole-body protein deposition (Moughan and Verstegen, 1988). This can be achieved by describing limits to the rates of protein synthesis and degradation, though, more commonly, a genetically based upper limit to whole-body protein deposition (Pdmax) is supposed. Pdmax is influenced by factors such as species, breed, genotype, gender and age. In relation to the latter variable, the simplest proposition is that Pdmax remains constant during the growing period. Whereas this may be a reasonable approximation over relatively low body weight ranges in species such as the pig, it does not hold true for more rapidly growing species of animals, nor over extended body weight ranges. An improved simulation of growth is achieved by developing theories around the curvilinear incline of Pdmax from birth, ultimately leading to a maximum rate, which then declines towards maturity, at which point Pdmax equals zero (e.g. Emmans, 1981).

At least in the case of modelling growth in the pig, the concept of Pdmax as an important constraint on growth has been retained by modellers, but more sophisticated means of describing changes in Pdmax with the age of the animal have been devised (Pomar *et al.*, 1991; Black *et al.*, 1995; Schinckel and de Lange, 1996; Wellock *et al.*, 2004).

Protein digestion

Since the mid-1970s, major steps forward have been made in the measurement of dietary amino acid digestibility and the ability to predict daily amino acid absorption. We have moved from quite inaccurate assessments based on the faecal digestibility of crude protein, to standardized ileal amino acid digestibility coefficients (Stein *et al.*, 2007), whereby unabsorbed amino acids are measured at the end of the ileum and correction is made for amino acids of endogenous origin. Ileal amino acid digestibility coefficients have been shown in a number of studies to allow a reasonably accurate prediction of overall amino acid absorption from diverse mixtures of feedstuffs.

In the recent past, questions have been raised about the metabolic activity of the gastric/small intestinal microbial population and as to whether upper-tract microbes may make a net contribution to the amino acid supply of the host animal. It is now established beyond doubt that gut microbes do synthesize dietary essential amino acids such as lysine (Fuller and Tomé, 2005). What is uncertain is the quantitative significance of this process and whether there is a net production of any of the dietary essential amino acids, and what is the precursor material in the gut. These are important considerations requiring further research. Also, it has become clear that the bioavailability of dietary amino acids, and in particular the bioavailability of lysine, may be an important consideration. The processing of feedstuffs, storage and the feed manufacturing process itself can all adversely affect amino acid bioavailability. Commentators often emphasize, mistakenly, that chemically altered amino acids are released during digestion and are absorbed, but in a form that is unable to be utilized for protein synthesis. In fact, many of the altered amino acids which are unavailable are not absorbed before the end of the small intestine. The real problem in accurately predicting bioavailable amino acid contents in a feedstuff is one of chemical analysis. During amino acid analysis, which involves the hydrolysis of proteins in strong acid, amino acids that have been chemically altered (unavailable) can revert back to the parent amino acid and be determined as being 'available'. An improvement in predicting amino acid absorption *in vivo* can be secured by determining the amounts of absorbed (ileal digestible) 'chemically unaltered' amino acids, i.e. bioavailable amino acids (Moughan, 2005b).

To date, most models of animal growth have relied upon empirically derived mean coefficients of amino acid digestibility or availability to predict amino acid uptake from the gut. Such an approach, however, is clearly an approximation and does not allow any representation of the kinetics of amino acid and nutrient absorption. Bastianelli *et al.* (1996) have explicitly modelled the mechanisms underlying the digestive and absorptive processes. Importantly, this allows the varying rate of flux of amino acids following a meal to be simulated and potentially allows a description of factors (both dietary and animal) known to affect amino acid digestibility. Causal-based models that can predict the kinetics of amino acid absorption stand to improve the accuracy of prediction of animal growth. Modelling nutrient uptake kinetics will be particularly important in the modelling of protein metabolism in humans (as opposed to *ad libitum* fed farm animals), whereby discrete meals are consumed, often several hours apart.

Inevitable amino acid catabolism

It might be expected that, when an animal receives an amount of the first-limiting dietary amino acid below the amount required to meet maximal protein synthesis, and along with a surfeit of other nutrients and non-protein energy, the amino acid would be used with almost complete efficiency. However, it is well known, as demonstrated by many protein biological value (BV) measures for high quality proteins published over the years, that this is not so. Empirically determined BVs are usually below unity and the first-limiting amino acid is, invariably, incompletely utilized.

Our own studies, which have involved feeding well-defined high quality proteins first limiting in lysine to animals, determining lysine deposition in the whole body and carefully correcting for body lysine losses at maintenance, suggest that around 15–20% of ingested lysine is oxidized, even when the animal receives high amounts of non-protein energy (carbohydrate and fat) and other essential nutrients. More recent published findings using a similar indirect method (Möhn *et al.*, 2000; de Lange *et al.*, 2001) give marginal values of 0.75 for the efficiency of utilization of absorbed lysine and of approximately 0.73 for threonine. Möhn *et al.* (2004) reported a 17.4% disappearance of true ileal digested lysine in the growing pig and a comparable 13.4% loss of true ileal digested lysine based on a direct measure of lysine oxidation. The amino acid tryptophan appears to be particularly poorly used for protein deposition post-absorption (Baker, 2005). Heger *et al.* (2002), in nitrogen balance studies with the growing pig, also report relatively low utilization values for absorbed trytophan, but high (91%) utilization values for lysine. The detailed work of Heger *et al.* (2002) and results reported in an accompanying paper (Heger *et al.*, 2003) suggest that an absorbed first-limiting amino acid is used with a constant efficiency at suboptimal levels of intake, but different amino acids have quite different absolute efficiencies of utilization.

Various hypotheses have been promulgated to explain this loss to oxidation of the absorbed amino acid first limiting for growth. One of these hypotheses centres on the idea of an 'inevitable' catabolism of amino acids. This theory assumes that cellular catabolic activity is, to some extent, indiscriminate and that catabolism of amino acids, although amino acids may be limiting for protein synthesis, never shuts down completely. Rather, there is always a degree of catabolism, arising inevitably from this basal catabolic activity. Work from the group of the late Dr Peter Reeds (Stoll *et al.*, 1999) and a recent study from France (Le Floc'h and Sève, 2005) provide some empirical support for this hypothesis and suggest that there may be a considerable degree of amino acid catabolism, specifically in the gut tissues, post-absorption (first-pass metabolism). Alternative hypotheses, incorporating the idea of a role for the first-limiting amino acid in inducing an 'anabolic drive', have also been argued by Millward (1998).

Preferential amino acid catabolism

The process of preferential amino acid catabolism is at the heart of explaining the long-observed phenomenon of dietary protein–energy interaction. Energy in the form of ATP derived from nutrient catabolism is required to fuel protein synthesis and other metabolic processes but, at the same time, amino acids are a potential source of ATP. Thus, an amino acid is both a building block for protein synthesis and a potential source of energy.

The term 'preferential' amino acid catabolism is used in addition to that of 'inevitable' catabolism to make the distinction between background catabolism (inevitable) and the directed catabolism of amino acids for the express purpose of energy supply (ATP generation). Preferential catabolism will occur in metabolic states whereby the supply of ATP from non-protein compounds is limiting in relation to the animal's needs.

There are three important aspects to the modelling of preferential catabolism. First, it is necessary to be able to predict the rate of generation in the body of available dietary energy. Secondly, it is necessary to be able to describe the metabolic and other processes which give rise to daily energy expenditure. Thirdly, some rule is required to predict the degree of preferential catabolism, whenever dietary energy supply is limiting, and thus allow calculation of the amounts of body protein and lipid deposited daily or, alternatively, an empirical relationship is needed to predict directly rates of body protein deposition under conditions of energy deficit.

Earlier models relied upon estimates of dietary digestible energy (DE) or metabolizable energy (ME) to drive metabolism, whereas more recently, and appreciating that the ATP yield per mole of absorbed nutrient differs among nutrients, a net energy (NE) approach offers greater accuracy (Boisen and Verstegen, 2000; van Milgen, 2002; Green and Whittemore, 2003; de Lange and Birkett, 2005). Modellers have also moved away from a simplistic description of energy expenditure being dependent upon only a maintenance energy cost and the biochemical costs of protein and lipid deposition and have sought rather to model energy expenditure at a more fundamental mechanistic level whereby energy costs can be better apportioned between intrinsic animal processes and dietary influences (Bastianelli and Sauvant, 1997; Rivest *et al.*, 2000; Birkett and de Lange, 2001a,b,c; Green and Whittemore, 2003; Lovatto and Sauvant, 2003; van Milgen and Noblet, 2003).

It is more satisfying intellectually, and allows a greater generality of model predictions, to model processes on a causal, rather than a strictly empirical, basis. From early on, therefore, modellers sought to develop causal-based 'rules' to describe the process of preferential catabolism. A possible biological basis for the interaction between dietary protein and non-protein energy is captured in the idea that there is a physiological requirement for a certain minimum amount of body lipid. The minimum 'essential' amount of lipid that a growing animal would strive to attain would be affected by factors such as breed, gender and age. If, following the 'classic' approach to energy partitioning, residual energy (residual NE = NE intake – maintenance NE cost – total NE cost of depositing potential protein) is insufficient to meet the minimum lipid deposition requirement based, in turn, on the minimum body lipid content, then deamination of amino acids is triggered and amino acids are degraded to supply energy. This theory of growth is consistent with the pragmatic view that an animal is unlikely to sacrifice body protein growth (essential for vital organs and skeletal structure) for the sake of lipid growth in situations whereby the animal already possesses more than adequate lipid reserves. The concept allows for long-run zero or negative body lipid retention during growth, for animals with a high degree of body fatness. Our early work (Moughan *et al.*, 1987) stressed a minimum whole-body lipid to whole-body protein ratio (Lt:Pt min), though this has been mistakenly interpreted by several workers (e.g. de Greef, 1992) to mean a minimal ratio of daily lipid to protein deposition (Ld:Pd min). The two constraints are not synonymous. Although the minimum Lt constraint has been controversial, the constraint, or at least some variant of it, has been retained and expanded upon by several groups (e.g. Weis *et al.*, 2004; Green and Whittemore, 2005; Sandberg *et al.*, 2005a,b) as an apparently useful alternative to using empirical relationships between body protein deposition and dietary energy intake. Elsewhere in this book, a detailed assessment of the concept of an absolute physiological minimum Lt:Pt ratio is given (Chapter 14) and a related parameter of the ratio of targeted body lipid mass to targeted body protein mass is introduced.

Conclusion

Over the past 20 years, growth modelling has become a mainstream activity in the study of animal science. Scientists have developed concepts and intellectual frameworks to synthesize knowledge and to allow description of a complex biological system. Where rigorous testing of model concepts has ensued, progress has been made towards a more causal understanding of the growth processes. To some extent, experimentation has moved away from one-off descriptive types of experiments having no general application, to studies testing hypotheses based on the principle of cause-and-effect and offering the great advantage of generality of prediction. Simulation models have also played an important role in commercial animal production, whereby they are used to design economically optimal feeding and production regimens.

References

Baker, D.H. (2005) Comparative nutrition and metabolism: explication of open questions with emphasis on protein and amino acids. *Proceedings of the National Academy of Sciences* 102, 17897–17902.

Bastianelli, D. and Sauvant, D. (1997) Modelling the mechanisms of pig growth. *Livestock Production Science* 51, 97–107.

Bastianelli, D., Sauvant, D. and Rérat, A. (1996) Mathematical modeling of digestion and nutrient absorption in pigs. *Journal of Animal Science* 74, 1873–1887.

Birkett, S. and Lange, K. de (2001a) Limitations of conventional models and a conceptual framework for a nutrient flow representation of energy utilization by animals. *British Journal of Nutrition* 86, 647–659.

Birkett, S. and Lange, K. de (2001b) A conceptual framework for a nutrient flow representation of energy utlilization of growing monogastric animals. *British Journal of Nutrition* 86, 661–674.

Birkett, S. and Lange, K. de (2001c) Calibration of a nutrient flow model of energy utilization by growing pigs. *British Journal of Nutrition* 86, 675–689.

Black, J.L., Davies, G.T., Bray, H.J., Giles, L.R. and Chapple, R.P. (1995) Modelling the effects of genotype, environment and health on nutrient utilisation. In: Danfaer, A. and Lescoat, P. (eds) *Proceedings of the IVth International Workshop on Modelling Nutrient Utlisation in Farm Animals.* National Institute of Animal Science, Foulum, Denmark, pp. 85–105.

Boisen, S. and Verstegen, M.W.A. (2000) Developments in the measurement of the energy content of feeds and energy utilisation in animals. In: Moughan, P.J., Verstegen, M.W.A. and Visser-Reyneveld, M.I. (eds) *Feed Evaluation – Principles and Practice.* Wageningen Pers, Wageningen, The Netherlands, pp. 57–76.

Cole, D.J.A. (1980) The amino acid requirements of pigs. The concept of an ideal protein. *Pig News and Information* 1, 201–205.

Emmans, G.C. (1981) A model of the growth and feed intake of *ad libitum* fed animals, particularly poultry. In: Hillyer, G.M., Whittemore, C.T. and Gunn, R.G. (eds) *Computers in Animal Production, Occasional Publication No. 5.* British Society of Animal Production, Edinburgh, UK, pp. 103–110.

Fuller, M.H. and Tomé, D. (2005) *In vivo* determination of amino acid bioavailability in humans and model animals. *Journal of AOAC International* 88, 923–934.

Greef, K.H. de (1992) Prediction of production, nutrition induced tissue partitioning in growing pigs. PhD thesis, Wageningen University, The Netherlands.

Green, D.M. and Whittemore, C.T. (2003) Architecture of a harmonized model of the growing pig for the determination of dietary net energy and protein requirements and of excretions into the environment (IMS Pig). *Animal Science* 77, 113–130.

Green, D.M. and Whittemore, C.T. (2005) Calibration and sensitivity analysis of a model of the growing pig for weight gain and composition. *Agricultural Systems* 84, 279–295.

Heger, J., Van Phung, T. and Krizova, L. (2002) Efficiency of amino acid utilization in the growing pig at suboptimal levels of intake: lysine, threonine, sulphur amino acids and tryptophan. *Journal of Animal Physiology and Animal Nutrition* 86, 153–165.

Heger, J., Van Phung, T., Krizova, L., Sustala, M. and Simecek, K. (2003) Efficiency of amino acid utilization in the growing pig at suboptimal levels of intake: branched-chain amino acids, histidine and phenylalanine + tyrosine. *Journal of Animal Physiology and Animal Nutrition* 87, 52–65.

Lange, C.F.M. de and Birkett, S.H. (2005) Characterisation of useful energy content in swine and poultry feed ingredients. *Canadian Journal of Animal Science* 85, 269–280.

Lange, C.F. de, Gillis, A.M. and Simpson, G.J. (2001) Influence of threonine intake on whole-body protein deposition and threonine utilization in growing pigs fed purified diets. *Journal of Animal Science* 79, 3087–3095.

Le Floc'h, N. and Sève, B. (2005) Catabolism through the threonine dehydrogenase pathway does not account for the high first-pass extraction rate of dietary threonine by the portal drained viscera in pigs. *British Journal of Nutrition* 93, 447–456.

Lovatto, P.A. and Sauvant, D. (2003) Modeling homeorhetic and homeostatic controls of pig growth. *Journal of Animal Science* 81, 683–696.

Miller, D.S. and Payne, P.R. (1963) A theory of protein metabolism. *Theoretical Biology* 5, 398–411.

Millward, D.J. (1998) Metabolic demands for amino acids and the human dietary requirement: Millward and Rivers (1988) revisited. *Journal of Nutrition* 128, 2563S– 2576S.

Möhn, S., Gillis. A.M., Moughan, P.J. and Lange, C.F. de (2000) Influence of dietary lysine and energy intakes on body protein deposition and lysine utilization in the growing pig. *Journal of Animal Science* 78, 1510–1519.

Möhn, S., Ball, R.O., Fuller, M.F., Gillis, A.M. and Lange, C.F. de (2004) Growth potential, but not body weight or moderate limitation of lysine intake, affects inevitable lysine catabolism in growing pigs. *Journal of Nutrition* 134, 2287–2292.

Moughan, P.J. (1981) A model to simulate the utilization of dietary amino acids by the growing pig (20–100 kg). Research Bulletin, Massey University, Palmerston North, New Zealand.

Moughan, P.J. (1985) Sensitivity analysis on a model simulating the digestion and metabolism of nitrogen in the growing pig. *New Zealand Journal of Agricultural Research* 28, 463–468.

Moughan, P.J. (1989) Simulation of the daily partitioning of lysine in the 50 kg live weight pig – a factorial approach to estimating amino acid requirements for growth and maintenance. *Research and Development in Agriculture* 6, 7–14.

Moughan, P.J. (1991) Towards an improved utilization of dietary amino acids by the growing pig. In: Haresign, W. and Cole, D.J.A. (eds) *Recent Advances in Animal Nutrition*. Butterworths, Heinemann, Oxford, UK, pp. 45–64.

Moughan, P.J. (1994) Modelling amino acid absorption and metabolism in the growing pig. In: D'Mello, J.P.F. (ed.) *Amino Acids in Farm Animal Nutrition*. CAB International, Wallingford, UK, pp. 133–154.

Moughan, P.J. (2005a) Physiological processes underlying the dietary amino acid requirement in humans: the role of the gut. In: Vorster, H.H., Blaauw, R., Dhansay, M.A., Kuzwayo, P.M.N., Moeng, L. and Wentzel-Viljoen, E. (eds) *Proceedings of the 18th International Congress of Nutrition*, Durban, South Africa. CD publication (ISBN 3-8055-8015-0), 10 pp.

Moughan, P.J. (2005b) Absorption of chemically unmodified lysine from proteins in foods that have sustained damage during processing or storage. *Journal of AOAC International* 88, 949–954.

Moughan, P.J. and Smith, W.C. (1984) Prediction of dietary protein quality based on a model of the digestion and metabolism of nitrogen in the growing pig. *New Zealand Journal of Agricultural Research* 274, 501–507.

Moughan, P.J. and Verstegen, M.W.A. (1988) The modelling of growth in the pig. *Netherlands Journal of Agricultural Science* 36, 145–166.

Moughan, P.J., Smith, W.C. and Pearson, G. (1987) Description and validation of a model simulating growth in the pig (20–90 kg live weight). *New Zealand Journal of Agricultural Research* 30, 481–489.

Pomar, C., Harris, D.L. and Minvielle, F. (1991) Computer simulation model of swine production systems: modeling the growth of young pigs. *Journal of Animal Science* 69, 1468–1488.

Rivest, J., Bernier, J.F. and Pomar, C. (2000) A dynamic model of protein digestion in the small intestine of pigs. *Journal of Animal Science* 78, 328–340.

Sandberg, F.B., Emmans, G.C. and Kyriazakis, I. (2005a) Partitioning of limiting protein and energy in the growing pig: description of the problem, and possible rules and their qualitative evaluation. *British Journal of Nutrition* 93, 205–212.

Sandberg, F.B., Emmans, G.C. and Kyriazakis, I. (2005b) Partitioning of limiting protein and energy in the growing pig: testing quantitative rules against experimental data. *British Journal of Nutrition* 93, 213–224.

Schinckel, A.P. and Lange, C.F.M. de (1996) Characterization of growth parameters needed as inputs for pig growth models. *Journal of Animal Science* 74, 2021–2036.

Stein, H.H., Sève, B., Fuller, M.F., Moughan, P.J. and Lange, C.F.M. de (2007) Invited review: amino acid availability and digestibility in pig feed ingredients: terminology and application. *Journal of Animal Science* 85, 172–180.

Stoll, B., Burrin, D.G., Henry, J., Yu, H., Jahoor, F. and Reeds, P.J. (1999) Substrate oxidation by the portal drained viscera of fed piglets. *American Journal of Physiology* 277, 168–175.

van Milgen, J. (2002) Modeling biochemical aspects of energy metabolism in mammals. *Journal of Nutrition* 132, 3195–3202.

van Milgen, J. and Noblet, J. (2003) Partitioning of energy intake to heat, protein and fat in growing pigs. *Journal of Animal Science* 81, E86–E93.

Weis, R.N., Birkett, S.H., Morel, P.C.H. and Lange, C.F.M. de (2004) Effects of energy intake and body weight on physical and chemical body composition in growing entire male pigs. *Journal of Animal Science* 82, 109–121.

Wellock, I.J., Emmans, G.C. and Kyriazakis, I. (2004) Describing and predicting potential growth in the pig. *Animal Science* 78, 379–388.

Whittemore, C.T. and Fawcett, T.H. (1976) Theoretical aspects of a flexible model to simulate protein and lipid growth in pigs. *Animal Production* 22, 87–96.

12 Compartmental Models of Protein Turnover to Resolve Isotope Dilution Data

L.A. CROMPTON,[1] J. FRANCE,[2] R.S. DIAS,[2] E. KEBREAB[2,3] AND M.D. HANIGAN[4]

[1]Animal Science Research Group, School of Agriculture, Policy and Development, University of Reading, UK; [2]Centre for Nutrition Modelling, Department of Animal and Poultry Science, University of Guelph, Canada; [3]National Centre for Livestock and Environment, Department of Animal Science, University of Manitoba, Canada; [4]Department of Dairy Science, Virginia Tech, USA

Introduction

Most dynamic models appearing in the animal sciences literature are based on systems of ordinary differential equations (ODEs). There is a mathematically standard way of representing such models called the rate:state formalism:

$$\text{rate of process} = \text{function of state of system}. \tag{12.1}$$

An appreciation of this formalism is central to understanding the role of modelling in the animal sciences. According to the formalism, the system under investigation is defined at time t by q state variables: X_1, X_2, ..., X_q. These variables represent properties or attributes of the system (e.g. organ or tissue mass, quantity of substrate). The model then comprises q first-order ODEs which describe how the state variables change with time:

$$\frac{dX_i}{dt} = f_i(X_1, X_2, ..., X_q; P);\ i = 1, 2, ..., q, \tag{12.2}$$

where P denotes a set of parameters and the function f_i gives the rate of change of the state variable X_i. The function f_i comprises terms (flows) which represent the rates of component processes (e.g. tissue synthesis, substrate utilization) with dimensions of state variable per unit time. In this type of mathematical modelling, the differential equations are formed through direct application of scientific laws (e.g. for chemical kinetics or transport) or by application of a continuity equation derived from more fundamental scientific laws.

There are three types of solution to these dynamic models.

1. The system under investigation is in steady state (or partial steady state) and solutions are obtained by setting the relevant differentials to zero, then manipulating and solving the resultant algebraic expressions to obtain an expression for each flow (Type I solution).
2. The system is in non-steady state and the ODEs are linear and can be integrated analytically to give an expression for each state variable (Type II).
3. The system is in non-steady state, but the ODEs are non-linear and have to be integrated numerically (Type III).

In this chapter, we illustrate applications in the animal sciences of dynamic modelling, based on the rate:state formalism, with Type I solutions. This chapter deals with modelling animal processes, i.e. specific components or functions of an individual organ or tissue (or whole organism). The processes described are all concerned with amino acid and protein metabolism in the whole body and specific tissues (hindlimb and mammary gland). Examples of two-, three-, four- and eight-pool models are considered.

Protein Turnover

Changes in the mass of protein in the body or individual tissues occur as a result of the dynamic process of protein turnover. This is the balance between the components of protein synthesis (anabolism) and protein degradation (catabolism); the regulation of these two processes dictates the net mass of protein in the animal or tissue. Whole-body and tissue protein mass are regulated by a series of endocrine signals that integrate physiological, environmental, genetic and nutritional cues to bring about orchestrated changes in the rates of protein synthesis and protein degradation. Improved protein accretion can be achieved by altering synthesis or degradation independently or in concert, either in different directions or in similar directions, but to different extents if changes in accretion are to be observed.

Studies on the regulation of tissue protein metabolism require estimates of the rate of both protein synthesis and degradation. In ruminants, the rate of tissue protein synthesis has been measured *in vivo* using either a continuous infusion (e.g. Crompton and Lomax, 1993) or a flooding dose (e.g. Lobley *et al.*, 1992) of tracer amino acid and estimating the incorporation of tracer in tissue. All techniques for measuring the rate of protein synthesis, either in the whole body or individual tissues, require knowledge of tracer activity in the true precursor pool for protein synthesis (see Discussion).

Measurements of protein degradation *in vivo* have usually been calculated indirectly from the difference between the rates of protein synthesis and protein accretion. The rate of protein accretion is measured over a period of time by comparative slaughter (e.g. Bohorov *et al.*, 1987), but this measurement is not made simultaneously with protein synthesis and repeated measurements cannot be made in one animal. Measurements of the urinary excretion of N^{τ}-methylhistidine have been used as a specific index of muscle protein degradation; however, the technique is invalid in sheep (Harris and Milne, 1977, 1980) and is still criticized in other species (see Tomas and Ballard, 1987; Barrett and Gelfand, 1989).

During the past two decades, several laboratories have developed an alternative indirect approach using a combination of arteriovenous (AV) difference techniques, isotope dilution kinetics and blood flow rate procedures to estimate the rates of protein accretion, synthesis and degradation across tissue beds, with particular emphasis on limb metabolism, in pre-ruminants/ruminants (Oddy and Lindsay, 1986; Pell *et al.*, 1986; Harris *et al.*, 1992; Boisclair *et al.*, 1993; Crompton and Lomax, 1993; Hoskin *et al.*, 2001, 2003), dogs (Barrett *et al.*, 1987; Biolo *et al.*, 1992, 1994) and humans (Cheng *et al.*, 1985, 1987; Gelfand and Barrett, 1987; Thompson *et al.*, 1989; Biolo *et al.*, 1995). The AV kinetic methods use measurements of amino acid net mass balance and isotopic transfer and dilution across a tissue bed to derive estimates for tissue protein turnover and, in addition to limbs, the techniques have been successfully applied across the mammary gland (Oddy *et al.*, 1988; France *et al.*, 1995; Bequette *et al.*, 2002) and liver (France *et al.*, 1999) in lactating ruminants. The AV difference methods contain inherent assumptions relating to the choice of precursor pool for estimating protein synthesis, the heterogeneity of the tissue bed and metabolism of the tracer amino acid within the tissues (see Discussion; Harris *et al.*, 1992; Crompton and Lomax, 1993; Waterlow, 2006) and require an accurate measurement of blood flow rate. None the less, the major advantage offered by the approach is the simultaneous estimation of tissue protein accretion, synthesis and degradation *in vivo* and it can, therefore, be used serially for large animal studies.

Amino acid tracers used to study protein metabolism *in vivo* can be either radioisotopes or stable isotopes of the natural compound (see Discussion). The terms *activity* and *isotopic activity* will be used throughout this chapter as a generality for both specific radioactivity (SRA) in the case of radioactive tracers and isotopic abundance or enrichment for stable isotope tracers.

Whole-body Protein Synthesis (Two-pool Model)

The two-pool precursor–product model for protein turnover, attributable to Waterlow *et al.* (1978), is shown in Fig. 12.1. It consists of two pools (assumed to be homogeneous), namely the precursor amino acid pool (Q_1, μmol free amino acid) and the whole-body protein pool (Q_2, μmol protein-bound amino acid). The precursor pool is fully interchanging. The external and internal inflows are amino acid uptake (absorption, F_{10}) and protein degradation (F_{12}), respectively, and the respective external and internal efflows are oxidation (F_{01}) and protein synthesis (F_{21}). The product pool is fully interchanging with the precursor pool, with an internal inflow (synthesis, F_{21}) and efflow (degradation, F_{12}). No external inflow is permitted, but protein loss from this pool via export or sloughing is significant in the more biologically active tissues and is, therefore, given explicit representation (F_{02}). The scheme permits recycling

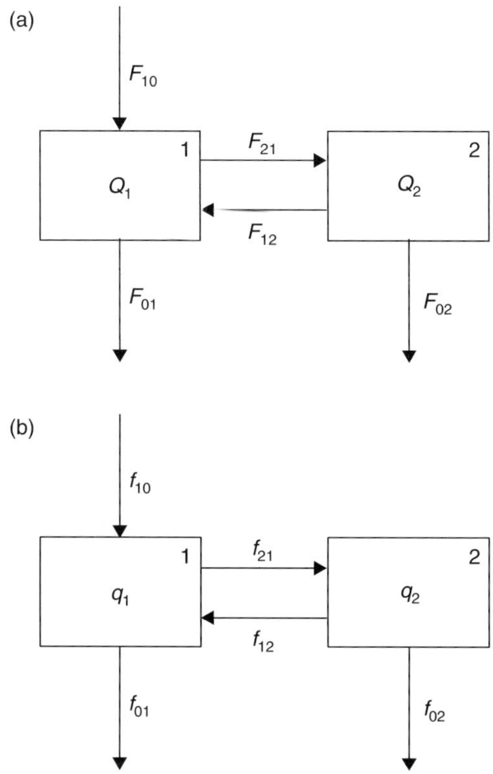

Fig. 12.1. Precursor–product model for protein turnover: (a) unlabelled material (tracee); (b) radio-labelled material (tracer). Q_1 and q_1 represent free amino acids in the blood/plasma pool; Q_2 and q_2 represent protein-bound amino acids. F_{ij} and f_{ij} represent flows to *i* from *j*; 0 denotes the environment (outside).

of radiolabel via the precursor pool, but not via the product pool, and it is assumed that radioactivity can be measured in both pools. Conservation of mass principles can be applied to each pool in Fig. 12.1a and b to generate differential equations that describe the dynamic behaviour of the system. For unlabelled amino acid, these differential equations are (mathematical notation is defined in Table 12.1 and Fig. 12.1):

$$\frac{dQ_1}{dt} = F_{10} + F_{12} - F_{01} - F_{21} \tag{12.3}$$

$$\frac{dQ_2}{dt} = F_{21} - F_{02} - F_{12} \tag{12.4}$$

and for the labelled amino acid:

$$\begin{aligned}\frac{dq_1}{dt} &= f_{10} + f_{12} - f_{01} - f_{21} \\ &= f_{10} + s_2 F_{12} - s_1(F_{01} + F_{21})\end{aligned} \tag{12.5a, b}$$

$$\begin{aligned}\frac{dq_2}{dt} &= f_{21} - f_{02} - f_{12} \\ &= s_1 F_{21} - s_2(F_{02} + F_{12})\end{aligned} \tag{12.6a, b}$$

Table 12.1. Principal symbols used for the kinetic models.

F_{ij}	Flow of tracee[a] to pool i from j; F_{i0} denotes an external flow into pool i and F_{0j} denotes a flow from pool j out of the system	μmol min^{-1} (nmol min^{-1} g^{-1} of tissue, Three-pool model)
f_{ij}	Flow of tracer to pool i from j; f_{i0} denotes an external flow into pool i and f_{0j} denotes a flow from pool j out of the system	Bq min^{-1} (radioisotope)[b] μmol min^{-1} (stable isotope)
I_i	Effective rate of constant infusion of primary tracer into primary pool i	Bq min^{-1} (radioisotope)[b] μmol min^{-1} (stable isotope)
Φ_i	Effective rate of constant infusion of secondary tracer into primary pool i	Bq min^{-1} (radioisotope) μmol min^{-1} (stable isotope)
Q_i	Quantity of tracee[a] in pool i	μmol (nmol g^{-1} of tissue, Three-pool model)
q_i	Quantity of primary tracer in pool i	Bq (radioisotope)[b] μmol (stable isotope)
ϕ_i	Quantity of secondary tracer in pool i	Bq (radioisotope) μmol (stable isotope)
s_i	Specific radioactivity of primary tracer in pool i: $(= q_i/Q_i)$	Bq μmol^{-1} (Bq nmol^{-1}, Three-pool model)
e_i	Enrichment of primary tracer in pool i: $(= q_i/Q_i)$	atoms % excess μmol^{-1}
ε_i	Enrichment of secondary tracer in pool i: $(= \phi_i/Q_i)$	atoms % excess μmol^{-1}
R	Dilution ratio	dimensionless
t	Time	min

[a]Total material (i.e. tracee + tracer) in the case of a stable isotope infusion.
[b]Scaled by g of tissue in Three-pool model.

The Waterlow equation for protein synthesis is derived from Eqn 12.5b by making a number of assumptions. First, the precursor pool is in steady state:

$$\frac{dq_1}{dt}\left(=\frac{dQ_1}{dt}\right)=0. \tag{12.7}$$

Secondly, radiolabel is continuously infused into the precursor pool at a constant rate I (Bq min^{-1}) and there is no recycling of label:

$$f_{10} = I. \tag{12.8}$$

Thirdly, the SRA of the product pool is negligible:

$$s_2 \approx 0. \tag{12.9}$$

Using Eqns 12.7–12.9, Eqn 12.5b simplifies to give the Waterlow equation:

$$F_{21} = I / s_1 - F_{01}. \tag{12.10}$$

Therefore, provided that rate of infusion and SRA of the precursor pool in steady state are measured, and provided that oxidation (F_{01}) can be estimated (or ignored), protein synthesis (F_{21}) can be calculated from Eqn 12.10. The rate protein synthesis (F_{21}, μmol min^{-1}) can be converted into whole-body protein synthesis (g day^{-1}) based on the amino acid contents of total body protein for the

Table 12.2. Whole-body protein synthesis rates for cattle and sheep.

Species	Body weight (kg)	Infusate	Protein synthesis (g day^{-1})	Reference
Cattle				
Growing heifer	250	[^{3}H]tyrosine	2925[a]	Lobley *et al.* (1980)
Growing heifer	368.5	[^{14}C]leucine	1239	Eisemann *et al.* (1986)
Dry cow	628	[^{3}H]tyrosine	2022[a]	Lobley *et al.* (1980)
Dry cow	628	[^{3}H]leucine	2919[a]	Lobley *et al.* (1980)
Growing steer	240	[^{3}H]tyrosine	3097[a]	Boisclair *et al.* (1993)
Growing steer	456	[^{2}H]phenylalanine	2334[a]	Lobley *et al.* (2000)
Sheep				
Ovine fetus	1.8	[^{14}C] or [^{3}H]tyrosine	112	Schaefer and Krishnamurti (1984)
Growing lamb	20.3	[^{3}H]tyrosine	241	Davis *et al.* (1981)
Growing lamb	29.3	[^{3}H]tyrosine	300	Crompton (1990)
Growing lamb	33.0	[^{3}H]phenylalanine	239	Harris *et al.* (1992)
Growing lamb	33.0	[^{13}C]leucine	281	Harris *et al.* (1992)
Growing lamb	32.5	[^{13}C]phenylalanine	386[a]	Savary-Auzeloux *et al.* (2003)
Growing lamb	32.5	[^{13}C]tyrosine	426[a]	Savary-Auzeloux *et al.* (2003)
Lactating ewe	56.9	[^{3}H]tyrosine	581[a]	Bryant and Smith (1982b)
Dry ewe	65.3	[^{3}H]tyrosine	470[a]	Bryant and Smith (1982b)
Mature wether	64.1	[^{3}H]tyrosine	293[a]	Bryant and Smith (1982a)

[a]Uncorrected for oxidation.

species being studied. The Waterlow equation has been used extensively in animal biology to determine the rate of whole-body protein synthesis; some of the values obtained for ruminant farm livestock are given in Table 12.2. Further mathematical analysis of the two-pool precursor–product model, its special cases and some three-pool variants for calculating protein turnover are given by France *et al.* (1988).

Tyrosine Kinetics in the Hindlimb Tissues (Three-pool Model)

Nutritional intake is known to be a potent modulator of protein turnover in many species (see Waterlow, 2006). Improved nutrition (both quantity and quality) alters the efficiency with which growing ruminants divert feed eaten to productive tissues such as muscle and results in faster growth rates and enhanced protein accretion, due to changes in whole-body and peripheral tissue protein synthesis and degradation (Oddy *et al.*, 1987; Harris *et al.*, 1992; Boisclair *et al.*, 1993; Crompton and Lomax, 1993; Thomson *et al.*, 1997; Hoskin *et al.*, 2001). Increases in feed intake are usually accompanied by elevated concentrations of certain amino acids (Hoskin *et al.*, 2001).

Lobley (1993b, 1998) proposed that peripheral tissue protein synthesis and degradation in ruminants both respond in a curvilinear manner to increasing feed intake between fasting and supra-maintenance levels, with synthesis being more sensitive to feed intake when linked to the action of anabolic hormones. In a study to test the curvilinear hypothesis, Hoskin *et al.* (2001) reported a significant linear relationship between increasing feed intake and hindlimb protein synthesis, with no evidence of a curvilinear response. However, protein synthesis did not change at lower intakes (0.5, 1.0 and 1.5 × maintenance) and the linear relationship was largely due to the increase at 2.5 × maintenance intake. There was no response in protein degradation with feed intake (Hoskin *et al.*, 2001).

Waterlow (1999) has suggested that amino acids could be the coordinating link between protein synthesis and degradation, being the substrate for one process and the product of the other. He proposed a curvilinear relationship to describe the effect of amino acid concentration on the rates of protein synthesis and degradation, termed the crossover model of coordination (Waterlow, 1999, 2006). In this model, synthesis increases and degradation decreases, both in a curvilinear relationship and, at a certain amino acid concentration, the lines for synthesis and degradation must cross; this is the point of zero protein accretion or balance. Waterlow (1999) suggests that each tissue may have a basal amino acid concentration at which the appearance (degradation + intake) and disappearance (synthesis + oxidation) of amino acids are equal and this will vary depending on tissue type, sensitivity and hormonal action. Any such changes would alter the position of the curves and their slopes.

The model described in this section was developed to resolve the data generated from trials with growing lambs which measured tyrosine (TYR) exchange and SRA across the hindlimb tissues over a range of feed intakes (France *et al.*, 2005; Crompton *et al.*, 2006). The trials were undertaken to investigate how changes in nutrition influence the control and coordination of protein metabolism in peripheral tissues.

The scheme adopted is shown in Fig. 12.2a. It contains one intracellular and two extracellular pools. The intracellular pool is free TYR (pool 2), while the extracellular pools are arterial and venous TYR (pools 1 and 3, respectively). The flows of TYR between pools and into and out of the system are shown as arrowed lines. The intracellular free TYR pool has two inflows, i.e. from the degradation of constitutive hindlimb protein, F_{20}, and from the extracellular arterial pool, F_{21}, and two efflows, i.e. synthesis of constitutive hindlimb protein, F_{02}, and outflow into the venous pool, F_{32}. The extracellular arterial TYR pool has a single inflow, entry into the pool, F_{10}, and two efflows, uptake by the hindlimb, F_{21}, and outflow into the venous pool, F_{31}. The extracellular venous TYR pool has two inflows, bypass from the arterial pool, F_{31}, and release from the intracellular TYR pool, F_{32}, and one efflow out of the system, F_{03}.

The scheme adopted for movement of label is shown in Fig. 12.2b. [side chain 2,3-^{3}H]TYR is infused systemically at a constant rate (e.g. 7.5 kBq min^{-1})

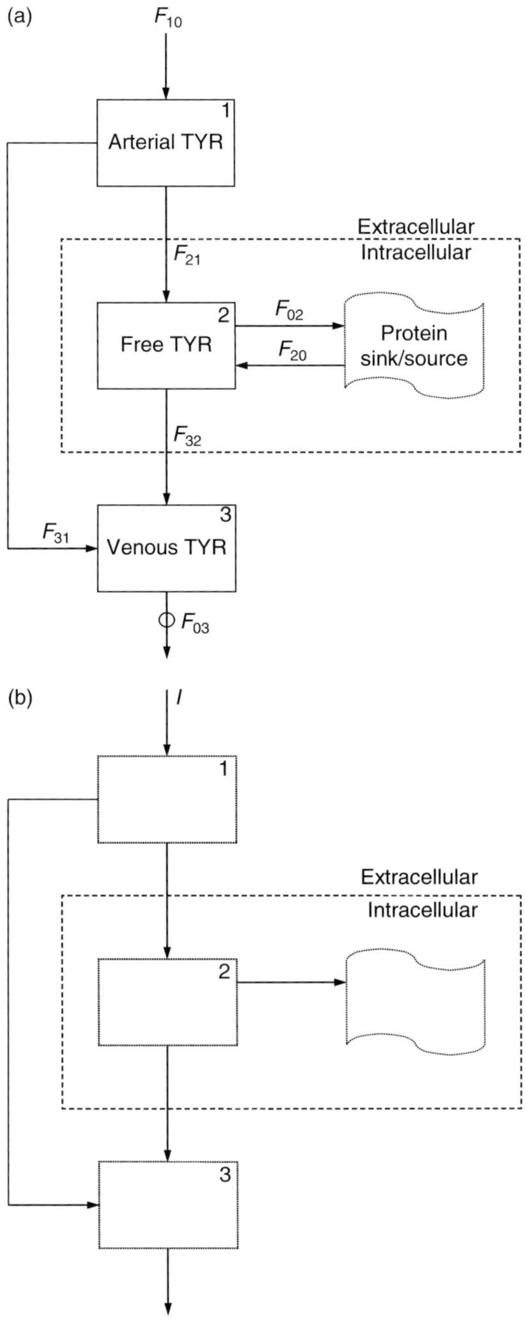

Fig. 12.2. Scheme for the uptake and utilization of tyrosine by the tissues of the hindlimb in lambs: (a) unlabelled tyrosine, (b) labelled tyrosine. The small circle in Fig. 12.2a indicates a flow out of the system that needs to be measured experimentally.

for a period of time (e.g. 6 h) and the SRA of all three pools monitored. The SRA of the extracellular pools is measured by taking blood samples from the carotid artery and deep femoral vein during the isotope infusion. The SRA of the intracellular pool is measured directly in muscle tissue samples taken at the end of the infusion. Blood flow rate across the hindlimb is measured using the diffusion equilibrium technique (Crompton and Lomax, 1993), which yields plasma flow rates as ml min^{-1} g^{-1} of tissue being drained (necessitating that pool sizes and flows are scaled by g of tissue, see Table 12.1). The scheme assumes that the only entry of label into the system is into the arterial TYR pool via the effective infusion rate, flow I (e.g. 10 Bq min^{-1} g^{-1}), and that the duration of the infusion is such that the SRA of constitutive protein can be regarded as negligible.

Conservation of mass principles can be applied to each pool in Fig. 12.2a and b to generate differential equations that describe the dynamic behaviour of the system. For unlabelled TYR, these differential equations are (mathematical notation is defined in Table 12.1):

$$\frac{dQ_1}{dt} = F_{10} - F_{21} - F_{31} \tag{12.11}$$

$$\frac{dQ_2}{dt} = F_{20} + F_{21} - F_{02} - F_{32} \tag{12.12}$$

$$\frac{dQ_3}{dt} = F_{31} + F_{32} - F_{03} \tag{12.13}$$

and for labelled TYR:

$$\frac{dq_1}{dt} = I - s_1 (F_{21} + F_{31}) \tag{12.14}$$

$$\frac{dq_2}{dt} = s_1 F_{21} - s_2 (F_{02} + F_{32}) \tag{12.15}$$

$$\frac{dq_3}{dt} = s_1 F_{31} - s_2 F_{32} - s_3 F_{03}. \tag{12.16}$$

When the system is in steady state with respect to both unlabelled and labelled TYR, the derivative terms in Eqns 12.11–12.16 are all zero. Algebraic manipulation of Eqns 12.11–12.16 with the derivates set to zero gives:

$$F_{10} = I/s_1 \tag{12.17}$$

$$F_{32} = (s_1 - s_3)F_{03}/(s_1 - s_2);\ s_1 \neq s_2 \tag{12.18}$$

$$F_{31} = F_{03} - F_{32} \tag{12.19}$$

$$F_{21} = F_{10} - F_{31} \tag{12.20}$$

$$F_{02} = s_1 F_{21}/s_2 - F_{32} \tag{12.21}$$

$$F_{20} = F_{02} + F_{32} - F_{21}, \tag{12.22}$$

where the italics denote steady-state values of flows and SRAs in these equations. Note that the efflow of TYR from the venous blood pool (i.e. F_{03}) can be measured experimentally.

Example solutions to the model, to illustrate the magnitude of the calculated flows, are given in Table 12.3 for four wether lambs (average live weight 33 kg). The lambs were fed a range of feed intakes (a higher lamb number indicates a higher

Table 12.3. Tyrosine uptake and partition by the hindlimb tissues in growing lambs obtained using the three-pool model (symbols are defined in the text and Table 12.1).

		Lamb number			
		01	04	06	09
DM intake (g day^{-1})		311	529	933	1087
Flow (nmol min^{-1} g^{-1})	F_{10}	1.20	2.63	4.06	8.68
	F_{32}	1.10	2.14	1.72	2.05
	F_{31}	0.28	0.68	2.13	6.06
	F_{21}	0.92	1.95	1.93	2.63
	F_{02}	0.67	1.26	1.56	1.80
	F_{20}	0.85	1.44	1.35	1.22
Protein turnover	FSR	2.93	5.51	6.86	7.88
(% day^{-1})	FDR	3.72	6.32	5.93	5.33
	FAR	−0.79	−0.81	0.92	2.55

FSR, fractional synthesis rate; FDR, fractional degradation rate; FAR, fractional accretion rate.

intake; see Table 12.3) as described previously (Crompton and Lomax, 1993). The diet consisted of a barley-based concentrate and chopped hay in a 9:1 ratio on a DM basis. The crude protein content of the diet was 153 g kg^{-1} DM. The nitrogen intake of the lambs ranged from 7 to 27 g day^{-1} and plasma TYR concentration varied from 27 to 81 nmol ml^{-1}. The kinetic model outputs demonstrated that the flow of TYR into constitutive protein only accounted for on average 0.71 (range 0.65–0.81) of the TYR inflow into the hindlimb tissues. Comparison of hindlimb fractional synthesis rates (FSRs), with FSRs measured directly in muscle, showed that the contribution of non-muscular tissues to hindlimb tissue was 0.49 (see Discussion).

When the model is applied sequentially in the same animal to examine treatment effects, there is potential for different treatments to cause changes in model pool sizes that may be manifested as a change in the calculated flow rates between the pools. For example, a perceived treatment decrease in the flow F_{20} (from protein degradation) could be due to the treatment stimulating an increase in intracellular pool size. To eliminate potential errors with data interpretation, the size of the intracellular-free TYR pool, Q_2, is estimated using the following derivation. Consider the rise to plateau phase commencing at the start of infusion and assume non-isotopic steady state during this phase. Equation 12.15 yields:

$$Q_2 \frac{ds_2}{dt} = s_1 F_{21} - s_2 (F_{02} + F_{32}). \tag{12.23}$$

Therefore:

$$Q_2 = [s_1 F_{21} - s_2 (F_{02} + F_{32})] \Big/ \left(\frac{ds_2}{dt} \right). \tag{12.24}$$

Let the SRA of each pool rise to a plateau following an exponential time course, i.e.

$$s_1 = A_1[1 - \exp(-k_1 t)] \quad (12.25)$$

$$s_2 = A_2[1 - \exp(-k_2 t)] \quad (12.26)$$

$$s_3 = A_3[1 - \exp(-k_3 t)], \quad (12.27)$$

where the A_is (Bq nmol^{-1}) are plateau SRAs and the k_is (min^{-1}) are rate constants. Differentiating Eqn 12.26:

$$\frac{ds_2}{dt} = k_2 A_2 \exp(-k_2 t). \quad (12.28)$$

Using Eqns 12.25, 12.26 and 12.28 in Eqn 12.24 gives pool size calculated at time $t_{0.5}$ as:

$$Q_2 = \{A_1[1 - \exp(-k_1 t_{0.5})]F_{21} - A_2[1 - \exp(-k_2 t_{0.5})](F_{02} + F_{32})\} / [k_2 A_2 \exp(-k_2 t_{0.5})], \quad (12.29)$$

where $t_{0.5} = (\ln 2)/k_2$ is the time (min) taken for the SRA of pool 2 to reach half its plateau value. Therefore, the solution to the model for the steady-state flows is given by Eqns 12.17–12.22 and for the intracellular pool size by Eqn 12.29.

The outputs from the three-pool model can be used to estimate the fractional rates of hindlimb tissue protein turnover using the following equations:

Hindlimb protein synthesis (HLPS)(% day^{-1}) $= (144F_{02})/\mathrm{MUS_{TYR}}$

Hindlimb protein degradation (HLPD)(% day^{-1}) $= (144F_{20})/\mathrm{MUS_{TYR}}$

Hindlimb protein accretion (% day^{-1}) = HLPS – HLPD,

where 144 is the conversion factor used to convert flow rates (nmol min^{-1} g^{-1}) to fractional rates (% day^{-1}) and $\mathrm{MUS_{TYR}}$ is the TYR content of muscle tissue from the hindlimb. The TYR content of the hindlimb tissues contributing to the blood sampled in the deep femoral vein cannot be determined directly; therefore, the TYR content of muscle is used. The mean TYR content of sheep muscle was 32.811 (SEM 0.882; $n = 10$) mmol kg^{-1} wet weight (Crompton and Lomax, 1993).

Response functions were developed to describe the relationship between the plasma TYR concentration (x axis, nmol ml^{-1}) and the fraction rates of hindlimb constitutive protein synthesis and accretion (y axis, % day^{-1}) for ten lambs. Both functions were sigmoidal in shape. For synthetic rate, the equation was:

$$\mathrm{FSR} = y_{max} / [1 + (k/x)^c]$$

and for accretion rate:

$$\mathrm{FAR} = a + \{b/[1 + (k/x)^c]\},$$

where a, b, c and k are parameters (note that c and k values for FSR differ from those for FAR). The fitted equations are shown in Fig. 12.3. Parameter estimates, residual sum of squares and Durbin–Watson statistics for both response functions are given in Table 12.4. The parameters of the two equations lend

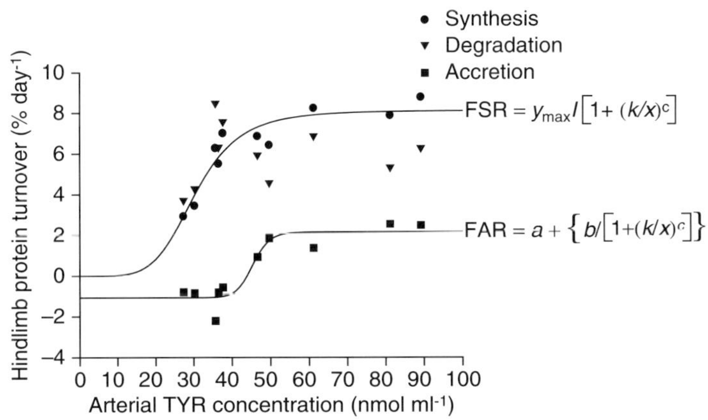

Fig. 12.3. Response functions to describe the relationship between plasma tyrosine concentration and the fraction rates of hindlimb constitutive protein synthesis and accretion in growing lambs.

Table 12.4. Parameter estimates (± standard error), residual sum of squares and Durbin–Watson statistics for the fractional synthetic rate and fractional accretion rate response functions (parameters are defined in the text).

Fractional synthesis rate FSR = $y_{max}/[1+(k/x)^c]$		Fractional accretion rate FAR = $a+\{b/[1+(k/x)^c]\}$	
y_{max} (% day^{-1})	8.11 ± 0.46	a (% day^{-1})	−1.07 ± 0.34
		b (% day^{-1})	3.22 ± 0.54
k (nmol ml^{-1})	30.5 ± 1.36	k (nmol ml^{-1})	45.4 ± 3.00
c	5.22 ± 1.50	c	21.4 ± 30.0
R^2	0.890	R^2	0.893
Durbin–Watson statistic	2.59	Durbin–Watson statistic	2.43
Residual sum of squares	3.67	Residual sum of squares	2.62

FSR, fractional synthesis rate; FAR, fractional accretion rate.

themselves to direct physiological interpretation. The maximum fractional rates for synthesis and accretion are described by the parameters y_{max} and b, respectively. The fractional accretion rate at zero amino acid concentration is given by the parameter a and the amino acid concentration at which half maximal rates are achieved is described by the k parameters. The steepness of each curve is described by the c parameter. Both response functions fit the data satisfactorily and provide a simple biological description for changes in peripheral tissue protein synthesis and accretion with increasing amino acid concentration. The functions support the concept of curvilinear relationships suggested by Lobley (1998) and Waterlow (1999) and emphasize the potential involvement of amino acids as a coordinator of protein turnover (Waterlow 1999, 2006).

Leucine Kinetics in the Mammary Gland of Dairy Cows (Four-pool Model)

Traditionally, dairy research has centred on the twin objectives of increasing milk output and improving efficiency of production. With the demand from consumers and industry to improve milk protein content, research has focused on identifying and understanding the factors and mechanisms regulating the partitioning of amino acids towards milk proteins. Much of the knowledge accrued to date on amino acid and protein metabolism in the lactating mammary gland has been derived from the perfused mammary gland (e.g. Roets *et al.*, 1979, 1983) and from *in vivo* measurements of tissue protein synthesis (e.g. Champredon *et al.*, 1990; Baracos *et al.*, 1991) using dairy goats. Such studies, while they have provided information on the metabolic pathways of milk synthesis, are generally limited by single measurements. The *in vivo* AV preparation of the mammary gland used, for example, by Linzell (1971) and Oddy *et al.* (1988) in goats overcomes this limitation. The preparation, used in conjunction with an infusion of isotopes of specific substrates, allows repeated measurements of the fates of metabolites in the mammary gland to be made *in vivo* throughout lactation. We have established an AV difference preparation for the bovine mammary gland to examine amino acid exchange and kinetic isotope transfers in a series of experiments.

Leucine (LEU) is an essential and potentially limiting amino acid in the synthesis of milk proteins. The model described in this section was developed to resolve the data generated from trials with lactating dairy cows which measured LEU exchange across the mammary gland plus the enrichment of [1-^{13}C]LEU in plasma and secreted milk (France *et al.*, 1995). The trials were undertaken to investigate the influence of diet on partitioning of this amino acid between milk protein output and other metabolic activities. It is also of interest in that a stable, rather than radioactive, isotope is used. Stable isotopes are not strictly tracers in that they have to be administered in non-trace amounts.

The scheme adopted is shown in Fig. 12.4a. It contains two intracellular and two extracellular pools. The intracellular pools are free LEU and LEU in milk protein (pools 2 and 3, respectively), while the extracellular pools are arterial and venous LEU (pools 1 and 4). The flows of LEU between pools and into and out of the system are shown as arrowed lines. The intracellular free LEU pool (pool 2) has three inflows: from the degradation of constitutive mammary gland protein, F_{20}; from the extracellular arterial pool, F_{21}; and from the degradation of milk protein, F_{23}. The pool has five efflows: secretion in milk, $F_{02}^{(m)}$; oxidation, $F_{02}^{(o)}$; synthesis of constitutive mammary gland protein, $F_{02}^{(s)}$; incorporation into milk protein, F_{32}; and outflow into the venous LEU pool, F_{42}. The milk protein-bound LEU pool has one inflow, from free LEU, F_{32}, and two efflows, secretion of protein in milk, F_{03}, and degradation, F_{23}. The extracellular arterial LEU pool also has a single inflow, entry into the pool, F_{10}, and two efflows, uptake by the mammary gland, F_{21}, and outflow to the venous pool, F_{41}. The extracellular venous LEU pool has two inflows, bypass from the arterial pool, F_{41}, and release from the intracellular LEU pool, F_{42}, and one efflow out of the system, F_{04}.

The scheme adopted for movement of label is shown in Fig. 12.4b. [1-^{13}C]LEU is infused systemically at a constant rate (e.g. 90 μmol min^{-1}) and the enrichment of all four pools monitored. The enrichment of the extracellular pools is measured directly by taking blood samples from the external pudic

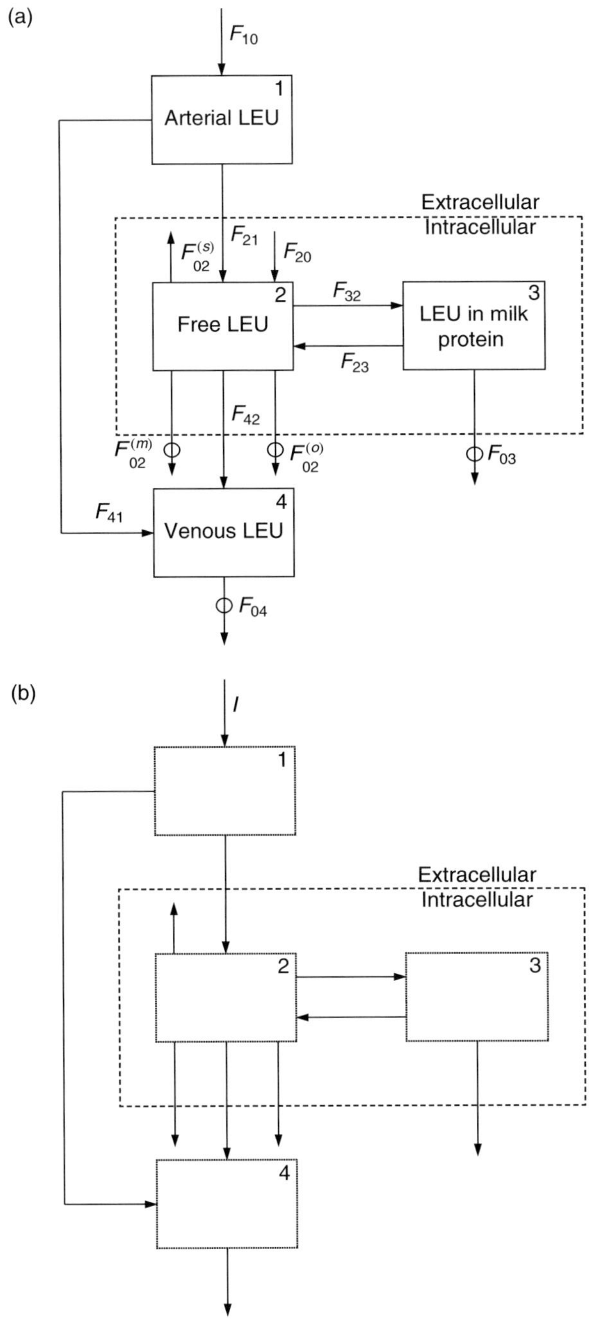

Fig. 12.4. Scheme for the uptake and utilization of LEU by the mammary gland of lactating dairy cows: (a) total LEU, (b) labelled LEU. The small circles in Fig. 12.4a indicate flows out of the system that need to be measured experimentally.

artery and subcutaneous abdominal vein during the isotope infusion. The enrichment of the intracellular free and milk protein-bound LEU pools is not measured directly and is, therefore, assumed to be equivalent to the respective enrichments of free and protein-bound LEU in secreted milk at the end of the infusion (see France *et al.*, 1995). Blood flow rate across the mammary gland was measured by downstream dye dilution with *p*-amino hippuric acid (PAH). The scheme assumes that the only entry of label into the system is into the arterial LEU pool via the effective infusion rate, flow I (e.g. 40 μmol min^{-1}), and that the duration of the infusion is such that the enrichment of constitutive protein can be regarded as negligible.

Conservation of mass principles can be applied to each pool in Fig. 12.4a and b to generate differential equations which describe the dynamic behaviour of the system. For total LEU, these differential equations are (mathematical notation as defined in Table 12.1):

$$\frac{dQ_1}{dt} = F_{10} - F_{21} - F_{41} \tag{12.30}$$

$$\frac{dQ_2}{dt} = F_{20} + F_{21} + F_{23} - F_{02}^{(m)} - F_{02}^{(o)} - F_{02}^{(s)} - F_{32} - F_{42} \tag{12.31}$$

$$\frac{dQ_3}{dt} = F_{32} - F_{03} - F_{23} \tag{12.32}$$

$$\frac{dQ_4}{dt} = F_{41} + F_{42} - F_{04} \tag{12.33}$$

and for ^{13}C-labelled LEU:

$$\frac{dq_1}{dt} = I - e_1(F_{21} + F_{41}) \tag{12.34}$$

$$\frac{dq_2}{dt} = e_1F_{21} + e_3F_{23} - e_2(F_{02}^{(m)} + F_{02}^{(o)} + F_{02}^{(s)} + F_{32} + F_{42}) \tag{12.35}$$

$$\frac{dq_3}{dt} = e_2F_{32} - e_3(F_{03} + F_{23}) \tag{12.36}$$

$$\frac{dq_4}{dt} = e_1F_{41} + e_2F_{42} - e_4F_{04}. \tag{12.37}$$

When the system is in steady state with respect to both unlabelled and labelled LEU, the derivative terms in Eqns 12.30–12.37 are zero, and these equations become:

$$F_{10} - F_{21} - F_{41} = 0 \tag{12.38}$$

$$F_{20} + F_{21} - F_{23} - F_{02}^{(m)} - F_{02}^{(o)} - F_{02}^{(s)} - F_{32} - F_{42} = 0 \tag{12.39}$$

$$F_{32} + F_{03} - F_{23} = 0 \tag{12.40}$$

$$F_{41} + F_{42} - F_{04} = 0 \tag{12.41}$$

$$I - e_1(F_{21} + F_{41}) = 0 \tag{12.42}$$

$$e_1F_{21} - e_3(F_{02}^{(m)} + F_{02}^{(o)} + F_{02}^{(s)} + F_{32} - F_{23} + F_{42}) = 0 \tag{12.43}$$

$$e_1F_{41} + e_3F_{42} - e_4F_{04} = 0. \tag{12.44}$$

Note that, for the scheme assumed, the enrichment of intracellular milk protein-bound LEU pool equalizes with that of the free LEU pool in steady state (i.e. $e_2 = e_3$), otherwise Eqns 12.32 and 12.36 are inconsistent, so these equations yield Eqn 12.40 and e_2 can be written as e_3 in Eqns 12.43 and 12.44, respectively. To obtain steady-state solutions to the model, it is assumed that free LEU in milk, LEU secreted in milk protein and LEU removal from the venous pool (i.e. $F_{02}^{(m)}$, F_{03} and F_{04}, respectively) can be measured experimentally. Algebraic manipulation of Eqns 12.38–12.44 gives:

$$F_{02}^{(o)} + F_{02}^{(s)} = I/e_3 - F_{02}^{(m)} - F_{03} - e_4F_{04}/e_3 \tag{12.45}$$

$$F_{10} = I/e_1 \tag{12.46}$$

$$F_{20} = (1/e_3 - 1/e_1)I + (e_3 - e_4)F_{04}/e_3 \tag{12.47}$$

$$F_{21} = I/e_1 - (e_3 - e_4)F_{04}/(e_3 - e_1);\ e_3 \neq e_1 \tag{12.48}$$

$$F_{32} - F_{23} = F_{03} \tag{12.49}$$

$$F_{41} = (e_3 - e_4)F_{04}/(e_3 - e_1);\ e_3 \neq e_1 \tag{12.50}$$

$$F_{42} = (e_1 - e_4)F_{04}/(e_1 - e_3);\ e_1 \neq e_3, \tag{12.51}$$

where the italics denote steady-state values of flows and enrichments for these equations. Note that the model solution requires the value of e_4 to lie between those of e_1 and e_3. This can be ascertained from inspection of Eqns 12.50 and 12.51 or of Fig. 12.4.

The model solution as given by Eqns 12.45–12.51 does not allow separation of $F_{02}^{(o)}$ and $F_{02}^{(s)}$, the LEU oxidation flow and LEU utilization for constitutive mammary gland protein synthesis (see Eqn 12.45). However, as the rate of accretion (i.e. synthesis minus degradation) of constitutive mammary protein in the lactating ruminant is likely to be small compared with oxidation, an indicator of LEU oxidation can be derived by subtracting Eqns 12.45 and 12.47 to give:

$$\begin{aligned} \text{oxidation} \approx \text{oxidation} + \text{(accretion)} &= F_{02}^{(o)} + (F_{02}^{(s)} - F_{20}) \\ &= I/e_1 - F_{02}^{(m)} - F_{03} - F_{04}. \end{aligned} \tag{12.52}$$

Equation 12.52 states that the difference between apparent uptake of LEU by the mammary gland and LEU losses in milk serves as an indicator of its oxidation in the glands. Alternatively, oxidation can be determined directly by measuring trans-organ evolution of isotopically labelled CO_2 arising during a labelled amino acid infusion (e.g. Bequette *et al.*, 2002).

Furthermore, model solution does not allow separation of milk protein synthesis and degradation flows F_{32} and F_{23}, but merely permits calculation of their difference, i.e. net synthesis (Eqn 12.49). However, separation can be achieved by assuming that a fixed proportion (≈ 0.1) of the nascent milk protein is cleaved and degraded during the docking and secretory processes (Razooki Hasan *et al.*, 1982).

The model can also be used to obtain a dilution ratio for identifying whether or not an amino acid, such as LEU, is limiting protein synthesis in the mammary gland by considering the venous amino acid pool (pool 4). Its steady-state flow equations are Eqns 12.41 and 12.44:

$$F_{41} + F_{42} = F_{04} \tag{12.53}$$

$$e_1 F_{41} + e_3 F_{42} = e_4 F_{04}. \tag{12.54}$$

Eliminating flow F_{41} by multiplying Eqn 12.53 by e_1 and subtracting Eqn 12.54 yields:

$$\begin{aligned} F_{42} &= \frac{(e_1 - e_4)}{(e_1 - e_3)} F_{04};\ e_1 \neq e_3 \\ &= RF_{04}, \end{aligned} \tag{12.55a,b}$$

where R, the dilution ratio, is defined by:

$$R = \frac{(e_1 - e_4)}{(e_1 - e_3)};\ e_1 \neq e_3.$$

R cannot lie outside the range 0 to 1 as the model solution requires e_4 to lie in the range e_1 to e_3. Equations 12.55 give F_{42} entry of LEU into the venous pool from the mammary glands. This cannot exceed F_{04} (see Eqn 12.53). If LEU limits protein synthesis, it is likely that little will leave the cell and so flow F_{42} will be negligible. From an inspection of Eqn 12.55b, it is apparent that F_{42} is negligible if the dilution ratio R or the flow F_{04} tends to zero. F_{04} will be negligible if venous LEU concentration is insignificant. Note that calculation of R requires enrichment in secreted milk to be a reliable proxy for intracellular enrichment. Venous concentration and index R, used in conjunction with a series of infusions of different amino acids, therefore provide, in theory at least, a means of ranking individual

Table 12.5. Leucine uptake and partition by the mammary gland for three lactating dairy cows obtained using the four-pool model (symbols are defined in the text and Table 12.1).

		Cow number		
		1	2	3
Dietary CP (g kg^{-1})		130	130	155
Flow (µmol min^{-1})	$F_{02}^{(o)}$	0	0	73
	$F_{02}^{(s)}$	91	62	256
	F_{10}	785	874	1156
	F_{20}	146	67	256
	F_{21}	524	607	755
	F_{23}	42	48	42
	F_{32}	421	478	421
	F_{41}	260	267	401
	F_{42}	200	182	303
	R	0.43	0.40	0.43

amino acids and identifying the most limiting under particular dietary and physiological conditions.

Example solutions to the model, to illustrate the magnitude of the calculated flows, are given in Table 12.5 for three Holstein-Friesian dairy cows in mid-lactation (average live weight 670 kg, average milk yield 23.7 kg day^{-1}). The cows were fed hourly at two levels of dietary crude protein (CP). Their daily intake was 20 kg dry matter (DM). The diet comprised grass silage (40% by DM) and a protein concentrate (60%) (see France *et al.*, 1995 for further details). Dilution ratio R suggests that LEU is not a limiting amino acid in any of the three cases.

Phenylalanine and Tyrosine Kinetics in the Mammary Gland of Dairy Cows (Eight-pool Model)

Phenylalanine (PHE) and, to a lesser extent, TYR are two of the most commonly used amino acid tracers for measuring protein metabolism in a variety of species and tissues. Their extensive use is due to the fact that neither amino acid is thought to be synthesized or degraded to any major degree in any tissue of the body other than the liver, where PHE can be converted to TYR by hydroxylation and both PHE and TYR are catabolized. The model described in this section was developed to resolve trans-organ and isotope dilution data collected from experiments with lactating dairy cows. The experiments were undertaken to investigate the effects of high and low protein diets on the partitioning of PHE and TYR between milk protein synthesis and other metabolic fates. Once again, as for the model of LEU metabolism, stable isotopes were used as the tracer.

The scheme adopted is shown in Fig. 12.5a. It contains four intracellular and four extracellular pools. The intracellular pools are free PHE (pool 4), PHE in milk protein (pool 3), free TYR (pool 5) and TYR in milk protein (pool 6), while the extracellular ones represent arterial PHE and TYR (pools 1 and 2) and venous PHE and TYR (pools 7 and 8). The flows of PHE and TYR between pools and into and out of the system are shown as arrowed lines. The milk protein-bound PHE pool has a single inflow: from free PHE, F_{34}; and two efflows: secretion of protein in milk, F_{03}, and degradation, F_{43}. The intracellular free PHE pool has three inflows: from the degradation of constitutive mammary gland protein, F_{40}; from the extracellular arterial pool, F_{41}; and from degradation of milk protein, F_{43}. The pool has five efflows: secretion in milk, $F_{04}^{(m)}$; synthesis of constitutive mammary gland protein, $F_{04}^{(s)}$; incorporation into milk protein, F_{34}; hydroxylation to the intracellular free TYR pool, F_{54}; and outflow to the extracellular venous PHE pool, F_{74}. The intracellular free TYR pool has four inflows: from the degradation of constitutive mammary gland protein, F_{50}; from the extracellular arterial TYR pool, F_{52}; from the intracellular PHE pool, F_{54}; and from the degradation of milk protein, F_{56}. The pool has five efflows: secretion in milk, $F_{05}^{(m)}$; oxidation and TYR degradation products, $F_{05}^{(o)}$; synthesis of constitutive mammary gland protein, $F_{05}^{(s)}$; incorporation into milk protein, F_{65}; and outflow to the extracellular venous TYR pool, F_{85}. The milk protein-bound TYR pool has one inflow: from the intracellular free TYR pool, F_{65}; and two efflows: secretion of protein in milk, F_{06}; and degradation, F_{56}. The extracellular arterial PHE pool has a single inflow: entry into the

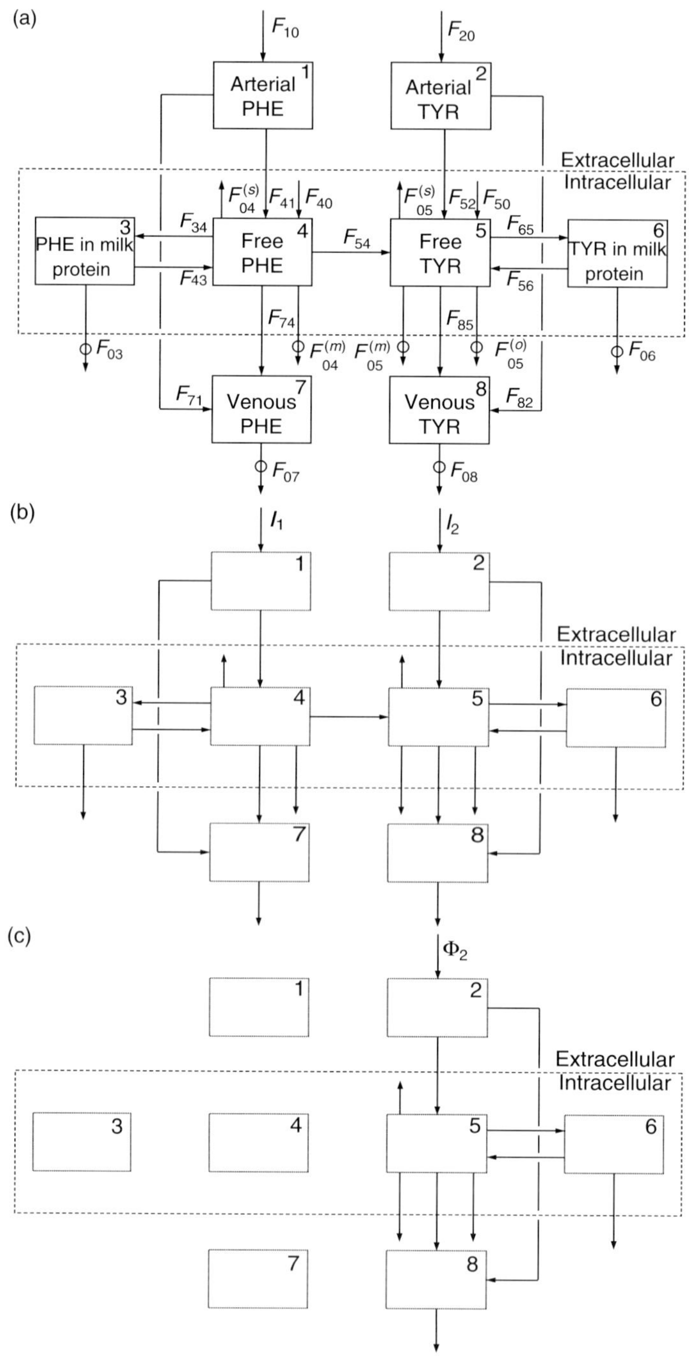

Fig. 12.5. Scheme for the uptake and utilization of PHE and TYR by the mammary gland of lactating dairy cows: (a) total PHE and TYR, (b) [^{13}C]-labelled PHE and TYR and (c) [^{2}H]-labelled TYR. The small circles in Fig. 12.5a indicate flows out of the system that need to be measured experimentally.

pool, F_{10}; and two efflows: uptake by the mammary gland, F_{41}; and release into the extracellular venous PHE pool, F_{71}. The extracellular arterial TYR pool also has a single inflow: entry into the pool, F_{20}; and two efflows: uptake by the mammary gland, F_{52}; and release into the extracellular venous TYR pool, F_{82}. The extracellular venous PHE pool has two inflows: bypass from the arterial PHE pool, F_{71}, and release from the intracellular PHE pool, F_{74}; and one efflow out of the system, F_{07}. The extracellular venous TYR pool also has two inflows: bypass from the arterial TYR pool, F_{82}; and release from the intracellular TYR pool, F_{85}; and one efflow out of the system, F_{08}.

The schemes adopted for the movement of label are shown in Fig. 12.5b and c. [1-^{13}C]PHE and [2,3,5,6-^{2}H]TYR were infused into the jugular vein at a constant rate (e.g. 35 and 10 μmol min^{-1}, respectively) and the enrichment of all eight pools monitored. The enrichments of the extracellular pools are measured directly by taking blood samples from the external pudic artery and subcutaneous abdominal vein during the isotope infusion. The enrichments of the intracellular free and milk protein-bound PHE and TYR pools can only be measured directly using invasive procedures. To avoid such procedures, the enrichments of the intracellular pools are assumed equivalent to their respective enrichments of free and protein-bound PHE and TYR in secreted milk at the end of the infusion (see France *et al.*, 1995). Blood flow rate across the mammary gland is measured by downstream dye dilution using PAH. The scheme assumes that the only entry of label into the system is into the PHE and TYR arterial pools via the effective infusion rates, flows I_1, I_2 and Φ_2 (e.g. 12.5, 0.75 and 5 μmol min^{-1}, respectively), and that the duration of the infusion is such that the enrichment of constitutive protein can be regarded as negligible.

Conservation of mass principles can be applied to each pool in Fig. 12.5a, b and c to generate differential equations that describe the dynamic behaviour of the system. For total (isotopic plus non-isotopic) PHE and TYR, these differential equations are (mathematical notation is defined in Table 12.1):

$$\frac{dQ_1}{dt} = F_{10} - F_{41} - F_{71} \tag{12.56}$$

$$\frac{dQ_2}{dt} = F_{20} - F_{52} - F_{82} \tag{12.57}$$

$$\frac{dQ_3}{dt} = F_{34} - F_{03} - F_{43} \tag{12.58}$$

$$\frac{dQ_4}{dt} = F_{40} + F_{41} + F_{43} - F_{04}^{(m)} - F_{04}^{(s)} - F_{43} - F_{54} - F_{74} \tag{12.59}$$

$$\frac{dQ_5}{dt} = F_{50} + F_{52} + F_{54} + F_{56} - F_{05}^{(m)} - F_{05}^{(o)} - F_{05}^{(s)} - F_{65} - F_{85} \tag{12.60}$$

$$\frac{dQ_6}{dt} = F_{65} - F_{06} - F_{56} \tag{12.61}$$

$$\frac{dQ_7}{dt} = F_{71} + F_{74} - F_{07} \tag{12.62}$$

$$\frac{dQ_8}{dt} = F_{82} + F_{85} - F_{08} \tag{12.63}$$

and for [^{13}C]-labelled PHE and TYR:

$$\frac{dq_1}{dt} = I_1 - e_1(F_{41} + F_{71}) \tag{12.64}$$

$$\frac{dq_2}{dt} = I_2 - e_2(F_{52} + F_{82}) \tag{12.65}$$

$$\frac{dq_3}{dt} = e_4F_{34} - e_3(F_{03} + F_{43}) \tag{12.66}$$

$$\frac{dq_4}{dt} = e_1F_{41} + e_3F_{43} - e_4(F_{04}^{(m)} + F_{04}^{(s)} + F_{34} + F_{54} + F_{74}) \tag{12.67}$$

$$\frac{dq_5}{dt} = e_2F_{52} + e_4F_{54} + e_6F_{56} - e_5(F_{05}^{(m)} + F_{05}^{(o)} + F_{05}^{(s)} + F_{65} + F_{85}) \tag{12.68}$$

$$\frac{dq_6}{dt} = e_5F_{65} - e_6(F_{06} + F_{56}) \tag{12.69}$$

$$\frac{dq_7}{dt} = e_1F_{71} + e_4F_{74} - e_7F_{07} \tag{12.70}$$

$$\frac{dq_8}{dt} = e_2F_{82} + e_5F_{85} - e_8F_{08} \tag{12.71}$$

and for [^{2}H]-labelled TYR:

$$\frac{d\phi_2}{dt} = \Phi_2 - \varepsilon_2(F_{52} + F_{82}) \tag{12.72}$$

$$\frac{d\phi_5}{dt} = \varepsilon_2F_{52} + \varepsilon_6F_{56} - \varepsilon_5(F_{05}^{(m)} + F_{05}^{(o)} + F_{05}^{(s)} + F_{65} + F_{85}) \tag{12.73}$$

$$\frac{d\phi_6}{dt} = \varepsilon_5F_{65} - \varepsilon_6(F_{06} + F_{56}) \tag{12.74}$$

$$\frac{d\phi_8}{dt} = \varepsilon_2F_{82} + \varepsilon_5F_{85} - \varepsilon_8F_{08}. \tag{12.75}$$

When the system is in steady state with respect to both total and labelled PHE and TYR, the derivative terms in Eqns 12.56–12.75 are zero. For the scheme assumed, the enrichment of intracellular milk protein-bound pools equalizes with that of the respective free pool in steady state (i.e. $e_3 = e_4$, $e_6 = e_5$, $\varepsilon_6 = \varepsilon_5$), otherwise Eqns 12.58 and 12.66, and 12.61, 12.69 and 12.74 are inconsistent. After equating intracellular enrichments and eliminating redundant equations, etc., Eqns 12.64–12.75 yield the following useful identities:

$$I_1 - e_1(F_{41} + F_{71}) = 0 \tag{12.76}$$

$$e_1F_{41} - e_3(F_{04}^{(m)} + F_{04}^{(s)} + F_{34} + F_{54} + F_{74} - F_{43}) = 0 \tag{12.77}$$

$$e_2F_{52} + e_3F_{54} - e_6(F_{05}^{(m)} + F_{05}^{(o)} + F_{05}^{(s)} + F_{65} + F_{85} - F_{56}) = 0 \tag{12.78}$$

$$e_1F_{71} + e_3F_{74} - e_7F_{07} = 0 \tag{12.79}$$

$$\Phi_2 - \varepsilon_2(F_{52} + F_{82}) = 0 \tag{12.80}$$

$$\varepsilon_2F_{52} - \varepsilon_6(F_{05}^{(m)} + F_{05}^{(o)} + F_{05}^{(s)} + F_{65} + F_{85} - F_{56}) = 0 \tag{12.81}$$

$$\varepsilon_2F_{82} + \varepsilon_6F_{85} - \varepsilon_8F_{08} = 0. \tag{12.82}$$

To obtain steady-state solutions to the model, it is assumed that free PHE and TYR secreted in milk, PHE and TYR secreted in milk protein, CO_2 production and PHE and TYR removal from the venous pools (i.e. $F_{04}^{(m)}$, $F_{05}^{(m)}$, F_{03}, F_{06}, $F_{05}^{(o)}$, F_{07} and F_{08}, respectively) can all be measured experimentally. Algebraic manipulation of Eqns 12.56–12.63 with the derivatives set to zero, together with Eqns 12.76–12.82, gives:

$$F_{10} = I_1 / e_1 \tag{12.83}$$

$$F_{20} = \Phi_2 / \varepsilon_2 \tag{12.84}$$

$$\overline{F_{34} - F_{43}} = F_{03} \tag{12.85}$$

$$\overline{F_{65} - F_{56}} = F_{06} \tag{12.86}$$

$$F_{71} = \left(\frac{e_7 - e_3}{e_1 - e_3}\right)F_{07};\ e_1 \neq e_3 \tag{12.87}$$

$$F_{41} = F_{10} - F_{71} \tag{12.88}$$

$$F_{74} = F_{07} - F_{71} \tag{12.89}$$

$$F_{82} = \left(\frac{\varepsilon_8 - \varepsilon_6}{\varepsilon_2 - \varepsilon_6}\right)F_{08};\ \varepsilon_2 \neq \varepsilon_6 \tag{12.90}$$

$$F_{52} = F_{20} - F_{82} \tag{12.91}$$

$$F_{85} = F_{08} - F_{82} \tag{12.92}$$

$$F_{05}^{(s)} = \left(\frac{\varepsilon_2}{\varepsilon_6}\right)F_{52} - F_{05}^{(m)} - F_{05}^{(o)} - \overline{F_{65} - F_{56}} - F_{85} \tag{12.93}$$

$$F_{54} = \left(\frac{e_6\varepsilon_2 - e_2\varepsilon_6}{e_3\varepsilon_6}\right)F_{52} \tag{12.94}$$

$$F_{04}^{(s)} = \left(\frac{e_1}{e_3}\right)F_{41} - F_{04}^{(m)} - \overline{F_{34} - F_{43}} - F_{54} - F_{74} \tag{12.95}$$

$$F_{40} = F_{04}^{(m)} + F_{04}^{(s)} + \overline{F_{34} - F_{43}} + F_{54} + F_{74} - F_{41} \tag{12.96}$$

$$F_{50} = F_{05}^{(m)} + F_{05}^{(o)} + F_{05}^{(s)} + \overline{F_{65} - F_{56}} + F_{85} - F_{52} - F_{54}, \tag{12.97}$$

where, for these equations, the italics denote steady-state values of flows and enrichments and the over-lining indicates coupled flows (which cannot be separately estimated).

Table 12.6. Phenylalanine and tyrosine uptake and partition by the mammary gland for four lactating dairy cows obtained using the eight-pool model (symbols are defined in the text and Table 12.1).

		Cow number			
		A	B	C	D
Flow (μmol min⁻¹)	F_{10}	202	238	250	241
	F_{20}	184	182	269	240
	$\overline{F_{34} - F_{43}}$	69.4	89.2	98.6	86.1
	$\overline{F_{65} - F_{56}}$	71.2	91.3	101	88.2
	F_{71}	127	137	142	153
	F_{41}	74.8	102	108	87.9
	F_{74}	8.9	24.0	4.7	22.0
	F_{82}	101	91.2	142	158
	F_{52}	83.3	90.6	126	81.9
	F_{85}	21.3	16.3	17.2	26.5
	$F_{05}^{(s)}$	50.8	59.9	116	40.1
	F_{54}	5.5	5.9	10.5	5.8
	$F_{04}^{(s)}$	25.2	40.1	61.1	40.3
	F_{40}	34.2	57.8	67.1	66.3
	F_{50}	54.6	70.9	97.2	67.1

Example solutions to the model, to illustrate the magnitude of the calculated flows, are given in Table 12.6 for four Holstein-Friesian dairy cows in mid-lactation (average live weight 634 kg, average milk yield 23.3 kg day^{-1}). The cows were fed two levels of dietary CP hourly. The diet consisted of chopped lucerne hay (12.8% CP) and concentrate (10.8% or 20.6% CP) in a 50:50 ratio on a DM basis. Their daily intake was 20.2 kg DM.

The model can also be solved by decomposing it into two four-pool schemes (i.e. a PHE submodel and a TYR submodel), then linking the two schemes. The PHE and TYR submodels are both very similar structurally to the model of LEU kinetics (cf. Figs 12.6, 12.7 and 12.4).

PHE submodel

The schemes adopted for the movement of total and labelled PHE in the PHE submodel are shown in Fig. 12.6a and b, respectively.

$$\frac{dQ_1}{dt} = F_{10} - F_{41} - F_{71} \tag{12.56}$$

$$\frac{dQ_3}{dt} = F_{34} - F_{03} - F_{43} \tag{12.58}$$

$$\frac{dQ_4}{dt} = F_{40} + F_{41} + F_{43} - F_{04}^{(m)} - F_{04}^{(s)} - F_{34} - F_{54} - F_{74} \tag{12.59}$$

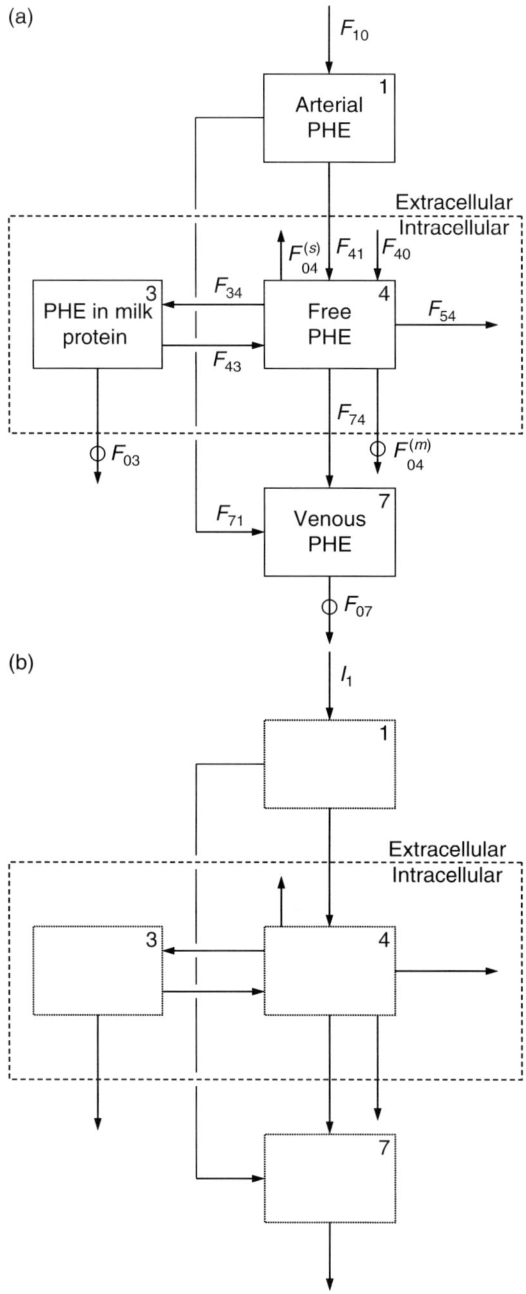

Fig. 12.6. Scheme for the uptake and utilization of PHE by the mammary gland of lactating dairy cows: (a) total PHE, (b) labelled PHE. The small circles in Fig. 12.6a indicate flows out of the system that need to be measured experimentally.

$$\frac{dQ_7}{dt} = F_{71} + F_{74} - F_{07} \tag{12.62}$$

and for ^{13}C-labelled PHE:

$$\frac{dq_1}{dt} = I_1 - e_1(F_{41} + F_{71}) \tag{12.64}$$

$$\frac{dq_3}{dt} = e_4F_{34} - e_3(F_{03} + F_{43}) \tag{12.66}$$

$$\frac{dq_4}{dt} = e_1F_{41} + e_3F_{43} - e_4(F_{04}^{(m)} + F_{04}^{(s)} + F_{34} + F_{54} + F_{74}) \tag{12.67}$$

$$\frac{dq_7}{dt} = e_1F_{71} + e_4F_{74} - e_7F_{07}. \tag{12.70}$$

When the system is in steady state with respect to both total and labelled PHE, the derivative terms in these eight differential equations are zero. For the scheme assumed, the enrichment of the intracellular milk protein-bound pool equalizes with that of the free pool in steady state (i.e. $e_3 = e_4$). After equating intracellular enrichments and eliminating redundant equations, the four differential equations for labelled PHE yield the following three identities:

$$I_1 - e_1(F_{41} + F_{71}) = 0 \tag{12.76}$$

$$e_1F_{41} - e_3(F_{04}^{(m)} + F_{04}^{(s)} + F_{34} + F_{54} + F_{74} - F_{43}) = 0 \tag{12.77}$$

$$e_1F_{71} + e_3F_{74} - e_7F_{07} = 0. \tag{12.79}$$

To obtain steady-state solutions to the model, it is assumed that free PHE in milk, PHE secreted in milk protein and PHE removal from the venous pool (i.e. $F_{04}^{(m)}, F_{03}$ and F_{07}, respectively) can be measured experimentally. Algebraic manipulation of Eqns 12.56, 12.58, 12.59 and 12.62 with the derivatives set to zero, together with Eqns 12.76, 12.77 and 12.79, gives:

$$F_{10} = I_1/e_1 \tag{12.83}$$

$$\overline{F_{34} - F_{43}} = F_{03} \tag{12.85}$$

$$F_{71} = \left(\frac{e_7 - e_3}{e_1 - e_3}\right)F_{07};\ e_1 \neq e_3 \tag{12.87}$$

$$F_{41} = F_{10} - F_{71} \tag{12.88}$$

$$F_{74} = F_{07} - F_{71} \tag{12.89}$$

$$F_{40} = \left(\frac{e_1 - e_3}{e_3}\right)F_{41} \tag{12.98}$$

$$\overline{F_{04}^{(s)} + F_{54}} = F_{40} + F_{41} - F_{04}^{(m)} - \overline{F_{34} - F_{43}} - F_{74}, \tag{12.99}$$

where the italics denote steady-state values of flows and enrichments for these equations and the over-lining indicates coupled flows (which cannot be separately estimated).

TYR submodel

The schemes adopted for the movement of total and labelled TYR in the TYR submodel are shown in Fig. 12.7a and b, respectively.

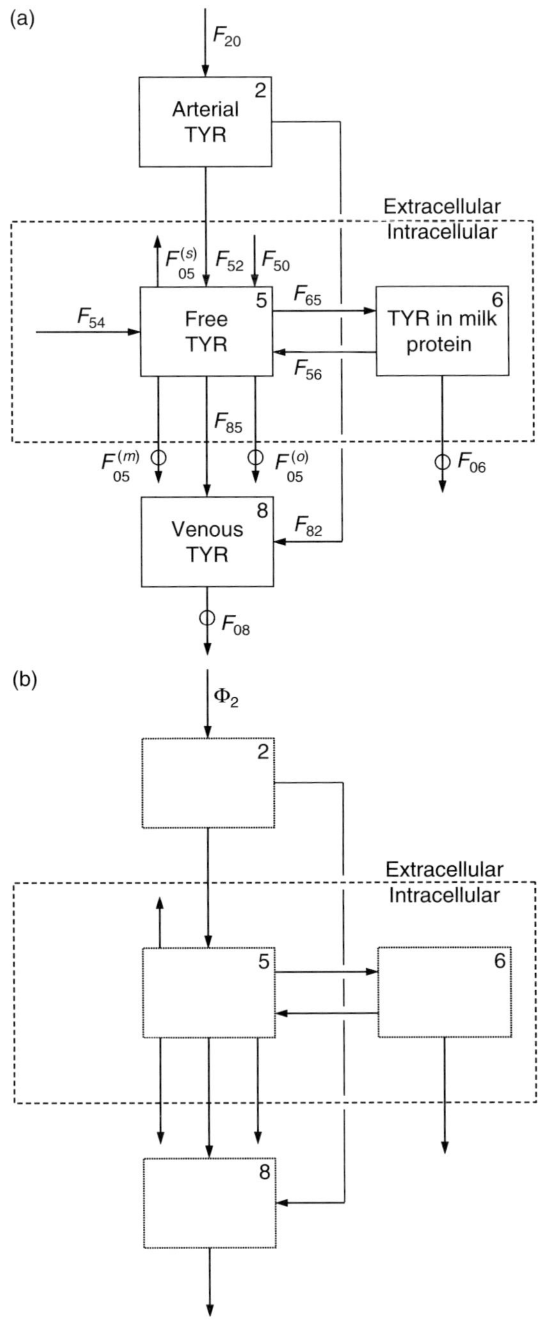

Fig. 12.7. Scheme for the uptake and utilization of TYR by the mammary gland of lactating dairy cows: (a) total TYR, (b) labelled TYR. The small circles in Fig. 12.7a indicate flows out of the system that need to be measured experimentally.

$$\frac{\mathrm{d}Q_2}{\mathrm{d}t} = F_{20} - F_{52} - F_{82} \tag{12.57}$$

$$\frac{\mathrm{d}Q_5}{\mathrm{d}t} = F_{50} + F_{52} + F_{54} + F_{56} - F_{05}^{(m)} - F_{05}^{(o)} - F_{05}^{(s)} - F_{65} - F_{85} \tag{12.60}$$

$$\frac{dQ_6}{dt} = F_{65} - F_{06} - F_{56} \tag{12.61}$$

$$\frac{dQ_8}{dt} = F_{82} + F_{85} - F_{08} \tag{12.63}$$

and for ^2H-labelled TYR:

$$\frac{d\phi_2}{dt} = \Phi_2 - \varepsilon_2 (F_{52} + F_{82}) \tag{12.72}$$

$$\frac{d\phi_5}{dt} = \varepsilon_2 F_{52} + \varepsilon_6 F_{52} - \varepsilon_5 (F_{05}^{(m)} + F_{05}^{(o)} + F_{05}^{(s)} + F_{65} + F_{85}) \tag{12.73}$$

$$\frac{d\phi_6}{dt} = \varepsilon_5 F_{65} - \varepsilon_6 (F_{06} + F_{56}) \tag{12.74}$$

$$\frac{d\phi_8}{dt} = \varepsilon_2 F_{82} + \varepsilon_5 F_{85} - \varepsilon_8 F_{08}. \tag{12.75}$$

When the system is in steady state with respect to both total and labelled TYR, the derivative terms in these eight differential equations are zero. For the scheme assumed, the enrichment of the intracellular milk protein-bound pool equalizes with that of the free pool in steady state (i.e. $\varepsilon_6 = \varepsilon_5$). After equating intracellular enrichments and eliminating redundant equations, the four differential equations for labelled TYR yield the following three identities:

$$\Phi_2 - \varepsilon_2 (F_{52} + F_{82}) = 0 \tag{12.80}$$

$$\varepsilon_2 F_{52} - \varepsilon_6 (F_{05}^{(m)} + F_{05}^{(o)} + F_{05}^{(s)} + F_{65} + F_{85} - F_{56}) = 0 \tag{12.81}$$

$$\varepsilon_2 F_{82} + \varepsilon_6 F_{85} - \varepsilon_8 F_{08} = 0. \tag{12.82}$$

To obtain steady-state solutions to the model, it is assumed that free TYR in milk, TYR secreted in milk protein and TYR removal from the venous pool (i.e. $F_{05}^{(m)}$, F_{06} and F_{08}, respectively) can be measured experimentally. Algebraic manipulation of Eqns 12.57, 12.60, 12.61 and 12.63 with the derivatives set to zero, together with Eqns 12.80–12.82, gives:

$$F_{20} = \Phi_2 / \varepsilon_2 \tag{12.84}$$

$$\overline{F_{65} - F_{56}} = F_{06} \tag{12.86}$$

$$F_{82} = \left(\frac{\varepsilon_2 - \varepsilon_6}{\varepsilon_2 - \varepsilon_6} \right) F_{08};\ \varepsilon_2 \neq \varepsilon_6 \tag{12.90}$$

$$F_{52} = F_{20} - F_{82} \tag{12.91}$$

$$F_{85} = F_{08} - F_{82} \tag{12.92}$$

$$\overline{F_{50} + F_{54}} = \left(\frac{\varepsilon_2 - \varepsilon_6}{\varepsilon_6} \right) F_{52} \tag{12.100}$$

$$\overline{F_{05}^{(o)} + F_{05}^{(s)}} = \overline{F_{50} + F_{54}} + F_{52} - F_{05}^{(m)} - \overline{F_{65} - F_{56}} - F_{85}, \tag{12.101}$$

where the italics denote steady-state values of flows and enrichments for these equations and the over-lining indicates coupled flows (which cannot be separately estimated).

Linking the PHE and TYR submodels

The two submodels can be linked by considering constitutive mammary protein. Assuming a fixed protein composition for this tissue, then the ratio of TYR to PHE in constitutive tissue, $R_{TYR:PHE}$ (μmol TYR/μmol PHE), is constant. This assumption allows Eqns 12.99–12.101 to be uncoupled:

$$F_{50} = R_{TYR:PHE} F_{40} \tag{12.102}$$

$$F_{54} = \overline{F_{54} + F_{50}} - F_{50} \tag{12.103}$$

$$F_{04}^{(s)} = \overline{F_{04}^{(s)} + F_{54}} - F_{54} \tag{12.104}$$

$$F_{05}^{(s)} = R_{TYR:PHE} F_{04}^{(s)} \tag{12.105}$$

$$F_{05}^{(o)} = \overline{F_{05}^{(o)} + F_{05}^{(s)}} - F_{05}^{(s)}. \tag{12.106}$$

Example solutions to the linked two four-pool models, to illustrate the magnitude of the calculated flows, are given in Table 12.7 for the same four animals used to illustrate the eight-pool model (Table 12.6). The results demonstrate that the two linked four-pool models give similar values for the flows of PHE and TYR when compared with the values calculated from the eight-pool model.

Discussion

Compartmental models

Compartmental analysis has been widely applied in the biological sciences for many years (Godfrey, 1983; Thornley and France, 2007), permitting more mechanistic interpretation of experimental data. In animal science, it has proved useful in kinetic investigations based on the use of tracers in studying glucose metabolism (Kronfeld *et al*., 1971; Shipley and Clark, 1972) and volatile fatty acid production (Leng and Brett, 1966; France and Dijkstra, 2005). Since 1980, tracer methods have gained increasing popularity in estimating protein turnover (i.e. synthesis and degradation) at the tissue and whole-animal levels, initially using radioactive tracers (Lobley *et al*., 1980; Reeds *et al*., 1987) and, more recently, stable isotopes (Bequette *et al*., 2002; Hoskin *et al*., 2003). This follows the pioneering work of Waterlow and co-workers (Waterlow *et al*., 1978; Waterlow, 2006) on turnover in laboratory animals.

Compartmental systems consist of a finite number of well-mixed, lumped subsystems called compartments or pools, which exchange with each other and with the environment so that the quantity or concentration of material within each pool can be described by a first-order differential equation. A

Table 12.7. Phenylalanine and tyrosine uptake and partition by the mammary gland for four lactating dairy cows obtained using the two four-pool models (symbols are defined in the text and Table 12.1).

		Cow number			
		A	B	C	D
Flow (μmol min^{-1})					
PHE submodel	F_{10}	202	238	250	241
	$\overline{F_{34} - F_{43}}$	69.4	89.2	98.6	86.1
	F_{71}	127	137	142	153
	F_{41}	74.8	102	108	87.9
	F_{74}	8.9	24.0	4.7	22.0
	F_{40}	34.2	57.8	67.1	66.3
	$\overline{F_{04}^{(s)} + F_{54}}$	30.7	46.0	71.6	46.1
TYR submodel	F_{20}	184	182	269	240
	$\overline{F_{65} - F_{56}}$	71.2	91.3	101	88.2
	F_{82}	101	91.2	142	158
	F_{52}	83.3	90.6	126	81.9
	F_{85}	21.3	16.3	17.2	26.5
	$\overline{F_{50} + F_{54}}$	60.0	76.9	108	72.9
	$\overline{F_{05}^{(o)} + F_{05}^{(s)}}$	50.8	59.9	116	40.1
Linking submodels	$R_{TYR:PHE}$	1.5	1.5	1.5	1.5
	F_{50}	51.4	86.6	101	99.4
	F_{54}	8.7	*	7.0	*
	$F_{04}^{(s)}$	22.0	55.8	64.6	72.6
	$F_{05}^{(s)}$	33.0	83.7	96.9	109
	$F_{05}^{(o)}$	17.8	*	18.6	*

*Non-physiological (negative) value obtained.

compartmental system may be used to model either the kinetics of one substance or the kinetics of two or more substances. In the former case, the pools occupy different spaces and the interpool transfers represent flow of material from one location to another. In the latter case, different pools can occupy the same space and some of the interpool transfers represent transformation from one substance to another (Godfrey, 1983).

In compartmental modelling, there are no hard and fast rules as to how many compartments to represent, though importance and accessibility are key considerations. A compartment refers to a collection of material that is separable, anatomically or functionally from other compartments. The term 'pool' refers to the contents of a compartment and implies that the contents are homogeneous. In studies of whole-body protein turnover, we refer to the pools of free and protein-bound amino acids, but this is an oversimplification of the real situation (see Waterlow, 2006). The animal body may be viewed as an assortment of pools or compartments, each made up of identical molecules, which tend, more or less, to be enclosed by anatomical boundaries. Body pools tend to remain constant in size while undergoing replacement by equal input and output flows. This dynamic equilibrium is known as steady state. The constancy applies to all rates, rate constants and the amount of unlabelled material in all pools and regions. If any of these change during the period of observation, the condition is non-steady state.

In a kinetic study, tracers are employed, permitting a further set of first-order differential equations for each tracer. The term 'isotopic steady state' is used to refer to the tracer when, for example, it reaches equilibrium either in a closed system or during a constant infusion in an open system, i.e. the rate of entry of tracer into the sampled compartment is equal to the rate at which it leaves. If the unlabelled material is in steady state, but the tracer has yet to reach equilibrium, the condition is termed non-isotopic steady state. All the biological systems described in this chapter are assumed to be in steady state with respect to both unlabelled and labelled material, with the exception of the precursor–product model, where steady-state assumptions are limited to the precursor pool.

In addition to measuring rates of chemical transfer or physical transport such as blood flow, compartmental analysis is also concerned with measuring pool size, i.e. the mass or volume of natural material which constitutes the pool. An important concept is that of fractional loss from the pool. The fraction of tracer lost per unit time is known as the fractional rate constant, or rate constant in linear systems.

A tracer has the same properties of interest as the natural counterpart (the tracee), but it presents a characteristic that enables its detection in the system where the tracee is also present. The production of an isotopic tracer involves the substitution of one or more naturally occurring atoms in specific positions in the tracee molecule with an isotope of that atom with a less common abundance. Isotopic elements have the same number of protons (same atomic number), but different numbers of neutrons (different atomic mass) from the naturally abundant element. Some isotopes are radioactive, where the neutrons decay to produce an electron and a proton, whereas other isotopes are stable. Tracers are assumed to behave chemically and physiologically exactly like the tracee, save for the slight differences in mass. When using radioactive tracers, the dose administered is normally very small in comparison to the number of existing natural atoms, the added tracer material does not perturb the system under observation; however, this is not true for stable isotope tracers (see below). Tracers have several potential uses in the intact whole animal. One of these is to study pathways of chemical conversion by identifying tracer in the product after introduction into the precursor. If the pathway is already known, then the tracer serves to assess the rate of conversion.

Using radioactive isotopes as tracers involves a health risk to the subjects and investigators which must be calculated and compared to the acceptable dosage from commonly encountered routes of exposure. Determination of beta radioactivity in the sample is done by scintillation counting. This technique allows simultaneous counting of ^{3}H and ^{14}C isotopes. Account must be taken of quenching when converting counts per second measured to actual nuclear disintegrations per second (becquerels).

Stable isotopes have now become the tracer of choice for metabolic studies in humans and animals as there are no known physiological risks associated with tracer doses. They have the advantage that several similarly labelled tracers can be given simultaneously and it is increasingly possible to determine the enrichment in specific positions of the tracer molecule. The major disadvantage of stable isotopes is that they are not strictly tracers, as they have to be administered in non-tracer amounts to achieve analytical precision, which, in turn, may affect the endogenous kinetics of the tracee.

Administration of isotope

An isotopic tracer can be delivered to a compartmental pool system over an extended period by continuous infusion at a constant rate or delivered as a single, abruptly administered dose.

When using the continuous infusion technique, an intravenous infusion of tracer is started and continued at a constant rate for 6–8 h into animals maintained in a metabolic steady state. Beyond 8 h, recycling of tracer from rapidly turning over proteins may become a problem. Under these conditions, the isotopic activity of the tracer in the extracellular and intracellular pools rises to a plateau by a curve (see Fig. 12.8), which can be approximately described by a monomolecular equation:

$$s = s_{max}[1 - \exp(-kt)],$$

where s is the activity of the tracer, s_{max} is the activity of tracer at plateau, k is a rate constant and t is the time since commencement of the infusion. The plateau is really a pseudoplateau at which, for practical purposes, the rate of entry of tracer into the sampled compartment is equal to the rate at which it leaves, which for radioactive isotopes is a product of the tracee flow and its activity or total flow (tracee + tracer) and its enrichment for stable isotopes. At the end of the infusion, the activity of the intracellular free pool is measured directly in tissue samples (e.g. three-pool model) or estimated from the activity of the most

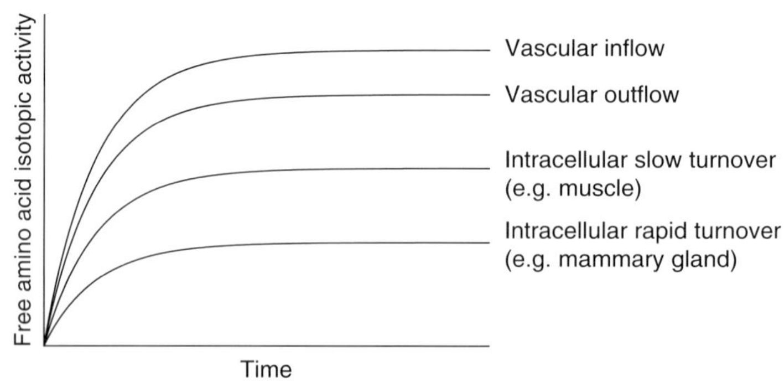

Fig. 12.8. Schematic representation of free amino acid isotopic activity in various pools during a continuous infusion of tracer at a constant rate.

appropriate accessible pool (e.g. milk in the four- and eight-pool models). Over the period of infusion, the area under the curve for isotopic activity needs to be estimated (see Fig. 12.8). For the extracellular pool, this is usually done empirically, while, for tissues, either a rate constant is assumed or calculated iteratively based on transfer rates into protein (see Waterlow, 2006). The large differences between isotopic activities in the extracellular and intracellular pools (see Fig. 12.8) are due to dilution of the intracellular free pool by non-labelled amino acids released during protein degradation (see Waterlow *et al.*, 1978; Waterlow, 2006). This is especially true for tissues with a high rate of protein turnover, such as the mammary gland, liver and gastrointestinal tract.

When using a continuous infusion of tracer amino acid, the choice of which precursor pool best represents the isotopic activity of the true precursor, from which aminoacyl-transfer-RNA(s) (tRNA) are charged, has to be made based on the tissue type being studied and the biological pools that are readily accessible for sampling. Surrogate precursor pools include the extracellular free pools (blood/plasma; vascular inflow or outflow), the intracellular free pool (usually estimated from the homogenate pool), or the extracellular transamination product (α-ketoisocaproate) pool, during tracer LEU infusions (Matthews *et al.*, 1982). Since isotopic activity or area under the curve of the assumed precursor pool is commonly the divisor in protein synthesis calculations, the lowest rates of synthesis will be based on the precursor pool with the highest activity, i.e. the extracellular pool. Conversely, the highest rates of synthesis will be based on the precursor pool with the lowest tracer activity, i.e. the intracellular pool. In muscle, for example, the ratio of tracer activity in the intracellular:extracellular pools was 0.5 and, consequently, synthetic rates calculated using the extracellular pool isotopic activity were 50% lower than those calculated using the intracellular activity (Crompton and Lomax, 1993).

To date, we have only discussed measuring kinetics using a continuous infusion of tracer at a constant rate. This is the popular approach because sampling can be minimized if the tracer is infused until isotopic steady state is achieved. Therefore, a few samples at the isotopic plateau are sufficient to calculate the rate of exit from a pool. However, if there are circumstances which preclude the use of a continuous infusion, then the entry rate can be calculated using a bolus injection of tracer.

In an ideal single pool, a single injection of tracer will result in an initial increase in the tracer:tracee ratio, which is assumed to be instantaneous, and then the ratio will decline over time in a curve that might be described by a single exponential equation. The SRA of tracer in the pool at any given time is:

$$s = s_0[\exp(-kt)],$$

where s is the isotopic activity of the tracer, s_0 is the activity of tracer at zero time, k is the rate constant for elimination and t is the time since isotope administration. Conventional curve-fitting programmes are often used to determine s_0 and k, given the input data of tracer isotopic activity versus time.

The problems associated with accurately determining isotopic activity in the true precursor pool can be minimized by using the large or flooding dose technique. With this method, the labelled amino acid is injected with a large or flooding dose of the unlabelled amino acid, (5–50 times the total body free amino acid content), with the aim of flooding all amino acid pools (extracellular, intracellular and aminoacyl-tRNA) to the same isotopic activity. The activity of the intracellular pool depends on the relative inflows of labelled amino acid from the extracellular pool and unlabelled amino acids from protein degradation. It is assumed that the flooding dose increases the entry from the extracellular pool to a point where the relative contribution from protein degradation becomes negligible. The large dose procedure results in rapid equilibration across all body pools and isotopic activity is equalized within a short period of time (min to 1.5 h); therefore, the precursor problem is overcome. Although the large dose method eliminates the major concern about isotopic activity in the precursor pool, in doing so it introduces other potential disadvantages. Besides the short study period, the injection of such a large amount of unlabelled amino acid greatly increases pool size of the unlabelled amino acid, which may cause alterations in intracellular transport and metabolism (Rocha *et al.*, 1993) and changes in hormonal secretions (e.g. insulin; see Lobley *et al.*, 1990). The flooding dose method is not suitable for amino acid oxidation studies and is expensive and, consequently, there are few measurements on large animals. The procedure has been thought more suited for measuring protein synthesis in tissues with a high fractional synthetic rate or rapidly turning over export proteins. However, recent evidence has demonstrated that the flooding dose method does not alter the rate of muscle protein synthesis in the post-absorptive state or the response to feeding, when compared with the continuous infusion method (Caso *et al.*, 2006). The mathematical ramifications of flood dosing with regard to application of the precursor–product model are considered in France *et al.* (1988).

Precursor pool

The major problem involved in using tracer amino acid kinetics to measure protein synthesis, whether in the whole body or in individual tissues, arises from a failure to measure directly the isotopic activity of the tracer amino acid in the charged aminoacyl-tRNA, the actual precursor pool for protein synthesis. Direct measurement of tracer activity in the aminoacyl-tRNA pool requires a sample of tissue and is technically difficult due to the extremely labile nature of aminoacyl-tRNA species (0.3–3 s for rodent valyl-tRNA; Smith and Sun, 1995). Furthermore, the values obtained represent only a mean value for the tissue and do not distinguish between different aminoacyl-tRNA pools which may support constitutive and export protein synthesis. Consequently, the isotopic activity of the aminoacyl-tRNA pool is usually estimated from the activity of more readily accessible pools, such as the extracellular free pool (blood/plasma) or the intracellular free pool within the tissue (tissue homogenate). The use of these surrogate pools to estimate the true precursor labelling is based on the assumption that the experimental treatment does not alter the relationship between labelling in the sampled pool and that of the aminoacyl-tRNA (Caso *et al.*, 2002).

Early studies measuring the activity of the aminoacyl-tRNA pool directly suggested compartmentation of amino acids for protein synthesis within the transport system of the cell membrane (Airhart *et al.*, 1974), i.e. there was preferential acylation of amino acids transported into cells, by plasma membrane bound aminoacyl-tRNA synthetases. In a further study, the same group (Vidrich *et al.*, 1977) were able to demonstrate that the activity of the aminoacyl-tRNA pool was proportional to the concentration gradient across the cell membrane. Fern and Garlick (1976) extended the concept of compartmentation from different sites for synthesis and oxidation to different sites of synthesis of individual proteins. There is limited evidence which suggests that proteins destined for export are probably synthesized on the rough endoplasmic reticulum and preferentially utilize amino acids as they enter the cell (Fern and Garlick, 1976; Connell *et al.*, 1997). Such cellular compartmentalization is achieved, at least in part, by the selectivity conferred by the 3′ untranslated region of mRNAs (Hesketh, 1994). As the endoplasmic reticulum is associated with extracellular components of the cell, the isotopic activity of free amino acids in this part of the cell will be closer to that of blood. Data in ruminants have supported this theory, demonstrating that the enrichment of hepatic apolipoprotein B-100 is most closely represented by the enrichment in the hepatic vein plasma pool (Connell *et al.*, 1997). In contrast, constitutive proteins are synthesized on polysomes within the cell cytosol and the precursor pool would include intracellular free amino acids, or perhaps preferential use of amino acids released from protein degradation (e.g. Smith and Sun, 1995).

To date, all published studies that have attempted to measure isotopic activity directly in the aminoacyl-tRNA pool have shown that the activity of the aminoacyl-tRNA pool lies between that of the tracer activity in the extracellular and intracellular pools (see Waterlow, 2006). Rather than discrete intracellular compartments, it is now thought that, as amino acids penetrate through the cytoplasmic gel, they create a gradient or series of gradients in isotopic activity of the tracer amino acid, with labelling of the tracer highest at points near the cell surface and lowest at points near the sites of degradation (Waterlow, 2006). The rates at which the amino acid moves through the cell will control the size of the gradient. Therefore, the isotopic activity of the aminoacyl-tRNA species will depend on the cellular location of the synthetic machinery, relative to this series of cytoplasmic gradients. The concept of cellular gradients and intracellular organization for tracer amino acid activity may need to be incorporated in the future into compartmental models of protein turnover.

Due to the uncertainty regarding the activity of the precursor pool, protein synthetic rates are generally given as a range of values with upper and lower estimates based on the isotopic activity in the various surrogate precursor pools that are sampled. More detailed and extensive consideration of the problems associated with using tracer amino acids to measure mammalian protein metabolism can be found in two comprehensive texts by Waterlow (Waterlow *et al.*, 1978; Waterlow, 2006).

Arteriovenous difference models

The final three models described in this chapter all use a combination of traditional AV difference techniques coupled with kinetic isotope transfers and compartmental modelling to measure amino acid exchange and estimate the rates of protein accretion, synthesis and degradation across the hindlimb and mammary gland in ruminants. In addition, amino acid oxidation can also be determined with the appropriate tracer. The AV difference models have two major assumptions which need to be considered when interpreting the data. The first assumption, as with all isotope tracer techniques, relates to the choice of pool to sample as being representative of tracer activity in the true precursor pool for protein synthesis. It is assumed that all kinetic inflows and efflows pass through this common precursor pool. Surrogate precursor activity can be measured directly in the intracellular (homogenate) free pool from tissue biopsy, but is more commonly estimated from tracer activity in the vascular inflow, vascular outflow or export protein pools.

The AV kinetic models described in this chapter assume the activity of the intracellular free pool is the best indicator of precursor pool activity, with the exception of the two-pool model, which uses the extracellular pool. Even for closely allied tissues, use of a common precursor pool may be inappropriate (Lobley *et al.*, 1992). Some evidence has suggested that, for ovine muscle, the precursor may be well represented by the intracellular amino acid free pool for LEU and PHE, but that the extracellular free pool (blood/plasma) may be the better choice for other tissues, such as skin (Lobley *et al.*, 1992). This further complicates the choice of precursor pool, since the vascular drainage from the hindlimb and mammary gland will include a contribution from other tissues. For AV preparations containing mixed tissue types, the correct approach would be to measure blood flow and metabolic activity for each tissue (Biolo *et al.*, 1994) and then apply a weighted average for the entire tissue bed. In practice, a measure of intracellular isotopic activity from the most abundant tissue type is usually assumed to reflect the mean for the composite tissues (e.g. Crompton and Lomax, 1993; Hoskin *et al.*, 2003). Often, the extracellular pool is the only reasonably accessible pool and, in comparative experiments, the assumption is made that the relationship between isotopic activities of the amino acid in the extracellular and various aminoacyl-tRNA pools is unchanged (Lobley, 1993a). The use of a chosen precursor often does not alter the qualitative nature of the information, but can affect its absolute magnitude.

The second assumption associated with AV difference models relates to the heterogeneity of the tissue bed being sampled. This is a particular problem for the hindlimb model. When using the hindlimb preparation, careful placement of the venous sampling catheter tip in the deep femoral vein should ensure that muscle tissue makes by far the largest contribution (approximately 90%) to the blood sampled, with only a 10% contribution from non-muscular sources (i.e. subcutaneous and intramuscular adipose tissue, skin, cartilage and bone) (Domanski *et al.*, 1974; Oddy *et al.*, 1981; Teleni and Annison, 1986; Crompton, 1990). However, in adult sheep the relative contributions of muscle, bone, skin and adipose tissue to the blood sampled in the deep femoral vein have been estimated at 61, 22, 12 and 5%, respectively (Oddy *et al.*, 1984). The protein metabolic activity of skin and bone is considerably higher than that for muscle (e.g. Seve *et al.*, 1986; Abdul-Razzaq and Bickerstaffe, 1989; Lobley *et al.*, 1992; Ponter *et al.*, 1994; Liu *et al.*, 1998), and drainage from these tissues will increase hindlimb protein synthesis above that for muscle. Assuming a minimum contribution from non-muscular tissues of 10%, protein synthetic rates of 3% day^{-1} in muscle and 15% day^{-1} in skin and bone would result in a value for hindlimb protein synthesis of 4.2% day^{-1}. Therefore, the theoretical contribution from non-muscular tissues to the values for hindlimb protein synthesis will be a minimum of approximately 36%. The data obtained using the three-pool model, when compared with values for muscle protein synthesis from tissue analysis, has shown that the actual contribution from non-muscular tissues is 49%. The problems of tissue heterogeneity are less pronounced in the mammary gland due to the high rate of synthesis in mammary tissue (Oddy *et al.*, 1988; Baracos *et al.*, 1991; France *et al.*, 1995).

Although AV procedures require extensive surgery and are technically demanding, once established, the preparations allow repeated simultaneous measurements to be made on the same animal, with the opportunity to reduce between-animal variation. The AV kinetic models have been able to provide valuable information on the nutritional and hormonal control of protein metabolism in ruminants and humans (see Lobley, 1998, 2003; Waterlow, 2006).

The ability to predict accurately dietary nitrogen utilization for production in the ruminant depends on a clear understanding of amino acid flows from the gut to productive tissues, i.e. it depends on an accurate description of the regulation of intestinal amino acid supply, absorption of these products from the gut, metabolism by gut and liver tissues and subsequent use by peripheral tissues. While each of these processes is important, a major site of net loss of digested and absorbed amino acids (and peptides) in a lactating dairy cow is the liver (Reynolds *et al.*, 1988; Danfaer, 1994). We have constructed and solved an isotope dilution model for partitioning LEU uptake by the liver of the lactating dairy cow in the steady state (see France *et al.*, 1999). If assumptions are made concerning the enrichment of the intracellular and export protein pools, model solution permits calculation of the rate of LEU uptake from portal and hepatic arterial blood supply, LEU export into the hepatic vein, LEU oxidation and transamination, and synthesis and degradation of hepatic constitutive and export proteins. The model requires the measurement of plasma flow rate through the liver in combination with LEU concentrations and plateau isotopic enrichments in arterial, portal and hepatic plasma during a constant infusion of [1-^{13}C]LEU tracer. The model can be applied to other amino acids with similar metabolic fates and will provide a means for assessing the impact of hepatic metabolism on amino acid availability to peripheral tissues. This is of particular importance when considering the dairy cow and the requirements of the mammary gland for milk protein synthesis.

Despite some limitations, the models described herein are useful tools for obtaining information on the uptake and partitioning of amino acids by the ruminant hindlimb and mammary gland, indicating aspects of metabolic regulation that could be manipulated to direct more amino acid towards muscle or milk protein synthesis. The level of representation adopted means that the models could be applied to other amino acids with similar metabolic fates within the hindlimb and the mammary gland. Linking the models consecutively and dynamically (including hepatic models) will allow quantitative description of the effects of liver metabolism on amino acid availability to peripheral tissues and simultaneously quantify the partition of amino acids between the mammary gland and peripheral tissues (hindlimb) and within the mammary gland between milk protein synthesis, constitutive protein turnover and other metabolic fates. If the models are to be rigorously applied, future *in vivo* studies must attempt to directly measure the isotopic activity of the precursor pool for protein synthesis or the closest surrogate pool for the tissue in question and should consider cellular organization.

References

Abdul-Razzaq, H.A. and Bickerstaffe, R. (1989) The influence of rumen volatile fatty acids on protein metabolism in growing lambs. *British Journal of Nutrition* 62, 297–310.

Airhart, J., Vidrich, A. and Khairallah, E.A. (1974) Compartmentation of free amino acids for protein synthesis in rat liver. *Biochemical Journal* 140, 539–548.

Baracos, V., Brun-Bellut, J. and Marie, M. (1991) Tissue protein synthesis in lactating and dry goats. *British Journal of Nutrition* 66, 451–465.

Barrett, E.J. and Gelfand, R.A. (1989) The *in vivo* study of cardiac and skeletal muscle protein turnover. *Diabetes/Metabolism Reviews* 5, 133–148.

Barrett, E.J., Revkin, J.H., Young, L.H., Zaret, B.L., Jacob, R. and Gelfand, R.A. (1987) An isotopic method for measurement of muscle protein synthesis and degradation *in vivo*. *Biochemical Journal* 245, 223–228.

Bequette, B.J., Kyle, C.E., Crompton, L.A., Anderson, S.E. and Hanigan, M.D. (2002) Protein metabolism in lactating goats subjected to the insulin clamp. *Journal of Dairy Science* 85, 1546–1555.

Biolo, G., Chinkes, D., Zhang, X.-J. and Wolfe, R.R. (1992) A new model to determine *in vivo* the relationship between amino acid transmembrane transport and protein kinetics in muscle. *Journal of Parenteral and Enteral Nutrition* 16, 305–315.

Biolo, G., Gastaldelli, A., Zhang, X.-J. and Wolfe, R.R. (1994) Protein synthesis and breakdown in skin and muscle: a leg model of amino acid kinetics. *American Journal of Physiology* 267, E467–E474.

Biolo, G., Fleming, R.Y., Maggi, S.P. and Wolfe, R.R. (1995) Transmembrane transport and intracellular kinetics of amino acids in human skeletal muscle. *American Journal of Physiology* 268, E75–E84.

Bohorov, O., Buttery, P.J., Correia, J.H.R.D. and Soar, J.B. (1987) The effect of the β-2-adrenergic agonist clenbuterol or implantation with oestradiol plus trenbolone acetate on protein metabolism in wether lambs. *British Journal of Nutrition* 57, 99–107.

Boisclair, Y.R., Bell, A.W., Dunshea, F.R., Harkins, M. and Bauman, D.E. (1993) Evaluation of the arteriovenous difference technique to simultaneously estimate protein synthesis and degradation in the hindlimb of fed and chronically underfed steers. *Journal of Nutrition* 123, 1076–1088.

Bryant, D.T.W. and Smith, R.W. (1982a) Protein synthesis in muscle of mature sheep. *Journal of Agricultural Science, Cambridge* 98, 639–643.

Bryant, D.T.W. and Smith, R.W. (1982b) The effect of lactation on protein synthesis in ovine skeletal. *Journal of Agricultural Science, Cambridge* 99, 319–323.

Caso, G., Ford, G.C., Nair, K.S., Garlick, P.J. and McNurlan, M.A. (2002) Aminoacyl-tRNA enrichment after a flood of labelled phenylalanine: insulin effect on muscle protein synthesis. *American Journal of Physiology* 282, E1029–E1038.

Caso, G., Garlick, P.J., Ballou, L.M., Vosswinkle, J.A., Gelato, M.C. and McNurlan, M.A. (2006) The increase in human protein synthesis induced by food intake is similar when assessed with the constant infusion and flooding techniques. *Journal of Nutrition* 136, 1504–1510.

Champredon, C., Debras, E., Mirand, P.P. and Arnal, M. (1990) Methionine flux and tissue protein synthesis in lactating and dry goats. *Journal of Dairy Research* 120, 1006–1015.

Cheng, K.N., Dworzak, F., Ford, G.C., Rennie, M.J. and Halliday, D. (1985) Direct determination of leucine metabolism and protein breakdown in humans using L-[1-^{13}C,^{15}N]-leucine and the forearm model. *European Journal of Clinical Investigation* 15, 349–354.

Cheng, K.N., Pacy, P.J., Dworzak, F., Ford, G.C. and Halliday, D. (1987) Influence of fasting on leucine and muscle protein metabolism across the forearm determined using L-[1-^{13}C,^{15}N]-leucine as the tracer. *Clinical Science* 73, 241–246.

Connell, A., Calder, A.G., Anderson, S.E. and Lobley, G.E. (1997) Hepatic protein synthesis in the sheep: effect of intake as monitored by use of stable-isotope-labelled glycine, leucine and phenylalanine. *British Journal of Nutrition* 77, 255–271.

Crompton, L.A. (1990) Acute nutritional signals in the control of hindlimb protein turnover in lambs *in vivo*. PhD thesis, University of Reading, UK.

Crompton, L.A. and Lomax, M.A. (1993) Hindlimb protein turnover and muscle protein synthesis in lambs: a comparison of techniques. *British Journal of Nutrition* 69, 345–358.

Crompton, L.A., France, J. and Lomax, M.A. (2006) Modelling protein metabolism by the hindlimb tissues in lambs. *Journal of Agricultural Science, Cambridge* 144, 465.

Danfaer, A. (1994) Nutrient metabolism and utilization in the liver. *Livestock Production Science* 39, 115–117.

Davis, S.R., Barry, T.N. and Hughson, G.A. (1981) Protein synthesis in tissues of growing lambs. *British Journal of Nutrition* 46, 409–419.

Domanski, A., Lindsay, D.B. and Setchell, B.P. (1974) Blood flow and substrate uptake and oxidation in the hindlimb muscles of sheep. *Journal of Physiology* 242, 28P–29P.

Eisemann, J.H., Hammond, A.C., Bauman, D.E., Reynolds, P.J., McCutcheon, S.N., Tyrrell, H.F. and Haaland, G.L. (1986) Effect of bovine growth hormone administration on metabolism of growing Hereford heifers: protein and lipid metabolism and plasma concentrations of metabolites and hormones. *Journal of Nutrition* 116, 2504–2515.

Fern, E.B. and Garlick, P.J. (1976) Compartmentation of albumin and ferritin synthesis in rat liver *in vivo*. *Biochemical Journal* 156, 189–192.

France, J. and Dijkstra, J. (2005) Volatile fatty acid production. In: Dijkstra, J., Forbes, J.M. and France, J. (eds) *Quantitative Aspects of Ruminant Digestion and Metabolism*, 2nd edn. CAB International, Wallingford, UK, pp. 157–175.

France, J., Calvert, C.C., Baldwin, R.L. and Klasing, K.C. (1988) On the application of compartmental models to radioactive tracer kinetic studies of *in vivo* protein turnover in animals. *Journal of Theoretical Biology* 133, 447–471.

France, J., Bequette, B.J., Lobley, G.E., Metcalf, J.A., Wray-Cahen, D., Dhanoa, M.S., Backwell, F.R.C., Hanigan, M.D., MacRae, J.C. and Beever, D.E. (1995) An isotope dilution model for partitioning leucine uptake by the bovine mammary gland. *Journal of Theoretical Biology* 172, 369–377.

France, J., Hanigan, M.D., Reynolds, C.K., Dijkstra, J., Crompton, L.A., Maas, J.A., Bequette, B.J., Metcalf, J.A., Lobley, G.E., MacRae, J.C. and Beever, D.E. (1999) An isotope dilution model for partitioning leucine uptake by the liver of the lactating dairy cow. *Journal of Theoretical Biology* 198, 121–133.

France, J., Crompton, L.A. and Lomax, M.A. (2005) Modelling tyrosine uptake and protein turnover by the hindlimb tissues in lambs. *Canadian Journal of Animal Science* 85, 549–550.

Gelfand, R.A. and Barrett, E.J. (1987) Effect of physiologic hyperinsulinemia on skeletal muscle protein synthesis and breakdown in man. *Journal of Clinical Investigation* 80, 1–6.

Godfrey, K. (1983) *Compartmental Models and Their Application*. Academic Press, London, 293 pp.

Harris, C.I. and Milne, G. (1977) The unreliability of urinary 3-methylhistidine excretion as a measure of muscle protein degradation in sheep. *Proceedings of the Nutrition Society* 36, 138A.

Harris, C.I. and Milne, G. (1980) The urinary excretion of N-methylhistidine in sheep: an invalid index of muscle protein breakdown. *British Journal of Nutrition* 44, 129–140.

Harris, P.M., Skene, P.A., Buchan, V., Milne, E., Calder, A.G., Anderson, S.E., Connell, A. and Lobley, G.E. (1992) Effect of food intake on hindlimb and whole-body protein metabolism in young growing sheep: chronic studies based on arteriovenous techniques. *British Journal of Nutrition* 68, 389–407.

Hesketh, J. (1994) Translation and the cytoskeleton: a mechanism for targeted protein synthesis. *Molecular Biology Reports* 19, 233–243.

Hoskin, S.O., Savary, I.C., Zurr, G. and Lobley, G.E. (2001) Effect of feed intake on ovine hindlimb protein metabolism based on thirteen amino acids and arteriovenous techniques. *British Journal of Nutrition* 86, 577–585.

Hoskin, S.O., Savary-Auzeloux, I.C., Calder, A.G., Zurr, G. and Lobley, G.E. (2003) Effect of feed intake on amino acid transfers across the ovine hindquarters. *British Journal of Nutrition* 89, 167–179.

Kronfeld, D.S., Ramberg, C.F. Jr and Shames, D.M. (1971) Multicompartment analysis of glucose kinetics in normal and hypoglycemic cows. *American Journal of Physiology* 220, 886–893.

Leng, R.A. and Brett, D.J. (1966) Simultaneous measurement of the rates of production of acetic, propionic and butyric acids in the rumen of sheep on different diets and the correlation between production rates and concentrations of these acids in the rumen. *British Journal of Nutrition* 20, 541–552.

Linzell, J.L. (1971) Techniques for measuring nutrient uptake by the mammary glands. In: Falconer, I.R. (ed.) *Lactation*. Butterworths, London, pp. 261–279.

Liu, S.M., Mata, G., Donoghue, H.O. and Masters, D.G. (1998) The influence of live weight, live-weight change and diet on protein synthesis in the skin and skeletal muscle in young Merino sheep. *British Journal of Nutrition* 79, 267–274.

Lobley, G.E. (1993a) Protein metabolism and turnover. In: Forbes, J.M. and France, J. (eds) *Quantitative Aspects of Ruminant Digestion and Metabolism*. CAB International, Wallingford, UK, pp. 313–339.

Lobley, G.E. (1993b) Species comparisons of tissue protein metabolism: effects of age and hormonal action. *Journal of Nutrition* 123, 337–343.

Lobley, G.E. (1998) Nutritional and hormonal control of muscle and peripheral tissue metabolism in farm species. *Livestock Production Science* 56, 91–114.

Lobley, G.E. (2003) Protein turnover – what does it mean for animal production? *Canadian Journal of Animal Science* 83, 327–340.

Lobley, G.E., Milne, V., Lovie, J.M., Reeds, P.J. and Pennie, K. (1980) Whole-body and tissue protein synthesis in cattle. *British Journal of Nutrition* 43, 491–502.

Lobley, G.E., Connell, A., Milne, E., Buchan, V., Calder, A.G., Anderson, S.E. and Vint, H. (1990) Muscle protein synthesis in response to testosterone administration in wether lambs. *British Journal of Nutrition* 64, 691–704.

Lobley, G.E., Harris, P.M., Skene, P.A., Brown, D., Milne, E., Calder, A.G., Anderson, S.E., Garlick, P.J., Nevison, I. and Connell, A. (1992) Responses in tissue protein synthesis to sub- and supra-maintenance intake in young growing sheep: comparison of large-dose and continuous-infusion techniques. *British Journal of Nutrition* 68, 373–388.

Lobley, G.E., Sinclair, K.D., Grant, C.M., Miller, L., Mantle, D., Calder, A.G., Warkup, C.C. and Maltin, C.A. (2000) The effect of breed and level of nutrition on whole-body and muscle protein metabolism in pure-bred Aberdeen Angus and Charolais beef steers. *British Journal of Nutrition* 84, 275–284.

Matthews, D.E., Schwarz, H.P., Yang, R.D., Motil, K.J., Young, V.R. and Bier, D.M. (1982) Relationship of plasma leucine and α-ketoisocaproate during a L-[1- ^{13}C] leucine infusion in man: a method for measuring human intracellular leucine tracer enrichment. *Metabolism* 31, 1105–1112.

Oddy, V.H. and Lindsay, D.B. (1986) Determination of rates of protein synthesis, gain and degradation in intact hindlimb muscle of lambs. *Biochemical Journal* 233, 417–425.

Oddy, V.H., Brown, B.W. and Jones, A.W. (1981) Measurement of organ blood flow using tritiated water. I. Hindlimb muscle blood flow in conscious ewes. *Australian Journal of Biological Sciences* 34, 419–425.

Oddy, V.H., Gooden, J.M. and Annison, E.F. (1984) Partitioning of nutrients in Merino ewes. I. Contribution of skeletal muscle, the pregnant uterus and the lactating mammary gland to total energy expenditure. *Australian Journal of Biological Sciences* 37, 375–388.

Oddy, V.H., Lindsay, D.B., Barker, P.J. and Northrop, A.J. (1987) Effect of insulin on hindlimb and whole-body leucine and protein metabolism in fed and fasted lambs. *British Journal of Nutrition* 58, 437–452.

Oddy, V.H., Lindsay, D.B. and Fleet, L.R. (1988) Protein synthesis and degradation in the mammary gland of goats. *Journal of Dairy Research* 55, 143–154.

Pell, J.M., Caldarone, E.M. and Bergman, E.N. (1986) Leucine and α-ketoisocaproate metabolism and interconversions in fed and fasted sheep. *Metabolism* 35, 1005–1016.

Ponter, A.A., Cortamira, N.O., Seve, B., Salter, D.N. and Morgan, L.M. (1994) The effect of energy source and tryptophan on the rate of protein synthesis and on hormones of the entero-insular axis in the piglet. *British Journal of Nutrition* 71, 661–674.

Razooki Hasan, H., White, D.A. and Mayer, R.J. (1982) Extensive destruction of newly synthesized casein in mammary explants in organ culture. *Biochemical Journal* 202, 133–138.

Reeds, P.J., Nicholson, B.A. and Fuller, M.F. (1987) Contribution of protein synthesis to energy expenditure *in vivo* and *in vitro*. In: Moe, P.W., Tyrrell, H.F. and Reynolds, P.J. (eds) *Energy Metabolism of Farm Animals, EAAP Publication No. 32*. Rowan and Littlefield, Totowa, New Jersey, pp. 6–9.

Reynolds, C.K., Huntington, G.B., Tyrrell, H.F. and Reynolds, P.J. (1988) Net portal-drained visceral and hepatic metabolism of glucose, L-lactate and nitrogenous compounds in lactating Holstein cows. *Journal of Dairy Science* 71, 1803–1812.

Rocha, H.J.G., Nash, J.E., Connell, A. and Lobley, G.E. (1993) Protein synthesis in ovine muscle and skin: sequential measurements with three different amino acids based on the large-dose procedure. *Comparative Biochemistry and Physiology* 105B, 301–307.

Roets, E., Massart-Leen, A.-M., Verbeke, R. and Peeters, G. (1979) Metabolism of [U-^{14}C;2,3-^{3}H]-L-valine by the isolated perfused goat udder. *Journal of Dairy Research* 46, 47–57.

Roets, E., Massart-Leen, A.-M., Verbeke, R. and Peeters, G. (1983) Metabolism of leucine by the isolated perfused goat udder. *Journal of Dairy Research* 50, 413–424.

Savary-Auzeloux, I., Hoskin, S.O. and Lobley, G.E. (2003) Effect of intake on whole body plasma amino acid kinetics in sheep. *Reproduction Nutrition Development* 43, 117–129.

Schaefer, A.L. and Krishnamurti, C.R. (1984) Whole-body and tissue fractional protein synthesis in the ovine fetus *in utero*. *British Journal of Nutrition* 52, 359–369.

Seve, B., Reeds, P.J., Fuller, M.F., Cadenhead, A. and Hay, S.M. (1986) Protein synthesis and retention in some tissues of the young pig as influenced by dietary protein intake after early weaning. Possible connection to the energy metabolism. *Reproduction, Nutrition, Development* 26, 849–861.

Shipley, R.A. and Clark, R.E. (1972) *Tracer Methods for* In Vivo *Kinetics*. Academic Press, New York, 239 pp.

Smith, C.B. and Sun, Y. (1995) Influence of valine flooding on channelling of valine into tissue pools and on protein synthesis. *American Journal of Physiology* 268, E735–E744.

Teleni, E. and Annison, E.F. (1986) Development of a sheep hindlimb muscle preparation for metabolic studies. *Australian Journal of Biological Sciences* 39, 271–281.

Thompson, G.N., Pacy, P.J., Merritt, H., Ford, G.C., Read, M.A., Cheng, K.N. and Halliday, D. (1989) Rapid measurement of whole-body and forearm protein turnover using a [$^{2}H_5$]phenylalanine model. *American Journal of Physiology* 256, E631–E639.

Thomson, B.C., Hosking, B.J., Sainz, R.D. and Oddy, V.H. (1997) The effect of nutritional status on protein degradation and components of the calpain system in skeletal muscle of weaned wether lambs. *Journal of Agricultural Science, Cambridge* 129, 471–477.

Thornley, J.H.M. and France, J. (2007) *Mathematical Models in Agriculture: Quantitative Methods for the Plant, Animal and Ecological Sciences*, 2nd edn. CAB International, Wallingford, UK, 906 pp.

Tomas, F.M. and Ballard, F.J. (1987) Applications of the N-methylhistidine technique for measuring myofibrillar protein breakdown *in vivo*. In: Glaumann, H. and Ballard, F.J. (eds) *Lysosomes: Their Role in Protein Breakdown*. Academic Press, London, pp. 679–711.

Vidrich, A., Airhart, J., Bruno, M.K. and Khairallah, E.A. (1977) Compartmentation of free amino acids for protein biosynthesis. *Biochemical Journal* 162, 257–266.

Waterlow, J.C. (1999) The mysteries of nitrogen balance. *Nutrition Research Reviews* 12, 25–54.

Waterlow, J.C. (2006) *Protein Turnover*. CAB International, Wallingford, UK, 301 pp.

Waterlow, J.C., Millward, D.J. and Garlick, P.J. (1978) *Protein Turnover in Mammalian Tissues and the Whole Body*. North-Holland, Amsterdam, 804 pp.

13 Assessment of Protein and Amino Acid Requirements in Adult Mammals, with Specific Focus on Cats, Dogs and Rabbits

A.K. SHOVELLER AND J.L. ATKINSON

Centre for Nutrition Modelling, Department of Animal and Poultry Science, University of Guelph, Canada

Introduction

Defining protein requirements and the physiological implications of long-term dietary protein adequacy or excess is fraught with difficulty and remains a controversial aspect of nutrition in all animals. The disagreement over amino acid requirements, even in species where multiple techniques have been used, such as the pig, has been the subject of numerous reviews. To our knowledge, only one has attempted an interspecies comparison (McLarney *et al.*, 1996). However, no attempt was made to reason why the amino acid recommendations varied, whereas we have attempted to explain some of the apparent differences. Understanding a comparative approach to protein and amino acid requirements necessitates information on: (i) the animals' natural food preferences; (ii) differences in digestive anatomy and physiology; (iii) differences in protein and amino acid metabolism; and (iv) details on the experimental design that has been used to investigate protein and amino acid requirements. This review will specifically discuss potential differences in protein and amino acid metabolism and requirements, as well as details on experimental design. Details of the experimental design include such factors as: the technique used to quantify the requirement or effect, the diet composition and the species, breed and anthropometric details of the animals studied. This review will focus on the broad base of knowledge available on rabbits (herbivores), dogs (omnivores) and cats (obligate carnivores).

A requirement for dietary protein actually represents the need for indispensable amino acids and the provision of adequate dispensable amino acids to maintain whole-body protein turnover and replace endogenous nitrogen losses, such as hair, skin and gut cells. It is generally accepted that adult animals need a much lower amount of indispensable amino acids, as a per cent of total protein, than growing animals (Young, 1987). Whole-body protein turnover represents the synthesis and breakdown of a variety of proteins such as skeletal muscle, enzymes, hormones and transport proteins, while protein losses such as skin and hair are likely different between animals and vary depending on the environment to which the animal is exposed (Young, 1987). Changes in turnover and protein loss of individual proteins contribute to changes in total whole-body protein synthesis and therefore affect dietary amino acid requirements. The present recommendations for cats and dogs, but not rabbits, are based on the assumption that good quality proteins, with the appropriate amounts (g day^{-1}) and proportions (% of diet or % of crude protein) of available indispensable and dispensable amino acids, are provided, but these recommendations may prove inadequate or inappropriate when applied to commercially formulated diets fed to animals in a broad population such as the rabbit, canine and feline populations. Furthermore, the disparity between the approach taken by the National Research Council (NRC) (2006) and the Association of American Feed Control Officials (AAFCO) (2005) for dogs and cats and the relative paucity of information on normal, free-living rabbits kept predominantly as pets can be misleading and confusing.

The traditional methods of assessing protein and amino acid requirements and availability have focused on outcome measures such as nitrogen balance (Table 13.1), growth and blood concentrations of urea nitrogen and plasma amino acids in studies where animals were adapted to the diets over a week or more. However, to demonstrate nutritional adequacy of a given commercial dog food, AAFCO assesses adequacy of the dietary protein content for dogs and cats at maintenance based only on body weight change over a 6-month feeding trial and monitoring of basic blood chemistry parameters. To our knowledge, there are no assessment procedures for rabbits and only the NRC (1977) is available to guide the formulation of diets for these animals. These methods are lagging behind the current state-of-the-art techniques to assess nutrition. The possible effects of different ingredients, their inclusion level and the extent of processing of commercial diets need to be considered, as well as appropriate adaptation times for diets differing in protein content or quality. Furthermore, it is controversial whether previous nutrition (i.e. long-term low protein intake) results in permanent alterations in metabolism and, if so, how do researchers quantify this? The selection of outcome parameters and the relevance of physiological (i.e. growth versus maintenance), physical (i.e. athletic training versus sedentary) and

Table 13.1. Interpretation of nitrogen balance.

Nitrogen balance	Physiological or nutritional stage
Zero where nitrogen intake = nitrogen excretion	Maintenance and no indispensable amino acid deficiency
Positive where nitrogen intake > nitrogen excretion	Growth, gestation or deposition of lean body mass (i.e. resistance exercise), recovery from illness and no indispensable amino acid deficiency
Negative where nitrogen intake < nitrogen excretion	Severe disease or injury, urinary nitrogen loss during renal failure, inadequate nutrition or a limitation in an indispensable amino acid

immunological (disease state differences) status have only recently begun to be addressed.

For the purpose of this chapter, only protein and amino acid requirements at *maintenance* will be discussed, as this is the status most pertinent to the majority of dogs, cats and rabbits kept as pets and because there is limited information at other life stages other than growth, where the majority of information on protein and amino acid adequacy of cats, dogs and rabbits exists. Dietary amino acids during growth (Pencharz *et al.*, 1996; Moughan, 2003) have been reviewed in humans and pigs, respectively. However, researchers are only now starting to look at how health affects metabolism and, ultimately, nutritional requirements.

Physiologically, the most meaningful estimates of protein requirements must be based on amino acid requirements supplied by defined protein sources with a specified level of processing, since both of these factors may affect results. However, the mode of expression of protein and amino acid requirements needs to be standardized for ease of comparison between diets with varying ingredients, and also needs to reflect potential genetic and body composition differences between animals. Clearly, we have much to learn about protein and amino acid requirements and the diversity of our companion animal population makes this an even more challenging endeavour. Since information specifically derived from studies with dogs, cats and especially rabbits is often limited, we should also draw on concepts from nutritionally similar species which have been more extensively studied to guide our way, such as pigs and humans. Currently, scientists are moving towards the use of isotopic approaches to define amino acid requirements while attempting to take into account the effects of dietary ingredient inclusion, physiological stage, body composition differences and experimental design differences. These methods will allow more rapid and less invasive determination of amino acid adequacy in healthy animals and can more easily be adapted in order to investigate changing requirements in response to a variety of disease states.

Protein and Amino Acid Requirements and Metabolism

The concept of dietary protein requirements for animals at maintenance

Although often a primary consideration when balancing diets, the requirement for protein represents the need for the 22 amino acids, both dispensable and indispensable, for which t-RNA exists and which are, therefore, components from which all proteins are synthesized (Crim and Munro, 1994). If they cannot be endogenously synthesized in sufficient amounts, then they are necessary in the diet and considered to be dietarily indispensable, also termed essential (Pencharz *et al.*, 1996). For mature healthy dogs and cats there are ten amino acids that are considered to be indispensable: phenylalanine, histidine, isoleucine, leucine, valine, lysine, methionine, arginine, tryptophan and threonine (Case *et al.*, 2000). Cats additionally require the β-amino acid, taurine, which is *not* incorporated in protein and is the metabolic product of sulfur amino acid metabolism and is required for bile acid conjugations, retinal development and osmoregulation. Rabbits are similar, but they do not have a requirement for arginine or taurine (NRC, 1977). The remaining amino acids that are utilized for protein synthesis are synthesized endogenously within the body and are not required unless their direct precursors are limiting, either metabolically or in the diet. If dietary indispensable amino acids and sufficient dispensable amino acids are not provided in the correct proportions, the protein providing these amino acids is considered to be of poor quality because whole-body protein synthesis will be reduced if this is the sole protein source (Crim and Munro, 1994). When the dietary amino acids are provided in the correct ratios in a protein source and are adequate to maintain maximal protein synthesis, the protein is considered to be of good quality. However, the way in which the food is processed can either increase or decrease the digestibility and cellular availability of these amino acids, consequently influencing the capacity for whole-body protein synthesis. For example, using a rat bioassay, Hendriks *et al.* (1999) found that incremental increases in heat treatment of canned cat food were associated with decreased amino acid digestibility. Therefore, the proportion of the indispensable amino acids and the level of processing can affect the protein quality of a given ingredient.

Minimal amino acid requirements, as presented in NRC (2006), are the lowest level of amino acid intake at which nitrogen balance can be achieved and maintained. Millward *et al.* (1990) presented three levels of amino acid requirement that they felt were appropriate to discuss when considering human amino acid requirements: the minimal, optimal and operational. The Minimal Requirement and Recommended Allowance (NRC, 2006) are similar to the minimal and operational theories, respectively. The Minimal Requirement has been the focus of numerous studies and is defined as the lowest level of protein or amino acid intake at which N balance can be achieved and maintained (Millward *et al.*, 1990). These requirements have been estimated based on one animal representing one data point and therefore will meet 50% of that given population's requirement. The Recommended Allowance, or operational theory, takes into account that nitrogen balance can be achieved at a wide range of protein intakes, although the reason for this remains unclear (Waterlow, 1994). NRC (2006) estimated the Adequate Intake, which falls between the Minimal Requirement and the Recommended Allowance, from the quantity of each amino acid in the digestible protein of commercial dry diets that were known to support normal maintenance, when no minimum requirement has been defined. The Recommended Allowance is defined as the concentration or amount of a nutrient to support maintenance with consideration of the bioavailability of the nutrient in typical quality feed ingredients. Alternatively, AAFCO (2005) makes recommendations for all nutrients supplied to cats and dogs and ultimately represents the state organizations regulating the sale of commercial animal feeds. Although the AAFCO (2005) guidelines have been largely based on the NRC recommendations, arbitrary safety factors have been applied to the suggested target inclusion rates of the amino acids. Morris and Rogers (1994) stated, 'Until the AAFCO allowances are adequately referenced citing experimental data, they lack scientific veracity. Although these allowances may be dismissed on a scientific basis, they have legal implications, and pet food manufacturers are disinclined to formulate diets below the AAFCO profile allowances as a protection against possible litigation.' Furthermore, as stated in NRC (2006) for the Nutrient Requirements of Dogs and Cats, there are no dose response data for any amino acid for any species of adult dog and one dose response for lysine in cats (Burger and Smith, 1987). With dietary protein being one of the more financially and metabolically expensive nutrients, it is clear that well-designed experiments on the amino acid requirements of cats, dogs and rabbits are needed to ensure nutrient adequacy without providing large excesses.

The AAFCO regulations to demonstrate protein adequacy in a commercial feed

Though not mandatory, AAFCO regulations and protocols are widely employed in the labelling of commercial dog and cat food in North America. In Canada, the Canadian Veterinary Medical Association (CVMA) also has guidelines for nutritional adequacy and these currently follow the AAFCO values. Other than meeting formulation targets as recommended by the NRC (1977), which are only suggestions and require a nutritionist to apply safety margins that they deem sufficient, rabbit food does not undergo similar testing procedures as AAFCO and CVMA have applied to dog and cat food.

There are many commercial feeds on the market and these may employ one of two AAFCO claims on dog and cat food labels. The first is 'This product is formulated to meet the nutritional levels established by the AAFCO dog/cat nutrient profiles for all ages' and simply means that all recommendations for energy, protein, essential fatty acid and vitamins and minerals have been met or exceeded. Simply put, this first nutritional claim means that the essential nutrients are met or exceeded by analysis, but offers no idea of the quality or digestibility of the primary protein source. The second statement that may appear on dog or cat food labels is: 'Animal feeding tests using Association of American Feed Control Officials procedures substantiate that this product provides complete and balanced nutrition for this given physiological stage.' For maintenance diets (appropriate for dogs and cats that are no longer growing and are not gestating or lactating), this means that appropriate measures of blood serum biochemistry, and whole blood taurine for cats, and weight maintenance have been achieved in a 6-month feeding trial with eight animals. The outcome measures for protein adequacy, other than weight loss, which can occur in a protein deficiency, are generally serum albumin, packed cell volume and haemoglobin. If the values of these parameters drop below what are considered normal values, the diet does not pass feeding trials. Although the AAFCO feeding test provides a practical method for assessing nutritional adequacy, there are several procedural and interpretative limitations.

Plasma albumin is slow to respond to a dietary restriction of protein and is not considered to be a good indicator of protein adequacy by the nutrition research community outside that of companion animal nutrition. In human nutrition, prealbumin is often used as a more sensitive indicator of protein sufficiency and should be considered for testing of protein and amino acid adequacy. For example, Arnold *et al.* (2001) found that plasma albumin was normal in all children and not adequately sensitive to detect protein depletion that was sufficient to cause anaemia or decreased growth; however, these researchers found that prealbumin was significantly correlated with protein depletion. Furthermore, albumin is also considered both a negative and positive acute phase protein and, as such, its synthesis may initially be upregulated during an immune response and later downregulated, resulting in profound differences in its plasma concentration during an acute phase immune response (Morley and Kushner, 1982). Therefore, either increased or decreased albumin may not be an adequately sensitive marker to detect dietary protein sufficiency, but rather that its plasma concentrations are compounded by possible immune status changes. Though the AAFCO maintenance protocol requires that the test cohort remains 'healthy' for the duration of the trial, this does not preclude the presence of subclinical disease, which may affect outcomes. Last, to use albumin or prealbumin appropriately as an indicator of protein adequacy, animals are required to stay on the test diets for long periods of time, and this may further perturb protein and amino acid metabolism due to an unbalanced diet. Clearly, a shorter test period with more sensitive markers of protein and amino acid adequacy would be beneficial.

Methods to determine amino acid requirements

Since the concept of protein requirement is predicated on an appropriate supply of the constituent amino acids, it is imperative that estimates of amino acid requirements are determined appropriately. To assess amino acid requirements properly, careful consideration must be given to the experimental design, statistical analysis implemented and interpretation of the results. Most experiments that have defined protein and amino acid requirements have measured growth, feed efficiency, plasma urea, plasma amino acids or nitrogen balance. To allow sufficient statistical power, both requirement and bioavailability studies necessitate feeding graded levels of the amino acid in question (Baker, 1986; Pencharz and Ball, 2003). A minimum of three, but preferably six or more, dietary levels of the amino acid in question are required, such that the data can be fitted to a descriptive response, which allows objective assessment of the requirement (Baker, 1986; Pencharz and Ball, 2003). The statistical differences, or lack thereof, between any two adjacent diet levels are essentially meaningless (Baker, 1986). Therefore, applying a continuous broken line model (the breakpoint model) or a quadratic or second-order polynomial regression is the most appropriate statistical method to apply to requirement studies (Baker, 1986; Pencharz and Ball, 2003).

To assess properly the data produced from a requirement study, the method of expression of the data should also be considered. Presenting requirements on a g kg^{-1} body weight day^{-1} basis avoids the complication of heavier animals requiring greater absolute amounts of the nutrient (g day^{-1}). Also commonly used in the presentation of an amino acid requirement is g 1000 $kcal^{-1}$ metabolizable energy (Baker, 1986; AAFCO, 2005) as the relationship between dietary energy and protein inclusion is well supported in the nutrition literature, but this raises the problem of precise estimates of the metabolizable energy content of the complete feed. The relationship between dietary energy and protein is maintained, as all amino acid requirements presented by NRC include a note about the dietary energy content. Although not included in the presentation of amino acid requirements, the food composition and the levels must also be considered. For example, the threonine requirement in grower pigs is higher when they are fed a barley diet versus a casein diet (Myrie *et al.*, 2003), due to the higher fibre content of the barley diet. In this case, the threonine requirement was greater in pigs receiving more dietary fibre because dietary fibre is a potent stimulator of intestinal mucin synthesis and these have large threonine concentrations. Conversely, microbes also contribute to amino acid synthesis and, thus, overall metabolic availability (Metges, 2000). Clearly, when determining the protein and amino acid requirements of dogs, cats and rabbits, the protein source needs to be reported and the presence of substances such as fibre needs to be quantified.

Presently, the greatest controversies in the design of amino acid requirement studies is the use of only a short period of adaptation to a new dietary level of the test amino acid that may be inadequate and that data have generally only been collected from animals in the fed state. The dietary adaptation issue arose because nitrogen balance studies required a long adaptation period (7–10 days) to stabilize urinary nitrogen excretion and thus it came to be believed that all aspects of amino acid metabolism required a long adaptation period to respond fully to dietary changes. However, alterations in dietary amino acid intake change the aminoacyl t-RNA expression in less than 4 h (Crim and Munro, 1994). Consequently, the oxidation of an amino acid changes and stabilizes within 4 h of altered dietary amino acid intake in adult humans (Zello *et al.*, 1995; Pencharz and Ball, 2003) and oxidation rate is similar whether measured at 16 h or 10 days after a dietary change in amino acids (Moehn *et al.*, 2004). Similarly, Young and Marchini (1990) reported that leucine oxidation changed within the course of 24 h due to an alteration from a low leucine to a high leucine intake. These results demonstrate that, although other factors can alter amino acid oxidation, substrate availability is a primary factor.

The second issue is whether amino acid oxidation studies can be conducted only in the fed state, or whether both fed and fasting periods must be measured. Although amino acid oxidation is higher in the fed state, calculation of the lysine requirement in human adults was not different when breath and blood measurements were taken over either a 24 h fed and fasted period or a 6 h fed period only (Kurpad *et al.*, 2001). The rapid change in oxidation response to a change in intake of a limiting amino acid is due to the lack of a storage compartment for free amino acids and the short half-life of the plasma free amino acid pool. This phenomenon has been associated primarily with the negative effects seen when excess levels of free amino acids accumulate, as often seen in inborn errors of metabolism, such as phenylketonuria. These require an immediate response of metabolism to an influx of nutrients. Therefore, a short adaptation period will result in changes in amino acid oxidation without the depletion of the whole-body pool of the test amino acid, which may cause further metabolic changes that may affect the estimate of the requirement. Ultimately, by properly designing requirement studies, any such biases can be removed and, with proper analysis of the data, an objective estimate of the requirement can be made.

The concept that the most limiting amino acid determines overall protein metabolism is the basis for most amino acid oxidation techniques and for the current state-of-the-art techniques to examine amino acid adequacy and requirements. Early work from Bayley's lab revealed a close relationship between the dietary concentration of amino acids and their catabolism (Kim *et al.*, 1983). When the test amino acid is isotopically labelled, oxidation of the isotopic tracer remains low until the requirement for that amino acid has been reached, and then its oxidation increases linearly. When the isotope is not the test amino acid but another indispensable amino acid, oxidation starts high and decreases until the requirement for the test amino acid has been reached, and then oxidation plateaus. The latter technique is called the indicator amino acid oxidation technique and has been applied to assess amino acid requirements in humans by Pencharz and Ball (2003) and the group at MIT (Kurpad *et al.*, 2001), in pigs by Brunton *et al.* (2000) and in poultry by Tabiri *et al.* (2002). Furthermore, the technique has been adapted to assess amino acid sufficiency (Brunton *et al.*, 2003) and lysine availability (Moehn *et al.*, 2005) and can rapidly detect an individual amino acid inadequacy, despite the provision of diets remaining equal in crude protein or total nitrogen. The adaptation of the isotopic techniques highlights the trend to move to rapid, minimally invasive techniques to assess amino acid requirements in a variety of species provided with a variety of different protein sources.

Despite the lack of information in the specific requirements of amino acids, and how these are affected by the multiple variables that can influence them, commercial pet foods are typically more than capable of meeting maintenance needs. However, the long-term health effects of providing diets that exceed requirements has not been elucidated, although an abundance of literature indicating that caloric restriction can lead to a longer life may suggest that protein restriction may, in part, play a role in enhancing longevity. In addition to understanding the amino acid availability in commonly used protein sources, such as meat, fish and soy, there is rising interest in using novel protein sources for pet foods and supplying balanced vegetarian diets. The use of these ingredients will require a better understanding of amino acid bioavailability in ingredients that contain much higher levels of other nutritional factors, such as fibre, which affect amino acid availability. The introduction of isotopic techniques provides an effective tool for investigating factors which influence amino acid availability. Moehn *et al.* (2005) demonstrated that the oxidation of an indicator amino acid responds to differences in amino acid availability due to differences in processing and, more specifically, heating. It would be interesting to apply this technique to examine the amino acid availability and protein adequacy in herbivores, omnivores and obligate carnivores given a variety of protein sources. Defining the amino acid requirements based on protein source would allow nutritionists to set nutrient inclusion rates more precisely and eliminate both nutrient inadequacy and excess.

The present recommendations for protein and amino acid inclusion for dogs, cats and rabbits

Presently, there are few estimates of protein synthesis and breakdown in adult, healthy free-living dogs and cats using more sensitive techniques than nitrogen balance. To our knowledge, there are no estimates of protein kinetics in the rabbit. Although a pioneering technique in the study of protein and amino acid metabolism, nitrogen balance represents the difference between nitrogen intake (protein and non-protein nitrogen present in the diet) and nitrogen excretion (both urinary and faecal) and cannot elucidate anything concerning individual amino acid adequacy (Table 13.1). For nitrogen balance, a stepwise increase in the most dietary limiting amino acid will result in a progressive increase in nitrogen balance until the requirement is reached, and then there is no further increase. However, nitrogen balance is an indirect measure of whole-body protein synthesis and can be insensitive to minor changes in dietary amino acid content. Furthermore, to conduct a nitrogen balance study properly, adult animals need to be adapted to the test diet for up to 10 days, and this level of dietary restriction is considered unacceptable for companion animal research. The majority of the estimates of protein or amino acid requirements using sound experimental designs have been based on nitrogen balance or growth studies in growing baby rabbits, puppies and kittens.

There have been no dose–response studies on any amino acid for adult dogs and rabbits, and only lysine and the sulfur amino acids have been reported in the cat, albeit as a proceedings paper and not a peer-reviewed manuscript (Burger and Smith, 1987).

The present Recommended Allowances for protein are based on meeting crude protein targets of 12, 10 and 20% for rabbits, dogs and cats, respectively (Table 13.2; NRC, 2006). These recommendations also come with recommendations for the indispensable amino acids (Table 13.2, Fig. 13.1). Given that rabbits are herbivorous, it is logical that this species would have lower protein requirements than dogs, which are omnivorous, although included in the zoological order Carnivora. However, this does not appear to be the case when we contrast these recommended nutrient targets because the data from NRC (2006) result from studies that were conducted on animals receiving a high quality protein that is highly available, unlike the rabbit data. Due to the ingestion of caecotrophs, a faecal pellet that is considered an integral part of the rabbit's digestive process (Cheeke, 1987), the intake and excretion of protein and amino acids is difficult to quantify. Low levels of dietary protein stimulate coprophagy or caecotroph consumption, while high protein diets decrease coprophagy (Cheeke, 1987). This additional source of protein and amino acids is difficult to quantify and will need to be controlled if quantitative measurements of amino acid requirements are going to be made. The cat, which is considered an obligate or true carnivore, has the highest protein requirements due to its apparent inability to regulate the catabolic enzymes for the amino acids (Rogers *et al.*, 1977). This has recently been questioned by Russell *et al.* (2002), who found, using indirect calorimetry, that cats oxidized significantly more protein when fed 52 versus 35%, suggesting cats can adapt net protein catabolism. However, it

Table 13.2. Recommended crude protein and indispensable amino acid (IAA) for NRC (2006, Recommended Allowances for cats and dogs) recommendations, average commercial supply and proportion as a measure of dietary crude protein. All numbers are for dogs and cats at maintenance and mature rabbits in the fattening period.

Nutrient as fed basis	Dog (Omnivore)				Cat (Carnivore)				Rabbit (Herbivore)		
	NRC (2006)[a]	AAFCO (2005)[b]	Commercial supply	% free IAA[c] g^{-1} of crude protein[f]	NRC (2006)[a]	AAFCO (2005)[b]	Commercial supply	% free IAA g^{-1} of crude protein[f]	Lebas (1988)[d]	% free IAA g^{-1} of crude protein[f]
ME (kcal ME g^{-1})	4	3.5	–	NA[e]	4.0	4.0	–	NA	–	NA
CP (%)	10	18	–	NA	20	26	–	NA	12	NA
Arginine (%)	0.35	0.51	–	3.50	0.77	1.04	–	3.85	0.64	4.89
Histidine (%)	0.19	0.18	0.44	1.90	0.26	0.31	0.47	1.30	0.28	2.17
Isoleucine (%)	0.38	0.37	0.50	3.80	0.43	0.52	0.77	2.15	0.46	3.53
Leucine (%)	0.68	0.59	2.00	6.80	1.02	1.25	1.80	5.10	0.85	6.52
Lysine (%)	0.35	0.63	0.90	3.50	0.34	0.83	1.20	1.7	0.53	4.07
Methionine + cystine (%)	0.65	0.43	0.62	6.50	0.34	1.10	0.70	1.70	0.42	3.26
Phenylalanine + tyrosine (%)	0.74	0.73	1.23	7.40	1.53	0.88	1.58	7.65	0.88	6.79
Threonine (%)	0.43	0.48	0.85	4.30	0.52	0.73	1.08	2.55	0.42	3.26
Tryptophan (%)	0.14	0.16	0.22	1.40	0.13	0.16	0.19	0.65	0.11	0.81
Valine (%)	0.49	0.39	0.90	4.90	0.51	0.62	1.00	2.55	0.56	4.34
Total % IAA	4.40	4.47	7.66	–	5.85	7.44	8.79	–	5.15	–

[a]The National Research Council Nutrient Requirements of Dogs and Cats (NRC, 2006) are *Recommended Allowances* and are based on feeding high quality protein.
[b]The Association of American Feed Control Officials (AAFCO, 2005) assumes a dietary energy density of 3.5 kcal g^{-1} and suggests that the numbers are adjusted for diets providing over 4.0 kcal g^{-1} for the diets of dogs and cats.
[c]IAA: indispensable amino acids.
[d]Maintenance requirements as presented by Lebas (1988).
[e]NA: not applicable.
[f]Calculated using NRC for Dogs and Cats (2006) and NRC for Rabbits (1977).

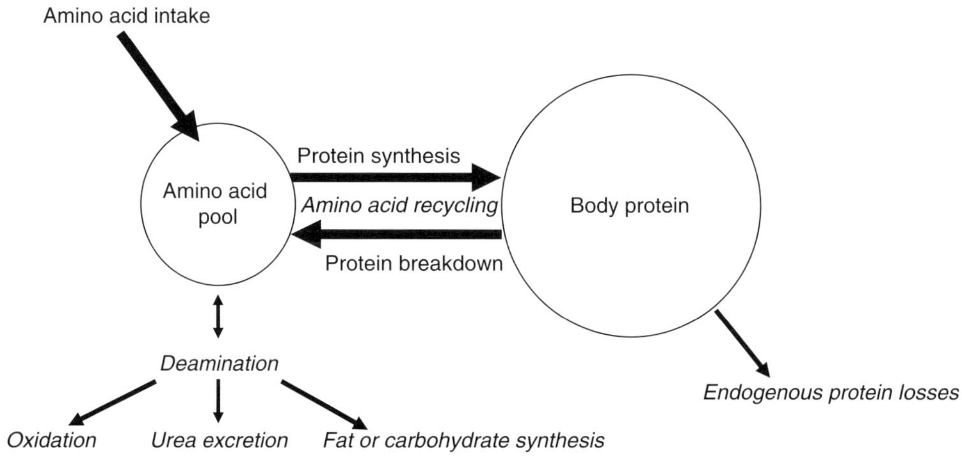

Fig. 13.1. Model of indispensable amino acid metabolism. Terminal output of an amino acid can only occur via oxidation through its respective catabolic pathway where the carbon backbone enters the TCA cycle and the nitrogen is excreted via the urine as urea. However, the carbon backbone may be conserved through conversion to fat or, if needed, carbohydrate.

should be noted that both of these diets were far above the requirement for crude protein and the question of the control of protein oxidation below 35%, which is greater than the amount of protein required to maintain nitrogen balance, remains unanswered. Rogers and Morris (2002) commented on the problems with the interpretation of the data made by Russell *et al.* (2002). The inability of cats to conserve protein or nitrogen is due to their apparent high obligatory endogenous protein losses when compared to other mammals that are considered omnivorous. Alternatively, Lester *et al.* (1999) suggested that feline protein oxidation did not respond to manipulation of dietary protein intake when protein oxidation was measured and cats that were fed a high fat–intermediate protein diet were compared to cats that were fed a low fat–high protein diet. However, given that the entire macronutrient content of the diet changed, it is difficult to attribute the lack of difference in protein oxidation solely to differences in protein intake. Clearly, more sensitive whole-body techniques need to be employed to come to a better understanding of the control of protein oxidation in the cat and to be able to compare adequately whole-body results between species.

For adult dogs at maintenance, nitrogen balance studies have resulted in estimates of the crude protein requirement in diets containing 4.0 kcal metabolizable energy g^{-1} of between 35 and 90 g kg^{-1} (Wannemacher and McCoy, 1966). The high variability in previous examinations of the dietary crude protein requirement is likely due to differences in breed, body composition, diet ingredients used and the method of experimental design and statistical analyses. The Minimum Requirement for cats is based on a study by Burger *et al.* (1984) where 17 out of 18 cats attained positive nitrogen balance and the protein intake was calculated to be 160 g kg^{-1} diet that contained 4 kcal metabolizable energy g^{-1}. In both the cat and the rabbit, variation appears to be lower than in the dog (NRC, 1977, 2006);

however, there are very few estimates of the crude protein requirement in the cat and rabbit and the variation is likely misleading if the recommendation were to be applied across different breeds and sizes of cats and rabbits.

To further compound the variability within the population and the relative effects on requirement estimates, at least two things must be taken into account, namely, what the previous nutritional status of the animals used was and how that could have affected the animals' baseline response to the dietary treatments. Baseline protein, or amino acid status, has most often been unstated, unmeasured or unstandardized. It is only common sense that protein or amino acid supplementation is most likely to improve outcomes if you compare deficient to excess levels of protein and/or amino acids. However, recent data from Sanderson *et al.* (2001) suggested that, although mature beagles maintained body weight and otherwise normal blood biochemistries when receiving a diet containing 82 g kg^{-1} highly digestible crude protein and 4.0 kcal metabolizable energy g^{-1}, they had low plasma taurine concentrations despite the diet containing adequate taurine precursors, the indispensable amino acid methionine and the conditionally indispensable amino acid cyst(e)ine. Interestingly, when a group of privately owned Newfoundlands were examined for possible taurine deficiency, 12 of 19 dogs had low plasma taurine concentrations when fed a specific lamb and rice diet, suggesting a possible dietary total sulfur amino acid restriction (Backus *et al.*, 2003). When these dogs were given supplemental methionine, a taurine precursor, the taurine deficiency was corrected, which indicates that the inclusion level of methionine was inadequate. There are no AAFCO recommendations for taurine provision in dog foods, unlike cats, so this deficiency occurred despite the AAFCO recommendations having been met and dogs remaining apparently healthy throughout the feeding trial. These studies suggest significant differences in amino acid metabolism between dog breeds and possible influences of the protein source chosen, two areas that need further investigation. Although the need for taurine in cats is well accepted, possible breed and size differences and dietary composition have not been considered. Taurine concentrations in whole blood is used as an indication of taurine sufficiency for AAFCO (2005) feeding trials for cat food, who state that concentrations at the end of a feeding trial must not be below 200 nmol ml^{-1}. Further indices of amino acid sufficiency, such as whole-blood taurine concentrations, should be added to demonstrate dietary amino acid sufficiency in animals other than cats. Other indices that we feel may be valuable are plasma amino acid, ammonia, urea, nitric oxide and whole-blood glutathione concentrations, and numerous intermediates and products from amino acid metabolic pathways in both plasma and tissue. These data demonstrate the need for more sensitive and accurate estimates of *individual* amino acid requirements and a measure of the variability within and between different dog breeds for a particular diet to maintain not only protein status, but health status in free-living dogs, cats and rabbits.

Differences in amino acid requirements

The free amino acid requirements (NRC, 2006) as a percentage of crude protein are presented in Fig. 13.2 and do not reflect that the sum of the free total

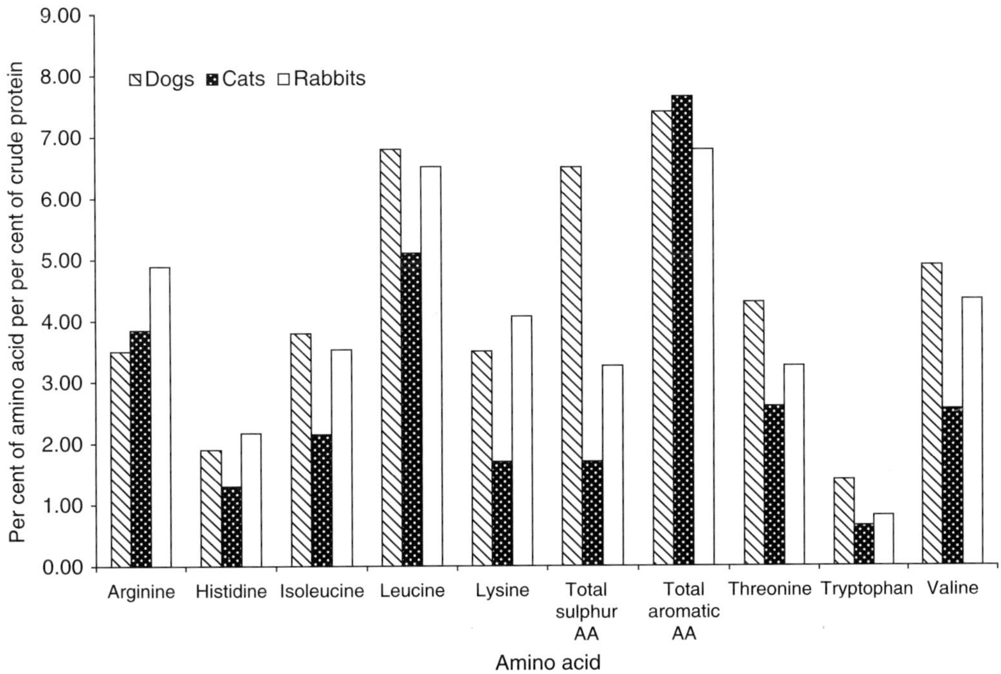

Fig. 13.2. Recommended amino acid supply represented as the per cent of free amino acid per per cent of recommended crude protein (total sulfur AA = methionine + cystine, total aromatic AA = phenylalanine + tyrosine).

indispensable amino acids recommended is 5.85, 4.4 and 5.15% of diet for cats, dogs and rabbits, respectively. It does not make sense why herbivores, namely rabbits, would have higher recommendations for indispensable amino acids and one must remember that the Recommended Allowances for cats and dogs (NRC, 2006) are based on high quality proteins, whereas those for the rabbit are not (NRC, 1977). Given the present recommendations, there is little difference in the percentage of arginine and histidine required as a percentage of crude protein, which is surprising considering that only the cat will respond with acute (~1 h post-feeding) hyperammonaemia due to receiving an arginine-free meal (MacDonald *et al.*, 1984). This is due to a limitation in arginine synthesis. Both dogs and rabbits will not respond as quickly to an arginine-free diet, as demonstrated by Czarnecki and Baker (1984). However, when recommendations are presented as a per cent of diet, cats do have a higher arginine requirement than dogs and rabbits. The indispensable amino acids (percentage of AA per percentage of CP) that are different between rabbits, dogs and cats include the following: (i) the lysine requirement is marginally greater in rabbits and dogs than in cats, likely due to the fact that lysine is commonly the first limiting amino acid in most plant sources that are included at a higher rate in omnivore and herbivore diets; (ii) the methionine + cysteine requirement (total sulfur amino acids) is greatest in dogs, intermediate in rabbits and lowest in cats; (iii) the phenylalanine + tyrosine (total aromatic amino acids) requirement is greatest in cats, intermediate in dogs and lowest in rabbits; (iv) the threonine requirement is greatest and similar in dogs and rabbits as compared to cats; and (v) the branched chain amino acid requirements are greater in dogs and rabbits, as compared to the cat. These amino acids will be discussed in further detail.

Despite the common belief that the total sulfur amino acid (TSAA) requirement is greater in cats than in omnivores or herbivores, the TSAA requirement is lowest in cats as compared to dogs and rabbits whether presented on a per cent protein basis or as a percentage of diet. The methionine + cyst(e)ine requirement was first thought to be greater in cats than in other animals because cats excrete felinine, a unique branched chain amino acid containing sulfur, in urine; however, Rogers (1963) initially showed that neither [^{35}S]methionine nor [^{35}S]cysteine was incorporated in felinine. Similarly, Roberts (1963) did not detect any radioactively labelled felinine after intravenously injecting [^{35}S]-cystine into a male cat; however, these data included an $n = 1$ and there are methodological problems to using [^{35}S]-cystine. Avizonis and Wriston (1959) found that cats that received supplemental dietary cystine had increased urinary felinine concentrations as compared to their unsupplemented counterparts, suggesting that dietary sulfur amino acid supply and urinary felinine were correlated. More recently, Hendriks *et al.* (2001) demonstrated that the incorporation rates of radioactivity into felinine by entire male cats ($n = 3$) receiving [^{35}S]-cysteine and [^{35}S]-methionine were 11.6 ± 1.6 and $8.6 \pm 0.6\%$, respectively, after 9 days. These data demonstrate that cysteine and methionine may both be precursors for felinine, and cysteine is quantitatively more important. Therefore, it is possible that the greater TSAA requirement is, in part, due to increased losses of the sulfur amino acids via felinine excretion in the urine. Further research where [^{35}S]-cysteine was administered to one entire male cat and urine was collected at 1, 4 and 8 h post-injection suggested that urine contains several other felinine-containing metabolites, including N-acetyl felinine, felinylglycine and unaltered γ-glutamylfelinylglycine. These results suggest that reported estimates may need to be increased by as much as 54%; however, resting conclusions on one entire male cat only indicates that further research is needed and neutered and spayed females should be investigated in light of the fact that they comprise the majority of our pet population. Indeed, free felinine concentrations in the urine have been found to be gender-dependent and are likely under hormonal control (Hendriks *et al.*, 1995; Rutherfurd *et al.*, 2002), further supporting the need to investigate whether differences in gender result in different estimates of amino acid requirements.

Very little methionine + cyst(e)ine is used for taurine synthesis in cats, which require the majority of their taurine supply preformed in the diet; therefore, taurine synthesis does not account for the greater requirement in cats (Morris and Rogers, 1992) and, in fact, this may in part explain the apparent lower TSAA requirement in cats that we observed in the present comparison. MacDonald *et al.* (1984) suggested that the increased requirement might be due to the additional sulfur needed for cats' dense fur; however, no one has investigated this using a hairless cat versus a domestic cat. Indeed, the mid-size hair growth rate of male and female domestic short-haired cats follows a sinusoidal pattern throughout the year, similar to day length and daily mean air temperature, with a maximum hair growth rate of 289 mg (cm^2 day)$^{-1}$ in the summer and a minimum hair growth rate of 62 mg (cm^2 day)$^{-1}$ in the winter (Hendriks *et al.*, 1997). It is likely that the seasonal differences in growth rate may also affect the TSAA requirement during the year, another area that requires investigation. MacDonald *et al.* (1984) also speculated that the requirement might be increased due to a higher demand in the first intermediate of methionine metabolism, S-adenosylmethionine. The methyl donating capacity of S-adenosylmethionine is involved in the production of many compounds, as well as an important mechanism to inactivate a number of active compounds such as catecholamines (phenylethanolamines, adrenaline, thymidine, lecithin and other compounds). Although methionine is a net donor of methyl groups, glycine and serine are quantitatively the largest methyl donors. The major use of methionine methyl groups is the formation of creatine from guanidinoacetate (Mudd and Poole, 1975) and methyl group donation for the formation of phosphatidylcholine from phosphatidylethanolamine has been shown (Noga *et al.*, 2003). However, these data are from experiments in the rat and should be compared cautiously to the cat as methyl donation in the cat may be different. Lastly, glutathione is a tripeptide of glycine, glutamate and cysteine and is mainly thought to protect red cells from oxidative damage. It is possible that glutathione synthesis is different in cats, which partially accounts for differences in the requirement for methionine + cyst(e)ine, but this question remains to be tested.

The phenylalanine + tyrosine requirement is higher in cats than in dogs and rabbits. The phenylalanine + tyrosine requirement for the cat was increased for the updated NRC (2006) due to data demonstrating that cats receiving less than 16 g kg^{-1} of diet (1.63% of diet) showed neurological and behavioural abnormalities, including vocalization, abnormal posture and gait and changes in coat colour (Dickinson *et al.*, 2004). Therefore, the minimum requirement for cats was increased to 1.53% of diet when 4 kcal ME g^{-1} was supplied. Thus, the maintenance of neurological and coat health in the cat requires a greater amount of phenylalanine and tyrosine than that which is supplied to dogs and rabbits.

The threonine requirement in rabbits, as a per cent of CP, is higher than in cats and dogs, although why is not as clear. De Blas *et al.* (1998) demonstrated that rabbit does fed 5.4 g kg^{-1} threonine had lower milk production than rabbit does fed 7.2 g kg^{-1}. These researchers concluded that adult does required a minimum of 6.4 g kg^{-1} diet; however, the reason for choosing this specific level was not apparent. Another aspect to consider is that threonine is a major component of mucins and diets that increase mucin production, such as those higher in fibre content, are related to decreased retention of threonine due to increased endogenous losses (Myrie *et al.*, 2003). It is therefore reasonable to assume that rabbits, due to the fibrous nature of their diets, require more threonine than cats and dogs, whose diets are substantially lower in fibre content.

Cats and dogs have a greater requirement than rabbits for the branched chain amino acids: leucine, valine and isoleucine. The reasons for this are unclear. The branched chain amino acids are considered together because they have a common enzyme initiating their catabolism, branched chain α-keto acid dehydrogenase kinase, which leucine is known to regulate. Consequently, the ratio of the three is similar between the NRC (2006) and AAFCO (2005) recommendations. In addition, this apparently high requirement is of little concern because the branched chain amino acids are rarely limiting in normal diet formulations; therefore, the minimum requirement of these three amino acids is easily met in diets formulated for either cats or dogs.

The effects of dietary protein inclusion

Another possible outcome parameter that has received a lot of attention has been the effect of dietary protein level on maintenance of lean body mass in dogs. The maintenance of whole-body protein mass and, more specifically, skeletal muscle mass represents the difference between protein synthesis and degradation (Fig. 13.1). In the adult dog, a balance between protein synthesis and degradation is what maintains body protein mass and this has been the focus of some current research in light of the interest in incipient muscle wasting in geriatric populations. The 'metabolic pool' represents amino acids derived from the diet or protein breakdown and it is the relative size of the metabolic pool that controls the fate of the amino acids, namely incorporation into body protein or catabolism (Fig. 13.1). In the normal healthy adult dog receiving adequate dietary amino acids, the difference between protein synthesis and breakdown is equal and body lean mass is maintained. If we revisit the nitrogen balance concept here, maintenance of lean body mass and a constant intake of dietary indispensable amino acid intake would mean that there is no change in nitrogen balance.

Wakshlag *et al.* (2003) compared lean body mass changes in dogs fed diets containing either 12 or 28% protein diets over 10 weeks. While the 12% diets met the published requirement for protein per se (NRC, 1985), the requirements for individual indispensable amino acids were not met and, in the most severe case, one 12% CP treatment contained 28% of the recommended dietary lysine and, as such, produced the largest decrease in lean body mass as compared to initial body mass. In this case, the limitation of dietary lysine would have limited protein synthesis and the other amino acids would be broken down, with the carbon backbone of those amino acids entering the TCA cycle for oxidation as an energy source or being converted to stored energy, and thus being deposited as fat. Wakshlag *et al.* (2003) consequently demonstrated that, where there was significant loss of lean body mass due to protein inadequacy or amino acid imbalance at the fundamental level of metabolic control, this was associated with decreased expression of the p31 subunit of the 26S proteasome, resulting in a shift towards lipogenesis and a consequent increase in fat mass and decrease in skeletal muscle protein breakdown in an attempt to conserve body protein. Protein or nitrogen balance primarily reflects the difference between protein synthesis and protein degradation and, in this case, the limitation in total protein synthesis was compromised to a greater extent than protein degradation, resulting in a loss of lean body mass. Increases in dietary protein (16, 24, or 32%), as assessed using a ^{15}N-glycine tracer, resulted in a quadratic response in whole-body protein synthesis and breakdown, but no significant difference in nitrogen balance in adult beagles

(Williams *et al.*, 2001). When the levels of individual indispensable amino acids in the diets used in this study were examined, only one diet contained limiting amino acids, and only at a moderate level; therefore, as the dietary crude protein was increased and amino acids were provided in excess of the requirement, whole-body protein synthesis and breakdown were both increased and this resulted in a correlation between protein intake and protein turnover, leading to a higher rate of urinary excretion and no difference in nitrogen balance (Williams *et al.*, 2001). Similarly, Humbert *et al.* (2001) fed adult dogs a control, protein deficient and protein–lysine–tryptophan deficient diet in random order, each being fed over a 2-week period. At the end of each 2-week feeding period, a ^{13}C-leucine tracer study was conducted. When dogs were fed a protein deficient diet, they had significantly lower rates of both protein synthesis and oxidation than the control group, but, when dogs were fed the protein–lysine–tryptophan deficient diets, they produced the lowest rates of both protein synthesis and oxidation (Humbert *et al.*, 2001). Further examination of the effects of protein source on protein kinetics demonstrated that dogs fed a diet containing a higher percentage of chicken protein than dogs receiving a higher percentage of maize gluten meal had a greater potential to regulate calpain-mediated degradation of protein (Helman *et al.*, 2003). These data clearly show that an individual limitation in an indispensable amino acid produces profound changes in lean body mass and these decreases in lean body mass are positively correlated with increases in fat mass due to the repartitioning of the carbon skeletons of other amino acids away from protein synthesis and towards fat deposition. To our knowledge, no similar data are available for cats or rabbits. Data examining lean tissue maintenance in cats would be especially interesting, considering their dependence on high protein diets.

It is important to note at this stage that these protein turnover rates are represented as a percentage of body weight, which is a potential source of bias. When comparing animals with different body composition, whether due to breed, sex or age, these values must be compared as a percentage of lean mass rather than body weight. For example, Morais *et al.* (1997) found no differences between old and young men when measurements of whole-body protein synthesis and degradation rates were compared as a percentage of lean body mass, but there were significant differences when these values were compared as percentage of body weight. Therefore, it would be more applicable to represent protein and amino acid requirements as a percentage of lean body mass rather than body mass, especially in light of the potential variation in this respect between breeds and the prevalence of obesity in the pet population (Crane, 1991).

Conclusions

Protein and, more importantly, amino acids are necessary in the diet of all pets, whether they are defined as herbivores, omnivores or carnivores. Both the amount of protein in a given ingredient and the ratio of the amino acids need to be considered when providing different protein sources. Although there is adequate information from growing animals, there is limited information from adult animals and, considering that adult pets comprise the majority of our pet population, it is important to continue to investigate amino acid requirements and bioavailability using sensitive, minimally invasive techniques. This knowledge will bring us to a better understanding of animals at maintenance, but will allow us a starting point for comparison when we begin to examine the effects of other nutrients and physiological and/or disease states on amino acid requirements.

References

Arnold, G.L., Kirby, R., Presto, C. and Blakely, E. (2001) Iron and protein sufficiency and red cell indices in phenylketonuria. *Journal of the American College of Nutrition* 20, 65–70.

Association of American Feed Control Officials (AAFCO) (2005) *AAFCO Manual*. AAFCO, Inc., Minnesota.

Avizonis, P.V. and Wriston, J.C. (1959) On the biosynthesis of felinine. *Biochimica et Biophysica Acta* 34, 279–281.

Backus, R.C., Cohen, G., Pion, P.D., Good, K.L., Rogers, Q.L. and Fascetti, A.J. (2003) Taurine deficiency in Newfoundlands fed commercially available complete and balanced diets. *Journal of the American Veterinary Medical Association* 223, 1130–1136.

Baker, D.H. (1986) Problems and pitfalls in animal experiments designed to establish dietary requirements for essential nutrients. *Journal of Nutrition* 116, 2339–2349.

Blas, J.C. de, Taboada, E., Nicodemus, N., Campos, R., Piquer, J. and Mendez, J. (1998) Performance response of lactating and growing rabbits to dietary threonine content. *Animal Feed Science and Technology* 70, 151–160.

Brunton, J.A, Pencharz, P.B. and Ball, R.O. (2000) Current total parenteral nutrition solutions for the neonate are inadequate. *Current Opinion in Clinical Nutrition and Metabolic Care* 3, 299–304.

Brunton, J.A, Shoveller, A.K., Brand, O., Pencharz, P.B. and Ball, R.O. (2003) Identification of limiting amino acids in parenteral solutions (TPN) by indicator amino acid oxidation. *FASEB Journal* 17, A702 Part 1 Supplement S.

Burger, I.H. and Smith, P.M. (1987) Amino acid requirements of adult cats. In: Edney, A.T.B. (ed.) *Nutrition, Malnutrition and Dietetics in the Dog and Cat, Proceedings of an International Symposium held in Hannover*. British Veterinary Association, London, pp. 49–51.

Burger, I.H., Blaza, S.E., Kendall, P.T. and Smith, P.M. (1984) The protein requirement of adult cats for maintenance. *Feline Practice* 14, 8–14.

Case, L.P., Carey, D.P., Hirakawa, D.A. and Daristotle, L. (2000) Protein and amino acids. In: *Canine and Feline Nutrition, 2nd edn*. Mosby, Inc., Toronto, Canada, pp. 99–116.

Cheeke, P.R. (1987) *Rabbit Feeding and Nutrition*. Academic Press, New York.

Crane, S.E. (1991) Occurrence and management of obesity in companion animals. *The Journal of Small Animal Practice* 32, 275–282.

Crim, M.C. and Munro, H.N. (1994) Proteins and amino acids. In: Shils, M.E., Olson, J.A. and Shike, M. (eds) *Modern Nutrition in Health and Disease*, 8th edn. Lea and Febiger, Philadelphia, Pennsylvania, pp. 3–35.

Czarnecki, G.L. and Baker, D.H. (1984) Urea cycle function in the dog with emphasis on the role of arginine. *Journal of Nutrition* 114, 581–590.

Dickinson, P.J., Anderson, P.J., Williams, D.C., Powell, H.C., Shelton, G.D., Morris, J.G. and LeCouteur, R.A. (2004) Assessment of the neurological effects of dietary deficiencies of phenylalanine and tyrosine in cats. *American Journal of Veterinary Research* 65, 671–680.

Helman, E.E., Huff-Lonergan, E., Davenport, G.M. and Lonergan, S.M. (2003) Effect of dietary protein on calpastatin in canine skeletal muscle. *Journal of Animal Science* 81, 2199–2205.

Hendriks, W.H., Tarttelin, M.F. and Moughan, P.J. (1995) Twenty-four hour felinine excretion patterns in entire and castrated cats. *Physiology and Behaviour* 58, 467–469.

Hendriks, W.H., Tarttelin, M.F. and Moughan, P.J. (1997) Seasonal hair growth in the adult domestic cat (*Felis catus*). *Comparative Biochemistry and Physiology* 116A, 29–35.

Hendriks, W.H., Emmens, M.M.A., Trass, B. and Pluske, J.R. (1999) Heat processing changes the protein quality of canned cat foods as measured with a rat bioassay. *Journal of Animal Science* 77, 669–676.

Hendriks, W.H., Rutherfurd, S.M. and Rutherfurd, K.J. (2001) Importance of sulfate, cysteine and methionine as precursors to felinine synthesis by domestic cats (*Felis catus*). *Comparative Biochemistry and Physiology. Toxicology and Pharmacology* 129, 211–216.

Humbert, B., Bleis, P., Martin, L., Dumon, D. and Nguyen, P. (2001) Effects of dietary protein restriction and amino acid deficiency on protein metabolism in dogs. *Journal of Animal Physiology and Animal Nutrition* 85, 255–261.

Kim, K.I., McMillan, I. and Bayley, H.S. (1983) Determination of amino acid requirements of young pigs using an indicator amino acid. *British Journal of Nutrition* 50, 369–382.

Kurpad, A.V., Raj, T., el-Khoury, A.E., Beaumier, L., Kuriyan, R., Srivasta, A., Borgonha, S., Selvaraj, A., Regan, M.M. and Young, V.R. (2001) Lysine requirements of healthy adult Indian subjects, measured by an indicator amino acid balance technique. *American Journal of Clinical Nutrition* 73, 900–907.

Lebas, F. (1988) Rabbits. In: De Boer, F. and Bickel, H. (eds) *Livestock Feed Resources and Feed Evaluation in Europe*. Elsevier, Amsterdam, pp. 289–298.

Lester, T., Czarnecki-Maulden, G. and Lewis, D. (1999) Cats increase fatty acid oxidation when isocalorically fed meat-based diets with increasing fat content. *American Journal of Physiology* 277, R878–R886.

MacDonald, M.L., Rogers, Q.R. and Morris, J.G. (1984) Nutrition of the domestic cat, a mammalian carnivore. *Annual Review of Nutrition* 4, 521–562.

McLarney, M.J., Pellett, P.L. and Young, V.R. (1996) Pattern of amino acid requirements in humans: an interspecies comparison using published amino acid recommendations. *Journal of Nutrition* 126, 1871–1882.

Metges, C.C. (2000) Contribution of microbial amino acids to amino acid homeostasis of the host. *Journal of Nutrition* 130, 1857S–1864S.

Millward, D.J., Price, G.M., Pacy, P.J.H. and Halliday, D. (1990) Maintenance protein requirements: the need for conceptual re-evaluation. *Proceedings of the Nutrition Society* 49, 473–487.

Moehn, S., Bertolo, R.F.P, Pencharz, P.B. and Ball, R.O. (2004) Indicator amino acid oxidation responds rapidly to changes in lysine or protein intake in growing and adult pigs. *Journal of Nutrition* 134, 836–841.

Moehn, S., Bertolo, R.F., Pencharz, P.B. and Ball, R.O. (2005) Development of the indicator amino acid oxidation technique to determine the availability of amino acids from dietary protein in pigs. *Journal of Nutrition* 135, 2866–2870.

Morais, J.A., Gougeon, R., Pencharz, P.B., Jones, P.J.H., Ross, R. and Marliss, G.B. (1997) Whole body protein turnover in the healthy elderly. *American Journal of Clinical Nutrition* 66, 880–889.

Morley, J.J. and Kushner, J. (1982) Serum C-reactive protein levels in disease. *Annals of the New York Academy of Science* 389, 406–418.

Morris, J.G. and Rogers, Q.R. (1992) The metabolic basis for the taurine requirement of cats. In: Lombardine, J.B., Schaeffer, S.W. and Azuma, J. (eds) *Taurine: Nutritional Value and Mechanisms of Action. Advances in Experimental Medicine and Biology 315*. Plenum Press, New York, pp. 33–44.

Morris, J.G. and Rogers, Q.R. (1994) Assessment of the nutritional adequacy of pet foods through the life cycle. *Journal of Nutrition* 124, 2520S–2534S.

Moughan, P.J. (2003) Simulating the partitioning of dietary amino acids: new directions. *Journal of Animal Science* 81 (Supplement 2), E60–E67.

Mudd, S.H. and Poole, J.R. (1975) Labile methyl balances for normal humans on various dietary regimens. *Metabolism* 24, 721–735.

Myrie, S.B., Bertolo, R.F.P., Sauer, W.C. and Ball, R.O. (2003) Diets that increase mucin production in pigs reduce threonine and amino acid retention. *Advances in Pork Production* 14, Abstract No. 9.

National Research Council (NRC) (1977) *Nutrient Requirements of Rabbits*. National Academy Press, Washington, DC.

National Research Council (NRC) (1985) *Nutrient Requirements of Dogs and Cats*. National Academy Press, Washington, DC.

National Research Council (NRC) (2006) *Nutrient Requirements of Dogs and Cats*. National Academy Press, Washington, DC.

Noga, A.A., Stead, L.M., Zhao, Y., Brosnan, M.E., Brosnan, J.T. and Vance, D.E. (2003) Plasma homocysteine is regulated by phospholipid methylation. *Journal of Biological Chemistry* 278, 5952–5955.

Pencharz, P.B. and Ball, R.O. (2003) Different approaches to define individual amino acid requirements. *Annual Review of Nutrition* 23, 101–116.

Pencharz, P.B., House, J.D., Wykes, L.J. and Ball, R.O. (1996) What are the essential amino acids for the preterm and term infant? In: *10th International Nutrition Symposium*. Kluwer, Dordrecht, The Netherlands, pp. 278–296.

Roberts, R.N. (1963) A study of felinine and its excretion by the cat. PhD thesis, State University of New York, Buffalo, New York.

Rogers, Q.R. (1963) A study of felinine and its excretion in the cat. PhD thesis, State University of New York, Buffalo, New York.

Rogers, Q.R. and Morris J.G. (2002) Up-regulation of nitrogen catabolic enzymes is not required to readily oxidize excess protein in cats. *Journal of Nutrition* 132, 2819–2820.

Rogers, Q.R., Morris, J.G. and Freedland, R.A. (1977) Lack of hepatic enzyme adaptation to low and high levels of dietary protein in the adult cat. *Enzyme* 22, 348–356.

Russell, K., Murgatroyd, P.R. and Batt, R.M. (2002) Net protein oxidation is adapted to dietary protein intake in domestic cats (*Felis silvestris catus*). *Journal of Nutrition* 132, 456–460.

Rutherfurd, K.J., Rutherfurd, S.M., Moughan, P.J. and Hendriks, W.H. (2002) Isolation and characterization of a felinine containing peptide from the blood of the domestic cat (*Felis catus*). *Journal of Biological Chemistry* 277, 114–119.

Sanderson, S.L., Gross, K.L., Ogburn, P.N., Calvert, C., Jacobs, G., Lowry, S.R., Bird, K.A., Koehler, L.A. and Swanson, L.L. (2001) Effects of dietary fat and L-carnitine on plasma and whole blood taurine concentrations and cardiac function in healthy dogs fed protein-restricted diets. *American Journal of Veterinary Science* 62, 1616–1623.

Tabiri, H.Y., Bertolo, R.F., Ball, R.O. and Korver, D.R. (2002) Development of the indicator amino acid oxidation technique in chickens: L-[1-^{14} C]phenylalanine infusion dose and phenylalanine oxidation. *Poultry Science* 81, 1516–1521.

Wakshlag, J.J., Barr, S.C., Ordway, G.A., Kallfelz, F.A., Flaherty, C.E., Christensen, B.W., Shepard, L.A., Nydam, D.V. and Davenport, G.M. (2003) Effect of dietary protein on lean body wasting in dogs: correlation between loss of lean mass and markers of proteasome-dependent proteolysis. *Journal of Animal Physiology and Animal Nutrition* 87, 408–420.

Wannemacher, R.W. and McCoy, J.R. (1966) Determination of optimal dietary protein requirements of young and old dogs. *Journal of Nutrition* 88, 66–74.

Waterlow, J.C. (1994) Emerging aspects of amino acid metabolism: where do we go from here? *Journal of Nutrition* 124, 1524S–1528S.

Williams, C.C., Cummins, K.A., Hayek, M.G. and Davenport G.M. (2001) Effects of dietary protein on whole-body protein turnover and endocrine function in young-adult and aging dogs. *Journal of Animal Science* 79, 3128–3136.

Young, V.R. (1987) McCollum Award Lecture: Kinetics of human amino acid metabolism: nutritional implications and some lessons. *American Journal of Clinical Nutrition* 46, 709–725.

Young, V.R. and Marchini, J.S. (1990) Mechanisms and nutritional significance of metabolic responses to altered intakes of protein and amino acids, with reference to nutritional adaptation in humans. *American Journal of Clinical Nutrition* 51, 270–289.

Zello, G.A., Wykes, L.J., Ball, R.O. and Pencharz, P.B. (1995) Recent advances in methods of assessing dietary amino acid requirements for adult humans. *Journal of Nutrition* 125, 2907–2915.

14 Mathematical Representation of the Partitioning of Retained Energy in the Growing Pig

C.F.M. de Lange,[1] P.C.H. Morel[2] and S.H. Birkett[3]

[1]*Centre for Nutrition Modelling, Department of Animal and Poultry Science, University of Guelph, Canada;* [2]*Institute of Food, Nutrition and Human Health, Massey University, New Zealand;* [3]*Department of Systems Design Engineering, University of Waterloo, Canada*

Introduction

In the growing pig body, energy is retained primarily in the form of body protein deposition (Pd) and body lipid deposition (Ld), which are closely associated with muscle and fat tissue growth, respectively. A mathematical representation of animal, feed and environmental factors that control or influence Pd and Ld is extremely useful for the manipulation of body composition and nutrient utilization efficiency in growing–finishing pigs. In previous reviews, the material and energetic efficiencies of converting dietary protein and energy-yielding nutrients to Pd and Ld in pigs have been discussed extensively (Black *et al.*, 1986; Moughan, 1999; Birkett and de Lange, 2001a,b,c; Whittemore *et al.*, 2001; van Milgen and Noblet, 2003). The focus of this review is the assessment of calculation rules to represent the partitioning of retained energy between Pd and Ld when Pd is driven by energy intake. During this energy-dependent phase, Pd is not limited by the animals' upper limit to Pd or the intake of balanced protein. In modern pig genotypes with improved lean tissue growth potentials, energy intake will drive Pd for most of the growing–finishing period.

Basic Principles of Nutrient Utilization for Body Protein and Body Lipid Deposition

Six basic principles are required to define a framework for the detailed assessment of partitioning of retained energy between Ld and Pd. Some of these principles may be considered conceptual, but they are based on extensive experimental evidence and allow for a simplified, quantitative and flexible representation of the complex biological processes that determine growth in different pig types and under varying conditions. The six basic principles are:

1. Among nutritional factors, Pd and Ld are influenced by intake of energy-yielding nutrients (starch, sugars, other carbohydrates, fat, protein) and balanced protein only (NRC, 1998; Moughan, 1999; Whittemore *et al.*, 2001; van Milgen and Noblet, 2003). Balanced protein reflects the dietary supply of the first limiting essential amino acid or total nitrogen when the intake of nitrogen is insufficient to cover needs for endogenous synthesis of non-essential amino acids.
2. Growing pigs have an upper limit to daily Pd (Pdmax) (Black *et al.*, 1986; Emmans and Kyriazakis, 1997; Moughan, 1999; Whittemore and Green, 2002). This Pdmax represents the maximum difference between body protein synthesis and body protein degradation and is ultimately determined by the pig's genotype. The expression of Pdmax will be influenced by environmental factors, such as the presence of pathogens, social interactions among pigs housed in groups, the thermal environment and nutrient intake. The pig's Pdmax varies with stage of maturity; in pigs approaching maturity, Pdmax will decline towards zero. There is still uncertainty about the relationship between body weight (BW) and Pdmax in young growing pigs before they start to mature. One view is that Pdmax is best represented by a sigmoidal relationship between body protein mass (P) and time (Black *et al.*, 1986; Emmans and Kyriazakis, 1997), implying that Pdmax increases with P until the inflexion point in the P growth curve is reached. An alternative view is that Pdmax is constant and independent of BW and P until pigs start to mature (Moughan, 1999). Based on a careful review of the literature, Whittemore and Green (2002) concluded that the concept of a Pdmax that was independent of BW and P in young growing pigs could not be rejected. In this review, it will be assumed that Pdmax is constant and independent of BW and P in pigs between 20 kg BW and until they start to mature.
3. The pig's desired feed intake is determined by nutrient needs for the various body functions, including expression of Pdmax and a desired Ld and body maintenance functions (Black *et al.*, 1986; Emmans and Kyriazakis, 1997; Nyachoti *et al.*, 2004). The first priority is to satisfy nutrient needs for body functions that are not related to Pd and Ld (Birkett and de Lange, 2001a,b,c), while energy intake above requirements for expression of Pdmax will all be used for Ld only. It is implied that pigs have a desire to express Pdmax and some target Ld. The realized feed intake of pigs is determined by various constraints, such as the pigs' physical feed intake and digestive capacity, maximum body heat loss, feed availability and feed palatability.
4. Dietary intakes of balanced protein and energy-yielding nutrients have independent effects on Pd (Campbell *et al.*, 1985; Möhn *et al.*, 2000). During the energy-dependent phase of Pd, the intake of the first limiting dietary amino acid does not influence Pd, and vice versa. This principle is supported by experimental observations such as those presented in Fig. 14.1.
5. There is maximum marginal efficiency of using metabolically available balanced protein intake for Pd, which is constant and independent of BW and pig type (e.g. Batterham *et al.*, 1990; Fuller *et al.*, 1995; Ferguson and Gous, 1997). The maximum efficiency of balanced protein utilization is a reflection of minimum

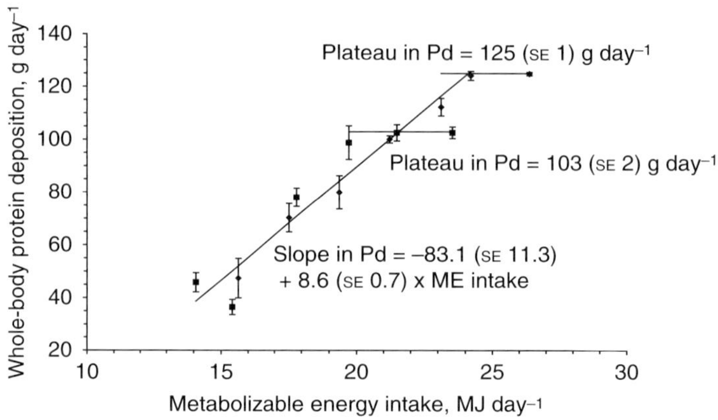

Fig. 14.1. Relationship between whole-body protein deposition (Pd) and metabolizable energy (ME) intake in growing pigs at available lysine intakes of either 11.7 (■) or 13.5 (◆) g day^{-1} (derived from Möhn *et al.*, 2000).

plus inevitable amino acid catabolism (Moughan, 1999) and varies slightly depending on which of the essential amino acids is first limiting in the diet (Heger *et al.*, 2002).

6. The marginal energetic efficiencies of utilizing dietary nutrients for Pd and Ld are not influenced by BW and pig type, but by dietary nutrient source (e.g. Birkett and de Lange, 2001a,b,c; Green and Whittemore, 2003).

These six principles are sufficient to predict marginal Pd and marginal Ld response of pigs to changing intakes of available energy or available amino acids, except when energy intake determines Pd. In this situation, some rules are needed to represent the partitioning of retained energy between Pd and Ld. For prediction of absolute Pd and Ld responses, estimates of maintenance nutrient requirements are needed.

Experimental Observations

Relatively few well-controlled studies have been conducted to relate Pd and Ld to energy intake of growing pigs during the energy-dependent phase of Pd, while even fewer studies have been conducted aimed at evaluating the impact of pig genotype, BW, nutritional history and environmental conditions on these relationships. However, in modern pig genotypes, Pdmax is not expressed, even at close to *ad libitum* feed intakes of diets that do not appear to be limiting in essential amino acids (Campbell and Taverner, 1988; Rao and MacCracken, 1991; de Greef *et al.*, 1994; Bikker *et al.*, 1995, 1996a,b; Weis *et al.*, 2004). This highlights the need for an accurate mathematical representation of the partitioning of retained body energy between Pd and Ld during the energy-dependent phase of Pd for manipulating growth and nutrient utilization in the pig.

Studies involving five or more energy intake levels and in which amino acid intake was unlikely to limit Pd indicate a highly linear relationship between energy intake and Pd (Close *et al.*, 1983; Dunkin and Black, 1987; Campbell and Taverner, 1988; Dunkin, 1990; Bikker *et al.*, 1995; Möhn *et al.*, 2000; Fig. 14.1). These studies indicate that both Ld and Pd in growing pigs increase with energy intake level and that the maximum efficiency of balanced protein utilization is not achieved during the energy-dependent phase of Pd. Apparently, some amino acids are preferentially catabolized to provide energy to support Ld during the energy-dependent phase of Pd (Moughan, 1999). Clearly, some mechanism exists that governs the partitioning of retained energy between Pd and Ld that is not reflected in the basic principles that were presented in the previous section.

By mathematical extrapolation of the linear relationships between energy intake and Pd or Ld to maintenance energy intake levels, and when body energy retention is zero, pigs appear to mobilize body lipid to support Pd. This extrapolation is consistent with the experimental observations of negative or zero Ld and positive Pd following a sudden and substantial drop in energy intake in young growing pigs (Close *et al.*, 1983; Kyriazakis and Emmans, 1992a; Bikker *et al.*, 1995). Obviously, pigs cannot sustain continued negative Ld to support Pd at low energy intake levels. Therefore, some time after pigs are kept at their maintenance energy intake levels, body fatness is reduced to a new equilibrium or minimum body fatness (minL/P), at which time both Pd and Ld must become zero. No direct estimates of minL/P have been made (Green and Whittemore, 2003), but it may be as low as 0.10 according to Wellock *et al.* (2003). These observations indicate that the composition of growth (Ld/Pd) varies with energy intake level and that pigs will increase in fatness with increasing energy intake level, even during the energy-dependent phase of Pd. This is supported by experimental observations, such as those reported by Bikker *et al.* (1995), who measured the composition of growth and body composition in growing gilts exposed to five levels of energy intake between 20 and 45 kg BW (Table 14.1).

Based on N-balance studies, the marginal response of Pd to increasing energy intake level (slope in Pd) is reduced with increasing BW (Dunkin and Black, 1987; Dunkin, 1990; Quiniou *et al.*, 1995; Bikker *et al.*, 1996a,b; Möhn and de Lange, 1998; Weis *et al.*, 2004; Fig. 14.2). This indicates that pigs get fatter with increasing BW, even during the energy-dependent phase of Pd. It should be noted that Sandberg *et al.* (2005b) recently argued that there was no BW effect on the slope in Pd, based on alternative interpretations of data such as those from Quiniou *et al.* (1995). Sandberg *et al.* (2005a,b) argued that the use of a constant slope in Pd across the four BW (45, 65, 80 and 94 kg) yielded an equally good fit to the data of Quiniou *et al.* (1995), as compared with a statistical model where the slope was allowed to vary with BW. However, the interpretation of observations by Quiniou *et al.* (1995) – as well as those by Möhn and de Lange (1998) and Möhn *et al.* (2000) – is influenced substantially by the lower slope in Pd at the lowest BW, as compared to those at higher BW. These observations reflect a higher Pd when energy intake is first reduced, apparently until a new equilibrium L/P is achieved. Eliminating the first N-balance periods from these data sets yields a better defined effect of BW on the slope in Pd in

Table 14.1. Whole-body protein deposition (Pd), whole-body lipid deposition (Ld), as well as composition of growth (Ld/Pd) and the whole-body lipid to whole-body protein ratio at final body weight (L/P) in growing gilts exposed to six levels of digestible energy (DE) intake between 20 and 45 kg live body weight.[a]

	Energy intake, fraction of maintenance energy						Pooled	Effects of
	1.7	2.2	2.7	3.2	3.7	Ad lib	SEM	DE intake
DE intake, MJ day^{-1}	11.3	14.1	17.4	20.5	23.8	27.2	0.57	–
Pd, g day^{-1}	75.3	98.8	113	134	160	172	4.95	L[b]
Ld, g day^{-1}	28.1	49.5	96.9	131	142	193	11.9	L[b]
Ld/Pd	0.32	0.52	0.87	0.98	0.89	1.13	0.089	L[b]
L/P[c]	0.42	0.55	0.74	0.81	0.76	0.87	–[c]	–[c]

[a]Derived from Bikker *et al.* (1995).
[b]Linear effect of daily DE intake ($P < 0.001$), while quadratic effects were not observed ($P > 0.10$).
[c]Values were calculated from whole-body protein mass and whole-body lipid mass data presented by Bikker *et al.* (1995) and not analysed statistically.

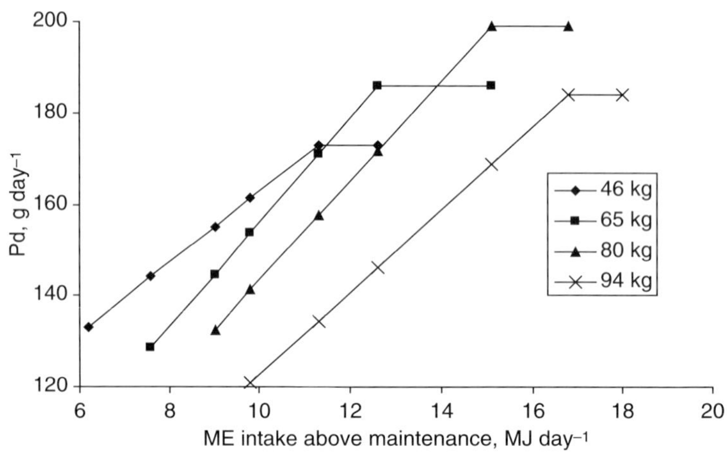

Fig. 14.2. Whole-body protein deposition (Pd) derived from N-balance measurements as influenced by metabolizable energy (ME) intake over maintenance at four stages of growth (46, 65, 80 and 94 kg body weight) in growing boars (derived from Quiniou *et al.*, 1995).

these studies. For example, based on N-balance observations, Möhn and de Lange (1998) reported slopes in Pd of 7.7 and 6.0 (SEM 0.6) g MJ^{-1} digestible energy (DE) intake in Yorkshire gilts at 40 and 70 kg BW, respectively. Finally, decreases in the slope of Pd with increasing BW are consistent with the increase in L/P with BW observed in serial slaughter studies and when pigs were in the energy-dependent phase of Pd (e.g. de Greef *et al.*, 1994).

Across studies, the slope in Pd during the energy-dependent phase appears to vary between pig genotypes (Möhn and de Lange, 1998). Moreover, when slopes in Pd were established for different genotypes within studies, clear genotype effects were also observed. For example, based on N-balance observations, Quiniou *et al.* (1996) observed slopes of 6.0, 4.0 and 3.4 g MJ^{-1} metabolizable energy (ME) intake for entire males and castrates of Large White × Pietrain crosses and castrates of a Large White line of pigs. Because of BW effects on the slope in Pd, pig genotype effects on slopes in Pd are likely to increase with BW. The latter may explain why Kyriazakis *et al.* (1994) observed such high values for slopes in Pd that did not differ between a cross of Large White × Landrace and Chinese Meisham pigs in a serial slaughter study conducted between 13 kg and about 25 kg (Meisham) or about 36 kg (Large White × Landrace) BW: 9.93 (SE 2.55) and 9.65 (SE 0.16), respectively. Moreover, in the study of Kyriazakis *et al.* (1994), pig type and BW effects were somewhat confounded.

In some studies, effects of nutritional history on Ld/Pd have been observed (Kyriazakis *et al.*, 1991; de Greef *et al.*, 1992; Bikker *et al.* 1996b), while no effects have been observed in other studies (Hogberg and Zimmerman, 1978; Martinez and de Lange, 2004). For example, in young growing pigs with high Pdmax and following a period of protein intake restriction, Pd was higher and the Ld/Pd was lower, as compared to control animals that were not subjected to previous protein intake restriction (Kyriazakis *et al.*, 1991). This catch-up or compensatory Pd following a period of balanced protein intake restriction influences the Pd response to energy intake during the energy-dependent phase of Pd and may also be related to minL/P. It is of interest to note that, following a period of compensatory Pd, L/P was similar for pigs that were previously fed protein-limiting or protein-adequate diets in the study by Kyriazakis *et al.* (1991). However, in that study, pigs were fed *ad libitum* during and after the period of balanced protein intake restriction, which complicates the interpretation of relationships between Pd and energy intake. In recent studies conducted at the University of Guelph, and when entire male pigs were scale-fed controlled levels of energy intake during and after a period of balanced protein intake restriction, complete compensatory Pd was achieved and body composition (L/P) at the final BW was identical to pigs that were scale-fed non-limiting diets (Martinez and de Lange, 2004; Martinez, 2005). In these studies, and based on N-balance observations, Pd was not dependent on BW in pigs that showed compensatory Pd, while Pd increased with BW in the control pigs. These observations provide some support that Pdmax is not related to BW or P in young growing pigs and indicate that compensatory Pd is more likely to occur during the energy-dependent phase of Pd. Moreover, induced increases in L/P due to amino acid intake restriction, as compared to L/P in control animals that were fed amino acid-adequate diets, were associated with increased plasma leptin levels. Observed differences in plasma leptin levels between these two groups of pigs diminished with increasing BW and when pigs expressed compensatory Pd (Martinez and de Lange, 2005), suggesting some physiological mechanisms whereby pigs can sense and control body composition (Houseknecht *et al.*, 1998; Horvath *et al.*, 2004). Such observation supports the presence of a causal link between body composition and nutrient partitioning that may be represented mathematically.

Unfortunately, insufficient solid information is available about the impact of environmental stresses on the partitioning of retained energy between Pd and Ld (Black *et al.*, 1995). It has, however, been suggested that environmental stresses such as exposure to pathogens will reduce the slope in Pd (Black *et al.*, 1995; Williams *et al.*, 1997).

Mathematical Representations

A variety of approaches have been used to represent mathematically the partitioning of retained energy between Pd and Ld during the energy-dependent phase of Pd in growing pigs. These approaches include constraints on Ld/Pd (minLd/Pd; Whittemore and Fawcett, 1976), empirical relationships between Pd and energy intake (Black *et al.*, 1986; NRC, 1998), direct effects of energy intake or dietary energy to protein ratios on the efficiency of using available balanced protein intake for Pd (Fuller and Crofts, 1977; Kyriazakis and Emmans, 1992a,b), or constraints on L/P (minL/P; Moughan *et al.*, 1987; de Lange, 1995; Whittemore, 1995). In approaches based on empirical relationships between Pd and energy intake or direct control of the efficiency of using available balanced protein intake for Pd, energy intake that is not used for Pd or body maintenance functions is used for Ld. In addition, Halas *et al.* (2004) recently attempted to represent energy utilization in the growing pig based on biochemical principles, and saturation kinetics in particular. Some of these approaches have been refined further, for example by applying constraints to the ratio of marginal Ld to marginal Pd (minδLd/δPd; de Greef and Verstegen, 1995), or partitioning of energy available for growth (MEp) between Pd ('X' × MEp) and Ld ([1 – 'X'] × MEp) (van Milgen and Noblet, 1999). Furthermore, mathematics has been applied to represent the impacts of pig genotype and BW (Black *et al.*, 1986; TMV, 1994; NRC, 1998) on the partitioning rules, which increases the number of parameters required to relate Pd to energy intake for different pig states. In the approach used by van Milgen and Noblet (1999), additional parameters were required to represent energy intake effects on the calculation rules.

According to Whittemore (1995) and Sandberg *et al.* (2005a,b), some of these approaches can be rejected outright, because they no longer represent our current understanding of energy partitioning in the growing pig (minLd/Pd; Whittemore and Fawcett, 1976) or because of the large number of empirical parameters needed to apply these approaches to specific conditions (Fuller and Crofts, 1977; van Milgen and Noblet, 1999). As discussed in the previous section, Ld/Pd is a function of energy intake level. Therefore, constraints on δLd/δPd, rather than Ld/Pd, should be used to represent the observed linear relationship between Pd and energy intake during the energy-dependent phase of Pd (de Greef and Verstegen, 1995). Obvious concerns with empirical approaches involving several parameters that do not represent biology are the extrapolation of the predictions outside the set of conditions used to establish mathematical relationships and parameter values and the inability to relate parameter values to underlying biological principles, such as gene expression.

In spite of differences in mathematical formats, some approaches yield similar predicted relationships between energy intake and Pd. The approach suggested by de Greef and Verstegen (1995), based on increases in minδLd/δPd with increasing BW, results in predicted changes in relationships between Pd and energy intake with increasing BW that are similar to the empirical approach used by Black *et al.* (1986). These two approaches have subsequently been adopted by TMV (1994) and NRC (1998), respectively. In NRC (1998), the approach suggested by Black *et al.* (1986) was adjusted to represent the effects of mean Pd between 20 and 120 kg BW (PdMean, g day^{-1}) and environmental temperature (T, °C) on the slopes in Pd per unit of extra energy intake (g Mcal^{-1} DE intake) at various BW (kg):

$$\text{Slope in Pd} = (17.5 \times e^{-0.0192 \times \text{BW}}) + 16.25) \times (\text{PdMean}/125) \times (1 + (0.015 \times (20 - T)) \quad (14.1)$$

A concern with the approach adopted by TMV (1994) is the assumption that across BW Ld is zero when metabolizable energy intake is equivalent to 1.3 times the energy requirements for maintenance. In this manner, positive Pd and negative Ld at maintenance energy intake levels are represented. However, as a result, and in combination with the increase in slope in Pd with BW, the difference between positive Pd and negative Ld at maintenance energy intake levels increases with BW. This is opposite to the approach suggested by Black *et al.* (1986) and conflicts with the observations that negative Ld at maintenance energy intake levels has been observed in young growing pigs only. Therefore, at extreme BW in particular, predicted Pd as determined by energy intake will differ between the approaches used by TMV (1994) and NRC (1998), and the approach used by NRC (1998) is preferred.

Relating the efficiency of available protein utilization for Pd to the energy to protein ratio in the diet, as suggested by Kyriazakis and Emmans (1992a,b; Fig. 14.3), yields relationships between Pd and energy intake that are similar to approaches used by TMV (1994) and NRC (1998). In fact, when both the efficiency of protein utilization and the energy to protein ratio in the diet (dependent and independent variables in Fig. 14.3) are multiplied by dietary available balanced protein level, it results in the linear–plateau relationship between Pd and energy intake. The main advantage of this approach is that the relationship between efficiency of protein utilization and dietary energy to protein ratios will hold across different feeding levels, which is consistent with some experimental observations. For example, based on the data presented in Fig. 14.1, the dietary lysine to energy ratio at which protein utilization is maximized is similar for both energy intake levels, simply because an increase in Pd requires both additional energy and additional balanced protein intake. However, Kyriazakis and Emmans (1992a,b; 1995) suggest that the relationship between the efficiency of protein utilization and dietary energy to protein ratio is also constant across pig types and BW. This is based on the notion that there is no effect of BW on the relationship between Pd and energy intake (Sandberg *et al.*, 2005a,b). The latter is not consistent with observations that were discussed in the previous section (Fig. 14.2; Quiniou *et al.*, 1996; Möhn and de Lange, 1998). Moreover, the notion that the maximum efficiency of protein utilization is achieved at the same

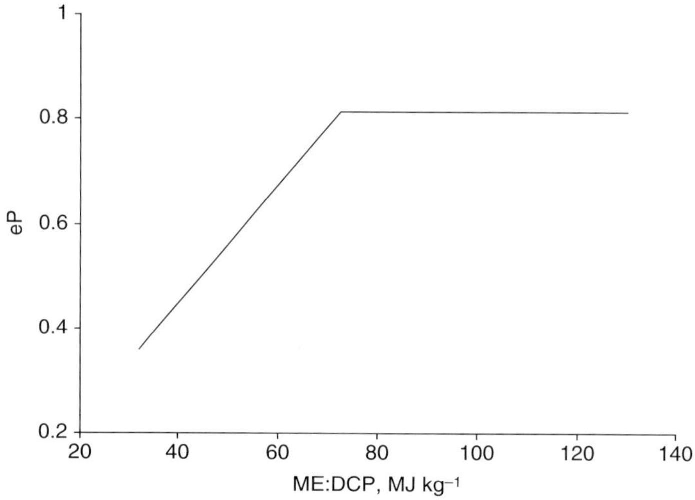

Fig. 14.3. Relationship between efficiency of available protein utilization for whole-body protein deposition (eP) and the metabolizable energy to digestible crude protein ratio (ME:DCP; MJ:kg N × 6.26) in the diet, as suggested by Kyriazakis and Emmans (1992a,b).

protein to energy ratio in the diet is not compatible with the well-documented increase in the optimum dietary energy to balanced protein ratio with BW (NRC, 1998) and a constant maximum marginal efficiency of balanced protein utilization for Pd across BW (starting principle 5).

All of the aforementioned approaches are not sufficiently flexible to reflect compensatory Pd following a period of balanced protein intake restriction. For this reason, Black *et al.* (1986) suggested some additional empirical adjustment to energy partitioning rules to accommodate the phenomenon of compensatory growth.

Constraints on body composition (L/P) are closely related to those on growth (Ld/Pd), simply because L/P is the result of cumulative Ld/Pd. An important advantage of imposing constraints on L/P rather than Ld/Pd is that the impact of nutritional history on compensatory Pd can be represented. As mentioned in the previous section, when L/P is increased due to a period of balanced protein intake restriction, pigs can demonstrate compensatory Pd and reduced Ld/Pd to achieve an L/P which is similar to that of pigs that were not exposed to balanced protein intake restriction. This observation provides a strong argument to impose constraints on L/P rather than Ld/Pd. However, the use of a constant value for minL/P to represent effects of energy intake or BW on the partitioning of retained energy between Ld and Pd during the energy-dependent phase of Pd should also be rejected. The use of a constant value implies that minLd/Pd is the same as minδLd/δPd, which is not consistent with experimental observations. For this reason, Schinckel and de Lange (1996) suggested that minL/P should vary with energy intake level and BW, as well as pig type. Given that there is a physiological absolute minL/P (Whittemore and Green, 2002), it is probably more appropriate to use the term 'targetL/P', which is dependent on energy intake and/or BW. If the actual L/P is higher than the targetL/P, pigs may increase Pd, provided that Pd is not constrained by the animal's Pdmax or balanced protein intake, while Ld is zero or possibly even negative. As discussed by Weis *et al.* (2004), energy intake in growing pigs is generally confounded with BW, making it difficult to differentiate direct effects of body weight and energy intake on targetL/P. Based on experimental observations, Weis *et al.* (2004) concluded that the effects of BW on targetL/P could be fully attributed to the effect of BW on energy intake. As a result, both energy intake and BW effects on the partitioning of retained energy during the energy-dependent phase of Pd can be represented using a simple (linear) relationship between daily energy intake and targetL/P. Further support for this simple energy partitioning rule is provided in the next section.

Metabolically, the partitioning of retained energy between Pd and Ld reflects the relative affinity of using absorbed nutrients for the synthesis and deposition of body protein versus synthesis and deposition of body lipid. For this reason, Halas *et al.* (2004) applied biochemical principles to represent intermediary metabolism in a mechanistic model of nutrient utilization in the growing pig. The rate of body protein deposition was chosen to follow saturation kinetics depending on the availability of lysine, as an approximation of balanced protein intake, and acetyl-CoA, as an approximation of energy intake. The model parameters were calibrated using experimental data from Bikker *et al.* (1995), who observed a clear linear relationship of both Pd and Ld with energy intake. In contrast to experimental observations, the biochemical model yielded highly non-linear muscle Pd and Ld responses to changes in energy intake during the energy-dependent phase of Pd (Figs 6 and 7 in Halas *et al.*, 2004). The discrepancy between experimental observations and model-generated predictions indicated that the mechanisms involved in energy partitioning in the growing pig were not represented adequately in the model of Halas *et al.* (2004). It appears that an improved understanding of physiological mechanisms, in addition to the explicit representation of intermediary metabolism, may provide more insight into animal and nutritional history effects on energy partitioning in growing pigs during the energy-dependent phase of Pd.

Empirical Support for a Simple Target L/P Dependent on Daily Energy Intake Only

Only a few pig studies have been conducted in which the impacts of both energy intake and BW on partitioning of retained energy between Pd and Ld are evaluated during the energy-dependent phase of Pd. A meaningful statistical investigation of the relationships between energy intake, BW and L/P in growing pigs requires independent observations of L/P at multiple energy intake levels and a range of (at least two) BW. Published experimental results which provide appropriate data for such analysis include: de Greef *et al.* (1994); Bikker *et al.* (1995, 1996a,b); Quiniou *et al.* (1995, 1996), supplemented by Quiniou (1995);

Coudenys (1998); and Weis *et al.* (2004). In these studies, experimental methodology and observations are clearly presented and, within studies, there is no apparent confounding effect of diet composition with feeding level or BW. The last of these studies was designed specifically to test our hypothesis that both energy intake and BW effects on the partitioning of retained energy during the energy-dependent phase of Pd can be represented using a simple (linear) relationship between daily energy intake and targetL/P, by minimizing confounding effects of energy intake and BW on target L/P. Three other studies (Kyriazakis and Emmans, 1992a,b; Kyriazakis *et al.*, 1994) yield relationships between energy intake and target L/P for three different pig types. However, in these studies, energy intake levels are very closely confounded with BW. Other published experimental studies which provide values for target L/P at multiple energy intake levels, but only at one BW, include: Campbell *et al.* (1985); Campbell and Taverner (1988); Möhn and de Lange (1998); Rao and McCracken (1991); and Möhn *et al.* (2000).

Having identified potential studies for testing our hypothesis, the next consideration was the accurate characterization of the data points (i.e. combinations of energy intake, BW and L/P) from the reported information. The absolute daily digestible energy intake (DEI) just prior to slaughter was chosen to represent energy intake, because this parameter was relatively easily obtained, was an important determinant of nutrient utilization in most dynamic biological models of pig growth and likely represented an important component of the physiological control of nutrient utilization in pigs on a particular day. The use of DEI implies that the relative partitioning of retained energy between Pd and Ld is determined by total daily energy intake, while the absolute Pd and Ld response to energy intake is determined by energy intake over and above energy requirements for body 'maintenance' functions. The latter should be explored further and other measures of energy intake, including diet nutrient composition, may be related to the (relative) partitioning of retained energy between Pd and Ld during the energy-dependent phase of Pd.

The whole empty body (including blood, skin and hair) L to P ratio (L/P) was chosen as a standardized variable to represent body composition. In most data sets, either the final P and L values were reported directly, or indirectly, as a proportion of empty BW, or they could be calculated from reported mean Pd and Ld by accumulating these over the growth period and using initial body composition. In some cases, neither of these calculations was possible due to missing information (Campbell *et al.*, 1985; Campbell and Taverner, 1988). In these last two studies, the empty body pool (not clearly defined) used for reporting Ld and Pd may also have excluded blood from the empty body definition, a factor which would have a significant impact on calculated L/P.

In practice, final weights were not always reported explicitly (Campbell *et al.*, 1985; Campbell and Taverner, 1988; Rao and McCracken, 1991), in which case nominal target weights had to be used for BW. In most of the studies, a value for DEI could be obtained (with a suitable conversion from metabolizable to digestible energy if necessary), although this was not possible when only mean intake data were reported for the growth period (Campbell *et al.*, 1985; Campbell and Taverner, 1988). In some instances, data points were omitted because factors other than energy intake determined Pd, such as balanced protein intake (Kyriazakis and Emmans, 1992b; Möhn *et al.*, 2000) or Pdmax (Möhn and de Lange, 1998). In our analysis, and after careful consideration, 5 out of 101 potential data points were eliminated from the data, as documented and explained in Table 14.2. The data from Campbell *et al.* (1985) and Campbell and Taverner (1988) were excluded entirely for the reasons described earlier. Thirteen unique combinations of sex × breed × study (pig populations) were defined for statistical analyses (Table 14.2; Fig. 14.4).

Regression analyses of data from the first seven pig populations (Table 14.3) indicate that BW does not affect ($P > 0.05$) L/P in a statistical model including both linear and quadratic effects of DEI, except for pig populations 'Coudenys' and 'QLWc', for which a small effect of BW contributes to the fit of the overall model. Excluding BW from the regression analyses reduces the degree of fit (R^2) from 0.959 to 0.892 and 0.999 to 0.851, respectively (data not shown). Thus, in at least five of these seven studies, BW effects on targetL/P can be attributed fully to the confounding of BW and DEI, as suggested by Weis *et al.* (2004).

Non-linear effects ($P < 0.05$) of DEI on L/P were observed for pig populations 'Weis' and 'QLWc' only. According to Weis *et al.* (2004), these quadratic effects can be attributed largely to the increased L/P at the highest DEI; as noted above, possibly pigs on the highest DEI level were no longer in the energy-dependent phase of Pd, resulting in L/P exceeding targetL/P. Based on analyses of the first seven pig populations (Fig. 14.4; Table 14.3), a simple linear relationship between targetL/P and daily energy intake is sufficient to represent partitioning of retained energy between Ld and Pd during the energy-dependent phase of Pd. In six of the seven pig populations, the intercept in the linear regression analyses was not different from zero. Alternatively, forcing a common intercept in the linear relationships between energy intake and L/P across the seven pig populations yields an extrapolated L/P of 0.062 (SE 0.055) at zero energy intake. This value is not different from zero or from 0.1, the value for minL/P suggested by Wellock *et al.* (2003).

The remaining six pig populations in Table 14.2 can be used to provide further support for a linear relationship between L/P and DEI (Table 14.4). As was determined for the first seven pig populations, in almost all of these six pig populations, the relationships between DEI and L/P model were also linear ($P < 0.05$ for slope). Across all of the 13 pig populations, a significant linear relationship was found between L/P and DEI, in 12 cases $P < 0.05$ (one P value is 0.15 for pig population Mohn97). This is a strong statistical argument to generalize the concept that targetL/P = $a + b \times$ DEI, with b being genotype specific.

Analysis of variance on the combined 13 pig populations establishes that targetL/P is related linearly to DEI with slope and intercept different between pig populations ($P < 0.0001$); however, closer examination of the data shows that the variation in intercept can be attributed entirely to QLWc data (intercept –0.69). Fitting a model with common intercept across the combined 13 pig populations (targetL/P = DEI × pig populations) gives a pig population's specific slope ($P < 0.0001$) and common intercept of 0.027 (SE 0.042) ($P = 0.6$), which is not different from zero. Results of a linear regression with the 13 combined pig populations and forced zero intercept are shown in Table 14.5, arranged in descending order of slope, i.e. fattest to leanest pig populations.

Table 14.2. Source and description of 13 sets of observations (pig populations) for statistical analyses of relationships between daily digestible energy intake (DEI) just prior to slaughter, body weight (BW) at slaughter, and body composition during the energy-dependent phase of body protein deposition in growing pigs. Each pig population represents a unique combination of gender × breed × study. All pig populations provide data for multiple DEI levels; the first seven pig populations provide data for (statistically) distinct multiple BW classes, as well as multiple DEI levels.

		Data range[a]					
Published source	Pig population label	BW (kg)	DEI (MJ day^{-1})	BW classes[b]	Data points[c]	Gender[d]	Breed
Multiple DEI × multiple BW							
Bikker *et al.*, 1996b	Bikker	45–85	14–49	2	8	G	Comm. hybrid
Coudenys, 1998	Coudenys	50–125	13–36	5	10	C	Yorkshire
de Greef *et al.*, 1994	De Greef	40–105	21–31	4	8	M	Comm. synth. cross
[e]Quiniou *et al.*, 1995, 1996	QLWc	40–100	27–38	2	5	C	LW
[e]Quiniou *et al.*, 1995, 1996	QLW × PPc	40–100	27–34	2	5	C	LW × Pietrain
[e]Quiniou *et al.*, 1995, 1996	QLW × PPm	40–100	23–39	2	5	M	LW × Pietrain
Weis *et al.*, 2004	Weis	40–105	13–29	4	14	M	Yorkshire

Multiple DEI × single BW							
Kyriazakis *et al.*, 1994	Kyria94	25–35	11–20	2	4	M	LW × Landrace
Kyriazakis and Emmans, 1992a,b	Kyria92g	30–53	14–26	3	10(1)[f]	M	LW × Landrace
Kyriazakis and Emmans, 1992a,b	Kyria92m	29–40	14–26	2	10(1)[f]	G	LW × Landrace
Möhn and de Lange, 1998	Mohn97	70	21–30	1	4(1)[g]	G	LW
Möhn *et al.*, 2000	Mohn	75	17–27	1	13(2)[g]	G	Yorkshire
Rao and McCracken, 1991	Rao	88	25–50	1	5	M	Landrace

[a]Range of values reported for BW and DEI excluding any points omitted. Note that not all DEI levels are represented at each LW class.

[b]Defined as the number of distinct BW clusters separated by at least 10 kg.

[c]Number of data points reported for each pig population. Any potential points which were omitted are indicated in parentheses.

[d]C = castrate; G = gilt; M = entire males.

[e]These three pig populations are compiled from the studies reported in Quiniou *et al.* (1995, 1996), as well as supplementary data from Quiniou (1995).

[f]This study includes treatments designed to vary in both energy and protein intake. At the lowest dietary P level (P1), balanced protein intake, rather than energy intake determined Pd; data for P1 were not considered in the analyses; for the same reason the data point at the highest intake level for the diet with the intermediate P level (P2) was also eliminated.

[g]SAL (semi-ad lib) treatment omitted in Mohn97. Highest intake levels (70/7 and 90/7) omitted in Mohn. The authors report that Pd is not limited by energy for these three treatments.

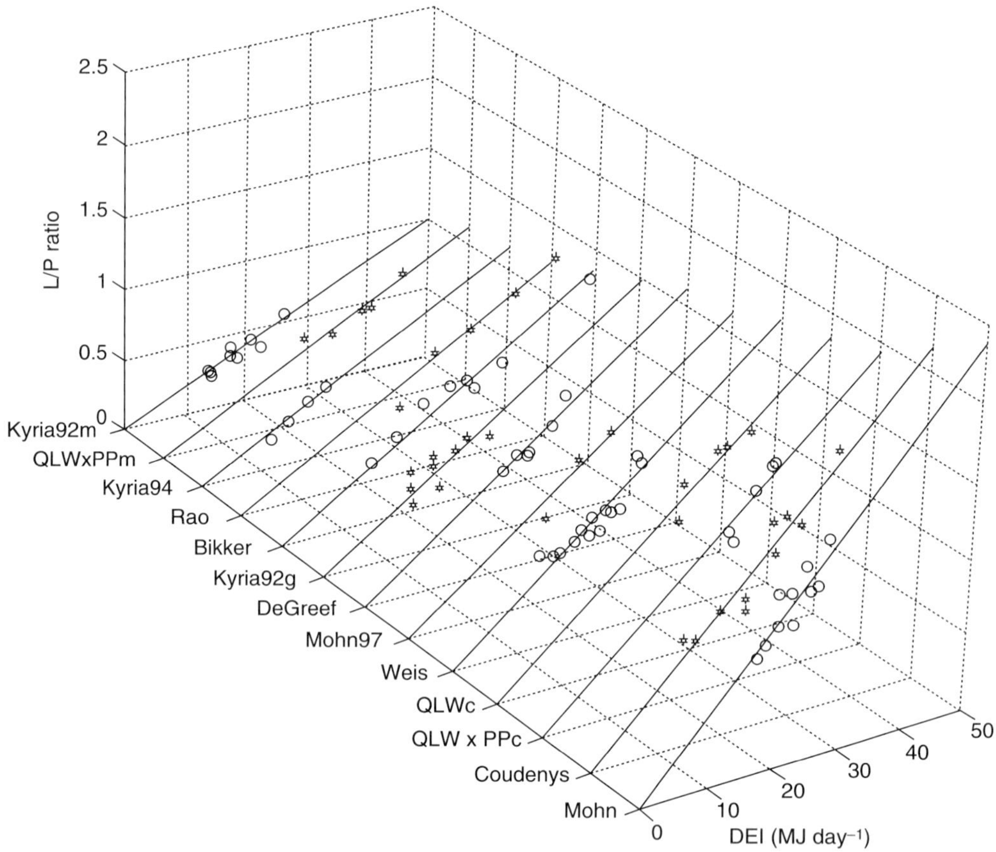

Fig. 14.4. Observed whole-body lipid to protein ratios (L/P) at varying levels of daily digestible energy intake (DEI, MJ day^{-1}) on the day prior to slaughter in studies where effects of body weight (BW) and DEI on L/P were evaluated in growing pigs during the energy-dependent phase of protein deposition. Data points for 13 pig populations, defined as a unique combination of sex × breed × source, are derived as detailed in Table 14.2 and discussed in the text. A statistical interpretation of these data is presented in Tables 14.3, 14.4 and 14.5. The regression lines shown were determined from a linear model of L/P versus DEI with zero intercept for all pig populations and pig population specific slopes ($P < 0.0001$). Data points for each pig population are plotted with alternating marker types (☆ and o) for clarity.

The use of a common or zero intercept implies that just one parameter is required to relate targetL/P to energy intake in different pig populations:

$$\text{targetL/P} = a \times \text{DEI} \tag{14.2}$$

Such an approach simplifies substantially the characterization of a key aspect of nutrient partitioning in the growing pig. In a one-parameter system, only one measurement of targetL/P is needed to characterize this aspect of nutrient partitioning in different pig populations. It is not critical at what BW or energy intake level measurements of targetL/P are made, as long as both L/P and energy intake are measured accurately and it is confirmed that measurements are made

Table 14.3. Level of significance of independent variables (*P*) and degree of fit of alternative statistical regression analysis models (R^2) for each of seven pig populations. Models represent effects of digestible energy intake (DEI) on the day prior to slaughter, and live body weight (BW) at slaughter on body composition as determined by empty body lipid to protein ratio (L/P) during the energy-dependent phase of body protein deposition in growing pigs. Individual data points are presented in Fig. 14.4.

	P				R^2	
		DEI				
Pig population[a]	Intercept	Linear	Quadratic	BW	Full model[b]	Linear function of DEI[c]
Bikker	0.65	0.0009	0.82	0.57	0.951	0.945
De Greef	0.07	0.0007	0.063	0.30	0.961	0.884
Coudenys	0.02	0.0001	0.11	0.02	0.959	0.869
QLWc	0.06	0.059	0.02	0.01	0.999	0.777
QLW × PPc	0.29	0.016	0.46	0.08	0.999	0.964
QLW × PPm	0.30	0.068	0.15	0.64	0.990	0.810
Weis	0.009	0.0001	0.007	0.08	0.910	0.751

[a]Pig population labels are defined and described in Table 14.2.
[b]Degree of fit of the models that include an intercept, linear and quadratic effects of DEI and linear effect of BW.
[c]Degree of fit of models that include an intercept and a linear effect of DEI only.

Table 14.4. Level of significance of independent variables (*P*) and degree of fit of alternative statistical regression analysis models (R^2) for six pig populations. Linear and quadratic effects of digestible energy intake (DEI) on the day prior to slaughter on body composition as determined by empty body lipid to protein ratio (L/P) were evaluated during the energy-dependent phase of body protein deposition in the growing pigs. Individual data points are presented in Fig. 14.4.

	P			R^2	
		DEI			
Pig population[a]	Intercept	Linear	Quadratic	Full model[b]	Linear model[c]
Kyria94	0.23	0.03	0.37	0.998	0.993
Kyria92g	0.90	0.06	0.74	0.480	0.470
Kyria92m	0.72	0.004	0.70	0.780	0.774
Mohn97	NA	NA	NA	NA	0.946
Mohn	0.86	0.0027	0.87	0.697	0.696
Rao	0.26	0.012	0.33	0.977	0.958

[a]Pig population labels are defined and described in Table 14.2.
[b]Degree of fit of the models that include an intercept, linear and quadratic effects of DEI.
[c]Degree of fit of models that include an intercept and a linear effect only of DEI.

Table 14.5. Results of a combined linear regression analysis ($R^2 = 0.937$) for data from all 13 pig populations.[a] The effect of digestible energy intake (DEI) on the day prior to slaughter on body composition as determined by empty body lipid to protein ratio (L/P) was evaluated during the energy-dependent phase of body protein deposition in the growing pigs using a model with a common zero intercept: targetL/P = $a \times$ DEI. The parameter 'a' (slope) is pig population specific ($P < 0.0001$) and was allowed to vary with pig population. The pig populations are arranged in decreasing order of slope, i.e. fattest to leanest pigs. Corresponding data points and regression lines for each pig population are shown in Fig. 14.4.

Pig population[a]	*n*	Slope	SE (slope)
Mohn	11	0.0475	0.0011
Coudenys	10	0.0433	0.0011
QLW × PPc	5	0.0389	0.0012
QLWc	5	0.0371	0.0012
Weis	14	0.0356	0.0011
Mohn97	3	0.0326	0.0019
DeGreef	8	0.0321	0.0012
Kyria92g	9	0.0295	0.0015
Bikker	8	0.0275	0.0010
Rao	5	0.0246	0.0010
Kyria94	4	0.0233	0.0027
QLW × PPm	5	0.0225	0.0012
Kyria92m	9	0.0199	0.0015

[a]Pig population labels are defined and described in Table 14.2.

during the energy-dependent phase of Pd. More observations are required relating energy intakes to L/P over wide ranges of (independent) energy intakes and live weights during the energy-dependent phase of Pd in order to confirm this simple linear relationship between DEI and targetL/P. Furthermore, variability in this relationship across pig populations should be assessed and may be related to physiological controls or indicators of body fatness, such as plasma leptin levels, leptin gene expression in fat tissue and leptin receptors in the hypothalamus (Houseknecht *et al.*, 1998; Horvath *et al.*, 2004). Also, the impact of sudden changes in energy intake on targetL/P and the dynamics of Pd and Ld should be explored further (Stamataris *et al.*, 1991; Bikker *et al.*, 1996a,b). However, under these conditions, Ld and Pd in visceral organs should be explicitly considered. It has been well established that the size of visceral organs is very responsive to changes in feeding level and diet characteristics (Bikker *et al.*, 1996a,b; de Lange and Fuller, 2000; de Lange *et al.*, 2003), while the control and extreme values for Pd and Ld in visceral organs have not been well characterized (Bikker *et al.*, 1996a,b).

Applications and Conclusions

A dynamic pig growth model (Birkett and de Lange, 2001a,b,c) was used to examine the theoretical implications of the proposed targetL/P concept for growth and Pd patterns. Two hypothetical pig types were created in the model, representing a range of body compositions observed in the analysis of published data sets above. Actual daily Pd during the energy-dependent phase of Pd was estimated for each day of growth where targetL/P was calculated daily from DEI according to Eqn 14.2. The targetL/P slope parameters for these pigs were set at 0.050 (fat) and 0.035 (lean), with a Pdmax of 150 g day^{-1}. Simulated daily Pd for each of these hypothetical pigs was calculated in response to two energy intake levels with daily DE intake at 80 and 100% of voluntary daily DE intakes according to NRC (1998). In these simulations, a fixed diet composition was used that was not limiting in any of the essential nutrients.

Figure 14.5 shows simulated Pd as a function of BW for the two pig types at the two energy intake levels. It can be seen that application of the targetL/P concept results in typical increases in Pd with increasing BW during the energy-dependent phase of Pd. During this phase of Pd, Pd increases in both pig types with energy intake and is higher for the pigs with the lower targetL/P. These patterns are consistent with previous observations (e.g. Quiniou *et al.*, 1995, 1996; Möhn *et al.*, 2000). Even though the relationship between targetL/P and DEI is linear, the simulations show a curvilinear increase in L/P with increasing BW, as a result of the curvilinear increase in energy intake with BW (Fig. 14.5). The observed change in L/P with increasing BW is also highly consistent with previous observations (de Greef *et al.*, 1994; Bikker *et al.*, 1995, 1996b; Coudenys, 1998). Among these scenarios, only the lean pig type on the higher energy intake level was able to achieve Pdmax, at about 70 kg BW. In all of these simulated scenarios, Pd is driven by energy intake for a substantial portion of the combined growing and finishing phases of growth in the pig.

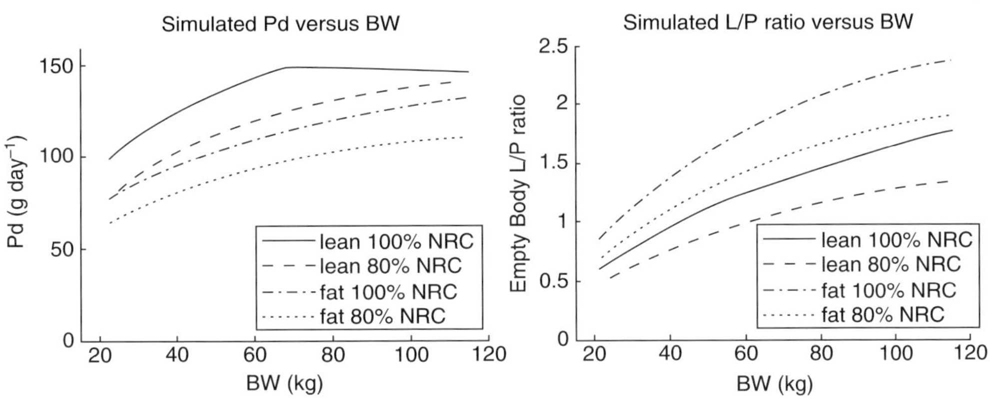

Fig. 14.5. Simulated results from a dynamic pig growth model (Birkett and de Lange, 2001a,b,c) illustrating changes in body protein deposition (Pd) and body composition (whole-body protein to whole-body lipid ratio; L/P) for two pig types and at two levels of digestible energy (DE) between 20 and 115 kg body weight (BW). Two hypothetical pig types were defined with targetL/P slopes MJ^{-1} day^{-1} DEI of 0.050 (fat) and 0.035 (lean), with a Pdmax of 150 g day^{-1}. A fixed high protein diet was used for simulated feed intakes at two energy intake levels of 80 and 100% of voluntary feed intake according to NRC (1998).

Largely because of continued genetic improvements in body protein deposition potentials of pigs, it is becoming increasingly important to characterize the partitioning of retained body energy during the energy-dependent phase of body protein deposition. During the energy-dependent phase of body protein deposition, the relationships between both body protein deposition and body lipid deposition and energy intake are highly linear. Based on extrapolation of these relationships to lower energy intake levels, pigs will mobilize body lipid to support body protein deposition when energy intake is reduced to satisfy maintenance energy requirements only. Because body protein deposition at the expense of body lipid loss is not sustainable, it is hypothesized that pigs have minimum body fatness, as well as a target body fatness that increases with energy intake level. This hypothesis is supported by experimental observations, including those on compensatory body protein deposition following a period of balanced protein intake restriction. It is concluded that current empirical approaches and approaches based on intermediary nutrient metabolism require too many parameters and are inaccurate or insufficiently flexible to represent partitioning of retained energy mathematically during the energy-dependent phase of body protein deposition. It is suggested that a simple linear relationship between daily digestible energy intake and target body fatness is sufficient to predict effects of energy intake, BW and previous balanced protein intake restriction on the partitioning of retained energy between body protein deposition and body lipid deposition during the energy-dependent phase of body protein deposition in growing pigs. In this approach, target fatness is represented by the target ratio between body lipid mass and body protein mass and only one parameter is required to reflect pig type effects on this aspect of nutrient partitioning. This approach will require further testing; in particular, further refinement will be required to represent the dynamics of body protein and body lipid deposition following sudden changes in energy intake. Moreover, physiological controls and indicators of body fatness should be explored further to improve our understanding and the mathematical representation of the complex biology of nutrient utilization for growth in the pig.

References

Batterham, E.S., Andersen, L.M., Braignent, D.R. and White, E. (1990) Utilization of ileal digestible amino acids by the growing pig: effect of dietary lysine concentration on efficiency of lysine retention. *British Journal of Nutrition* 64, 81–94.

Bikker, P., Karabinas, V., Verstegen, M.W.A. and Campbell, R.G. (1995) Protein and lipid accretion in body components of growing gilts (20 to 45 kilograms) as affected by energy intake. *Journal of Animal Science* 73, 2355–2363.

Bikker, P., Verstegen, M.W.A., Kemp, B. and Bosch, M.W. (1996a) Performance and body composition of finishing gilts (45 to 85 kilograms) as affected by energy intake and nutrition in earlier life: 1. Growth of the body and body components. *Journal of Animal Science* 74, 817–826.

Bikker, P., Verstegen, M.W.A. and Campbell, R.G. (1996b) Performance and body composition of finishing gilts (45 to 85 kilograms) as affected by energy intake and nutrition in earlier life: II. Protein and lipid accretion in body components. *Journal of Animal Science* 74, 817–826.

Birkett, S. and Lange, K. de (2001a) Limitations of conventional models and a conceptual framework for a nutrient flow representation of energy utilization by animals. *British Journal of Nutrition* 86, 647–659.

Birkett, S. and Lange, K. de (2001b) A computational framework for a nutrient flow representation of energy utilization by growing monogastric animals. *British Journal of Nutrition* 86, 661–674.

Birkett, S. and Lange, K. de (2001c) Calibration of a nutrient flow model of energy utilization by growing pigs. *British Journal of Nutrition*. 86, 675–689.

Black, J.L., Campbell, R.G., Williams, I.H., James, K.J. and Davies, G.T. (1986) Simulation of energy and amino acid utilization in the pig. *Research and Development in Agriculture* 3, 121–145.

Black, J.L., Davies, G.T., Bray, H.R. and Chapple, R.P. (1995) Modelling the effects of genotype, environment and health on nutrient utilization. In: Danafaer, A. and Lescoat, P. (eds) *Proceedings IVth International Workshop on Modelling Nutrient Utilization in Farm Animals.* National Institute of Animal Science, Tjele, Denmark, pp. 85–106.

Campbell, R.G. and Taverner, M.R. (1988) Genotype and sex effects on the relationship between energy intake and protein deposition in growing pigs. *Journal of Animal Science* 66, 676–686.

Campbell, R.G., Taverner, M.R. and Curic, D.M. (1985) The influence of feeding level on the protein requirements of pigs between 20 and 45 kg live weight. *Animal Production* 40, 489–496.

Close, W.H., Bershauer, F. and Heavens, R.P. (1983) The influence of protein: energy value of the ratio and level of feed intake on the energy and nitrogen metabolism of the growing pig. 1. Energy metabolism. *British Journal of Nutrition* 49, 255–269.

Coudenys, K. (1998) Effects of body weight and energy intake on physical and chemical body composition in growing pigs. MSc thesis, University of Guelph, Guelph, Ontario, Canada.

Dunkin, A.C. (1990) Responses to energy intake in the growing pig. *Pig News and Information* 11, 159–162.

Dunkin, A.C. and Black, J.L. (1987) The relationship between energy intake and nitrogen balance in the growing pig. In: Moe, P.W., Tyrrell, H.F. and Reynolds, P.J. (eds) *Energy Metabolism of Farm Animals*. European Association for Animal Production. Publication No 32. Rowman and Littlefield, Totowa, New Jersey, pp. 110–114.

Emmans, G.C. and Kyriazakis, I. (1997) Models of pig growth: problems and proposed solutions. *Livestock Production and Science* 51, 119–129.

Ferguson, N.S. and Gous, R.M. (1997) The influence of heat production on the voluntary food intake in growing pigs given protein deficient diets. *Animal Science* 64, 365–378.

Fuller, M.F. and Crofts, R.M.J. (1977) The protein-sparing effect of carbohydrate. 1. Nitrogen retention of growing pigs in relation to diet. *British Journal of Nutrition* 38, 479–488.

Fuller, M.F., Franklin, M.F., McWilliam, R. and Pennie, K. (1995) The response of growing pigs of different sex and genotype to dietary energy an protein. *Animal Science* 60, 291–298.

Greef, K. de and Verstegen M.W.A. (1995) Evaluation of a concept on energy partitioning in growing pigs. In: Moughan, P.J., Verstegen, M.W.A. and Visser-Reyneveld, M. (eds) *Modelling Growth in the Pig.* Pudoc, Wageningen, The Netherlands, pp. 137–149.

Greef, K. de, Kemp, B. and Verstegen, M.W.A. (1992) Performance and body composition of fattening pigs of two strains during protein deficiency and subsequent realimentation. *Livestock Production Science* 30, 141–153.

Greef, K. de, Verstegen, M.W.A., Kemp, B. and van der Togt, P.L. (1994) The effect of body weight and energy intake on the composition of deposited tissue in pigs. *Animal Production* 58, 263–270.

Green, D.M. and Whittemore, C.T. (2003) Architecture of a harmonized model of the growing pig for the determination of dietary net energy and protein requirements and of the excretions into the environment. *Animal Science* 77, 113–130.

Halas, V., Dijkstra, J., Babinszky, L., Verstegen, M.W.A. and Gerrits, W.J.J. (2004) Modelling of nutrient partitioning in growing pigs to predict their anatomical body composition. 1. Model description. *British Journal of Nutrition* 92, 707–723.

Heger, J., van Phung, T. and Krizova, L. (2002) Efficiency of amino acid utilization in the growing pig at sub-optimal levels of intake: lysine, threonine, sulphur amino acids and tryptophan. *Journal of Animal Physiology and Animal Nutrition* 86, 153–165.

Hogberg, M. and Zimmerman, D. (1978) Compensatory responses to dietary protein, length of starter period and strain of pig. *Journal of Animal Science* 47, 893–899.

Horvath, T.L., Diano, S. and Tschöp, M. (2004) Brain circuits regulating energy homeostasis. *Neuroscientist* 10, 235–246.

Houseknecht, K.L., Baile, C.A., Matteri, R.L. and Spurlock, M.E. (1998) The biology of leptin: a review. *Journal of Animal Science* 76, 1405–1420.

Kyriazakis, I. and Emmans, G.C. (1992a) The effects of varying protein and energy intakes on the growth and body composition of pigs: 1. The effects of energy intake at constant high protein intake. *British Journal of Nutrition* 68, 603–613.

Kyriazakis, I. and Emmans, G.C. (1992b) The effects of varying protein and energy intakes on the growth and body composition of pigs: 2. The effects of varying both energy and protein intake. *British Journal of Nutrition* 68, 615–625.

Kyriazakis, I. and Emmans, G.C. (1995) Do breeds of pigs differ in the efficiency with which they use a limiting protein supply? *British Journal of Nutrition* 74, 183–195.

Kyriazakis, I., Stamataris, C., Emmans, G.C. and Whittemore, C.T. (1991) The effects of food protein content on the performance of pigs previously given foods with low or moderate protein contents. *Animal Production* 52, 165–173.

Kyriazakis, I., Dotas, D. and Emmans, G.C. (1994) The effect of breed on the relationship between feed composition and the efficiency of protein utilization in pigs. *British Journal of Nutrition* 71, 849–859.

Lange, C.F.M. de (1995) A simplified framework for a growth model to demonstrate principles of nutrient utilization for growth in the pig. In: Moughan, P.J., Verstegen, M.W.A. and Visser-Reyneveld, M. (eds) *Modelling Growth in the Pig.* Pudoc, Wageningen, The Netherlands, pp. 71–86.

Lange, C.F.M. de and Fuller, M.F. (2000) Advances in feed evaluation for pigs. In: Moughan, P.J., Verstegen, M.W.A. and Visser-Reyneveld, M. (eds) *Feed Evaluation – Principles and Practice.* Wageningen Pers, Wageningen, The Netherlands, pp. 221–242.

Lange, C.F.M. de, Morel, P.C.H. and Birkett, S.H. (2003) Modeling chemical and physical body composition of the growing pig. *Journal of Animal Science*, Available at: http:// www.asas.org/symposia/03esupp2/jas2454.pdf

Martinez, H.R. (2005) Characterization of the dynamics of body protein deposition response following sudden changes in amino acid intake. MSc thesis, University of Guelph, Guelph, Ontario, Canada.

Martinez, H.R. and Lange, C.F.M. de (2004) Body protein deposition response following sudden changes in ideal protein intake differs between pig types. *Journal of Animal Science* 82 (Suppl. 1; Abstracts), 420.

Martínez, H.R. and Lange, C.F.M. de (2005) Nutrition induced variation in body composition, compensatory growth, cortisol and leptin in growing pigs. *Journal of Animal Science* 83 (Suppl. 1; Abstracts), 214.

Möhn, S. and Lange, C.F.M. de (1998) The effect of body weight on the upper limit to protein deposition in a defined population of growing gilts. *Journal of Animal Science* 76, 124–133.

Möhn, S., Gillis, A.M., Moughan, P.J. and Lange C.F.M. de (2000) Influence of dietary lysine and energy intakes on body protein deposition and lysine utilization in growing pigs. *Journal of Animal Science* 78, 1510–1519.

Moughan, P.J. (1999) Protein metabolism in the pig. In: Kyriazakis, I. (ed.) *A Quantitative Biology of the Pig*. CAB International, Wallingford, UK, pp. 299–331.

Moughan, P.J., Smith, W.C. and Pearson, G. (1987) Description and validation of a model simulating growth in the pig (20–90 kg live weight). *New Zealand Journal of Agricultural Research* 30, 481–489.

National Research Council (NRC) (1998) *Nutrient Requirements of Swine*, 10th rev. edn. National Academic Press, Washington, DC.

Nyachoti, C.M., Zijlstra, R.T., Lange, C.F.M. de and Patience, J.F. (2004) Voluntary feed intake in growing–finishing pigs: a review of the main determining factors and potential approaches for accurate predictions. *Canadian Journal of Animal Science* 84, 549–566.

Quiniou, N. (1995) Utilisation de l'énergie chez le porc selon son potentiel de croissance: contribution à la modélisation des besoins nutritionnels et de la composition corporelle. PhD thesis, L'Ecole National Supérieure Agronomique de Rennes, France.

Quiniou, N., Noblet, J., van Milgen, J. and Dourmand, J.-Y. (1995) Effect of energy intake on performance, nutrient and tissue gain and protein and energy utilization in growing boars. *Animal Science* 61, 133–143.

Quiniou, N., Dourmad, J.-Y. and Noblet, J. (1996) Effect of energy intake on the performance of different types of pigs from 45–100 kg body weight. 1. Protein and lipid deposition. *Animal Science* 63, 277–288.

Rao, D.S. and McCracken, K.J. (1991) Effect of energy intake on protein and energy metabolism of boars of high genetic potential for lean growth. *Animal Production* 52, 499–507.

Sandberg, F.B., Emmans, G.C. and Kyriazakis, I. (2005a) Partitioning of limiting protein and energy in the growing pigs: description of the problem, possible rules and their quantitative evaluation. *British Journal of Nutrition* 93, 205–212.

Sandberg, F.B., Emmans, G.C. and Kyriazakis, I. (2005b) Partitioning of limiting protein and energy in the growing pigs: testing quantitative rules against experimental data. *British Journal of Nutrition* 93, 213–224.

Schinckel, A.P. and Lange, C.F.M. de (1996) Characterization of growth parameters needed as inputs for pig growth models. *Journal of Animal Science* 74, 2021–2036.

Stamataris, C., Kyriazakis, I. and Emmans, G.C. (1991) The performance and body composition of young pigs following a period of growth retardation by food restriction. *Animal Production* 53, 373–381.

Technisch Model Varkensvoeding (TMV) (1994) *Research Station for Swine Husbandry*. PO Box 83, Rosmalen, The Netherlands.

van Milgen, J. and Noblet, J. (1999) Energy partitioning in growing pigs: the use of a multivariate model as an alternative for the factorial analyses. *Journal of Animal Science* 77, 2154–2162.

van Milgen, J. and Noblet, J. (2003) Partitioning of energy intake to heat, protein and fat in growing pigs. *Journal of Animal Science* 81, E86–E93.

Weis, R.N., Birkett, S.H., Morel, P.C.H. and de Lange, C.F.M. (2004) Independent effects of energy intake and body weight on physical and chemical body composition in growing entire male pigs. *Journal of Animal Science* 82, 109–121.

Wellock, I.J., Emmans, G.C. and Kyriazakis, I. (2003) Modelling the effects of thermal environment and dietary composition on pig performance: model logic and development. *Animal Science* 77, 255–266.

Whittemore, C.T. (1995) Modelling the requirements of the young growing pig for dietary protein. *Agricultural Systems* 47, 415–425.

Whittemore, C.T. and Fawcett, R.H. (1976) Theoretical aspects of a flexible model to simulate protein and lipid growth in pigs. *Animal Production* 22, 87–96.

Whittemore, C.T. and Green, D.M. (2002) The description of the rate of protein and lipid growth in pigs in relation to live weight. *Journal of Agricultural Research* 138, 415–423.

Whittemore, C.T., Green, D.M. and Knap, P.W. (2001) Technical review of the energy and protein requirements of growing pigs: protein. *Animal Science* 73, 363–373.

Williams, N.H., Stahly, T.S. and Zimmerman, D.R. (1997) Effect of level of chronic immune system activation on the growth and lysine needs of pigs fed from 6 to 112 kg. *Journal of Animal Science* 75, 2481–2496.

15 Aspects of Energy Metabolism and Energy Partitioning in Broiler Chickens

G. Lopez and S. Leeson

Centre for Nutrition Modelling, Department of Animal and Poultry Science, University of Guelph, Canada

Introduction

The modern commercial broiler chicken is capable of fast growth rate that is fuelled and sustained by its voracious appetite. Able to consume feed at the rate of 10% of body weight on a dry matter basis, there is the suggestion that appetite per se governs intake. This situation is invalid, since the broiler still adjusts its feed intake according to energy concentration of the diet (Leeson and Summers, 1996). The broiler exhibits a remarkably similar growth rate over a wide range of diet energy concentrations. Only at limits of physical capacity does energy intake decline with low energy diets, while an upper limit is often imposed by physical characteristics and associated organoleptics of high fat diets. While growth rate per se is sustained over a vast range of feeding scenarios, there are subtle changes in body composition associated with diet energy density and energy intake, while classical feed efficiency is predictably altered by change in diet energy. Energy intake fuels growth and development of the modern broiler and so, unlike with other farm species, it is surprising that so few data are available on energy metabolism and energy partitioning of modern broiler chickens. To some extent, the situation is confounded by the fact that the broiler chicken is now more difficult to categorize. Commercially, it can be grown as sexed flocks or as a mixed sex flock, while commercial market ages of from 35 to 70 days impose variance in inherent energy needs relative to other nutrients, such as amino acids, and the impact of inherent change in body composition on energy partitioning.

Classical Definitions of Energy Partitioning

It is expected that growing broilers deposit nutrients into body tissues, such as fat and protein, quite efficiently relative to other poultry species (Leeson and Summers, 2001). Metabolizable energy (ME) intake is generally partitioned into energy retained (ER) as fat and protein and as heat production (HP): ME = HP + ER (Close, 1990; Lawrence and Fowler, 2002). In thermoneutral conditions, HP represents heat associated with the utilization of ME intake for maintenance (MEm) and productive process, which in juvenile broilers represents 52–64% of intake (van Milgen *et al.*, 2001; Noblet *et al.*, 2003). Therefore, ER represents the difference between ME and HP in that ME – HP = ER. When evaluating ER, it is necessary to measure energy retained as both fat (ERF) and protein (ERP), along with their efficiency of utilization of ME, usually termed *kf* for fat and *kp* for protein deposition. Estimates of ERF and ERP in broilers have been determined using such methods as indirect calorimetry (Farrell, 1974; Fuller *et al.*, 1983; van Milgen *et al.*, 2001; Noblet *et al.*, 2003) and comparative slaughter (Fuller *et al.*, 1983; MacLeod, 1991). However, values for *kf* and *kp* have only been estimated using statistical models from experiments involving different feeding levels (Boekholt *et al.*, 1994).

There have been limitations in nutritional studies using growing broilers to define ME utilization adequately and, consequently, their energy requirements. There are surprisingly few estimates of HP and its components, namely fasting heat production (FHP), heat production due to physical activity and the thermic effect of feeding (TEF) (van Milgen *et al.*, 2001; Noblet *et al.*, 2003). Few studies have determined the efficiency of ME utilization for fat and protein deposition (Boekholt *et al.*, 1994). Currently, the model that is most commonly used to predict the effect of diet on growth (ERF and ERP) and efficiency is based on the equation of Kielanowski (1965). In this model, metabolizable energy intake is defined as: MEI = MEm + (1/*kf* × ERF) + (1/*kp* × ERP), where MEm represents ME for maintenance as a function of body weight BW^b, *kf* and *kp* efficiencies of utilization of ME for fat and protein deposition, respectively (Boekholt *et al.*, 1994; Birkett and de Lange, 2001a; Lawrence and Fowler, 2002). Requirements for maintenance are also influenced by the method used to express MEm. MEm of broilers is traditionally reported as a function of BW raised to the 0.75 power (Fuller *et al.*, 1983; MacLeod, 1990; Boekholt *et al.*, 1994; Buyse *et al.*, 1998). Recent information suggests that MEm in broilers is, in fact, more adequately described by BW exponents other than the exponent 0.75 (MacLeod, 1991, 1997; van Milgen *et al.*, 2001; Noblet *et al.*, 2003).

Metabolic Modifiers

We have conducted studies to determine energy utilization in broilers and birds of intermediate growth rate exemplified by pure-line strains of White Leghorn and Barred Rock and have analysed data using the assumption that maintenance energy requirements are proportional to body weight raised to either 0.75 or 0.60 power (Table 15.1). The models fitted were:

$$\text{ME} = a\,\text{BW}^{0.75} + (1/0.86)\ \text{ERF} + (1/0.66)\ \text{ERP} + \varepsilon$$

$$\text{ME} = a\,\text{BW}^{0.60} + (1/0.86)\ \text{ERF} + (1/0.66)\ \text{ERP} + \varepsilon.$$

The constants (0.86 and 0.66) are taken from the data of Boekholt *et al.* (1994), since these values seem to be reasonable and agree with commonly used data.

Table 15.1. Performance and nitrogen balance in growing broilers, Barred Rock and Leghorn birds.

	Broiler	BR[a]	Leghorn	SEM[b]	*P*
FI[c], g bird^{-1} day^{-1}	151*	50**	45**	4.46	< 0.001
Average BW[d], kg	2.100*	0.555**	0.476**	0.03	< 0.001
Average BWG[c], g bird^{-1} day^{-1}	72*	16**	15**	3.3	< 0.001
Nitrogen balance, g bird^{-1} day^{-1}					
Ingested	4.64*	1.55**	1.40**	0.13	< 0.001
Retained	2.31*	0.87**	0.70**	0.12	< 0.001
Excreted	2.33*	0.67**	0.69**	0.74	< 0.001
% N retained	51.0*	43.0*	50.0*	0.40	> 0.05
BWG[e] gN^{-1} retained	31*	25**	22**	1.74	< 0.01
MEI[f], kcal gN^{-1} retained	206*	243*	216*	13.91	> 0.05
MEI[f], kcal BWG^{-1} [e]	7**	10*	10*	0.53	< 0.001

*Significant difference ($P < 0.05$); **significant difference ($P < 0.01$).
[a]Barred Rock.
[b]SEM, standard error of the mean.
[c]FI, feed intake.
[d]BW, body weight.
[e]BWG, body weight gain.
[f]MEI, metabolizable energy intake.

As expected, the rate of growth in broilers was significantly different to that of Barred Rock and Leghorn birds. The average BW at 42 days was 2.1 kg, 0.55 kg and 0.48 kg for broilers, Barred Rock and Leghorns, respectively (Table 15.1). Feed intake of broilers was 2.5–3 times higher than for Leghorn and Barred Rock strains, although HP adjusted to $BW^{0.60}$ was not different.

Data adjusted to $BW^{0.60}$ showed ER, ERF and ERP to be different for broilers (Table 15.2). There was also a significant effect of bird type on all parameters relative to various ME ratios of energy, namely ME/GE, ER/ME, REF/ME and REP/ME ($P < 0.05$, Table 15.2), although broilers had higher relative energy losses in excreta. (GE is gross energy.)

Broilers ingested and retained more N than did the slower growing strains, largely as a result of their twofold increase in feed intake (Table 15.3). However, the percentage of retained N did not differ significantly at any time across strains. N excretion was elevated by more than 300% in broilers compared to the slower growing strains. Broilers also exhibited greater body weight gain g^{-1} of N retained and needed less ME intake g^{-1} BWG (Table 15.3).

Maintenance Energy Requirement

Estimates of maintenance requirements as a function of BW raised to the 0.75 and 0.60 power are shown in Table 15.4. The model using BW $^{0.60}$ showed the

Table 15.2. Utilization of ME in growing birds with different growth rates from 37–42 days.

	Broiler	BR[a]	Leghorn	SEM	P
ME intake kcal kg^{-1} $BW^{0.60}$ day^{-1}	305*	225**	231**	8.52	< 0.001
HP	183	171	182	6.91	> 0.05
ER	123*	53**	50**	11.55	< 0.001
ERF	57*	20**	15**	6.82	< 0.001
ERP	66*	33**	35**	6.34	< 0.01
[b]ME intake/GE intake	75.2**	74.8**	77.7*	0.58	< 0.01
[b]ER/ME intake	39.4*	23.4**	21.7**	3.53	< 0.01
[b]ERF/ME intake	18.3*	8.7**	6.6**	2.42	< 0.01
[b]ERP/ME intake	21.1*	14.7**	15.1**	1.86	< 0.10

*Significant difference ($P < 0.05$); **significant difference ($P < 0.01$).
[a]Barred Rock.
[b]Energetic efficiencies.

Table 15.3. Utilization of ME in broilers.

	10–15 days	23–28 days	37–42 days	SEM	P
ME intake kcal kg^{-1} $BW^{0.60}$ day^{-1}	368*	345*	305**	11.47	**
HP	228*	226*	183**	6.28	***
ER	139	120	123	13.04	NS
ERF	81	55	57	9.07	NS
ERP	58	65	66	6.36	NS
Energetic efficiencies:					
ER/ME intake	37.6	34.3	39.4	2.95	NS
ERF/ME intake	21.8	15.4	18.3	2.22	NS
ERP/ME intake	15.8	18.8	21.1	1.60	NS

NS – No significant difference ($P > 0.05$); *significant difference ($P < 0.05$); **significant difference ($P < 0.01$); ***significant difference ($P < 0.001$).

smallest residual variance and therefore appears to be more precise than the alternate $BW^{0.75}$ model. These results show that maintenance requirements for broilers kg^{-1} $BW^{0.75}$ are 8% lower compared to estimates based on $BW^{0.60}$. This difference changes as the value of BW^b increases, and vice versa. For example, if BW^b is 1.6, then the difference decreases by 2% and vice versa, indicating that the basis for estimating BW is more critical for younger and smaller birds. Maintenance requirements for the two strains, with inherent slower growth rate, were higher than those of commercial broilers, regardless of the model used (Table 15.4), although variance of the estimate was always less for $K = 0.60$.

Table 15.4. Summary of estimates in the non-linear regression model; $\hat{a}$ estimated using experimental data producing two models for each bird strain.

	$K = 0.60$		$K = 0.75$	
	$\hat{a}^a$	σ^2	$\hat{a}^a$	σ^2
Broiler	155.3	1331.8	143.0	2043.3
Barred Rock	182.1	686.6	204.1	981.7
Leghorn	189.5	473.6	217.8	749.3

[a]kcal (kg $BW^b)^{-1}$ day^{-1}, all estimates significant ($P < 0.01$).

HP in growing broilers represents 52–64% of total ME intake (Fuller *et al.*, 1983; van Milgen *et al.*, 2001; Noblet *et al.*, 2003) and is directly associated with the ME requirements for maintenance and productive processes. Using indirect calorimetry, van Milgen *et al.* (2001) showed that FHP and physical activity together represented 36–37% of ME intake. In their experiment, van Milgen *et al.* (2001) described physical activity as a major component of maintenance (8–10%). Requirements for daily maintenance (MEm), including both FHP and physical activity as main components, were established at 152–157 kcal kg^{-1} $BW^{0.60}$. These values are similar to the values 155 kcal kg^{-1} $BW^{0.60}$ for MEm as reported in the current experiment using comparative slaughter and using the same metabolic body modifier (kg $BW^{0.60}$).

Implications for Modelling Energy Requirements

Estimates for maintenance needs are greatly influenced by the method of calculating MEm and, consequently, such choices influence calculation of the partitioning of energy between maintenance and growth in terms of fat and protein deposition. Findings from the current experiment suggest that MEm as a function of $BW^{0.75}$ underestimates the energy requirements for growing broilers, and especially for younger birds. Maintenance requirements for broilers based on kg $BW^{0.75}$ are 8% lower than the values estimated using $BW^{0.60}$, and this difference becomes more obvious for younger and/or smaller birds. BW raised to the exponent 0.60 appears to be a more precise estimator, and this supposition implies higher energy requirements for maintenance. Other researchers have also proposed the use of exponents other than 0.75 in both broilers (MacLeod, 1991, 1997; van Milgen *et al.*, 2001, Noblet *et al.*, 2003) and pigs (van Milgen *et al.*, 1998; Noblet *et al.*, 1999). The underestimation of the maintenance requirements directly impacts estimates of efficiencies of fat and protein deposition. Estimates of maintenance and energy efficiencies are closely related, and so lower MEm implies more energy for production, and hence lower *kp* and *kf*. In growing broilers, there are few attempts at measuring or estimating such effects. Few studies have involved estimates of efficiencies for protein and fat deposition in poultry, and most such data are invariably based on $BW^{0.75}$ (Boekholt *et al.*, 1994), or data are extrapolated from studies with pigs (Noblet *et al.*, 1999; Birkett and de Lange, 2001b).

Close (1990) indicated that differences in MEm are mainly affected by changes in body composition. Since adipose tissue contributes little to heat production compared to that of muscle, it is suggested that maintenance energy requirements are lower in fat versus lean animals (Close, 1990). MacLeod *et al.* (1988) found significantly higher FHP and N retention in broiler lines selected for leanness, suggesting an increased maintenance energy requirement in lean birds. It is still unclear whether or not fat animals have lower MEm, or whether animals with a lower MEm become fatter (van Milgen *et al.*, 1998).

Regression analyses show a significant linear relationship for the ratio ERP/ME on ME intake, although this changes over time with higher efficiency of protein deposition as the bird ages. These data suggest that less protein (as a fraction of ME) will be deaminated and, therefore, birds are leaner during the very early growth phase. Alternatively, broilers may have a greater rate of protein synthesis and/or reduced protein degradation (Urdaneta and Leeson, 2004). It is important to consider that broilers growing to 42 days undergo a number of periods of moult and feather regeneration, and this more so in broilers than for the slower growing BR and Leghorn strains. In this regard, it is important to emphasize that carcass data in the present study included feathers and, where practical, moulted feathers were collected and included in carcass preparation.

Since MEm is more highly correlated with $BW^{0.60}$ than $BW^{0.75}$, it seems as though conventional estimates have been too low for small chicks. Data from this experiment show that, for a 400 g bird, the model $BW^{0.75}$ underestimates MEm by 20%, yet overestimates MEm for a 2600 g bird by 6%. Underestimation of the MEm for younger or smaller birds implies less energy for production and, therefore, by calculation, greater apparent efficiency for growth. The converse effect, but to a lesser degree, is expected for the overestimation of MEm for older or heavier birds. MEm requirements represent a large portion of the MEI in broilers, being in the order of 42–44% of MEI, and hence accurate assessment is critical for an understanding of energy metabolism in broilers.

As previously discussed, partitioning, and hence utilization of energy in the broiler, will be greatly impacted by body composition and to a particular degree by fatness. In most commercial feeding programmes, the desire for fast growth with *ad libitum* feeding invariably entails moderate levels of energy and high crude protein (CP) for the starter diets and high energy and lower CP for the later diets (Leeson and Summers, 2005). It is well documented that such changes to energy:protein (E:P) in the diet are associated with increased weight gain as fat (Bartov *et al.*, 1974; MacLeod, 1990, 1991; Wiseman and Lewis, 1998; Morris, 2004). Mathematical growth models have been used to study the influence of changes over time in dietary energy (Wiseman and Lewis, 1998) or dietary protein (Eits *et al.*, 2005) on body components such as fat (Wiseman and Lewis, 1998). These models are used as a tool to predict body weight (BW) with desired carcass characteristics. It is expected that mature animals retain energy mainly as fat, while growing animals retain energy as both fat and protein. Gross energy retained in the body as fat (TERF) and protein (TERP) together contributes most of the total energy retained (TER) in the body. TER is calculated from accumulation of fat and protein and by using corresponding energy values of 9.5 kcal g^{-1} fat and 5.7 kcal g^{-1} protein (Znaniecka, 1967; Hakansson and Svensson, 1984). Since fat and protein accretion probably differ in their efficiencies of transfer of energy from feed to tissue (Buttery and Boorman, 1976; Pullar and Webster, 1977), changes in the proportion of both fat and protein during growth influence the total energy in the body and the efficiency of such gain. Today's broilers reach commercial body weight very early at an 'immature' body weight and often without achieving maximum genetic potential for fat and protein deposition in terms of absolute quantities deposited each day.

Energy Deposition as Fat Versus Protein

Little information is available to help our understanding of how modern broilers quantitatively deposit energy as fat and/or protein and so this places limits on our understanding of the energy metabolism of commercial broilers. To study the effect of bird weight on TERF or TERP, a non-linear regression model was used. The model corresponds to the Gompertz equation given by:

$$Y = a \exp\{-\exp[-b(W - M)]\} + \varepsilon$$

where Y represents TERF and TERP, W is bird weight and a (the asymptotic of TERF and TERP), b (a measure of the decline in TERF and TERP growth rate) and M (BW at inflection) are regressions coefficients. The term ε is a random variable assumed to be normally distributed with mean 0 and variance σ^2. A separate model was fitted per bird strain. The estimated models were:

Broilers:

$$\text{TERF} = 3151.5 \exp\{-\exp[-1.0634(W - 1.1637)]\}$$

$$\text{TERP} = 3396.4 \exp\{-\exp[-1.0175(W - 1.2287)]\}$$

PBR:

$$\text{TERF} = 606.3 \exp\{-\exp[-3.6084(W - 0.3444)]\}$$

$$\text{TERP} = 1035.4 \exp\{-\exp[-3.2108(W - 0.3875)]\}$$

Leghorns:

$$\text{TERF} = 511.4 \exp\{-\exp[-3.6303(W - 0.2958)]\}$$

$$\text{TERP} = 851.6 \exp\{-\exp[-3.9168(W - 0.3235)]\}.$$

Figures 15.1–15.3 detail the significant quadratic relationship for deposition of energy in the body of birds growing to 42 days. In terms of total energy (TER) and energy as fat (TERF) and protein (TERP), the pattern of deposition was similar for the two slower growing strains. For broilers, the deposition of total energy in the EBW (empty body weight (feed in the digestive tract was removed and the birds were reweighed)) (Fig. 15.1) grew at an ever-increasing rate over time. The rate of energy deposition as protein over time in broilers was slightly greater than for the corresponding coefficient for fat deposition (Figs 15.2 and 15.3). The effect of TERF and TERP as a proportion of TER is detailed in Table 15.5, indicating that broilers deposited a constant proportion (50%) of body energy as fat and protein ($P < 0.001$). The high R^2 for both response variables indicates that most of the variability shown by the data, for both TERF and TERP, is explained by the simple linear regression model.

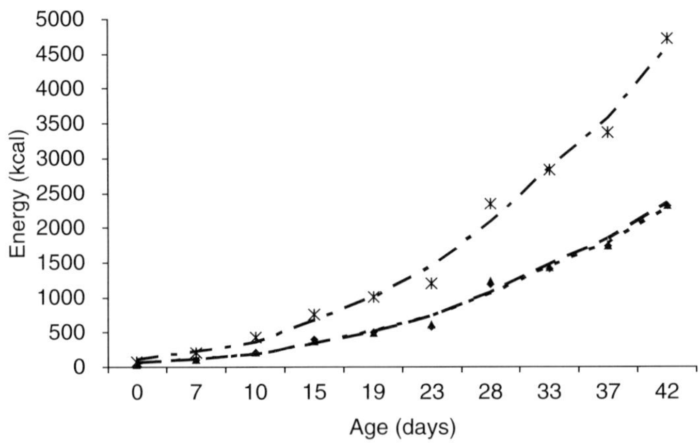

◆ TERF $y = 46.950 + 1.041 \pm 5.44(x) + 1.242 \pm 0.12(x)^2$ $R^2 = 0.96$***
▲ TERP $y = 52.925 - 1.344 \pm 5.01(x) + 1.337 \pm 0.11(x)^2$ $R^2 = 0.97$***
✳ TER $y = 108.4 - 0.982 \pm 9.45(x) + 2.565 \pm 0.21(x)^2$ $R^2 = 0.97$***

Fig. 15.1. Total energy deposition in growing birds.

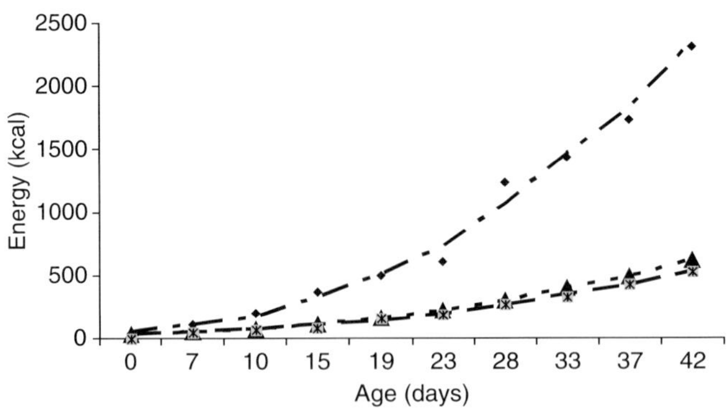

◆ Broiler $y = 52.925 - 1.344 \pm 5.01\ (x) + 1.337 \pm 0.11\ (x)^2$ $R^2 = 0.97$***
▲ PBR $y = 30.395 + 0.761 \pm 1.48\ (x) + 0.317 \pm 0.03\ (x)^2$ $R^2 = 0.96$***
✳ Leghorn $y = 32.208 + 1.006 \pm 1.074\ (x) + 0.257 \pm 0.02\ (x)^2$ $R^2 = 0.97$***

Fig. 15.2. Body energy deposition as protein.

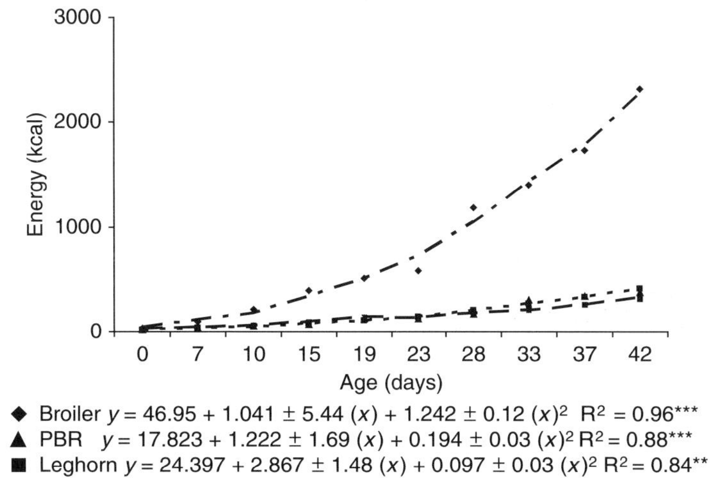

Fig. 15.3. Body energy deposition as fat.

Table 15.5. Summary of results from linear regression analyses of TERF and TERP on TER.[c]

	TERF[a]				
Bird type	R^2	β_0	β_1	SE β_0	SE β_1
Broiler	0.99	5.476NS	0.492***	8.643	0.0037
BR[d]	0.99	–1.191NS	0.4024***	4.004	0.0076
Leghorn	0.99	10.216*	0.377***	4.820	0.010
			TERP[b]		
Broiler	0.99	–5.476NS	0.5075***	8.643	0.0037
BR	0.99	1.191NS	0.5975***	4.004	0.0076
Leghorn	0.99	–10.21*	0.622***	4.820	0.010

Model linear in *X*; β_0 , β_1 = regression coefficient; SE β_0, SE β_1 are standard errors; *significant difference ($P < 0.05$); ***significant difference ($P < 0.001$).
[a]TERF, total gross energy as fat (kcal).
[b]TERP, total gross energy as protein (kcal).
[c]TER, total gross energy calculated (TERF + TERP).
[d]BR, Barred Rock.

Table 15.6 shows the effect of bird strain and body weight on the rate of energy deposition as TERF or TERP. The Gompertz model fits the observed data, for all strains, with a high coefficient of determination (R^2). According to the observed data, in broilers, the asymptotic values of TERP were higher than for TERF at 2.5 kg EBW. In broilers selected for fast growth, the maximum rate of TERF and TERP was reached at 1.16 kg and 1.22 kg of EBW, respectively,

Table 15.6. Coefficient estimates in male broilers for total gross energy as fat (TERF, kcal) and total gross energy as protein (TERP, kcal) versus body weight using the Gompertz equation.

	TERF	TERP
Broiler		
a	3151.5 ± 149.9	3396.4 ± 141.9
b	1.0634 ± 0.0606	1.0175 ± 0.0482
M	1.1637 ± 0.0556	1.2287 ± 0.0500
RSS	405,518	282,380
R^2	0.9946	0.9964
Barred Rock		
a	606.3 ± 82.084	1035.4 ± 66.9570
b	3.6084 ± 0.533	3.2108 ± 0.1991
M	0.3444 ± 0.0446	0.3875 ± 0.0228
RSS	65,980	22,886
R^2	0.9752	0.9961
Leghorn		
a	511.4 ± 100.2	851.6 ± 45.7027
b	3.6303 ± 0.7606	3.9168 ± 0.2154
M	0.2958 ± 0.06116	0.3235 ± 0.0157
RSS	66,625	13,712
R^2	0.9650	0.9961

RSS, residual sum of squares.
± SE, standard error.
R^2, coefficient of determination.

and then declined slowly as body weight increased, whereas, for the other strains, maximum values were not achieved until the birds reached a body weight of 0.30–0.35 kg for TERF and 0.32–0.38 for TERP.

Energy content in the body as fat and protein was relatively consistent throughout the 42-day growth period for all strains. Selection for reduced abdominal fat (Cahaner, 1988; Leclercq, 1988) and for improved feed efficiency (Leenstra, 1988; Buyse *et al.*, 1998) has produced leaner broilers, although this parameter will be affected by the diet energy level used in a given study.

Gompertz for Modelling Body Composition Changes

The Gompertz equation has been adopted in broiler studies to describe growth over time appropriately (Wilson, 1977; Emmans, 1995; Hurwitz and Talpaz, 1997; Darmani Kuhi *et al.*, 2002) and/or growth of body components in broilers (Tzeng and Becker, 1981; Peter *et al.*, 1997; Wiseman and Lewis, 1998; Gous *et al.*, 1999). This equation describes a sigmoidal biological growth pattern of growing broilers with a slow rate of initial growth, followed by acceleration up to a certain age (the inflection point), then by a subsequent decline in the rate as body weight approaches its maximum growth near to sexual maturity (Hurwitz and Talpaz, 1997). Tzeng and Becker (1981) fitted the non-linear Gompertz equation to abdominal fat, intending to predict total carcass fat over time (Becker *et al.*, 1979). Usually, the methods for evaluating the growth of body components in broiler studies using the Gompertz have been carried out for extended periods of time varying from 10 to 16 weeks (Tzeng and Becker, 1981; Peter *et al.*, 1997; Wiseman and Lewis, 1998; Gous *et al.*, 1999). Under these conditions, the asymptotic value of live weight and body components are obviously better estimated. However, as today's broilers reach commercial body weight earlier (approximately 6 weeks) without ever achieving maximum genetic potential for fat and protein deposition, the asymptotic value of live weight, or for various body components, is expected to be higher than for commercial application and so classical predictions of the response variable for 'mature' broilers could lead to unreliable predictions.

It is well documented that ME intake influences body composition (Hakansson and Svensson, 1984; Boekholt *et al.*, 1994; Wiseman and Lewis, 1998) and therefore body ER. Boekholt *et al.* (1994), feeding broilers from 60 to 100% of daily energy intake, reported that daily retention of fat and protein was linearly related to energy retention, suggesting that, in growing broilers, each additional unit of gain generated by energy intake over 43 kcal kg^{-1} $BW^{0.75}$ day^{-1} is composed of constant amounts of protein and fat, but different proportions of energy as protein (15%) and fat (85%). This situation indicates that, at an ER of 43 kcal kg^{-1} $BW^{0.75}$ day^{-1}, ERF is zero and only protein is retained, perhaps at the expense of fat mobilization (Boekholt *et al.*, 1994). In our studies, birds were fed *ad libitum*, and neither TERF nor TERP changed as broilers retained energy, suggesting that, during their early period of 'immature' commercial growth (0–42 days), broilers deposit a constant proportion (50%) of body energy as fat and protein. It is calculated that, within the commercial growing range of 0–42 days, broilers deposit body fat and protein that together represent 35–40% of their daily ME intake.

Previous studies indicate that the efficiency of protein deposition is lower than that for fat deposition (Petersen, 1970; De Groote, 1974; Boekholt *et al.*, 1994). De Groote (1974) reports that the efficiency of ME utilization above maintenance varies from 70 to 84% for lipid deposition in adult birds and from 37 to 85% in growing birds. Petersen (1970), using White Plymouth Rock birds, estimated efficiencies of 0.51 and 0.78 for protein and fat, respectively, indicating a need for 11.2 kcal ME g^{-1} protein and 12.2 kcal ME g^{-1} fat deposited. More recent information in growing broilers suggests higher efficiencies for protein (0.66) and fat (0.86) deposition (Boekholt *et al.*, 1994), indicating lower needs for protein (8.63 kcal ME g^{-1}) and fat (10.9 kcal ME g^{-1}). Similar efficiencies (0.65 and 0.83) are reported in comparable studies with growing pigs (Noblet *et al.*, 1999). These data suggest that broiler selection has indirectly increased the efficiency of lean meat deposition by increasing the efficiency of utilization of ME (Decuypere *et al.*, 2003). Broilers may also have been inadvertently selected for greater rate of protein synthesis and/or reduced protein degradation (Urdaneta and Leeson, 2004).

Conclusions

Our data suggest that, in immature birds fed *ad libitum*, total ME intake can be estimated with reasonable accuracy based on the actual TERF and TERP accretion rates and efficiency of utilization for fat and protein deposition. This approach also requires an estimate of maintenance energy requirements (MEm). For example, assuming MEm at 155 kcal kg^{-1} $BW^{0.60}$ and using efficiency values for *kf* (0.86) and *kp* (0.66) obtained by Boekholt *et al.* (1994), along with the gross energy content of the body fat of 9.5 kcal g^{-1} and protein of 5.7 kcal g^{-1}, the total energy costs for fat TERFk and protein TERPk deposition for a 42-day-old broiler weighing 2.3 kg are 2652 kcal and 3568 kcal ME, respectively, while 5607 kcal ME is the corresponding energy cost for maintenance. The calculated total fat and protein deposition represents about 38–40% of ME intake.

As broilers grow, accretion of fat and protein is the result of the interactions between bird strain, sex, environmental conditions, nutrition, body weight (BW) and degree of maturity. Quantifying and partitioning TER as TERF and TERP as major components of the requirement of ME in growing broilers can be used in the industry to establish useful models. Such models will have economic consequences and allow management decisions, taking into account the biological understanding of the growth of modern birds within the normal commercial range of 0–42 days. This is of interest to the industry since the economic cost of supplying energy versus protein often changes over time.

References

Bartov, I., Bornstein, S. and Lipstein, B. (1974) Effects of calorie to protein ratio on the degree of fatness in broilers fed on practical diets. *British Poultry Science* 15, 107–117.

Becker, W.A., Spencer, J.V., Mirosh, L.W. and Verstrate, J.A. (1979) Prediction of fat and fat-free live weight in broiler chickens using backskin fat, abdominal fat and live body weight. *Poultry Science* 58, 835–842.

Birkett, S. and Lange, K. de (2001a) Limitations of conventional models and a conceptual framework for a nutrient flow representation of energy utilization by animals. *British Journal of Nutrition* 86, 647–659.

Birkett, S. and Lange, K. de (2001b) Calibration of a nutrient flow model of energy utilization by growing pigs. *British Journal of Nutrition* 86, 675–689.

Boekholt, H.A., Van Der Grinten, P.H., Schreurs, V.V.A.M., Los, M.J.N. and Leffering, C.P. (1994) Effect of dietary energy restrictions on retention of protein, fat and energy in broiler chickens. *British Poultry Science* 35, 603–614.

Buttery, P.J. and Boorman, K.N. (1976) The energetic efficiency of amino acid metabolism. In: Cole, D.J.A., Boorman, K.N., Buttery, P.J., Lewis, D., Neal, R.J. and Swan, H. (eds) *Protein Metabolism and Nutrition*. Butterworths, London, pp. 197–206.

Buyse, J., Michels, H., Vloeberghs, J., Saevels, P., Aerts, J.M., Ducro, B., Berckmans D. and Decuypere, E. (1998) Energy and protein metabolism between 3 and 6 weeks of age male broiler chicken selected for growth rate or for improved food efficiency. *British Poultry Science* 39, 264–272.

Cahaner, A. (1988) Experimental divergent selection on abdominal fat in broilers – female and male type lines and their crosses. In: Leclercq, B. and Whitehead, C.C. (eds) *Leanness in Domestic Birds: Genetic, Metabolic and Hormonal Aspects*. Butterworths, London, pp. 71–86.

Close, W.H. (1990) The evaluation of feeds through calorimetry studies. In: Wiseman J. and Cole, D.J.A. (eds) *Feedstuff Evaluation*. Butterworths, Cambridge, UK, pp. 21–39.

Darmani Kuhi, H., Kebreab, E., Lopez, S. and France, J. (2002) A derivation and evaluation of the von Bertalanffy equation for describing growth in broilers over time. *Journal of Animal and Feed Science* 11, 109–125.

Decuypere, E., Bruggeman, V., Barbato, G.F. and Buyse, J. (2003) Growth and reproduction problems associated with selection for increased broiler meat production. In: Muir, W.M. and Aggrey, S.E. (eds) *Poultry Genetics, Breeding and Biotechnology*. CAB International, Wallingford, UK, pp. 13–28.

Eits, R.M., Kwakkel, R.P., Verstengen, M.W.A. and Den Hartog, L.A. (2005) Dietary balanced protein in broiler chickens. 1. A flexible and practical tool to predict dose–response curves. *British Poultry Science* 46, 300–309.

Emmans, G.C. (1995) Problems in modelling the growth of poultry. *World's Poultry Science Journal* 51, 77–89.

Farrell, D.J. (1974) General principles and assumptions of calorimetry. In: Morris, T.R. and Freeman, B.M. (eds) *Energy Requirements of Poultry*. British Poultry Science Ltd, Edinburgh, UK, pp. 1–24.

Fuller, H.L., Dale, N.M. and Smith, C.F. (1983) Comparison of heat production of chickens measured by energy balance and by gaseous exchange. *Journal of Nutrition* 113, 1403–1408.

Gous, R.M., Moran, E.T., Stilborn, H.R. Jr, Bradford, G.D. and Emmans, G.C. (1999) Evaluation of the parameters needed to describe the overall growth, the chemical growth, and the growth of feathers and breast muscle of broilers. *Poultry Science* 78, 812–821.

Groote, G. De (1974) Utilisation of metabolisable energy. In: Morris, T.R. and Freeman, B.M. (eds) *Energy Requirements of Poultry*. British Poultry Science Ltd, Edinburgh, UK, pp. 113–133.

Hakansson, J. and Svensson, S.A. (1984) Gross energy content of fat and protein in different tissues of male broiler chicks. *Swedish Journal of Agricultural Research* 14, 207–212.

Hurwitz, S. and Talpaz, H. (1997) Modelling of growth. In: *11th European Symposium on Poultry Nutrition*. Faaborg, Denmark, pp. 148–157.

Kielanowski, J. (1965) Estimates of the energy cost of protein deposition in growing animals. In: Blaxter, K.L. (ed.) *Proceeding of the 3rd Symposium on Energy Metabolism*. EAAP Publications No. 11, Academic Press, London, pp. 13–20.

Lawrence, T.L.L. and Fowler, V.R. (2002) Efficiency and growth. In: Lawrence T.L.J. and Fowler, V.R. (eds) *Growth of Farm Animals*. CAB International, Wallingford, UK, pp. 216–228.

Leclercq, B. (1988) Genetic selection of meat-type chickens for high or low abdominal fat content. In: Leclercq, B. and Whitehead, C.C. (eds) *Leanness in Domestic Birds: Genetic, Metabolic and Hormonal Aspects*. Butterworths, London, pp. 25–40.

Leenstra, F.R. (1988) Selection for leanness: results of the Spelderholt experiment. In: Leclercq, B. and Whitehead, C.C. (eds) *Leanness in Domestic Birds: Genetic, Metabolic and Hormonal Aspects*. Butterworths, London, pp. 59–70.

Leeson, S. and Summers, J.D. (1996) Broiler response to diet energy. *Poultry Science* 75, 529–535.

Leeson, S. and Summers, J.D. (2001) Energy. In: Leeson, S. and Summers, J.D. (eds) *Nutrition of the Chicken*. University Books, Guelph, Canada, pp. 34–99.

Leeson, S. and Summers, J.D. (2005) Feeding programs for broilers chickens. In: *Commercial Poultry Nutrition*, 3rd edn. University Books, Guelph, Canada, pp. 229–296.

MacLeod, M.G. (1990) Energy and nitrogen intake, expenditure and retention at 20° in growing fowl given diets with a wide range of energy and protein contents. *British Journal of Nutrition* 64, 625–637.

MacLeod, M.G. (1991) Fat deposition and heat production as response to surplus dietary energy in fowls given a wide range of metabolizable energy:protein ratios. *British Poultry Science* 32, 1097–1108.

MacLeod, M.G. (1997) Effects of amino acid balance and energy:protein ratios on energy and nitrogen metabolism in male broiler chickens. *British Poultry Science* 38, 405–411.

MacLeod, M.G., Whitehead, C.C., Griffin H.D. and Jewitt, T.R. (1988) Energy and nitrogen retention and loss in broiler chickens genetically selected for leanness and fatness. *British Poultry Science* 29, 285–292.

Morris, T.R. (2004) Nutrition of chicks and layers. *World's Poultry Science Journal* 60, 5–18.

Noblet, J., Karage, C., Dubois, S. and van Milgen, J. (1999) Metabolic utilization of energy and maintenance requirements in growing pigs: effects of sex and genotype. *Journal of Animal Science* 77, 1208–1216.

Noblet, J., van Milgen, J., Carré, B., Dimon, P., Dubois, S., Rademacher M. and van Cauwenberghe, S. (2003) Effect of body weight and dietary crude protein on energy utilization in growing pigs and broilers. In: Souffrant, W.B. and Metges C.C. (eds) *Progress in Research on Energy and Protein Metabolism*. EAAP Publications No. 109, Wageningen Academic Publishers, The Netherlands, pp. 205–208.

Peter, W., Danicke, S. and Jeroch, H. (1997) Description of growth of body weight and body protein of French label type chickens with Gompertz equations in dependence on the protein content of the diet. In: *11th European Symposium on Poultry Nutrition*. Faaborg, Denmark, pp. 400–402.

Petersen, C.B. (1970) Efficiency of protein and fat deposition in growing chickens determined by respiration experiments. In: Schürch, A. and Wenk, C. (eds) *Proceeding of the 5th EAAP Symposium on Energy Metabolism of Farm Animals*. Zurich, Switzerland, pp. 205–208.

Pullar, J.D. and Webster, A.J.F. (1977) The energy cost of fat and protein deposition in the rat. *British Journal of Nutrition* 37, 355–363.

Tzeng, R.Y. and Becker, W. (1981) Growth patterns of body and abdominal fat weights in male broiler chickens. *Poultry Science* 60, 1101–1106.

Urdaneta, M. and Leeson, S. (2004) Effect of dietary crude protein and lysine on feather growth in chicks to twenty-one days of age. *Poultry Science* 83, 1713–1717.

van Milgen, J., Bernier, J.F., Le Cozler, Y., Dubois, S. and Noblet, J. (1998) Major determinants of fasting heat production and energetic cost of activity in growing pigs of different body weight and breed/castration combination. *British Journal of Nutrition* 79, 509–517.

van Milgen, J., Noblet, J., Dubois, S., Carre, B. and Juin, H. (2001) Utilization of metabolizable energy in broiler chickens. *Poultry Science* 80 (Suppl.1), 170 (Abstr.).

Wilson, B.J. (1977) Growth curves: their analysis and use. In: Boorman, K.N. and Wilson, B.J. (eds) *Growth and Poultry Meat Production*. British Poultry Science Ltd, Edinburgh, UK, pp. 89–115.

Wiseman, J. and Lewis, C.E. (1998) Influence of dietary energy and nutrient concentration on the growth of body weight and carcass components of broiler chickens. *Journal of Agricultural Science* 131, 361–371.

Znaniecka, G. (1967) Calorific value of protein and fat of the chicken's body. In: Blaxter, K.L., Kielanowski, J. and Thorbek, G. (eds) *Proceeding of the 4th EAAP Symposium on Energy Metabolism of Farm Animals*. Oriel Press, Newcastle-upon-Tyne, UK, pp. 407–408.

16 Modelling Phosphorus Metabolism

E. KEBREAB,[1,3] D.M.S.S. VITTI,[2] N.E. ODONGO,[3]
R.S. DIAS,[3] L.A. CROMPTON[4] AND J. FRANCE[3]

[1]National Centre for Livestock and Environment, Department of Animal Science, University of Manitoba, Canada; [2]Animal Nutrition Laboratory, Centro de Energia Nuclear na Agricultura, Brazil; [3]Centre for Nutrition Modelling, Department of Animal and Poultry Science, University of Guelph, Canada; [4]Animal Science Research Group, School of Agriculture, Policy and Development, University of Reading, UK

Introduction

Phosphorus (P) is an essential nutrient involved not only with bone development, growth and productivity, but also with most metabolic processes in the body. Phosphorus constitutes 1% of the total body weight (BW), 80% of which is found in bones and the remaining 20% distributed within body cells, where it is involved in maintaining the structural integrity of cells and intracellular energy and protein metabolism (McDowell, 1992). Phosphorus and calcium (Ca) are the two most abundant minerals in the mammalian body. These elements are closely related, so that deficiency or over-abundance of one may interfere with the proper utilization of the other. Almost all of the Ca in ruminants (99%) is located in the bones and teeth, with the remaining 1% distributed in various soft tissues of the body. Phosphorus is present in bone in the hydroxyapatite molecule, where it occurs as tri-calcium phosphate and magnesium phosphate.

Phosphorus has become the focus of recent research due to concerns that overfeeding P to farmed livestock is contributing to environmental pollution. The NRC (1998) suggested that P rather than nitrogen (N) will limit land application of manure in intensive pig producing areas and successful management strategies for reducing P excretion will depend on accurate estimates of P requirements for all levels of production (Ekpe *et al.*, 2002). Therefore, research has focused on improving the efficiency of conversion of dietary P into animal products and accurate estimates of P requirements by the animal.

Quantitative aspects of P metabolism have been examined using balance studies and isotope dilution techniques in conjunction with compartmental and mechanistic models. The mathematical approaches can be broadly classified into empirical and mechanistic modelling (Kebreab and Vitti, 2005). For example, approaches based on regression analysis (e.g. Schulin-Zeuthen *et al.*, 2007a) are empirical, while mechanistic approaches are process-based (e.g. Kebreab *et al.*, 2004). Mechanistic models can be further divided into three types, depending on the solutions of the equation statements (Thornley and France, 2007). If the system is in steady state, Type I models obtain solutions by setting the relevant differentials to zero and manipulating to give algebraic expressions for each flow (e.g. Vitti *et al.*, 2000). In non-steady state, Type II models solve rate:state equations analytically. Type III models solve complex cases of rate:state equations numerically in non-steady state (e.g. Kebreab *et al.*, 2004). In this chapter, examples of empirical, kinetic and mechanistic models of P metabolism in ruminants and monogastric animals will be discussed.

Modelling Phosphorus Metabolism in Ruminants

Cattle

Factorial

Most of the models used for calculating P requirements are based on a factorial approach by adding requirements for various physiological processes such as maintenance, growth, pregnancy and lactation. Such models compute the requirement of an animal for minerals for a predetermined level of production. Most European and American national standards for P requirements are based on this approach. For example, in NRC (2001), P requirement for maintenance in growing cattle based on P balance studies was calculated to be 0.8 g kg^{-1} dry matter intake (DMI), with an allowance of 0.002 g kg^{-1} BW for urinary P. AFRC (1991) calculated P requirements for growth empirically (P_{reqg}; g day^{-1}) in cattle using the following equation:

$$P_{reqg} = [1.6\,(-0.06 + 0.693\,DMI) + WG\,(1.2 + 4.635\,A^{0.22}\,W^{-0.22})]/0.58$$

where DMI is in kg day^{-1}, WG is live weight gain (kg day^{-1}), A is mature body weight (kg) and W is the current live weight (kg). According to the German feeding standards, the recommended dietary P intake for a 600 kg cow producing 25 kg of milk is 61 g day^{-1} (GfE, 2001), which is slightly lower than the 67 g day^{-1} recommended by Kebreab *et al.* (2005a).

Estimation of minimum P requirements for cattle using empirical regression methods has been the subject of many studies (e.g. Challa and Braithwaite, 1988a,b). Pfeffer *et al.* (2005) used the results of Challa and Braithwaite (1988a,b) to estimate the inevitable faecal P losses from calves as a function of dietary P concentration. Challa and Braithwaite (1988a,b) fed a low P diet at a constant rate to ruminating calves and varied P supply to the animals either by supplementing P in the diet or by infusing P into the abomasum while varying the amounts of orthophosphate. Pfeffer *et al.* (2005) plotted P retention (y) against P concentration in dietary dry matter (DM) (x) (Fig. 16.1) and fitted the data to the equation:

$$y = b_0(1 - e^{-k(x-c)})$$

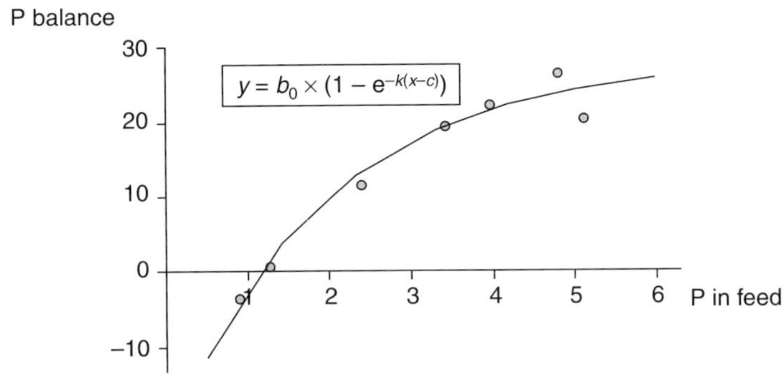

Fig. 16.1. Daily P balance (g day^{-1}) as a function of dietary P concentration (g kg^{-1} of DM). Adapted from Pfeffer *et al.* (2005).

where b_0 is maximum theoretical P retention, k is a shape constant and c is the point on the abscissa at which $y = 0$. The constants computed had the following values: $b_0 = 28.6$ g day^{-1}; $k = 0.48$ and $c = 1.17$, and they concluded that zero P balance could only be achieved at a dietary P concentration greater than ≈ 1.2 g kg^{-1} DM. The Pfeffer *et al.* (2005) results were supported by those of Spiekers *et al.* (1993), who also fed a low P diet of constant composition to dairy cows consuming either 16.9 or 10.0 kg DM daily and reported that, irrespective of dietary intake, cows excreted approximately 1.2 g P kg^{-1} DM ingested, in agreement with the results shown in Fig. 16.1 for calves.

Mechanistic

A mechanistic model of P metabolism in dairy cows was developed by Kebreab *et al.* (2004). The model contains ten state variables or pools, with inputs and outputs to the pools represented by arrows (see Fig. 16.2). The standard cow was assumed to weigh 600 kg with a rumen volume of 90 l and was non-pregnant. The input of P to the cow is via the diet and the outputs are in faeces, milk and urine. The model considers P passage through the rumen, small intestine (including duodenum), large intestine and extracellular fluid.

Dietary P input can be divided into potentially digestible and non-digestible P. The model uses the mechanistic rumen model of Dijkstra *et al.* (1992) and Dijkstra (1994) to estimate rumen microbial synthesis and microbial outflow to the duodenum. In the rumen, two forms of P are represented based on digestibility. Dietary potentially digestible P and salivary P are inputs to the digestible P pool in the rumen. On average, 45% of the P entering the rumen comes from saliva, as endogenous P (Kebreab *et al.*, 2005b). The majority of P in saliva is inorganic (Reinhardt *et al.*, 1988) and the amount secreted appears to be regulated by parathyroid hormone (Wasserman, 1981). Saliva plays a significant role as a buffer in the rumen and is an important source of P for rumen microorganisms (Care, 1994). The concentration of P in the saliva depends on the P status of the animal and, at steady state, the model calculations are influenced by P concentrations in the diet and the extracellular fluid. Phosphorus, as an important component of cell membranes, is essential for microbial growth. The rumen

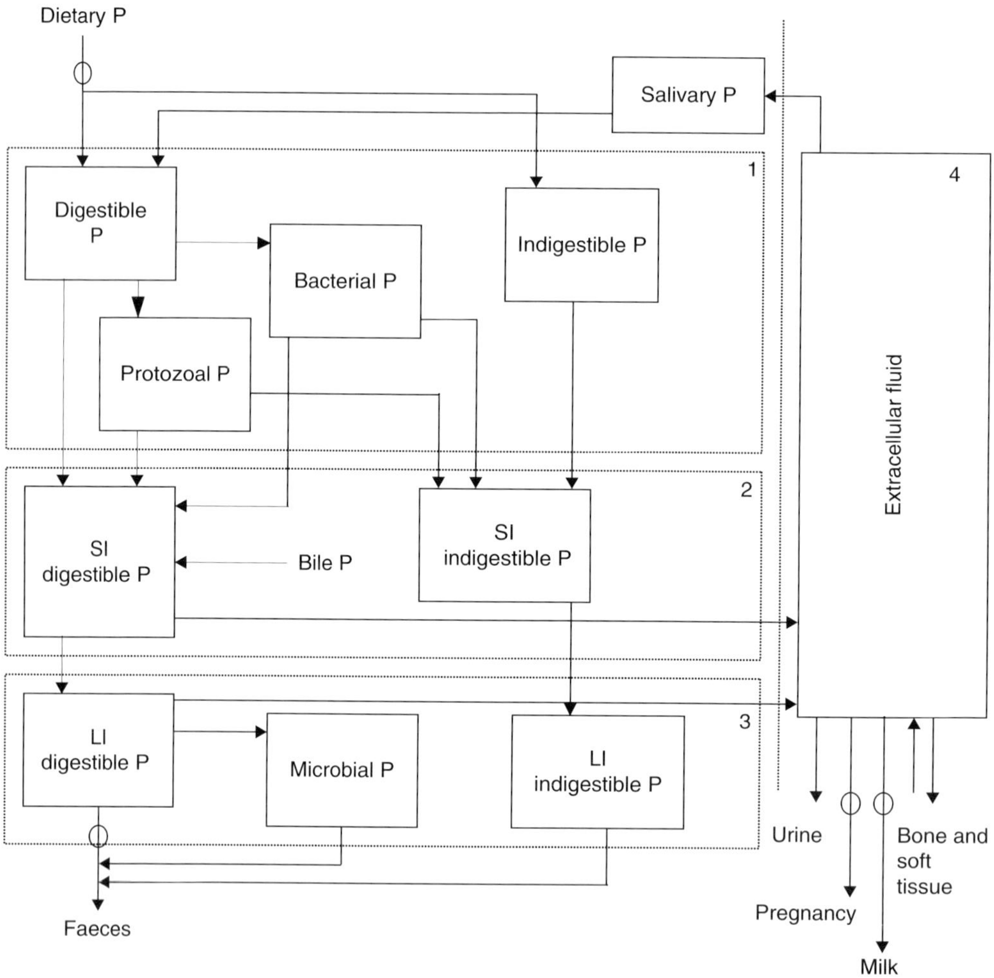

Fig. 16.2. Schematic representation of the model of P metabolism in the ruminant. The compartments were rumen (1), small intestine (2), large intestine (3) and extracellular fluid (4) (Kebreab and Vitti, 2005).

model of Dijkstra (1994) estimates protozoal and bacterial polysaccharide-free DM; therefore, P contents of 13.8 and 17.9 mg g^{-1} polysaccharide-free DM (assuming a ratio of 5:1 of small:large bacteria in the rumen liquor (Czerkawski, 1976)) for protozoa and bacteria, respectively, were used in the model by Kebreab *et al.* (2004). Ruminal P not incorporated into microbial cells is assumed to pass to the duodenum at a fractional outflow rate of fluid of 8.3% h^{-1}. Phosphorus from the indigestible P pool in the rumen is assumed to pass to the small intestine at a particulate fractional passage rate of 4.0% h^{-1}.

Microbial P constitutes a major proportion of the P entering the small intestine and it is generally accepted that the upper small intestine, where the pH of the digesta is acid, is the main site for P absorption (Breves and Schröder, 1991).

Studies examining how P is absorbed in ruminants have shown that two processes are involved, one a passive process, related to intake, and the other, an active process, related to demand (Braithwaite, 1984). A substantial portion of the active transport consists of a sodium-dependent P transport mechanism (Schröder *et al.*, 1995) and a Michaelis–Menten type saturation equation was used to describe the absorption of P from the small intestinal digestible P pool into the extracellular fluid (Kebreab *et al.*, 2004). Unabsorbed digestible P, which includes endogenous P, is assumed to pass into the large intestinal digestible P pool at the same fractional passage rate as for fluid. Endogenous P loss in faeces accounts for approximately 80% of the P excreted by the animal (McCaskill, 1990). Indigestible dietary P and undigested microbial P in the rumen are inputs to the indigestible P pool in the small intestines, which passes into the large intestine at a particulate matter passage rate of 4.0% h^{-1}.

Most of the P in the large intestine is present as insoluble P or nucleic acids (Poppi and Ternouth, 1979), so the model has a low affinity for P absorption in the large intestine, but there is some P utilization by microbes. The potentially digestible and indigestible P in the large intestine is excreted in faeces at a fractional passage rate of the large intestine.

Inputs to the extracellular fluid pool are from P absorbed post-ruminally and from bone resorption. The outputs are to the lower gastrointestinal tract (via bile), bone absorption, secretion in milk and excretion in urine. If the cow is pregnant, a figure for utilization by the fetus needs to be an output from this pool. Besides its structural function, bone represents a reserve of P and the model has bidirectional P flow to represent accretion and resorption. Milk P output is directly related to milk yield because the concentration of P in milk is constant (NRC, 2001). Ruminants fed roughage diets usually excrete very little P in their urine and it is generally accepted that the major variations in P balance are dependent on the digestive tract rather than the kidneys (Scott, 1988). Urinary P excretion was described by an exponential equation based on the experiments of Challa and Braithwaite (1988c), where at low P concentrations in the extracellular fluid (< 1.8 mmol l^{-1}), urinary P was relatively unimportant, but increased significantly as P concentration in extracellular fluid rose.

Phosphorus can be present in the soft tissues as lecithin, cephalin and sphingomyelin and in blood as phospholipids (Cohen, 1975). Blood constitutes the central pool of minerals that is readily available and red blood cells contain 350–450 mg P l^{-1}. Plasma P occurs mainly as organic compounds, with the remainder in inorganic forms, e.g. PO_4, HPO_4 and H_2PO_4 (Georgievskii, 1982). There is a correlation between inorganic P in plasma and P intake for animals fed deficient to moderate levels of P (Ternouth and Sevilla, 1990; Scott *et al.*, 1995). However, at high P intakes, the levels of inorganic P in plasma begin to stabilize. In cattle, P intake varying from 27.1 to 62.5 mg P kg^{-1} BW resulted in plasma P levels of 47 to 77 mg l^{-1}, respectively. In contrast, some reports have not observed a correlation between P intake and plasma P concentrations (Louvandini and Vitti, 1994; Louvandini, 1995).

Phosphorus homeostasis is normally maintained by the balance between P absorption from the digestive tract, excretion in the faeces, secretion in milk and the accretion or resorption from bone. Homeostasis was simulated in the model by estimating key parameters that controlled the movement of P in the different pools within the animal.

The model can be extended to other ruminant species by adjusting key parameters such as rumen and blood volume; however, there could be considerable intraspecies differences in P metabolism. Phosphorus also interacts with other minerals, especially Ca, and responds to vitamin D levels and endocrine factors, and these issues need to be addressed to improve our understanding of P metabolism.

Goats

Using data from balance and isotope tracer studies, a model of P metabolism in growing goats fed increasing levels of P was proposed by Vitti *et al.* (2000) (Fig. 16.3). The model has four pools (gut (1), blood (2), bone (3) and soft tissues (4)), and P enters the system via intake (F_{10}) and exits via faeces (F_{01}) and urine (F_{02}). The gut lumen, bone and soft tissue pools interchange bidirectionally with the blood pool, with fluxes F_{21} and F_{12}, F_{23} and F_{32}, and F_{24} and F_{42}, respectively. Labelled ^{32}P was administered as a single dose and the size and specific radioactivity of the blood, bone and soft tissues pools were measured 8 days after tracer administration. The scheme assumes there is no re-entry of label from external sources.

Vitti *et al.* (2000) postulated that, with P intakes insufficient to meet maintenance requirements, the input of P to the blood pool was maintained by increased bone P resorption and P mobilization from soft tissues. Compared to goats fed high P diets, those on a low P diet mobilized 74% more P from bone to the blood pool. Despite the low P intake leading to a negative P balance, an inevitable endogenous faecal loss of P occurs. The minimum endogenous loss of P from the goats was 67 mg day^{-1}, which must be absorbed to avoid being in negative balance. When P intake was increased to meet the maintenance requirements (zero P balance), the rate of absorption was increased in direct relation to P supply, so endogenous secretion in the digestive tract also increased. The maintenance requirement for P in Saanen goats was calculated to be 610 mg day^{-1} or 55 mg kg^{-1} metabolic body weight ($W^{0.75}$) day^{-1}. The model showed that bone resorption, faecal and endogenous P excretion and P absorption all play a part in P homeostasis in growing goats. Urinary P excretion did not influence the control of P metabolism, even in goats fed high P diets. At low P intakes, bone and tissue mobilization maintained P levels in blood. Vitti *et al.* (2002) adapted the model to illustrate the processes that occur in goats fed different levels of Ca and showed that Ca intake influenced absorption, retention and excretion of Ca. The model could be used to investigate P metabolism in other ruminants.

Sheep

Several studies have used sheep as a model for ruminants when studying P metabolism and have focused on empirical and kinetic methods.

Some steady-state models have been developed to resolve data from experiments with radioactive tracers (Schneider *et al.*, 1985, 1987; Dias *et al.*, 2006).

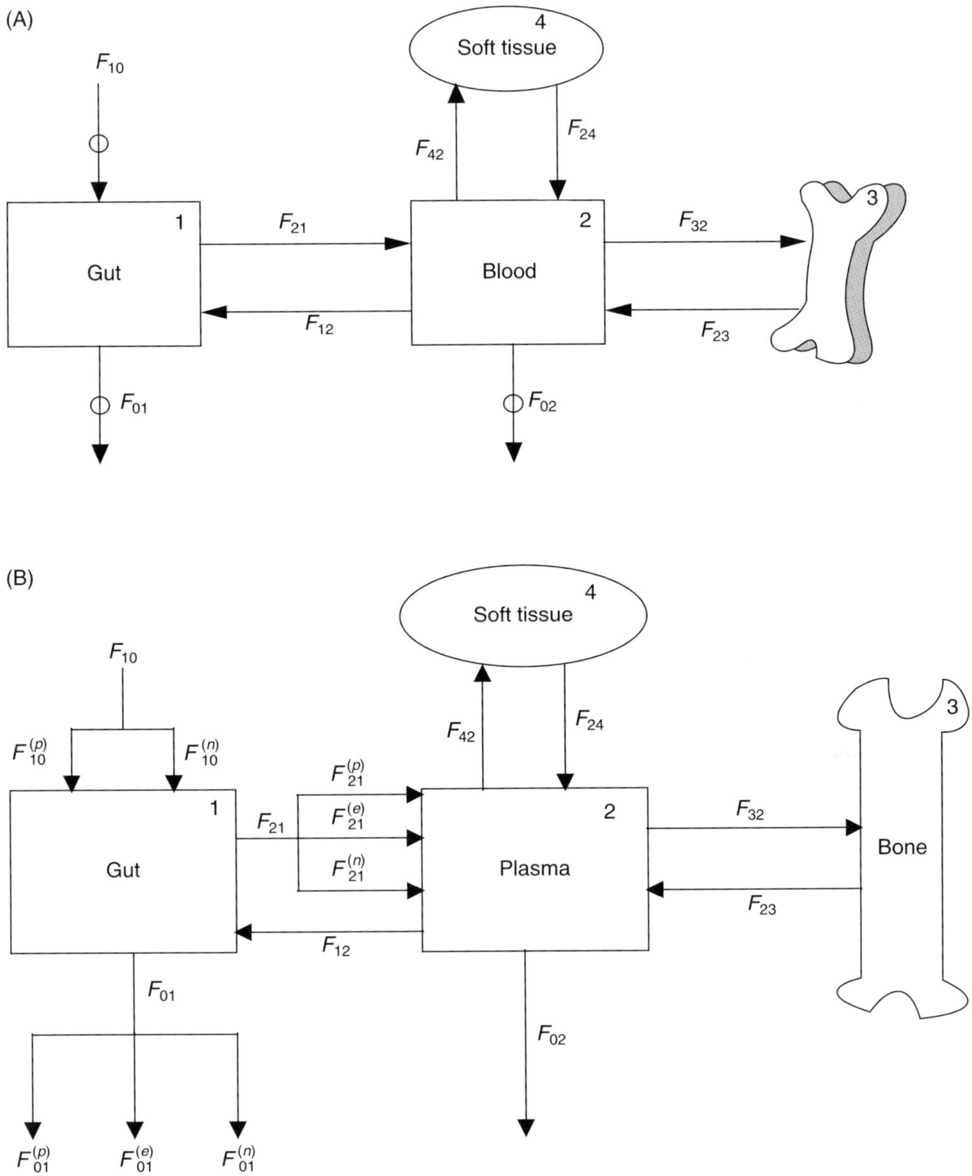

Fig. 16.3. (A) Schematic representation of the model of P metabolism in goats. F_{ij} is the total flux of pool *i* from *j*, F_{i0} is an external flux into pool *i* and F_{0j} a flux from pool *j* out of the system and circles denote fluxes measured experimentally (Vitti *et al.*, 2000). (B) Revised model of P metabolism in growing sheep showing phytate P. F_{10} denotes ingestion of P, F_{01} excretion of P in faeces, F_{02} excretion of P in urine. The flows F_{10}, F_{01} and F_{21} are partitioned as shown, with superscripts (*p*), (*e*) and (*n*) indicating P of dietary phytate, recycled endogenous and dietary non-phytate origin, respectively (Dias *et al.*, 2006).

The models are based on isotope dilution kinetics using ^{32}P as tracer, which is intravenously injected into the ruminant and its distribution within the body traced. The model of Schneider *et al.* (1987) used eight compartments to represent P pools within the body and analysed the tracer data using a compartmental analysis computer program (Boston *et al.*, 1981). Schneider *et al.* (1987) reported that the main control site for P excretion was the gastrointestinal tract and that model predictions were sensitive to parameters describing the absorption of P and salivation. Salivation rate was also found to be a major controlling factor in urinary P excretion, since decreasing salivation rate increased P concentrations in plasma and resulted in more P being excreted via urine.

Grace (1981) developed a compartmental model to represent P flow in sheep comprised of four pools, which together represented the total exchangeable P pool, the gut and non-exchangeable bone and soft tissues. Grace (1981) reported that most of the P was excreted via faeces, with only small amounts excreted in urine; however, as P intake increased, proportionally more of the P lost from the body was excreted in the urine rather than returned to the digestive tract via the saliva.

The model of P metabolism proposed by Vitti *et al.* (2000) in goats was revised and extended to include Ca flows in growing sheep (Dias *et al.*, 2006) (Fig. 16.3). Sheep weighing 32 kg were injected with ^{32}P and ^{45}Ca to trace the movement of P and Ca in the body. The revised model contained instantaneous values for pool derivatives rather than average values and was extended to represent absorption and excretion of phytate P. The revised model showed higher flows between plasma and bone than between plasma and tissue, which was a more accurate representation of observed values. Phosphorus and Ca metabolism were then assessed conjointly using the revised model. Dias *et al.* (2006) found that phytate P digestibility in the forage fed to the animals was only 47% and P retention was negative, suggesting that a feed characteristic impaired P utilization and led to P deficiency.

Modelling Phosphorus Metabolism in Non-ruminants

Phosphorus utilization in non-ruminants is markedly different to ruminants due to the absence of the rumen microorganisms which break down phytate P of plant origin using phytase enzymes. Cereal grains, oilseeds and grain by-products are major constituents of non-ruminant diets, but approximately two-thirds of their total P is present as phytate P (Eeckhout and De Paepe, 1994); therefore, research regarding P metabolism in non-ruminants is focused on determining P availability and improving P retention. This section discusses the modelling approaches that have been used to study P metabolism in pigs, poultry and, to a lesser extent, equines.

Pigs

The availability of P in feed ingredients for pigs is commonly evaluated using either digestibility studies or the slope–ratio assay technique (Jongbloed *et al.*, 1991).

Digestibility studies estimate P availability by measuring its digestive utilization, whereas the slope–ratio assay provides a combined estimate of digestive and post-absorptive utilization of P at the tissue level (Jongbloed *et al.*, 1991). In digestibility studies, determination of true P digestibility requires knowledge of endogenous P excretion and Fan *et al.* (2001) developed a linear regression analysis to determine true P digestibility and endogenous P excretion that was subsequently applied to maize-based (Shen *et al.*, 2002) and soybean meal-based (Ajakaiye *et al.*, 2003) diets for growing pigs. Methods of determining endogenous and faecal P losses are summarized by Fan *et al.* in Chapter 17 of this book. A concern with the approach of Fan *et al.* (2001) is whether the relationship between endogenous P output and dietary P intake is actually linear. Schulin-Zeuthen *et al.* (2007) addressed this concern by evaluating four functions. The functions chosen were a straight line, a diminishing returns function (monomolecular), a sigmoidal function with a fixed point of inflection (Gompertz) and a sigmoidal function with a flexible point of inflection (Richards) (Table 16.1). The non-linear functions were reparameterized to assign biological meaning to parameters and a meta-analysis of the data was used to estimate endogenous P excretion, maintenance requirement and efficiency of utilization. Phosphorus retention was regressed against either available P intake or total P intake (both variables scaled by $BW^{0.75}$). There was evidence of non-linearity in the data and the monomolecular function produced the best fit for the data. Estimates of endogenous P excretion of 14 and 17 mg kg^{-1} $BW^{0.75}$ day^{-1}, based on available and total P respectively, were predicted by the monomolecular equation, which agreed with Dilger and Adeola (2006), who summarized literature values and concluded that endogenous P excretion in pigs was likely to be less than 20 mg kg^{-1} $BW^{0.75}$ day^{-1}. Schulin-Zeuthen *et al.* (2007) estimated maintenance requirement as 15 and 37 mg P kg^{-1} $BW^{0.75}$ day^{-1} for available and total P based on the monomolecular equation, and average P conversion efficiency estimates were 65 and 36% for available and total P, respectively.

In a further study, Kebreab *et al.* (2007) used growth models and evaluated four mathematical functions (monomolecular, Gompertz, Richards and von Bertalanffy) to describe P utilization for growth. A meta-analysis found that the

Table 16.1. The functional forms used to describe the relationship between retained P, $y(x)$, and P intake, x.

Function[a]	$y(x)$	Value of x when $y = 0$
Straight line	$ax - b$	b/a
Monomolecular	$a - (a + b)e^{-cx}$	$c^{-1}\ln[(a+b)/a]$
Gompertz	$b\exp[(1-e^{-cx})\ln\frac{a+2b}{b}] - 2b$	$c^{-1}\ln\left\{\frac{\ln(a+2b)/b}{\ln[(a+2b)/(2b)]}\right\}$
Richards	$\frac{b(a+2b)}{\{b^n + [(a+2b)^n - b^n]e^{-cx}\}^{1/n}} - 2b$	$c^{-1}\ln\left\{\frac{2^n[(a+2b)^n - b^n]}{(a+2b)^n - (2b)^n}\right\}$

[a]The parameters a, b and c are positive entities, $n \geq -1$ and in non-linear models $y_{max} = a$ and $y_{min} = -b$.

monomolecular equation was best at determining efficiencies of P utilization for weight gain compared to the sigmoidal functions. Estimates for the rate constant parameters (change of P retention per unit time) in all functions decreased as available P intake increased. They also recommended that the Richards and monomolecular equations be included in growth and nutrient efficiency analyses. Furthermore, Schulin-Zeuthen *et al.* (2008) introduced the Schumacher growth function (Thornley and France, 2007) and evaluated its performance against well-known growth equations such as the Gompertz and Weibull. They reported that the Schumacher fits pig growth profiles well, especially those with lower inflection points than that predicted by the Gompertz equation and it is simpler than the Weibull, having only three parameters.

Isotope dilution techniques have been used to evaluate P metabolism in growing pigs fed a basal diet supplemented with increasing phytase levels using the model of Vitti *et al.* (2000) (Moreira, 2002). A single dose of radioactive ^{32}P was administered and blood samples taken for calculation of P flows. Total P absorbed was negatively related to total P excreted in faeces and decreased with increasing phytase level (Moreira, 2002). Phosphorus absorption and retention were highest at the lowest phytase inclusion level (157 mg kg^{-1} BW day^{-1} and 139 mg kg^{-1} BW day^{-1}, respectively). The model showed highest P flow from soft tissue to plasma at high phytase inclusion level, indicating that P was mobilized from soft tissue likely to attend P demand for bone growth. There was a strong correlation between total P absorbed and net bone P retention, suggesting that the main fate of P was bone deposition, regardless of total P absorption (Moreira, 2002).

Mechanistic models have been developed for pig nutrition (e.g. Birkett and de Lange, 2001; Halas *et al.* 2004), but they are focused on energy and protein metabolism and do not include a routine calculation for P transactions. Aarnink *et al.* (1992) developed a dynamic mathematical model to estimate the amount and composition of slurry, including P; however, retained P was empirically determined as a function of average daily gain (G, kg) and body weight (W), and was calculated as follows:

$$\text{Phosphorus retention} = 0.005467W^{-0.025}G$$

Birkett and de Lange (2001) described a computational framework for representing energy utilization in growing monogastric animals including the main biological and biochemical processes to estimate their contribution to energetic inefficiency. The model requires inputs such as DM intake, CP, crude fat, starch, simple sugars and ash. Outputs include undigested DM, N in urine and energy losses in methane. Recently, the model has been expanded to include a representation of P utilization (de Lange *et al.*, 2006).

Poultry

In poultry, P is required for replacement of tissue metabolites such as nucleotides and phospholipids, to maintain skeletal integrity, and, in hens, for production of the egg. There is a close relationship between P and Ca in the laying hen producing eggs. Calcium is the major structural element in eggshell and large amounts of Ca are required to synthesize the shell. The shell gland is usually active during the hours of darkness, but Ca stores in the gut may be low at this time since hens exhibit a nocturnal fast (Scanes *et al.*, 1987) and therefore rely on other sources of Ca, particularly mobilization from bone. The medullary bone is a specialized, highly mineralized bone containing a mobile source of Ca that acts as a temporary reserve, releasing Ca at times when supply from feed is insufficient (Etches, 1987). Calcium in bone is stored as calcium phosphate and, therefore, bone mobilization results in elevated concentrations of P in plasma and excretion of P, especially during times of shell formation (Hurwitz and Bar, 1965).

Several models have been developed to describe quantitative mineral flows in hens. Etches (1987) predicted intestinal Ca content, Ca retention, Ca deposition in eggshell and flows of Ca into and out of bone reserves on an hourly basis, but did not consider P in the model. Van Krieken (1996) and Tolboom and Kwakkel (1998) modelled Ca and P dynamics in hens partly based on the model of Etches (1987), also on an hourly basis, in which most transactions were linear.

Dijkstra *et al.* (2006) developed a dynamic, mechanistic model of Ca and P metabolism in layers using the rate:state formalism and non-linear kinetics to evaluate dietary and management strategies for reducing P excretion (Fig. 16.4). The model consists of eight state variables representing Ca and P pools in the crop (c), stomachs (proventriculus and gizzard) (s), plasma (p) and bone (b). P is defined as absorbable P at the terminal ileum. Zero pools are assigned to Ca and P in the duodenum (d), assuming that duodenal retention time for Ca and P is small.

Conte (2000) used isotope dilution techniques to determine endogenous faecal excretion, true P absorption and true P availability in broiler chickens fed

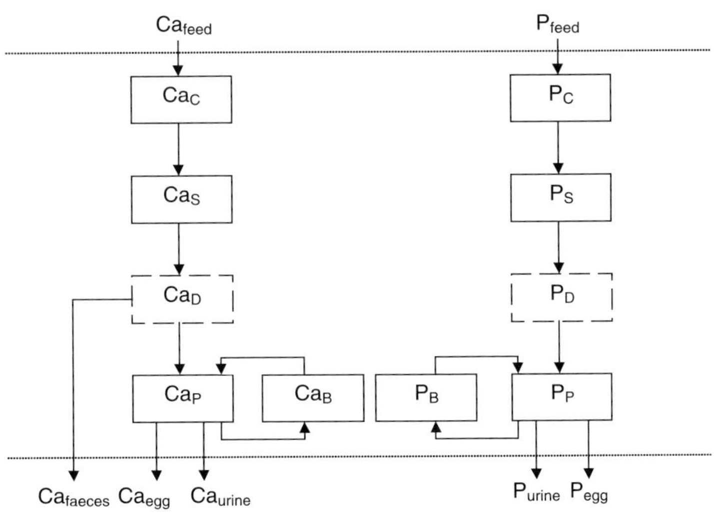

Fig. 16.4. Diagrammatic representation of the Ca and P model for laying hens. Boxes enclosed by solid lines denote state variables; boxes enclosed by dashed lines depict zero pools; arrows depict flows (Dijkstra *et al.*, 2006).

four levels of phytase in a diet containing 38% available P. He reported a linear increase in P availability up to a phytase inclusion level of 800 phytase units (FTU) kg^{-1} DM in the diet, which plateaued at an inclusion rate of 1200 FTU kg^{-1}. Endogenous faecal P and truly absorbed P also showed a linear increase with increasing phytase up to 800 FTU kg^{-1}. At low levels of phytase inclusion, endogenous P excretion was 12 mg day^{-1} and truly absorbed P was 273 mg day^{-1} (Conte, 2000).

Equine

Phosphorus constitutes 14–17% of the equine skeleton (El Shorafa *et al.*, 1979) and Schryver *et al.* (1971) estimated the daily endogenous P loss in mature horses at 10 mg kg^{-1} BW. NRC (1989) estimated the efficiency of true P absorption to range from 30 to 55%, depending on the age of the animal, the breed and concentration of dietary P. Assuming a P absorption efficiency of 35% for idle horses, gestating mares and working horses, the estimated P requirement for maintenance would be 28.6 mg kg^{-1} BW day^{-1} (10/0.35) (NRC, 1989). A mature, 500 kg horse would require 14.3 g P day^{-1} for maintenance. Although P in phytate was poorly absorbed, phytate P was partially available because there was some phytase in the equine lower gut (Hintz and Schryver, 1973).

Schryver *et al.* (1974) estimated that growing horses deposited approximately 8 g P kg^{-1} BW gain and the NRC (1989) assumed a P absorption efficiency of 45% for growing horses and lactating mares because their diets were typically supplemented with inorganic P. Therefore, the estimated P requirements for optimal bone development in a 215 kg foal gaining 0.85 kg day^{-1} would be 15.1 g P day^{-1} ((8 g $\times$ 0.85 kg)/0.45), in addition to its maintenance requirement of 4.8 g ((215 kg $\times$ 10 mg)/0.45) for a total of 19.9 g P day^{-1}.

During late gestation and lactation, P requirements increase. Although data on the rate of P deposition in the fetus are very limited, P requirements for the fetus of mares in months 9, 10 and 11 of pregnancy have been estimated to be 7, 12 and 6.7 mg kg^{-1} BW day^{-1}, respectively (Drepper and Drepper, 1982). Total daily P requirement for a 500 kg mare during the third trimester in months 9, 10 and 11 would therefore be 7.8, 13 and 7.4 g, respectively (NRC, 1989).

The concentration of P in mares' milk is 0.75 and 0.50 g kg^{-1} in early and late lactation, respectively (NRC, 1989). If the absorption efficiency is 45%, the daily P requirement above maintenance for lactation would be 25.0 g for a mare averaging 15 kg milk day^{-1} in early lactation and 11.1 g for the mare producing 10 kg milk day^{-1} during late lactation. At these rates of milk production, a 500 kg mare would require 36.0 and 22.2 g P day^{-1} in early and late lactation, respectively.

The Ca:P ratio is an important consideration for equine diets and ratios less than 1:1 (i.e. when P intake exceeds Ca intake) may be detrimental to Ca absorption (NRC, 1989). Schryver *et al.* (1971) have shown that, even when the Ca requirements are met, excessive P intake will cause skeletal malformations. However, Jordan *et al.* (1975) reported that Ca:P ratios as high as 6:1 in the diets of growing horses may not be detrimental if P intake is adequate.

Conclusions

Several types of modelling have been used to describe P flows in animals. Empirical models provide a quick and easy method for relating P input and outputs in different groups of animals. However, empirical models lack the necessary biological detail to evaluate different feeding strategies aimed at maximizing the efficiency of P utilization or reducing P excretion. The mechanistic models of P flow in ruminants and monogastric animals described in this chapter represent various processes within the animal and can be integrated with other extant models to provide a decision support tool that can lead to assessment of diets for their efficiency of utilization or pollution impact and suggest mitigation options. Mechanistic models provide an improved understanding of P metabolism and enable diets to be formulated to reduce environmental P pollution without compromising animal performance or health. This can be achieved by matching the animal's requirement for various physiological conditions with dietary P intake, which can be simulated using mechanistic models.

References

Aarnink, A.J.A., van Ouwekerk, E.N.J. and Verstegen, M.W.A. (1992) A mathematical model for estimating the amount of and composition of slurry from fattening pigs. *Livestock Production Science* 31, 133–147.

Agriculture and Food Research Council (AFRC) (1991) A reappraisal of the calcium and phosphorus requirements of sheep and cattle. *Nutrition Abstracts and Reviews (Series B)* 61, 573–612.

Ajakaiye, A., Fan, M.Z., Archbold, T., Hacker, R.R., Forsberg, C.W. and Phillips, J.P. (2003) Determination of true digestive utilization of phosphorus and the endogenous phosphorus outputs associated with soybean meal for growing pigs. *Journal of Animal Science* 81, 2766–2775.

Birkett, S.H. and Lange, C.F.M. de (2001) A computational framework for a nutrient flow representation of energy utilization by growing monogastric animals. *British Journal of Nutrition* 86, 661–674.

Boston, R.C., Greif, P.C. and Berman, M. (1981) Conversational SAAM – an interactive program for kinetic analysis of biological systems. *Computer Programs in Biomedicine* 13, 111–119.

Braithwaite, G.D. (1984) Some observations on phosphorus homoeostasis and requirements of sheep. *Journal of Agricultural Science, Cambridge* 102, 295–306.

Breves, G. and Schröder, B. (1991) Comparative aspects of gastrointestinal phosphorus metabolism. *Nutrition Research Reviews* 4, 125–140.

Care, A.D. (1994) The absorption of phosphate from the digestive tract of ruminant animals. *British Veterinary Journal* 150, 197–205.

Challa, J. and Braithwaite, G.D. (1988a) Phosphorus and calcium metabolism in growing calves with special emphasis on phosphorus homoeostasis. 1. Studies of the effect of changes in the dietary phosphorus intake on phosphorus and calcium metabolism. *Journal of Agricultural Science, Cambridge* 110, 573–581.

Challa, J. and Braithwaite, G.D. (1988b) Phosphorus and calcium metabolism in growing calves with special emphasis on phosphorus homoeostasis. 2. Studies of the effect of different levels of phosphorus, infused abomasally, on phosphorus metabolism. *Journal of Agricultural Science, Cambridge* 110, 583–589.

Challa, J. and Braithwaite, G.D. (1988c) Phosphorus and calcium metabolism in growing calves with special emphasis on phosphorus homoeostasis. 3. Studies of the effect of continuous intravenous infusion of different levels of phosphorus in ruminating calves receiving adequate dietary phosphorus. *Journal of Agricultural Science, Cambridge* 110, 591–595.

Cohen, R.D.H. (1975) Phosphorus and the grazing ruminant. An examination of the role of phosphorus in ruminant nutrition with particular reference to the beef cattle industry in Australia. *Animal Production* 11, 27–43.

Conte, A.J. (2000) Nutritive value of rice bran in broiler chicken diets supplemented with phytase and xylanase. PhD thesis, University of Lavras, Minas Gerais, Brazil.

Czerkawski, J.W. (1976) Chemical composition of microbial matter in the rumen. *Journal of the Science of Food and Agriculture* 27, 621–632.

Dias, R.S., Kebreab, E., Vitti, D.M.S.S., Roque, A.P., Bueno, I.C.S. and France, J. (2006) A revised model for studying phosphorus and calcium kinetics in growing sheep. *Journal of Animal Science* 84, 2787–2794.

Dijkstra, J. (1994) Simulation of the dynamics of protozoa in the rumen. *British Journal of Nutrition* 72, 679–699.

Dijkstra, J., Neal, H.D.St.C., Beever, D.E. and France, J. (1992) Simulation of nutrient digestion, absorption and outflow in the rumen: model description. *Journal of Nutrition* 122, 2239–2256.

Dijkstra, J., Kebreab, E., Kwakkel, R.P. and France, J. (2006) Development of a dynamic model of Ca and P flows in layers. In: Kebreab, E., Dijkstra, J., Gerrits, W.J.J., Bannink, A. and France, J. (eds) *Nutrient Utilization in Farm Animals: Modelling Approach*. CAB International, Wallingford, UK, pp. 192–210.

Dilger, R.N. and Adeola, O. (2006) Estimation of true phosphorus digestibility and endogenous phosphorus loss in growing pigs fed conventional and low-phytate soybean meals. *Journal of Animal Science* 84, 627–634.

Drepper, G. and Drepper, K. (1982) Isolation and identification of various bitter peptides from erythrocyte concentrates. *Zentralbl Veterinarmed Reihe A* 29, 237–252.

Eeckhout, W. and Paepe, M. De (1994) Total phosphorus, phytate–phosphorus and phytase activity in plant feedstuffs. *Animal Feed Science and Technology* 47, 19–29.

Ekpe, E.D., Zijlstra, R.T. and Patience, J.F. (2002) Digestible phosphorus requirement of grower pigs. *Canadian Journal of Animal Science* 82, 541–549.

Etches, R.J. (1987) Calcium logistics in the laying hen. *Journal of Nutrition* 117, 619–628.

Fan, M.Z., Archbold, T., Sauer, W.C., Lackeyram, D., Rideout, T., Gao, Y., Lange, C.F.M. de and Hacker, R.R. (2001) Novel methodology allows simultaneous measurement of true phosphorus digestibility and the gastrointestinal endogenous phosphorus outputs in studies with pigs. *Journal of Nutrition* 131, 2388–2396.

Georgievskii, V.I. (1982) The physiological role of macro elements. In: Georgievskii, V.I., Annenkov, B.N. and Samokhin, V.I. (eds) *Mineral Nutrition of Animals*. Butterworths, London, pp. 91–170.

GfE (Ausschuss für Bedarfsnormen der Gesellschaft für Ernährungsphysiologie) (2001) *Empfehlungen zur Energie- und Nährstoffversorgung der Milchkühe und Aufzuchtrinder*. DLG-Verlag, Frankfurt/Main, Germany.

Grace, N.D. (1981) Phosphorus kinetics in the sheep. *British Journal of Nutrition* 45, 367–374.

Halas, V., Dijkstra, J., Babinszky, L., Verstegen, M.W.A. and Gerrits, W.J.J. (2004) Modelling of nutrient partitioning in growing pigs to predict their anatomical body composition. 1. Model description. *British Journal of Nutrition* 92, 707–723.

Hintz, H.F. and Schryver, H.F. (1973) Magnesium, calcium and phosphorus metabolism in ponies fed varying levels of magnesium. *Journal of Animal Science* 37, 927–930.

Hurwitz, S. and Bar, A. (1965) Absorption of calcium and phosphorus along the gastrointestinal tract of the laying fowl as influenced by dietary calcium and egg shell formation. *Journal of Nutrition* 86, 433–438.

Jongbloed, A.W., Everts, H. and Kemme, P.A. (1991) Phosphorus availability and requirements in pigs. In: Heiemann, E.R. (ed.) *Recent Advances in Animal Nutrition.* Butterworths, London, pp. 65–80.

Jordan, R.M., Meyers, V.S., Yoho, B. and Spurrell, F.A. (1975) Effects of calcium and phosphorus levels on growth, reproduction, and bone development of ponies. *Journal of Animal Science* 40, 78–85.

Kebreab, E. and Vitti, D.M.S.S. (2005) Mineral metabolism. In: Dijkstra, J., Forbes, J.M. and France, J. (eds) *Quantitative Aspects of Ruminant Digestion and Metabolism.* CAB International, Wallingford, UK, pp. 469–486.

Kebreab, E., Mills, J.A.N., Crompton, L.A., Bannink, A., Dijkstra, J., Gerrits, W.J.J. and France, J. (2004) An integrated mathematical model to evaluate nutrient partition in dairy cattle between the animal and its environment. *Animal Feed Science and Technology* 112, 131–154.

Kebreab, E., France, J., Sutton, J.D., Crompton, L.A. and Beever, D.E. (2005a) Effect of energy and protein supplementation on phosphorus utilization in lactating dairy cows. *Journal of Animal and Feed Sciences* 14, 63–77.

Kebreab, E., Shah, M.A., Beever, D.E., Humphries, D.J., Sutton, J.D., France, J. and Mueller-Harvey, I. (2005b) Effects of contrasting forage diets on phosphorus utilisation in lactating dairy cows. *Livestock Production Science* 93, 125–135.

Kebreab, E., Schulin-Zeuthen, M., Lopez, S., Soler, J., Dias, R.S., Lange, C.F.M. de and France, J. (2007) Comparison of mathematical functions to describe growth and efficiency of phosphorus utilization in growing pigs. *Journal of Animal Science* 85, 2498–2507.

Lange, C.F.M. de, vanderVoort, G., Morel, P.C. and Visser, A. (2006) Current applications of pig growth models: assessing environmental and financial impacts. *Eastern Nutrition Conference*, Guelph, Ontario, Canada. Animal Nutrition Association of Canada, Ottawa.

Louvandini, H. (1995) Perda endógena de fósforo em ovinos suplementados com diferentes níveis do elemento na dieta. PhD thesis, Instituto de Pesquisas Energéticas e Nucleares, São Paulo, Brazil.

Louvandini, H. and Vitti, D.M.S.S. (1994) Perda endógena de fósforo em ovinos com diferentes níveis do elemento na dieta. *Pesquisa Agropecuária Brasileira* 29, 145–149.

McCaskill, M.R. (1990) Phosphorus and beef production in northern Australia: modeling phosphorus requirements of beef cattle. *Tropical Grassland* 24, 231–238.

McDowell, L.R. (1992) *Minerals in Animal and Human Nutrition*. Academic Press, New York, 524 pp.

Moreira, J.A. (2002) Use of radiophosphorus to study the bioavailability and endogenous losses, kinetic flow in tissues through a mathematical model associated with the performance of pigs fed diets containing phytase. PhD thesis, University of São Paulo, São Paulo, Brazil.

National Research Council (NRC) (1989) *Nutrient Requirement of Horses*, 5th edn. National Academy Press, Washington, DC.

National Research Council (NRC) (1998) *Nutrient Requirements of Swine*, 10th edn. National Academy Press, Washington, DC.

National Research Council (NRC) (2001) *Nutrient Requirement of Dairy Cattle*, 7th edn. National Academy Press, Washington, DC.

Pfeffer, E., Beede, D.K. and Valk, H. (2005) Phosphorus metabolism in ruminants and requirements of cattle. In: Pfeffer, E. and Hristov, A.N. (eds) *Nitrogen and Phosphorus Nutrition of Cattle*. CAB International, Wallingford, UK, pp. 195–231.

Poppi, D.P. and Ternouth, J.H. (1979) Secretion and absorption of phosphorus in the gastrointestinal tract of sheep fed on four diets. *Australian Journal of Agricultural Research* 30, 503–512.

Reinhardt, T.A., Horst, R.L. and Goff, J.P. (1988) Calcium, phosphorus, and magnesium homeostasis in ruminants. *Veterinary Clinics of North America: Food Animal Practice* 4, 331–350.

Scanes, C.G., Campbell, R. and Griminger, P. (1987) Control of energy balance during egg production in the laying hen. *Journal of Nutrition* 117, 605–611.

Schneider, K.N., Ternouth, J.H., Sevilla, C.C. and Boston, R.C. (1985) A short-term study of calcium and phosphorus absorption in sheep fed on diets high and low in calcium and phosphorus. *Australian Journal of Agricultural Research* 36, 91–105.

Schneider, K.M., Boston, R.C. and Leaver, D.D. (1987) Quantitation of phosphorus excretion in sheep by compartmental analysis. *American Journal of Physiology* 252, R720–R731.

Schröder, B., Happner, H., Failing, K., Pfeffer, E. and Breves, G. (1995) Mechanisms of intestinal phosphate transport in small ruminants. *British Journal of Nutrition* 74, 635–648.

Schryver, H.F., Hintz, H.F. and Craig, P.H. (1971) Phosphorus metabolism in ponies fed varying levels of phosphorus. *Journal of Nutrition* 101, 1257–1263.

Schryver, H.F., Hintz, H.F. and Lowe, J.E. (1974) Calcium and phosphorus in the nutrition of the horse. *Cornell Veterinary* 64, 493–515.

Schulin-Zeuthen, M., Kebreab, E., Gerrits, W.J.J., Lopez, S., Fan, M.Z., Dias, R.S. and France, J. (2007) Meta-analysis of phosphorus balance data from growing pigs. *Journal of Animal Science* 85, 1953–1961.

Schulin-Zeuthen, M., Kebreab, E., Dijkstra, J., Lopez, S., Bannink, A. and France, J. (2008) A comparison of the Schumacher with other functions for describing growth in pigs. *Animal Feed Science and Technology* (in press).

Scott, D. (1988) Control of phosphorus balance in ruminants. In: *Proceedings of the Satellite Symposium of the International Congress of the International Union of Physiological Sciences, 30, Aspects of Digestive Physiology in Ruminants*. Comstock Publishing Associates, Ithaca, New York, pp. 156–174.

Scott, D., Rajaratne, A.A.J. and Buchan, W. (1995) Factors affecting faecal endogenous phosphorus loss in the sheep. *Journal of Agricultural Science, Cambridge* 124, 145–151.

Shen, Y., Fan, M.Z., Ajakaiye, A. and Archbold, T. (2002) Use of the regression analysis technique to determine the true phosphorus digestibility and the endogenous phosphorus output associated with corn in growing pigs. *Journal of Nutrition* 132, 1199–1206.

El Shorafa, W.M., Feaster, J.P. and Ott, E.A. (1979) Metacarpal bone: age, ash content, cortical area and failure stress interrelationships. *Journal of Animal Science* 49, 979–982.

Spiekers, H., Brintrup, R., Balmelli, M. and Pfeffer, E. (1993) Influence of dry matter intake on faecal phosphorus losses in dairy cows fed rations low in phosphorus. *Journal of Animal Physiology and Animal Nutrition* 69, 37–43.

Ternouth, J.H. and Sevilla, C.C. (1990) The effects of low levels of dietary phosphorus upon the dry matter intake and metabolism of lambs. *Australian Journal of Agricultural Research* 41, 175–184.

Thornley, J.H.M. and France, J. (2007) *Mathematical Models in Agriculture*, 2nd edn. CAB International, Wallingford, UK, 910 pp.

Tolboom, J.G. and Kwakkel, R.P. (1998) Dynamic modelling of Ca and P flows in layers: prospects to reduce dietary digestible P levels. *British Poultry Science* (Supplement) 39, S43–S44.

Van Krieken, M.A. (1996) Calcium and phosphorus in layers [in Dutch]. MSc thesis, Wageningen University, The Netherlands.

Vitti, D.M.S.S., Kebreab, E., Abdalla, A.L., De Carvalho, F.F.R., De Resende, K., Crompton, L.A. and France, J. (2000) A kinetic model of phosphorus metabolism in growing goats. *Journal of Animal Science* 78, 2706–2712.

Vitti, D.M.S.S., Kebreab, E., Lopes, J.B., Dorigan, C.J., De Resende, K.T., Abdalla, A.L., Crompton, L.A. and France, J. (2002) Calcium metabolism in Saanen goats – a kinetic model. *Proceedings of the British Society of Animal Science*. BSAS, Penicuik, UK, 105 pp.

Wasserman, R.H. (1981) Intestinal absorption of calcium and phosphorus. *Federation Proceedings* 40, 68–72.

17 Methodological Considerations for Measuring Phosphorus Utilization in Pigs

M.Z. Fan,[1] Y. Shen,[1] Y.L. Yin,[2] Z.R. Wang,[3] Z.Y. Wang,[4] T.J. Li,[2] T.C. Rideout,[1] R.L. Huang,[2] T. Archbold,[1] C.B. Yang[1] and J. Wang[5]

[1]*Centre for Nutrition Modelling, Department of Animal and Poultry Science, University of Guelph, Canada;* [2]*Institute of Subtropical Agricultural Research, The Chinese Academy of Sciences, China;* [3]*College of Animal Science, Xinjiang Agricultural University, China;* [4]*College of Wildlife Resources, Northeast Forestry University, China;* [5]*National Institute of Animal Sciences, The Chinese Academy of Agricultural Sciences, China*

Introduction

Phosphorus (P) is an essential macromineral for all known life forms and is utilized by microorganisms, plants and animals in the form of inorganic phosphates (Pi) such as HPO_4^{2-}, $H_2PO_4^-$ and PO_4^{3-}, which are the basic functional units of P (Carpenter, 2005). Therefore, understanding P nutrition requires a knowledge of phosphate utilization and metabolism (Berner and Shike, 1988; Anderson, 1991).

At present, global pig production operates at a low P conversion efficiency of 30–60%, which contributes to the overall poor P recycling among the agrifood production system and human food chains, as summarized in Table 17.1. The poor efficiency of P utilization in pigs has the following three major concerns. First, P is the third most expensive nutrient after energy and protein in pig rations (NRC, 1998; Fan *et al.*, 2001). Thus, improving the efficiency of dietary P utilization will reduce feed costs and improve profitability. Secondly, Pi is a limited and non-renewable natural resource and the geological distribution (Forsberg *et al.*, 2005) and conservation of P have become global issues (Abelson, 1999). Finally, excessive P excretion in pig manure is a key pollutant responsible for surface-water eutrophication (Mallin, 2000). In addition to the adverse effect on marine life, eutrophication of surface water results in anaerobic biogenesis of odour compounds (Forsberg *et al.*, 2005) and greenhouse gas emission

Table 17.1. Efficiencies (% of total dietary intake) of major steps of whole-body phosphorus (P) utilization in weanling and growing pigs.

Items	Weanling pigs	Growing pigs
Without both inorganic P and microbial phytase supplementations:[a,b]		
Total faecal P loss	68	59
Apparent P digestibility	32	41
Total urinary loss	4	5
Apparent P retention	28	36
With inorganic P but no microbial phytase supplementation:[c,d]		
Total faecal P loss	51	42
Apparent P digestibility	49	59
Total urinary loss	5	5
Apparent P retention	44	54
Without inorganic P but with microbial phytase supplementation:[e,f]		
Total faecal P loss	36	43
Apparent P digestibility	64	58
Total urinary loss	4	3
Apparent P retention	61	55
Low-phytate cereals without both inorganic P and microbial phytase supplementations:[g,h]		
Total faecal P loss	49	44
Apparent P digestibility	51	56
Total urinary loss	7	2
Apparent P retention	43	48

Weanling pigs: [a]Lei *et al.* (1993a,b), Spencer *et al.* (2000) and Sands *et al.* (2001); [c]Lei *et al.* (1993a) and Spencer *et al.* (2000); [e]Lei *et al.* (1993a,b) and Sands *et al.* (2001); [g]Spencer *et al.* (2000) and Sands *et al.* (2001).
Growing pigs: [b]Mroz *et al.* (1994) and Fan *et al.* (2005); [d]Armstrong and Spears (2001), Rideout and Fan (2004) and Fan *et al.* (2005); [f]Mroz *et al.* (1994) and Fan *et al.* (2005); [h]Veum *et al.* (2001, 2002).

(Naqvi *et al.*, 2000), as illustrated in Fig. 17.1. The problems associated with poor P utilization have made research on improving the efficiency of P retention in pigs one of the most important issues in pig nutrition research.

This chapter will review the major processes of digestive and post-absorptive utilization of dietary P in pigs, examine the methodology for measuring whole-body P utilization and discuss the criteria developed for assessing P bioavailability in feed ingredients for formulating pig diets and strategies developed for improving the efficiency of P utilization in pigs.

Definitions of Digestive and Post-absorptive Use Processes

Whole-body P utilization can be partitioned into the two processes of digestion and post-absorptive utilization, as illustrated in Fig. 17.2.

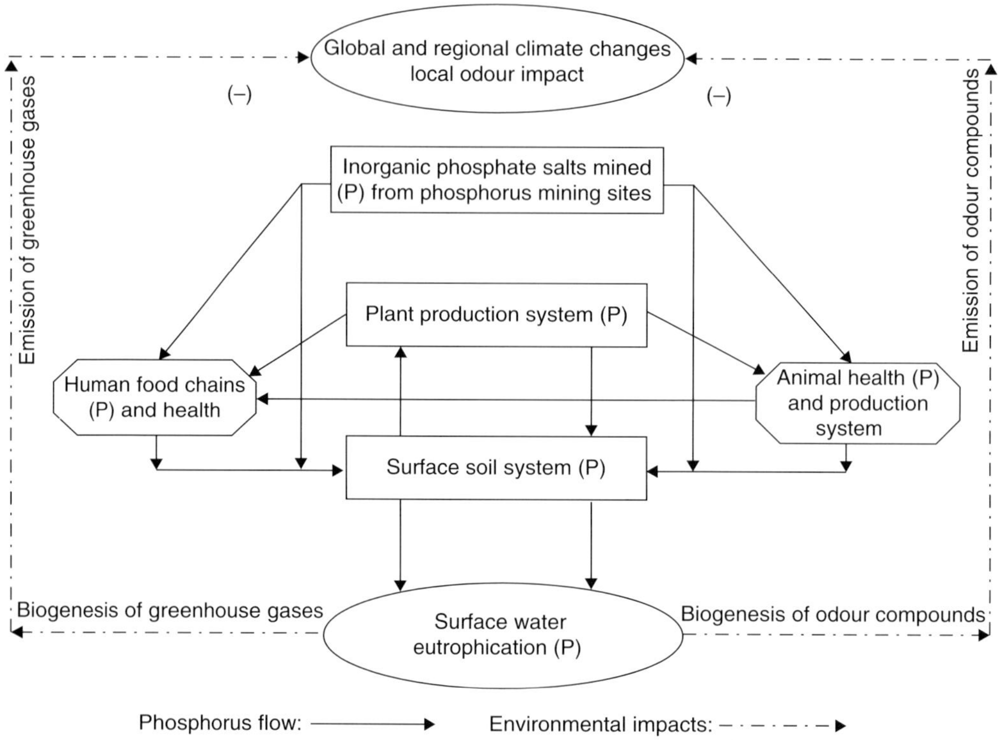

Fig. 17.1. Illustration of phosphorus (P) as a non-renewable natural resource essential to agricultural, plant and animal production systems and human food chains and health, as well as its potential detrimental impacts on the environment.

Digestive utilization

The major steps in the digestive utilization of dietary P are shown in Fig. 17.3. A large proportion of total P in feed ingredients of plant origin is present in the form of phytate (Jongbloed *et al.*, 1991). Digestion of dietary P includes gastric hydrolytic release of phytate P under an acidic environment by dietary supplementation of the exogenous phytase (Simons *et al.*, 1990) and the salivary endogenous phytase in the transgenic phytase pig (Golovan *et al.*, 2001), as well as the microbial degradation release of phytate P in the distal small intestinal region and, to a lesser extent, in the hindgut (Shen *et al.*, 2005d; Shen, 2006). Although Pi transport across the mucosal apical membrane in the large intestine has been reported in pigs, this process is likely to be limited to the maintaining of local mucosal tissue growth and metabolism (Shen, 2006; Shen and Fan, 2007). The large intestine contributes little to P absorption in the pig (Fan *et al.*, 2001; Schröder *et al.*, 2002; Shen *et al.*, 2005d; Shen, 2006). Other organic forms of P in phospholipids, nucleic acids and phosphorylated proteins are hydrolysed by exocrine pancreatic and intestinal mucosal phospholipases (Tso, 1994) and intestinal alkaline phosphatase (Fan *et al.*, 2002a), as well as by

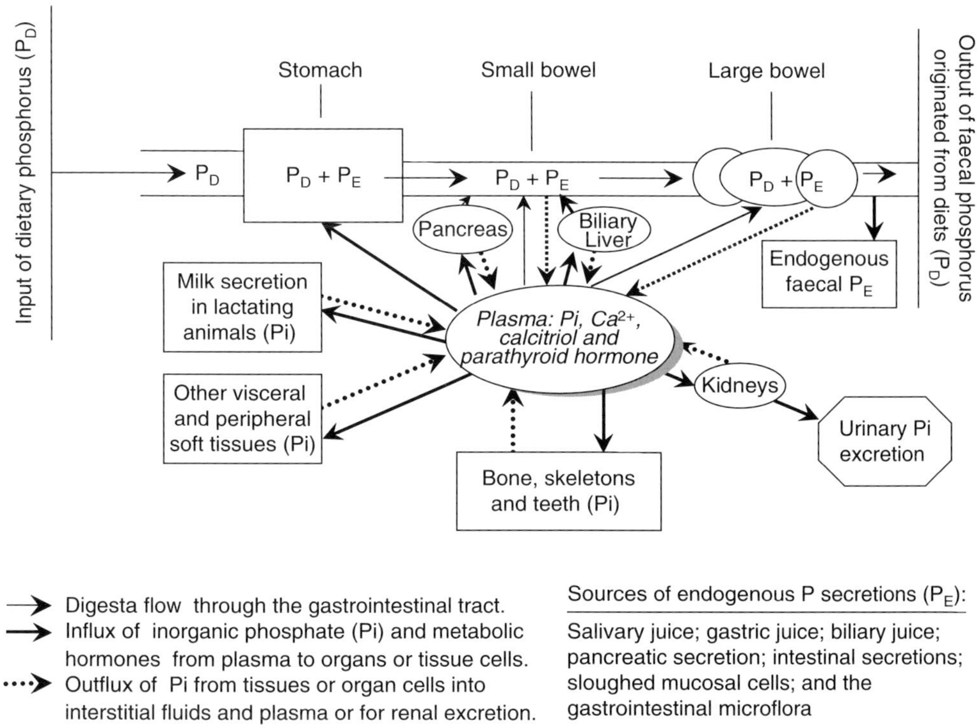

Fig. 17.2. Schematic representation of whole-body phosphorus (P) flow between organs and tissues and the major routes of P excretions in pigs. Adapted from Fan *et al.* (2001).

pancreatic nuclease, intestinal mucosal phosphodiesterases and nucleotidases (Newsholme and Leech, 1991), which are all unlikely to be limiting steps. The inorganic supplemental P salts, on the other hand, must be solubilized and ionized in the intestinal lumen in order to be absorbed (Fig. 17.3). Therefore, the gastric hydrolysis of phytate is thought to be the rate-limiting step in the absorption of dietary P in pigs consuming commercial diets (Shen *et al.*, 2005d).

Transport of the digestive end product Pi, from the intestinal lumen across the apical membrane of the brush border via the paracellular and transcellular routes, marks the end of the digestive process (Fig. 17.3) (Fan *et al.*, 2006). The intracellular environment of the intestinal epithelial cells is relatively more negatively charged compared with its extracellular environment. Therefore, transport of negatively charged ions or solutes across the apical membrane is against the membrane potential gradient and transcellular Pi uptake is operated by Na^+–Pi (NaPi) type-II co-transporters driven by an Na^+ gradient across the membrane. The solute carrier family SLC34 genes, including NaPi-IIa, b and c isomers, have been characterized in rodents and humans (Hilfiker *et al.*, 1998; Xu *et al.*, 1999; Murer *et al.*, 2004). Recently, the partial cDNA sequences for the NaPi-IIa, b and c isomers have been reported for the major visceral organs of pigs (Yang *et al.*, 2006). NaPi-IIa messenger RNA (mRNA) was expressed in kidney, NaPi-IIb mRNA

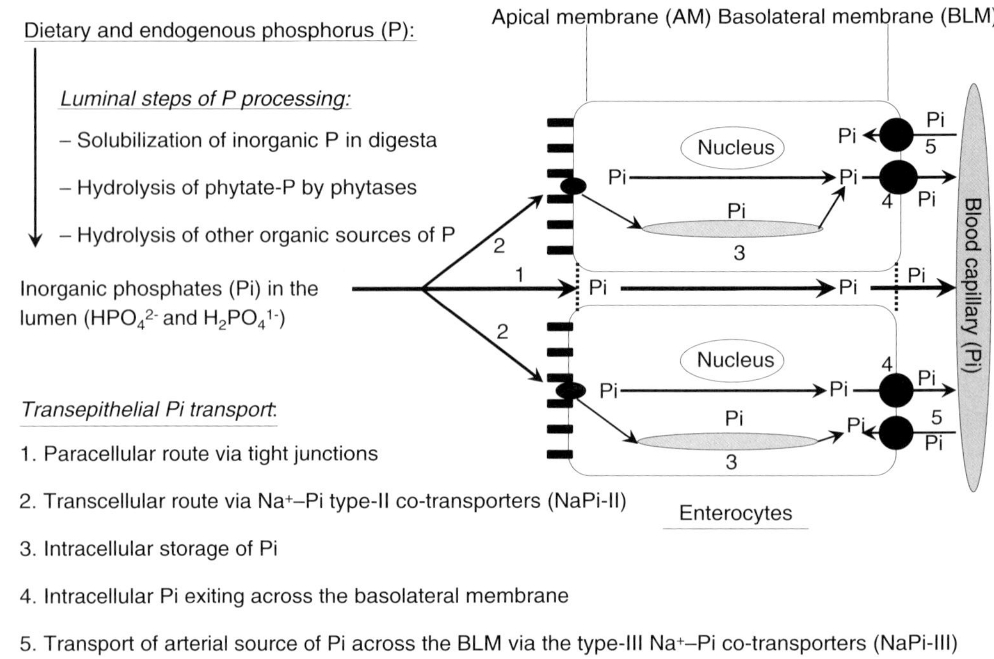

Fig. 17.3. Pathways of intestinal phosphorus (P) digestion and transport in pigs.

was detectable only in lung and NaPi-IIc mRNA was expressed in the intestines, kidney, lung, liver and heart (Yang *et al.*, 2006). The abundance of NaPi-IIc mRNA was low in the duodenum, high in the proximal jejunum and there was a decreasing gradient in the distal jejunum, ileum, caecum and colon (Yang *et al.*, 2006). The NaPi-IIb isomer is expressed in the gut of rodents and humans (Hilfiker *et al.*, 1998; Xu *et al.*, 1999). Thus, porcine gut expresses a different NaPi-II isomer for transcellular Pi uptake across the apical membrane. The paracellular transport of Pi is believed to be driven by both Pi and osmolarity gradients across the intestinal epithelia (Danisi and Murer, 1992; Schröder *et al.*, 2002). However, little is known regarding mechanisms of the paracellular regulation of Pi uptake in the gut. Recent studies in pigs have demonstrated that apical transcellular Na^+–Pi uptake activity occurs along the entire length of the small and the large intestines (Shen, 2006; Shen and Fan, 2007). However, this apical transcellular Na^+–Pi uptake capacity accounts for approximately 1% only of the total daily Pi requirement in the post-weaned pig, suggesting that apical transcellular Na^+–Pi uptake is only essential to obtain luminal Pi for maintaining gut mucosal growth and metabolism (Shen and Fan, 2007). Thus, the small intestinal paracellular transport of Pi may be the major route of intestinal P absorption in pigs and other mammalian species.

From the nutritional point of view, the disappearance of the digestive end products from the intestinal apical membrane surface at the end of an appropriate intestinal segment is measured as nutrient digestibility (Fan *et al.*, 2006). Several studies have shown no differences between the distal ileal and the faecal

P digestibility in pigs (Fan *et al.*, 2001; Shen *et al.*, 2002; Ajakaiye *et al.*, 2003). It has been recommended that true, rather than apparent, faecal P digestibility should be measured in feed ingredients or diets for pigs (Fan *et al.*, 2001; Shen *et al.*, 2002; Petersen and Stein, 2006; Fang *et al.*, 2007).

Post-absorptive utilization

Transport of the digestive end product Pi across the intestinal apical membrane is also the starting point of the post-absorptive utilization process (see Figs 17.2 and 17.3). Post-absorptive utilization of absorbed Pi includes utilization and metabolism inside the epithelia, movement through the intestinal epithelial intracellular environment, exit across the epithelial basolateral membrane, movement through the interstitial fluid and transport across the plasma membranes for utilization and metabolism by visceral organs and peripheral tissues (see Figs 17.2 and 17.3).

Intracellular metabolic fates for Pi include protein phosphorylation, biosynthesis of phospholipids and nucleotides (Newsholme and Leech, 1991), as well as biosynthesis of inositol molecules for signalling functions (Chi and Crabtree, 2000). Subcellular use of Pi in the mitochondria involves the transport of Pi across the mitochondrial inner membrane (Newsholme and Leech, 1991). Little is known about the mechanisms involved whereby Pi moves through the intracellular matrix to the basolateral membrane; none the less, an intracellular gradient of Pi or a channelling system must exist to facilitate the Pi movement through the cells. The exit of Pi across the basolateral membrane from the inside of the cell is, in principle, favoured by the membrane potential gradient and may include a Na^+-independent transporter driven by the Pi gradient; however, such a putative Na^+-independent Pi transporter has not been identified at this time. As shown in Fig. 17.2, an essential step for the subsequent utilization of the absorbed Pi is the transport of Pi across the plasma membrane from extracellular fluid. Two such Na^+–Pi co-transporter proteins have been identified in mammalian species and subsequently classified as type-III Na^+–Pi co-transporters (Collins *et al.*, 2004). These Na^+Pi-III co-transporters were originally described as retroviral receptors and are now also termed Pit-1 (SLC20A1) and Pit-2 (SLC20A2) (Collins *et al.*, 2004). Pit-1 and Pit-2 are known to be expressed on the basolateral membrane of polarized epithelial cells responsible for uptake of circulatory Pi into cells such as intestinal and renal epithelia. In addition, Pit-1 and Pit-2 are also expressed in bone, aortic smooth muscle cells and parathyroid glands (Collins *et al.*, 2004).

Endogenous gastrointestinal P secretions, recycling and losses are important steps in the post-absorptive metabolism of P, the major components of which are illustrated in Fig. 17.2. Methods for measuring the endogenous P losses are discussed in a later section of this chapter. Under normal nutritional and physiological conditions, endogenous P loss is the second largest route of P inefficiency after indigestible faecal P loss (Rideout and Fan, 2004; Fan *et al.*, 2005). The faecal endogenous P loss is the largest component of the daily P requirement for the maintenance determined by the factorial analysis approach (Schulin-Zeuthen *et al.*, 2007). Urinary P excretion is another major route of excretion for post-absorptive Pi inefficiency mediated by renal Na^+–Pi co-transporters (Fig. 17.2; Murer *et al.*, 2004). When pigs are fed within recommended P requirement levels, urinary P excretion is within 2% of the total manure P loss (e.g. Rideout and Fan, 2004; Pettey *et al.*, 2006).

Methods for Measuring P Utilization

Methods for measuring P utilization reviewed in this section include:

1. The assay of phytate-P content, phytase activity and *in vivo* phytate degradation rate.
2. Estimating intestinal apical transcellular Na^+–Pi co-transport kinetic parameters and using *in vitro* apical membrane vesicles and a system biology approach for calculating Pi transport capacity.
3. Measuring true P digestibility and gastrointestinal endogenous P loss associated with feed ingredients.
4. Quantifying urinary P excretion in the pig.

Assay of phytate-P content, phytase activity and *in vivo* phytate degradation rate

Vegetal ingredients are the major sources of dietary P and a large proportion of the total P in plant ingredients is phytate P. The hydrolysis of phytate by phytase is considered to be the rate-limiting step in the digestion of vegetal P in pigs, as demonstrated by Golovan *et al.* (2001). Phytase in pig diets comes from many sources, including vegetal ingredients (Reddy, 2002), feed additives (Lambrechts *et al.*, 1992), microbes in the lumen of the gastrointestinal tract of animals (Sreeramulu *et al.*, 1996) and gut mucosa of some animal species (Maenz and Classen, 1998). Two approaches are used in assaying phytase activity, including the one time-point method and the multiple time-point linearity analysis method (Maenz and Classen, 1998; Shen *et al.*, 2005d). The one time-point method measures phytase activity over one period of incubation time (e.g. 1 h) and assumes a constant velocity of inorganic P hydrolysis under the given assay conditions (Engelen *et al.*, 2001). The linearity analysis of multiple time-point incubations is also used for measuring phytase activity (Maenz and Classen, 1998). Recent studies by Shen *et al.* (2005d) have suggested that the one time-point method may underestimate intrinsic phytase activity for certain ingredients, such as oats, and that multiple time-point experiments need to be conducted to determine reliable intrinsic phytase activity from the slope of the linear relationship (Fig. 17.4).

Several other methods have been developed to measure the phytate-P content of samples, including the precipitation method (Vaintraub and Lapteva, 1988), high-performance liquid chromatography (HPLC) (Tangendjaja *et al.*, 1980),

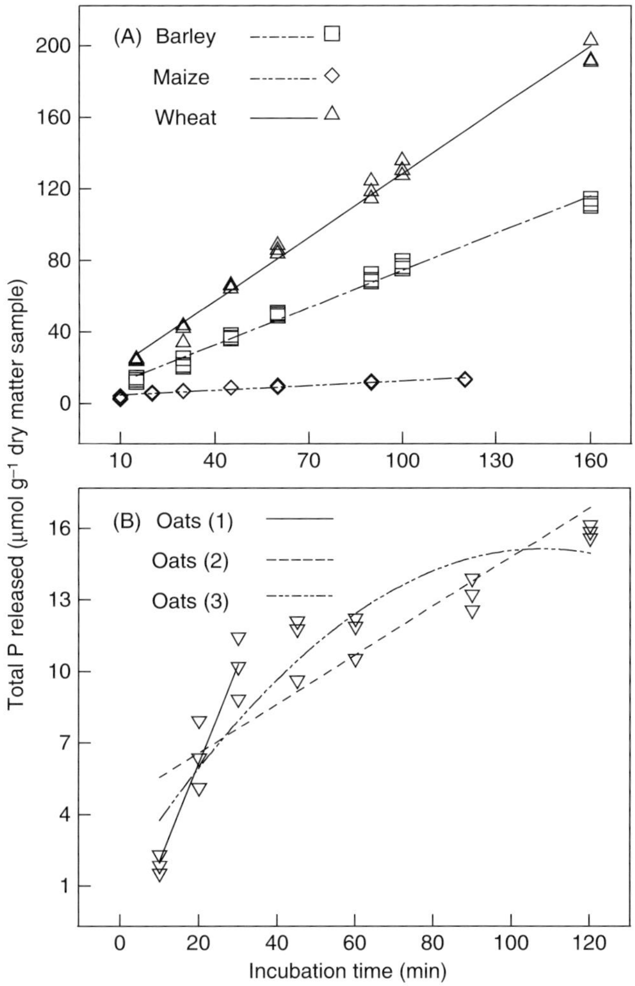

Fig. 17.4. Time-course monitoring the amount of phosphorus (P) released from selected cereal grains by intrinsic phytase hydrolysis. (A) Linear relationship: wheat, $y = 9.547 + 1.189x$, $R^2 = 0.99$; barley, $y = 5.006 + 0.693x$, $R^2 = 0.99$; and maize, $y = 3.926 + 0.086x$, $R^2 = 0.91$; $P < 0.05$ for all the parameter estimates; (B) curvilinear and linear relationships: (i) analysed linear relationship in the oat sample for up to 30 min of incubation, $y = -2.362 + 0.412x$, $R^2 = 0.99$, $P < 0.05$; (ii) analysed linear relationship in the oat sample for up to 2-h incubation, $y = 4.348 + 0.103x$, $R^2 = 0.77$, $P < 0.05$; and (iii) analysed quadratic relationship in the oat sample for up to 2-h incubation, $y = 1.130 + 0.257x - 0.001x^2$, $R^2 = 0.87$, $P < 0.05$ for all the parameter estimates. Adapted from Shen *et al.* (2005d).

ion-exchange chromatography (Skoglund and Sandberg, 2002) and the phytase incubation method (Wheeler and Ferrel, 1971). The precipitation and HPLC methods measure total phytic acid content and assume the inositol phosphate is associated with six phosphate groups (Skoglund and Sandberg, 2002). The ion-exchange chromatography method allows the analysis of inositol phosphate isomers with one to six phosphate groups (Skoglund and Sandberg, 2002), but application of the technique may be limited due to its relatively complicated procedures and the commercial supply of purified phytate isomers as standards. Although intrinsic plant phytase activity may not completely hydrolyse phytate P, microbial phytase is shown to completely dephosphorylate phytate with prolonged incubations (Newkirk and Classen, 1998). Studies by Shen *et al.* (2005d) indicated that there were quadratic with plateau relationships between the release of inorganic P from various sources of phytate using microbial phytases. The minimal incubation time required to reach the plateau level of phytate hydrolysis was affected by the sources of phytate (Fig. 17.5). It was concluded that multiple time-point experiments needed to be conducted with microbial phytases to determine phytate-P content in samples (Shen *et al.*, 2005d).

For the calculation of phytate-P content in samples, the maximum plateau value of net P released from the microbial phytase incubations can be obtained by using the segmented quadratic with plateau model (Eqn 17.1):

$$y = a + bx + cx^2, \text{ if } x < x_0 \tag{17.1}$$

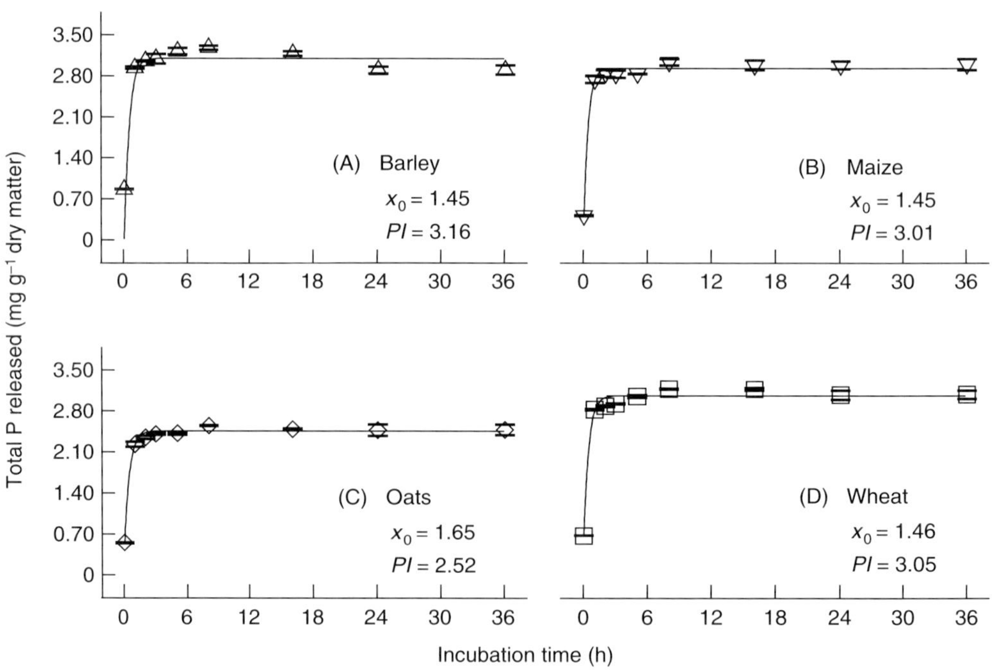

Fig. 17.5. Quadratic plateau relationships between the amount of phosphorus (P) released and incubation time from selected cereal grains after enzymatic hydrolysis by microbial phytase. (A) barley, $y = 0.98 + 3.64x - 1.26\ x^2$, $R^2 = 0.99$; (B) maize, $y = 0.48 + 4.05x - 1.38x^2$, $R^2 = 0.99$; (C) oats, $y = 0.60 + 2.71x - 0.82\ x^2$, $R^2 = 0.99$; and (D) wheat, $y = 0.75 + 3.82x - 1.31\ x^2$, $R^2 = 0.99$, $P < 0.05$ for all the parameter estimates. Adapted from Shen *et al.* (2005d). x_0, breakpoint between the quadratic and the plateau sections on the *x*-axis; *PI*, initial plateau value on the *y*-axis.

$$y = PI, \text{ if } x > x_0, \tag{17.2}$$

where y is the amount of P released; a is the intercept of the quadratic equation; b is the slope of the linear effect; x_0 is incubation time; c is the slope of the quadratic effect; x_0 is the breakpoint on the x-coordinate between the quadratic and the plateau sections and represents the minimal incubation time required for the maximal phytate hydrolysis; and PI is the initial plateau value of Pi released from microbial phytase hydrolysis.

When $x < x_0$, the equation relating y and x is quadratic; when $x > x_0$, the equation is a constant, i.e. the plateau value from Eqn 17.2. The two sections must meet at x_0 on the x-axis and the curve must be continuous and smooth. Thus, x_0 and PI can be obtained from Eqns 17.3 and 17.4:

$$x_0 = 0.5\ b/c \tag{17.3}$$

$$PI = a + bx_0 + cx_0^2 = a - b^2/(4c). \tag{17.4}$$

True *in vivo* degradability of phytate-P complex at the precaecal and faecal stages in the pig can be measured according to Eqn 17.5 by using the linear regression analysis described by Shen *et al.* (2002) and Shen (2006):

$$P_{Ai} = -P_E + [(D_T \times 100^{-1}) \times P_{Di}], \tag{17.5}$$

where P_{Ai} represents the apparent ileal or faecal degradable P content in the ith diet (g kg^{-1} dry matter intake (DMI)); P_E is the endogenous source of phytate originated from the endogenous secretions and gut microbes in the ileal digesta or faeces (g kg^{-1} DMI); D_T is the true ileal or faecal phytate degradation rate (%) in a test ingredient; and P_{Di} is the total phytate P content in the ith diet (g kg^{-1} DMI).

Shen *et al.* (2005c) compared true degradability values of phytate-P complex of oats using weanling and growing pigs (Fig. 17.6) and reported degradability of phytate-P complex to be 80.8% at the precaecal stage for weanling pigs and 97.8 and 96.9% at the faecal stage for weanling and growing pigs, respectively. Phytate degradability was significantly higher at the faecal compared with the ileal stage in growing pigs; however, there was no significant difference in phytate degradability between weanling and growing pigs at the faecal stage. On the other hand, significant intercepts of the linear regression give the estimated endogenous phytate outputs. As described in the legend to Fig. 17.6, no significant endogenous phytate output was observed for the weanling pigs at the ileal stage. However, significant endogenous phytate-P outputs were estimated for the weanling (0.084 g kg^{-1} DMI) and the growing (0.055 g kg^{-1} DMI) pigs at the faecal stage (see Fig. 17.6; Shen *et al.*, 2005c).

Estimating apical transcellular Na^+–Pi co-transport capacity

Intestinal apical membrane vesicles can be prepared by Mg^{2+}-precipitation and differential centrifugation and a rapid filtration procedure is adopted for measuring *in vitro* phosphate uptake using $[^{32}P]NaH_2PO_4$ as a tracer, as described by

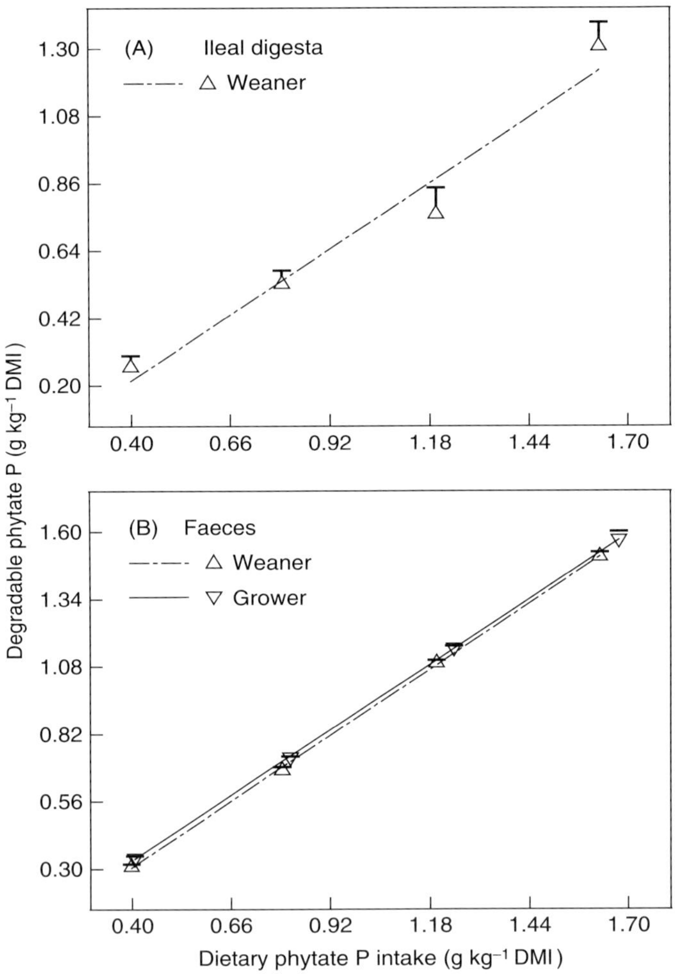

Fig. 17.6. Linear relationships between the degradable phytate phosphorus (P) associated with the oat sample in weanling and growing pigs. (A) At the ileal level of the weaned pigs: $y = -(0.103 \pm 0.084) + (0.808 \pm 0.080)x$, $n = 16$, $R^2 = 0.89$, $P = 0.22$ for the pig effect, $P = 0.17$ for the period effect, $P = 0.24$ for the intercept estimate, $P < 0.05$ for the slope estimate, $P = 0.13$ for the quadratic effect, and $P = 0.29$ for the cubic effect; and (B) at the faecal level; for the weaned pigs: $y = -(0.084 \pm 0.017) + (0.978 \pm 0.013)x$, $n = 16$, $R^2 = 0.99$, $P = 0.53$ for the pig effect, and $P = 0.78$ for the period effect; for the growing pigs, $y = -(0.055 \pm 0.015) + (0.969 \pm 0.016)x$, $n = 16$, $R^2 = 0.99$, $P = 0.12$ for the pig effect, $P = 0.21$ for the period effect, $P = 0.74$ for the quadratic effect, and $P = 0.64$ for the cubic effect. $P < 0.05$ for all the other parameter estimates unless specified otherwise. Adapted from Shen (2006).

Fan *et al.* (2004). The initial rate of [^{32}P]phosphate uptake is calculated according to Eqn 17.6:

$$J_{\text{initial}} = \{[(R_F - R_B) \times S]/R_I\}/(W \times T), \tag{17.6}$$

where $J_{initial}$ is the initial rate of [^{32}P]phosphate tracer uptake into the membrane vesicles (pmol mg^{-1} protein s^{-1}); R_F is radioactivity in counts per min (cpm) per filter (cpm $filter^{-1}$); R_B is radioactivity for non-specific binding to the cellulose membrane filters (cpm $filter^{-1}$); S is extravesicular [^{32}P]phosphate tracer concentrations (mM); R_I is radioactivity in the uptake media (cpm μl^{-1}); W is the amount of membrane protein provided for the incubations (mg protein $filter^{-1}$); and T is the time of incubation for the initial uptake (s) determined from the time-course experiments.

Kinetic parameter estimates of the Na^+-phosphate co-transporter maximal transport activity, affinity and the transmembrane diffusion rate constant are determined according to a previously established tracer inhibitory kinetic model (Fan *et al.*, 2004), shown in Eqn 17.7:

$$J_{initial} = (J_{max} \times S_{TRACER})/(K_m + S_{COLD} + S_{TRACER}) + J_{diffu}, \quad (17.7)$$

where $J_{initial}$ is initial rate of [^{32}P]phosphate tracer uptake into the membrane vesicle (pmol mg^{-1} protein s^{-1}); J_{max} is the maximal rate of phosphate transport into the membrane vesicle (pmol mg^{-1} protein s^{-1}); S_{TRACER} is the extravesicular concentration of [^{32}P]phosphate tracer (mM); K_m is the transporter affinity (mM); S_{COLD} is extravesicular concentrations of unlabelled phosphate (mM); and J_{diffu} is the transmembrane diffusion rate of the [^{32}P]phosphate tracer in the membrane vesicles (pmol mg^{-1} protein s^{-1}).

In order to determine the contribution of the intestinal Na^+-phosphate co-transporter activity capacity to the whole-body P requirement in the pig, the apical membrane protein recovered from the various intestinal segmental tissues is calculated from Eqn 17.8:

$$R_m = (P_m/P_H \times W_t) \times 100, \quad (17.8)$$

where R_m is the apical membrane recovery rate (%) from the corresponding intestinal tissues including duodenum, jejunum, ileum, caecum and colon; P_m is the amount of apical membrane protein recovered (mg) from the corresponding intestinal tissues weighed out; P_H is the protein content (mg g^{-1}) of the corresponding intestinal tissues; and W_t is the amount (g) of corresponding intestinal tissues weighed out for the apical membrane preparation.

The intestinal segmental Na^+-phosphate co-transport capacity was calculated according to Weiss *et al.* (1997), as described in Eqn 17.9:

$$J_{cap} = W_s \times R_m \times J_{max} \times 60 \times 60 \times 24/(1000 \times 1000) \times 31 \times W_B, \quad (17.9)$$

where J_{cap} is the calculated Na^+-phosphate co-transport activity capacity (μg P kg^{-1} BW day^{-1}) for each of the intestinal segments; W_s is the weight of the freshly frozen and pulverized intestinal segmental tissue protein weight (g protein pig^{-1}); J_{max} is as defined in Eqn 17.7; $60 \times 60 \times 24$ is to convert the J_{max} time unit to day^{-1} from s^{-1}; $1000 \times 1000 \times 31$ is to convert the J_{max} in pmol of phosphate ($H_2PO_4^{-1}$, $FW = 98$) unit to μg of P (atomic weight 31); R_m is the measured apical membrane protein recovery rate (%) from the corresponding intestinal segments; and W_B is the body weight (kg) of the experimental pigs.

Using this *in vitro* uptake approach, Shen (2006) observed significant Na^+–Pi co-transport activity on the apical membrane along the entire small and large intestines in the pig; however, the transcellular P transport capacity contributed very little to whole-body P requirements and homeostasis in the pig.

Measuring P digestibility, endogenous P loss and urinary P excretion

Apparent versus true digestibility

The apparent digestibility of P in experimental diets can be measured using the indicator technique according to Eqn 17.10:

$$D_{Ai} = 100\% - [(I_D \times P_I)/(I_I \times P_D)] \times 100\%, \tag{17.10}$$

where D_{Ai} is apparent P digestibility in the assay diets (%, on as-fed basis); I_D is digestibility marker concentration in the *i*th assay diet (%, on as-fed basis); P_I is P concentration in faeces (%, on as-fed basis); P_D is P concentration in the *i*th assay diet (%, on as-fed basis); and I_I is digestibility marker concentration in faeces (%, on as-fed basis).

As shown in Fig. 17.7, the apparent P digestibility values were more variable and lower than true digestive efficiency of dietary P utilization, thus the latter should be measured (Fan *et al.*, 2001; Ajakaiye *et al.*, 2003; Fang *et al.*, 2007). The true P digestibility can be calculated using apparent P digestibility and an estimate of endogenous faecal P loss according to Eqn 17.11:

$$D_{Ti} = D_{Ai} + (P_E/P_{Di}) \times 100\%, \tag{17.11}$$

where D_{Ti} is the true P digestibility of the diet (%); D_{Ai} is apparent P digestibility of the diet (%); P_E is endogenous faecal P loss (g kg^{-1} DMI); and P_{Di} is the P content of the diet (g kg^{-1} DM diet).

Alternatively, if the true P digestibility is known, endogenous P loss from individual diets can be calculated using Eqn 17.12:

$$P_E = [(D_{Ti} - D_{Ai}) \times P_{Di}]/100\%. \tag{17.12}$$

Methods of measuring true P digestibility and the endogenous P loss

Several methods have been developed for measuring true P digestibility and the endogenous P outputs associated with feed ingredients in pigs, including P-free feeding, the substitution method, linear regression analysis and multiple linear regression analysis.

P-FREE FEEDING METHOD. The P-free feeding method reported by Petersen and Stein (2006) is suitable for measuring basal faecal endogenous P output and assessing which dietary factors influence endogenous P loss in pigs. Once faecal endogenous P loss has been measured, true P digestibility in the diet or individual ingredients can be calculated using Eqn 17.11. This method has been used for measuring true P digestibility in the major inorganic P supplements (Petersen and Stein, 2006). However, the method may not be suitable for measuring true P digestibility in ingredients with other intrinsic components, such as fibre and anti-nutritional factors, which may affect the faecal endogenous P excretions (Fang *et al.*, 2007).

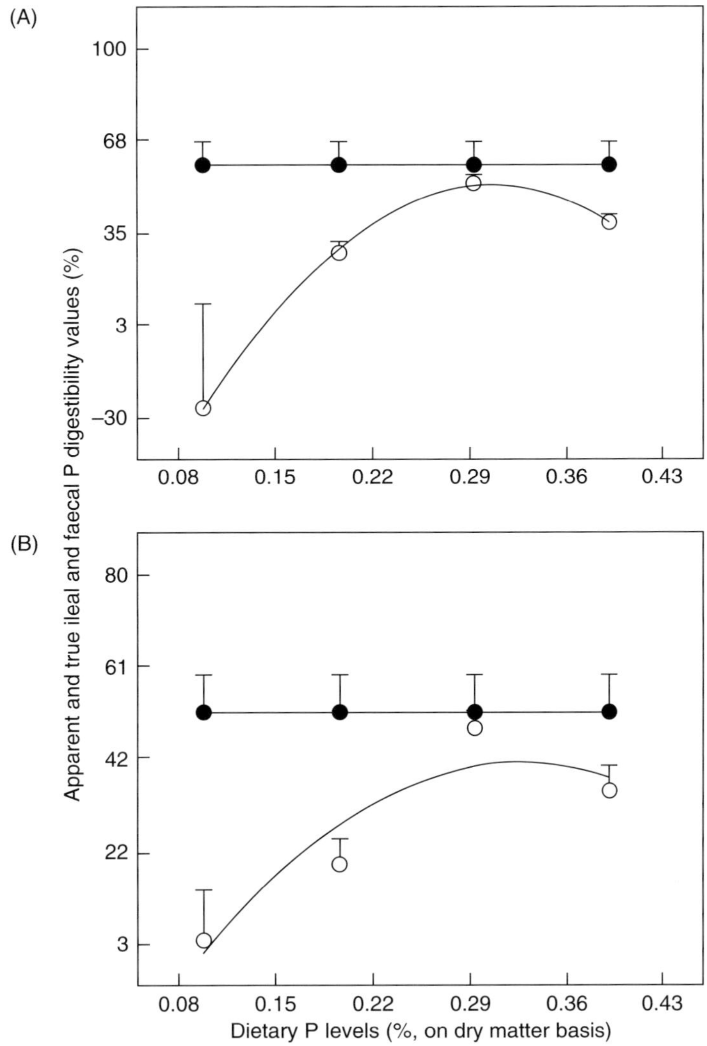

Fig. 17.7. Effects of dietary phosphorus (P) levels on apparent (○) and true (●) ileal and faecal P digestibility in growing pigs fed soybean meal-based diets varying from low to high in P content. (A) Ileal level; and (B) faecal level. Adapted from Ajakaiye *et al.* (2003).

THE SUBSTITUTION METHOD. The substitution method is based on the principle originally described by Ammerman *et al.* (1957) for ruminants, as illustrated in Fig. 17.8 and expressed mathematically in Eqn 17.13 (Fang *et al.*, 2007):

$$D_T = (P_{A2} - P_{A1}) \times 100\% \times (P_{D2} - P_{D1})^{-1}, \qquad (17.13)$$

where D_T is true P digestibility of the dietary ingredient (%); P_{A2} is the apparent digestible P content (g DMI^{-1}) from the higher-P diet; P_{A1} is the apparent digestible P content (g DMI^{-1}) from the lower-P diet; P_{D2} is total dietary P content from the higher-P diet; and P_{D1} is total dietary P content from the lower-P diet.

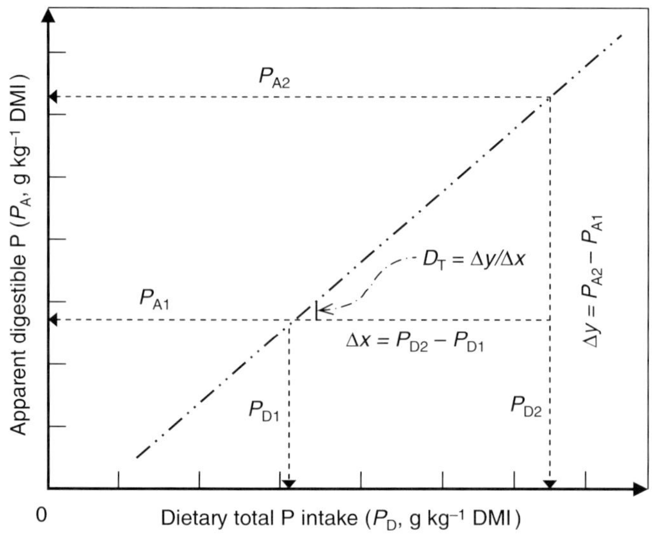

Fig. 17.8. Schematic illustration of the substitution method for measuring true phosphorus (P) digestibility (D_T) and endogenous P output associated with a test feed ingredient.

Once true P digestibility is determined, the endogenous P output can be calculated using Eqn 17.12. This method can be used for measuring true P digestibility and endogenous P loss for a wide variety of diets and test ingredients. In addition, the method is relatively simple, as it involves only two test diets and assumes that changes in the dietary inclusion levels of the individual ingredient(s) will not affect true P digestibility and endogenous P loss (Wang *et al.*, 2005).

LINEAR REGRESSION METHOD. Two types of linear regression analyses have been developed for measuring true P digestibility and endogenous P loss associated with a test ingredient (Fan *et al.*, 2001; Shen *et al.*, 2002).

The determination of true P digestibility and endogenous gastrointestinal P output by linear regression between total P output and dietary input is illustrated with soybean meal in weanling pigs (Fig. 17.9). To establish such a relationship, a series of test diets are formulated to contain graded amounts of the test nutrient, but only from the assay ingredient. The contents of other dietary factors, such as anti-nutritive factors that affect the test nutrient digestion and endogenous test nutrient output, should be controlled between the assay diets (Fan *et al.*, 2001). The total (dietary + endogenous) faecal P output (g kg^{-1} DMI) is calculated from Eqn 17.14:

$$P_{Oi} = P_I \times (I_D/I_I), \qquad (17.14)$$

where P_{Oi} is P output in faeces (g kg^{-1} DMI), P_I is P content of faeces (g kg^{-1} DM faeces), I_D is the concentration of digestibility marker (e.g. Cr_2O_3) in the test diets (g kg^{-1} DM diet) and I_I is the concentration of digestibility marker in faeces (g kg^{-1} DM faeces). If there are linear relationships between P output in faeces and the

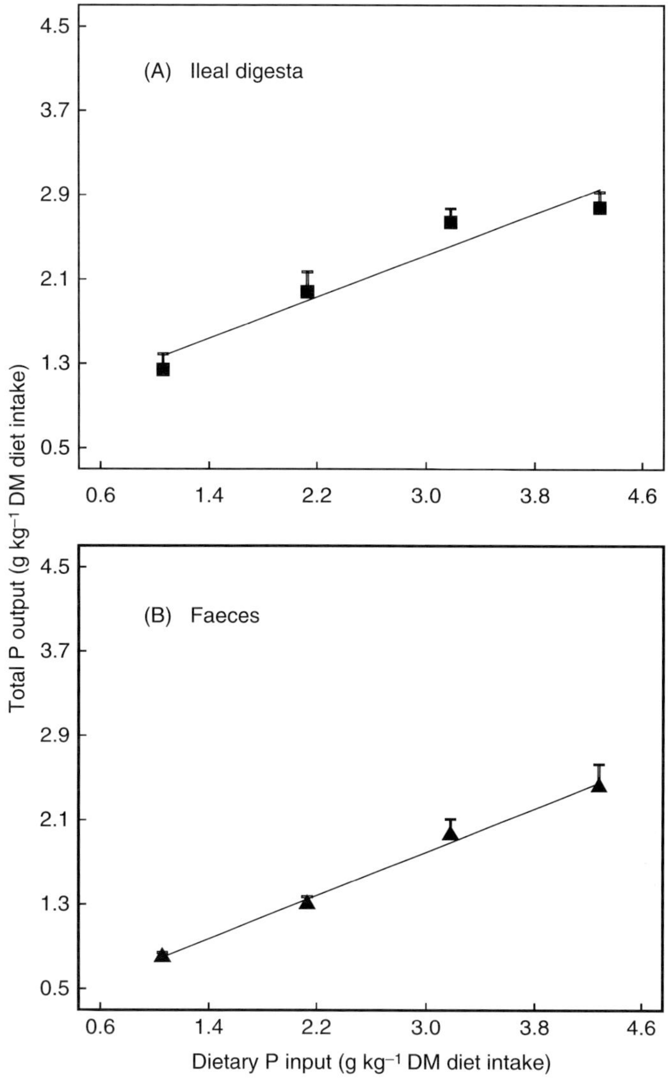

Fig. 17.9. Linear relationship between total phosphorus (P) outputs in ileal digesta and faeces and dietary P input in the weanling pig fed soybean meal-based diets varying from low to high in P content. (A) In ileal digesta, $y = 0.49x + 0.86$, $n = 16$, $R^2 = 0.78$, $P < 0.05$; and (B) in faeces, $y = 0.51x + 0.31$, $n = 16$, $R^2 = 0.87$, $P < 0.05$. Adapted from Fan *et al.* (2001).

graded levels of total dietary P input from diets (g kg^{-1} DMI), their relationships can be further expressed according to Eqn 17.15:

$$P_{Oi} = P_E + D_I \times P_{Di}, \tag{17.15}$$

where P_{Oi} is the output of P in faeces collected from animals fed the *i*th test diet, determined using Eqn 17.14 (g kg^{-1} DMI), P_E is endogenous faecal P (g kg^{-1}

DMI), D_I is indigestible P (%), P_{Di} is P content of the *i*th test diet (g kg^{-1} DM) and D_T is true P digestibility (%) in the test ingredient and can be calculated using Eqn 17.16, once D_I has been estimated from the linear regression analysis and Eqn 17.15:

$$D_T = 100\% - D_I \quad (17.16)$$

Equation 17.15 represents a simple linear regression model in which P_{Oi} and P_{Di} are the dependent and independent variables, respectively. P_E and D_I are the regression coefficients and are estimated by fitting a linear regression model. If there are linear relationships between P output in faeces and graded levels of P input from assay diets with significant intercepts, then the endogenous P level in faeces can be directly determined by extrapolating the dietary input of P to zero by obtaining the intercept of the linear regression equation (P_E) (Fan *et al.*, 2001).

The determination of true P digestibility and endogenous P output by establishing linear relationships between apparent digestible P intakes and total P intakes in test diets is illustrated for maize-using growing pigs in Fig. 17.10.

The apparent digestible P content of the diets (g kg^{-1} DMI) is calculated from Eqn 17.17 (Shen *et al.*, 2002):

$$P_{Ai} = P_{Di} \times D_{Ai}, \quad (17.17)$$

where P_{Ai} is the apparent digestible P content of the *i*th diet (g kg^{-1} DMI), P_{Di} is the total P content of the *i*th diet (g kg^{-1} DMI) and D_{Ai} is the apparent P digestibility of the *i*th diet (%) measured according to Eqn 17.10. If there is a linear relationship between the apparent digestible faecal P content and the graded levels of total P input from assay diets, when expressed as g kg^{-1} DMI, their relationships can be expressed according to Eqn 17.18:

$$P_{Ai} = -P_E + [(D_T \times 100^{-1}) \times P_{Di}], \quad (17.18)$$

where P_{Ai} is apparent digestible P content of the *i*th diet (g kg^{-1} DMI) determined from Eqn 17.17, P_E is the endogenous faecal P loss (g kg^{-1} DMI), D_T is the true P digestibility (%) of the diet ingredient and P_{Di} is the total P content of the *i*th diet (g kg^{-1} DMI). Equation 17.18 represents a linear regression model in which P_{Ai} is the dependent variable and P_{Di} is the independent variable. P_E and D_T are the regression coefficients and are estimated by fitting a linear regression (Shen *et al.*, 2002).

These linear regression models have been used for assessing true P digestibility and endogenous P loss for a wide variety of feed ingredients in weanling and growing pigs, as summarized in Tables 17.2 and 17.3. However, linear models may not be suitable for certain cereal grains in weanling pigs and other ingredients with poor palatability and limited levels of dietary inclusion (Shen, 2006).

A comparative study by Fang *et al.* (2007) did not observe any significant differences between the substitution method and the simple linear regression technique for measuring true P digestibility and endogenous P losses associated with soybean meal and wheat middlings in growing pigs.

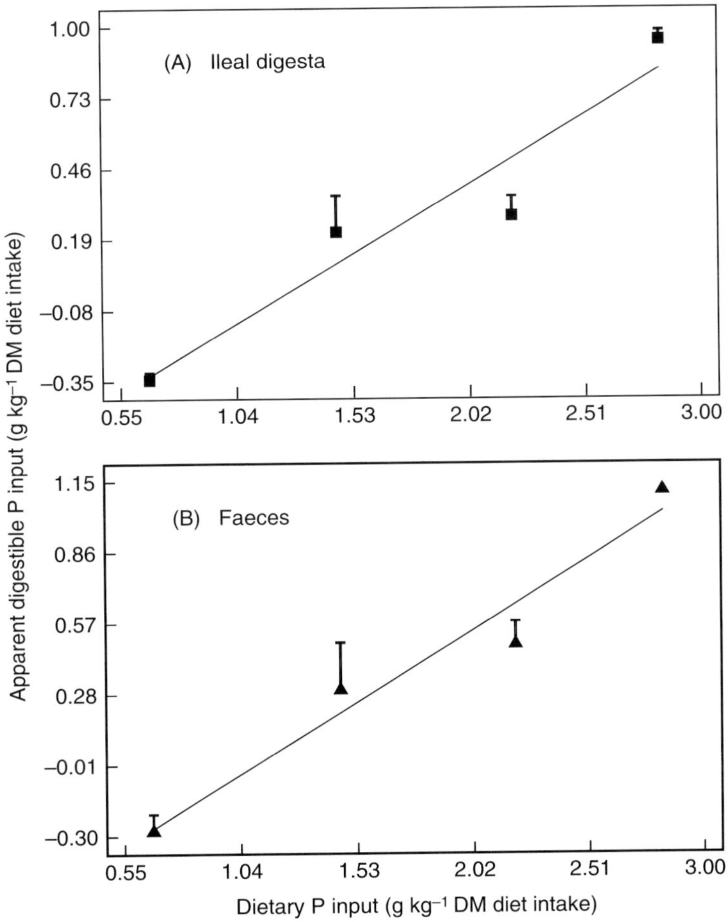

Fig. 17.10. Linear relationships between apparent ileal and faecal digestible dietary phosphorus (P) and the dietary total P input in growing pigs fed maize-based diets varying from low to high in P contents. (A) In ileal digesta, $y = 0.539x - 0.693$, $n = 16$, $R^2 = 0.83$, $P < 0.05$; and (B) in faeces, $y = 0.598x - 0.670$, $n = 16$, $R^2 = 0.78$, $P < 0.05$. Adapted from Shen *et al.* (2002).

MULTIPLE LINEAR REGRESSION METHOD. The determination of true P digestibility and the endogenous P output using multiple linear regression relies on establishing a multiple linear relationship between apparent digestible and total intake of P in test diets contributed from more than one test ingredient.

This method is expressed by using two test ingredients according to Eqn 17.19 derived from Eqn 17.18:

$$P_{Ai} = -P_E + [(D_{1-T} \times 100^{-1}) \times P_{1Di}] + [(D_{2-T} \times 100^{-1}) \times P_{2Di}], \quad (17.19)$$

where P_{Ai} is the apparent digestible P of the *i*th diet (g kg^{-1} DMI) contributed collectively from both test ingredients 1 and 2 and determined from Eqn 17.17, P_E is endogenous P in faeces associated with test ingredients 1 and 2 (g kg^{-1} DMI),

Table 17.2. Recommended available phosphorus (P) requirements (g kg^{-1} dry matter diet) and faecal endogenous P losses (g kg^{-1} dry matter intake) in pigs under various dietary conditions and stages of growth.

Items	Dietary conditions	Types of pigs and body weights (kg)	Methods of estimation and sources
P requirements:			
3.6–4.4	maize–soybean meal-based diets	weanling pigs (5–20)	growth and bone responses[1]
Endogenous P loss:			
0.507 ± 0.156 (*n* = 16)	barley-based diets	weanling pigs (25–38)	linear regression[2,3]
0.725 ± 0.083 (*n* = 36)	brown rice-based diets	weanling pigs (13)	simple linear regression analysis[4,5]
0.304 – 0.320 (*n* = 32)	oats-based diets	weanling pigs (7–11)	simple linear regression analysis[3,6]
0.800 ± 0.580 (*n* = 16)	canola meal-based diets	weanling pigs (8–14)	simple linear regression analysis[7]
0.310 ± 0.060 (*n* = 16)	soybean meal-based diets	weanling pigs (7–21)	simple linear regression analysis[8]
P requirements:			
1.7–2.6	maize–soybean meal-based diets	growing–finishing pigs (20–120)	growth and bone responses[1]

Endogenous P loss:			
0.07–0.08 ($n = 12$)	semi-purified diets	growing–finishing pigs (27–98)	P-free feeding[9]
0.139 ± 0.018 ($n = 7$)	semi-purified diets	growing–finishing pigs (27–79)	P-free feeding[10]
0.670 ± 0.160 ($n = 16$)	maize-based diets	growing pigs (25–45)	simple linear regression analysis[11]
0.304 ± 0.320 ($n = 32$)	oats-based diets	growing pigs (26–45)	simple linear regression analysis[3,6]
0.341 ± 0.086 ($n = 16$)	wheat-based diets	growing pigs (28–40)	simple linear regression analysis[3,12]
0.620–0.92 ($n = 16$)	wheat middling-based diets	growing pigs (21)	regression analysis/substitution[13]
0.280 ± 0.060 ($n = 16$)	canola meal-based diets	growing pigs (30–50)	simple linear regression analysis[14]
0.450 ± 0.210 ($n = 16$)	soybean meal-based diets	growing pigs (30–50)	simple linear regression analysis[15]
0.071 ($n = 64$)	soybean meal-based diets	growing pigs (18–44)	simple linear regression analysis[16]
0.450–1.02 ($n = 16$)	soybean meal-based diets	growing pigs (21)	regression analysis/substitution[13]
1.08 ± 0.01 ($n = 36$)	soybean meal-based diets	growing gilts (29)	simple linear regression analysis[17]
0.89 ± 0.007 ($n = 36$)	soybean meal-based diets	growing barrows (28)	simple linear regression analysis[17]
0.780 ± 0.170 ($n = 16$)	soybean meal-based diets	dry sows with 5–7 parities (200)	simple linear regression analysis[18,19]

[1]NRC (1998); [2]Shen *et al.* (2005b); [3]Shen (2006); [4]Yang (2005); [5]Yang *et al.* (2007); [6]Shen *et al.* (2005c); [7]Fan *et al.* (2003); [8]Fan *et al.* (2001); [9]Petersen and Stein (2006); [10]Pettey *et al.* (2006); [11]Shen *et al.* (2002); [12]Shen *et al.* (2005a); [13]Fang *et al.* (2007); [14]Fan *et al.* (2002b); [15]Ajakaiye *et al.* (2003); [16]Dilger and Adeola (2006); [17]Zhang (2004); [18]Kuang (2005); and [19]Kuang *et al.* (2006).

Table 17.3. True faecal phosphorus (P) digestibility values (% of total P content) in feed ingredients for various stages of growth in pigs.

True P digestibility	Ingredients	Types of pigs and body weights (kg)	Methods of estimation and sources
92.0 (n = 7)	monosodium phosphate	growing–finishing pigs (27–79)	P-free feeding[1]
88–89 (n = 7)	monocalcium phosphate	growing–finishing pigs (27–79)	P-free feeding[1]
82–83 (n = 7)	dicalcium phosphate	growing–finishing pigs (27–79)	P-free feeding[1]
49.9 ± 8.7 (n = 16)	conventional maize	weanling pigs (8)	linear regression[2,3]
59.8 ± 8.5 (n = 16)	conventional maize	growing pigs (25–45)	simple linear regression analysis[2,4]
64.7 ± 7.3 (n = 16)	conventional barley	growing pigs (25–38)	simple linear regression analysis[2,5]
28.5 ± 7.3 (n = 16)	conventional wheat	weanling pigs (8–12)	simple linear regression analysis[2,6]
41.2 ± 4.3 (n = 16)	conventional wheat	growing pigs (28–40)	simple linear regression analysis[2,6]
63.7 ± 5.0 (n = 16)	wheat middlings	growing pigs (21)	simple linear regression analysis[7]
81.2 ± 3.7 (n = 16)	conventional hulled oats	weanling pigs (7–11)	simple linear regression analysis[2,8]
83.5 ± 4.6 (n = 16)	conventional hulled oats	growing pigs (26–45)	simple linear regression analysis[2,8]
58.2 ± 5.9 (n = 36)	brown rice	weanling pigs (13)	simple linear regression analysis[9,10]
32.0 ± 9.0 (n = 12)	canola meal	weanling pigs (8–14)	simple linear regression analysis[11]
31.0 ± 4.1 (n = 16)	canola meal	growing pigs (30–50)	simple linear regression analysis[12]
48.5 ± 5.4 (n = 16)	soybean meal	weanling pigs (7–21)	simple linear regression analysis[13]
51.3 ± 7.9 (n = 16)	soybean meal	growing pigs (40–58)	simple linear regression analysis[14]
45.2 ± 7.1 (n = 64)	soybean meal	growing pigs (18)	simple linear regression analysis[15]
49.4 ± 3.5 (n = 64)	soybean meal	growing pigs (21)	simple linear regression analysis[8]
41.4 ± 5.9 (n = 36)	soybean meal	growing gilts (29)	simple linear regression analysis[16]
48.8 ± 9.1 (n = 36)	soybean meal	growing barrows (28)	simple linear regression analysis[16]
44.0 ± 4.5 (n = 36)	soybean meal	dry sows with 5–7 parities (200)	simple linear regression analysis[17,18]

[1]Petersen and Stein (2006); [2]Shen (2006); [3]Shen *et al.* (2003); [4]Shen *et al.* (2002); [5]Shen *et al.* (2005b); [6]Shen *et al.* (2005a); [7]Fang *et al.* (2007); [8]Shen *et al.* (2005c); [9]Yang (2005); [10]Yang *et al.* (2007); [11]Fan *et al.* (2003); [12]Fan *et al.* (2002b); [13]Fan *et al.* (2001); [14]Ajakaiye *et al.* (2003); [15]Dilger and Adeola (2006); [16]Zhang (2004); [17]Kuang (2005); [18]Kuang *et al.* (2006).

D_{1-T} and D_{2-T} are true P digestibilities (%) for test ingredients 1 and 2, respectively, which are to be estimated, and P_{1Di} and P_{2Di} are the total P contents of the *i*th diet (g kg^{-1} DMI) from test ingredients 1 and 2, respectively. Equation 17.19 represents a multiple linear regression model in which P_{Ai} is the dependent variable and P_{1Di} and P_{2Di} are the independent variables. P_E, D_{1-T} and D_{2-T} are the regression coefficients estimated by fitting the multiple linear regression model.

The multiple linear regression method has two main advantages; it allows the simultaneous estimation of P digestive parameters for two or more feed ingredients from one study and allows examination of their additivity at multiple levels of diet mixing. Zuo (2005) used the multiple linear regression method to measure true P digestibility and endogenous faecal P output with four types of diet mixtures using soybean meal–barley, soybean meal–sorghum, soybean meal–rapeseed meal and soybean meal–cottonseed meal at multiple levels of dietary inclusion according to Eqn 17.19. Under their test conditions, true P digestibility (38.9 versus 28.0% of dietary P) and endogenous faecal P output (0.53 g kg^{-1} DMI) associated with soybean meal–cottonseed meal were successfully estimated by the multiple linear regression approach (Zuo, 2005). Therefore, this method has the most potential for the measurement of multiple feed ingredients formulated at the range of levels on inclusions close to practical dietary levels used in pig production.

Urinary P excretion

Urinary P loss can be measured in animals adapted to the experimental diets using a total urine collection (Rideout and Fan, 2004). Total urinary P excretion can be calculated according to Eqn 17.20:

$$P_{\text{Urinary loss}} = C_{\text{Urinary conc}} \times V_{\text{Urine}}, \qquad (17.20)$$

where $P_{\text{Urinary loss}}$ is the daily urinary loss of P (g pig^{-1} day^{-1}), $C_{\text{Urinary conc}}$ is the concentration of P in urine (g l^{-1}) and V_{Urine} is the volume of urine produced (l day^{-1}). When pigs are fed diets with available P close to requirements, urinary P excretion is very low, accounting for only 1–2% of total P intake (Rideout and Fan, 2004).

Measuring Phosphorus Bioavailability in Feed Ingredients

Criteria for assessing P bioavailability

Accurate determination of bioavailable P in feed ingredients and complete diets is essential to ensure efficient utilization of dietary P (Jongbloed *et al.*, 1991). Digestibility studies and the slope–ratio method are the two major evaluation systems for assessing the bioavailability of P in feed ingredients for pigs (Jongbloed *et al.*, 1991; Cromwell, 1992; Fan *et al.*, 2001). Digestibility studies measure the digestive utilization of P, whereas the slope–ratio method provides a combined estimation of digestion and post-absorptive utilization of P at the tissue level (Weremko *et al.*, 1997; Fan *et al.*, 2001). Apparent P digestibility values in feed ingredients for pigs have commonly been reported by researchers from European countries, especially The Netherlands (Jongbloed *et al.*, 1991); however, the values are variable for the same ingredient and are affected by the P content of the test diet and the contribution of P from endogenous sources (Fan *et al.*, 2001; Shen *et al.*, 2002; Ajakaiye *et al.*, 2003). Bioavailability values determined by the slope–ratio method have been reported from the USA for pigs fed maize and soybean meal diets (Cromwell and Coffey, 1991) and are also variable and are affected by method criteria (Ketaren *et al.*, 1993a,b). It is now established that apparent P digestibility and P availability are variable and considerably underestimate true P bioavailability in feed ingredients for pigs (Fan *et al.*, 2001; Petersen and Stein, 2006; Fang *et al.*, 2007). Therefore, true P digestibility should be measured in feed ingredients and used to formulate pig diets. As an optimal dietary calcium (Ca):P ratio is essential to ensure efficient retention of Ca and P, true Ca digestibility in feed ingredients for pigs must also to be measured. In addition, true digestible Ca and P requirements should be determined for pigs for different stages of growth and production.

Strategies for improving efficiency of P utilization

The majority of P in feed ingredients of plant origin is present in the form of phytate that cannot be effectively digested by conventional pigs (Jongbloed *et al.*, 1991). Transgenic pigs that express higher levels of phytase activity have been developed to digest 90+% of plant P (Golovan *et al.*, 2001). New crop cultivars that produce grains with low levels of phytate P are also being developed (Spencer *et al.*, 2000; Raboy, 2002) and supplementing diets with exogenous microbial phytase is also effective at increasing dietary P utilization (Simons *et al.*, 1990). Thus, the ultimate goal of improving the efficiency of P utilization in global pig production is not likely to be limited by the presence of phytate P or the availability of phytase in pig production systems. Rather importantly, animals are fed in excess of their requirements, or the requirements are set too high. Only improving P bioavailability without reducing total P loading or flow, i.e. total P contents in feed or food ingredients, into the agrifood production system and the human food chain will not ultimately solve the P concerns (Fig. 17.1). Thus, developing low-phytate and low-P crops will lead to reduced crop requirements for P and reduce total P flow into the agrifood production system and human food chains.

Studies by Pettey *et al.* (2006) have demonstrated that growing–finishing pigs fed purified diets with a completely bioavailable Ca and P supply, a correct available Ca to P ratio (Ca/P = 2–2.5) and dietary P levels close to the recommended levels have been able to grow at 90+%. Using phytase or low-phytate feed ingredients and decreasing dietary total P input, it is hoped that future pig production systems can operate at a P retention efficiency in the upper 90% range, thereby minimizing pollution to the environment.

In conclusion, formulation of low-P pig diets based on true faecal digestible Ca and P supply, combined with the use of phytase and low-phytate ingredients, will considerably improve the efficiency of P utilization and address one of the major concerns from intensive pig production systems.

References

Abelson, P.H. (1999) A potential phosphate crisis. *Science* 283, 2015.

Ajakaiye, A., Fan, M.Z., Archbold, T., Hacker, R.R., Forsberg, C.W. and Phillips, J.P. (2003) Determination of true phosphorus digestibility and the endogenous loss associated with soybean meal for growing–finishing pigs. *Journal of Animal Science* 81, 2766–2775.

Ammerman, C.B., Forbes, R.M., Garrigus, U.S., Newmann, A.L., Norton, H.W. and Hatfield, E.E. (1957) Ruminant utilization of inorganic phosphorus. *Journal of Animal Science* 16, 796–810.

Anderson, J.J.B. (1991) Nutritional biochemistry of calcium and phosphorous. *The Journal of Nutritional Biochemistry* 2, 300–307.

Armstrong, T.A and Spears, J.W. (2001) Effect of dietary boron on growth performance, calcium and phosphorus metabolism, and bone mechanical properties in growing barrows. *Journal of Animal Science* 79, 3120–3127.

Berner, Y.N. and Shike, M. (1988) Consequences of phosphate imbalance. *Annual Review of Nutrition* 8, 121–148.

Carpenter, S.R. (2005) Eutrophication of aquatic ecosystems: bistability and soil phosphorus. *The Proceedings of the National Academy of Sciences of the USA* 102, 10002–10005.

Chi, T.H. and Crabtree, G.R. (2000) Inositol phosphates in the nucleus. *Science* 287, 1937–1939.

Collins, J.F., Bai, L. and Ghishan, F.K. (2004) The SLC20 family of proteins: dual functions and sodium-phosphate cotransporters and viral receptors. *European Journal of Physiology* 447, 647–652.

Cromwell, G.L. (1992) The biological availability of phosphorus in feedstuffs for pigs. *Pig News Inform*ation 13, 75 N–78 N.

Cromwell, G.L. and Coffey R.D. (1991) Phosphorus – a key essential nutrient, yet a possible major pollutant – its central role in animal nutrition. In: Lyons, T.P. (ed.) *Biotechnology in the Feed Industry*. Alltech Technical Publications, Nicholasville, Kentucky, pp. 133–145.

Danisi, G. and Murer, H. (1992) Inorganic phosphate absorption in small intestine. In: Schultz, S.G. and Field, M. (eds) *Handbook of Physiology. Section 6: The Gastrointestinal System IV. Intestinal Absorption and Secretion*. Oxford University Press, New York, pp. 323–335.

Dilger, R.N. and Adeola, O. (2006) Estimation of true phosphorus digestibility and endogenous phosphorus loss in growing pigs fed conventional and low-phytate soybean meals. *Journal of Animal Science* 84, 627–684.

Engelen, A.J., van der Heeft, F.C., Randsdorp, P.H.G. and Somer, W.A.C. (2001) Determination of phytase activity in feed by a colorimetric enzymatic method: collaborative interlaboratory study. *Journal of AOAC International* 84, 629–633.

Fan, M.Z., Archbold, T., Sauer, W.C., Lackeyram, D., Rideout, T., Gao, Y., Lange, C.F.M. de and Hacker, R.R. (2001) Novel methodology allows measurement of true phosphorus digestibility and the gastrointestinal endogenous phosphorus outputs in studies with pigs. *The Journal of Nutrition* 131, 2388–2396.

Fan, M.Z., Adeola, O., Asem, E.K. and King, D. (2002a) Postnatal ontogeny of kinetics of porcine jejunal brush border membrane-bound alkaline phosphatase, aminopeptidase N, and sucrase activities in pigs. *Comparative Biochemistry and Physiology A. Molecular and Integrated Physiology* 132, 599–607.

Fan, M.Z., Archbold, T., Ajakaiye, A., Shen, Y., Bregendahl, K., Atkinson, J.L. and Hacker, R.R. (2002b) True phosphorus digestibility and the endogenous phosphorus outputs associated with canola meal for growing pigs. *Journal of Animal Science* 80 (Supplement 1), 348 (Abstract).

Fan, M.Z., Archbold, T., Atkinson, J.L. and Hacker, R.R. (2003) True fecal phosphorus digestibility and the endogenous phosphorus output are determined with limited levels of canola meal intake in weanling pigs. In: Ball, R. (ed.) *The 9th International Symposium on Digestive Physiology in Pigs*. University of Alberta, Edmonton, Alberta, Canada, pp. 174–176.

Fan, M.Z., Matthews, J., Etienne, N.M.P., Stoll, B., Lackeyram, D. and Burrin, D.G. (2004) Expression of brush border L-glutamate transporters in epithelial cells along the crypt–villus axis in the neonatal pig. *American Journal of Physiology* 287, G385–G398.

Fan, M.Z., Li, T.J., Yin, Y.L., Fang, R.J., Tang, Z.Y., Hou, Z.P., Huang, R.L., Deng, Z.Y., Zhong, H.Y., Zhang, R.G., Zhang, J., Wang, B. and Schulze, H. (2005) Effect of phytase supplementation with two levels of phosphorus diets on ileal and faecal digestibilities of nutrients and phosphorus, calcium, nitrogen and energy balances in growing pigs. *Animal Science* 81, 67–75.

Fan, M.Z., Chiba, L.I., Matzat, P.D., Yang, X., Yin, Y.L., Mine, Y. and Stein, H. (2006) Measuring synthesis rates of nitrogen-containing polymers by using stable isotope tracers. *Journal of Animal Science* 84 (E. Supplement), E79–E93.

Fang, R.J., Yin, Y.L., Wang, K.N., He, J.H., Chen, Q.H., Li, T.J, Fan, M.Z. and Wu, G. (2007) Comparison of the regression analysis technique and the substitution method for the determination of true phosphorus digestibility and faecal endogenous phosphorus losses associated with feed ingredients for growing pigs. *Livestock Science* 109, 251–254.

Forsberg, C.W., Golovan, S.P., Ajakaiye, A., Phillips, J.P., Meidinger, R.G., Fan, M.Z., Kelly, J.M. and Hacker, R.R. (2005) Genetic opportunities to enhance sustainability of pork production in developing countries: a model for food animals. In: Makkar H.P.S. and Viljoen, G.J. (eds) *Applications of Gene-based Technologies for Improving Animal Production and Health in Developing Countries*. Springer, Dordrecht, The Netherlands, pp. 429–446.

Golovan, S., Meidinger, R.D., Ajakaiye, A., Cottrill, M., Weiderkehr, M.Z., Plante, C., Pollard, J., Fan, M.Z., Hayes, A., Jesper Laursen, A.C., Hjorth, J.P., Hacker, R.R., Barney, D., Phillips, J.P. and Forsberg, C. (2001) Enhanced phosphorus digestion and reduced pollution potential by pigs with salivary phytase. *Nature – Biotechnology* 19, 741–745.

Hilfiker, H., Hattenhauer, O., Traebert, M., Forster, I., Murer, H. and Biber, J. (1998) Characterization of a murine type II sodium-phosphate cotransporter expression in mammalian small intestine. *The Proceedings of the National Academy of Sciences of the USA* 95, 14564–14569.

Jongbloed, A.W., Everts, H. and Kemme P.A. (1991) Phosphorus availability and requirements in pigs. In: Heinemann, E.R. (ed.) *Recent Advances in Animal Nutrition*. Butterworths, London, pp. 65–80.

Ketaren, P.P., Batterham, E.S., Dettmann, E.B. and Farrell, D.J. (1993a) Phosphorus studies in pigs: 2. Assessing phosphorus availability for pigs and rats. *British Journal of Nutrition* 70, 269–288.

Ketaren, P.P., Batterham, E.S., Dettmann, E.B. and Farrell, D.J. (1993b) Phosphorus studies in pigs: 3. Effect of phytase supplementation on the digestibility and availability of phosphorus in soya-bean meal for grower pigs. *British Journal of Nutrition* 70, 289–311.

Kuang, C. (2005) Determination of true calcium and phosphorus digestibility and the endogenous calcium and phosphorus losses associated with soybean meal for pigs by the linear regression analysis. MSc thesis (in Chinese with an English abstract), Huazhong Agricultural University, Wuhan, China.

Kuang, C., He, R., Wang, J., Yin, Y.L. and Fan, M.Z. (2006) True calcium and phosphorus digestibility and the endogenous calcium and phosphorus outputs associated with soybean meal for multi-parity sows measured by the simple linear regression technique. *Journal of Animal Science* 84 (Supplement 1), 337 (Abstract).

Lambrechts, C., Boze, H., Moulin, G. and Galzy, P. (1992) Utilization of phytate by some yeasts. *Biotechnology Letter* 14, 61–66.

Lei, X.G., Ku, P.K., Miller, E.R. and Yokoyama, M.T. (1993a) Supplementing corn–soybean meal diets with microbial phytase linearly improves phytate phosphorus utilization by weanling pigs. *Journal of Animal Science* 71, 3359–3367.

Lei, X.G., Ku, P.K., Miller, E.R., Yokoyama, M.T. and Ullrey, D.E. (1993b) Supplementing corn–soybean meal diets with microbial phytase maximizes phytate phosphorus utilization by weanling pigs. *Journal of Animal Science* 71, 3368–3375.

Maenz, D.D. and Classen, H.L. (1998) Phytase activity in the small intestinal brush border membrane of the chicken. *Poultry Science* 77, 557–563.

Mallin, M. (2000) Impacts of industrial animal production on rivers and estuaries. *American Scientist* 88, 26–37.

Mroz, Z., Jongbloed, A.W. and Kemme, P.A. (1994) Apparent digestibility and retention of nutrients bound to phytate complexes as influenced by microbial phytase and feeding regimen in pigs. *Journal of Animal Science* 72, 126–132.

Murer, H., Forster, I. and Biber, J. (2004) The sodium phosphate cotransporter family SLC34. *European Journal of Physiology* 447, 763–767.

Naqvi, S.W.A., Jayakumar, D.A., Narvekar, P.V., Nalk, H., Sarma, V.V.S.S., D'Souza, W., Joseph, S. and George, M.D. (2000) Increased marine production of N2O due to intensifying anoxia on the Indian continental shelf. *Nature* 408, 346–349.

National Research Council (NRC) (1998) *Nutrient Requirements for Swine*, 10th edn. National Academy Press, Washington, DC.

Newkirk, R.W. and Classen, H.L. (1998) *In vitro* hydrolysis of phytate in canola meal with purified and crude sources of phytase. *Animal Feed Science and Technology* 72, 315–327.

Newsholme, E.A. and Leech, A.E. (1991) *Biochemistry for the Medical Sciences*. John Wiley & Sons, Chichester, UK.

Petersen, G.I. and Stein, H.H. (2006) Novel procedure for estimating endogenous losses and measurement of apparent and true digestibility of phosphorus by growing pigs. *Journal of Animal Science* 84, 2126–2132.

Pettey, L.A., Cromwell, G.L. and Lindemann, M.D. (2006) Estimation of endogenous phosphorus loss in growing and finishing pigs fed semi-purified diets. *Journal of Animal Science* 84, 618–626.

Raboy, V. (2002) Progress in breeding low phytate crops. *The Journal of Nutrition* 132, 503S–505S.

Reddy, N.R. (2002) Occurrence, distribution, content, and dietary intake of phytate. In: Reddy, N.R. and Sathe, S.K. (eds) *Food Phytates*. CRC Press, Boca Raton, Florida, pp. 25–61.

Rideout, T.C. and Fan, M.Z. (2004) Nutrient utilization in response to chicory inulin supplementation in studies with pigs. *Journal of the Science of Food and Agriculture* 84, 1005–1012.

Sands, J.S., Ragland, D., Baxter, C., Joern, B.C., Sauber, T.E. and Adeola, O. (2001) Phosphorus bioavailability, growth performance, and nutrient balance in pigs fed high available phosphorus corn and phytase. *Journal of Animal Science* 79, 2134–2142.

Schröder, B., Huber, K. and Breves, G. (2002) Comparative aspects of gastrointestinal calcium and phosphate absorption in pigs and small ruminants during early postnatal life. In: Zabielski, R., Gregory, P.C. and Weström, B. (eds) *Biology of the Intestine in Growing Animals*. Elsevier Science BV, Amsterdam, pp. 605–624.

Schulin-Zeuthen, M., Kebreab, E., Gerrits, W.J.J., Lopez, S., Fan, M.Z., Dias, R.S. and France, J. (2007) Meta-analysis of phosphorus balance data from growing pigs. *Journal of Animal Science* 85, 1953–1961.

Shen, Y. (2006) Digestive utilization of phosphorus in cereal grains by pigs. PhD thesis, University of Guelph, Guelph, Ontario.

Shen, Y. and Fan, M.Z. (2007) The intestinal transcellular Na^+-Pi co-transport contributes little to whole-body phosphorus absorption in the pig. *The FASEB Journal* 21, A724 (Abstract).

Shen Y., Fan, M.Z., Ajakaiye, A. and Archbold, T. (2002) True phosphorus digestibility and the endogenous phosphorus loss associated with corn for growing–finishing pigs are determined with the regression analysis technique. *The Journal of Nutrition* 132, 1199–1206.

Shen, Y., Fan, M.Z., Archbold, T., McBride, B.W. and Hacker, R.R. (2003) True phosphorus digestibility and the endogenous phosphorus outputs associated with conventional corn for weanling pigs. In: Ball, R. (ed.) *The 9th International Symposium on Digestive Physiology in Pigs*. University of Alberta, Edmonton, Alberta, Canada, pp. 395–397.

Shen, Y., Hacker, R.R. and Fan, M.Z. (2005a) Estimation of true phosphorus digestibility and the endogenous phosphorus losses associated with wheat for pigs. *Journal of Animal Science* 83 (Supplement 1), 155 (Abstract).

Shen, Y., Hacker, R.R. and Fan, M.Z. (2005b) True phosphorus digestibility and the endogenous phosphorus losses associated with barley for pigs. *Journal of Animal Science* 83 (Supplement 1), 155 (Abstract).

Shen, Y., Smith, T.K., Leeson, S., Hacker, R.R. and Fan, M.Z. (2005c) True digestibility and the endogenous output of phosphorus associated with oat grain in pigs measured by the regression analysis technique. *The FASEB Journal* 19(4), A92 (Abstract).

Shen, Y., Yin, Y.L., Chavez, E.R. and Fan, M.Z. (2005d) Methodological aspects of measuring phytase activity and phytate phosphorus content in selected cereal grains and digesta and feces of pigs. *Journal of Agricultural and Food Chemistry* 53, 853–859.

Simons, P.C.M., Versteegh, H.A.J., Jongbloed, A.W., Kemme, P.A., Slump, P., Box, K.D., Wolters, M.G.E., Beudeker, R.F. and Verschoor, G.J. (1990) Improvement of phosphorus availability by microbial phytase in broilers and pigs. *British Journal of Nutrition* 64, 525–529.

Skoglund, E. and Sandberg, A.S. (2002) Methods for analysis of phytate. In: Reddy, N.R. and Sathe, S.K. (eds) *Food Phytates*. CRC Press, Boca Raton, Florida, pp. 127–137.

Spencer, J.D., Allee, G.L. and Sauber, T.E. (2000) Phosphorus bioavailability and digestibility of normal and genetically modified low-phytate corn for pigs. *Journal of Animal Science* 78, 675–681.

Sreeramulu, G., Srinivasa, D.S., Nand, K. and Joseph, R. (1996) *Lactobacillus amylovorus* as a phytase producer in submerged culture. *Letters of Applied Microbiology* 23, 385–388.

Tangendjaja, B., Buckle, K.A. and Wootton, M. (1980) Analysis of phytic acid by high performance liquid chromatography. *Journal of Chromatography* 197, 274–277.

Tso, P. (1994) Intestinal lipid absorption. In: Johnson, L.R. (ed.) *Physiology of the Gastrointestinal Tract*, 3rd edn. Raven Press, New York, pp. 1867–1907.

Vaintraub, I.A. and Lapteva, N.A. (1988) Colorimetric determination of phytate in unpurified extracts of seeds and the products of their processing. *Analytical Biochemistry* 175, 227–230.

Veum, T.L., Ledoux, D.R., Raboy, V. and Ertl, D.S. (2001) Low-phytic acid corn improves nutrient utilization for growing pigs. *Journal of Animal Science* 79, 2873–2880.

Veum, T.L., Ledoux, D.R., Bollinger, D.W., Raboy, V. and Cook, A. (2002) Low-phytic acid barley improves calcium and phosphorus utilization and growth performance in growing pigs. *Journal of Animal Science* 80, 2663–2670.

Wang, Z.R., Yang, C.B., Shen, Y., Yin, Y.L., Archbold, T. and Fan, M.Z. (2005) True phosphorus digestibility and the endogenous phosphorus outputs in diets for weaned pigs determined by the substitution method. *Journal of Animal Science* 84 (Supplement 1), 39 (Abstract).

Weiss, S.L., Lee, E.A. and Diamond, J. (1997) Evolutionary matches of enzyme and transporter capacities to dietary substrate loads in the intestinal brush border. *Proceedings of the National Academy of Sciences of the USA* 95, 2117–2121.

Weremko, D., Fandrejewski, H., Zebrowska, T., Han, I.K., Kim, J.H. and Cho, W.T. (1997) Bioavailability of phosphorus in feeds of plant origin for pigs. *Asian–Australian Journal Animal Science* 10, 551–566.

Wheeler, E.L. and Ferrel, R.E. (1971) A method for phytic acid determination in wheat and wheat fractions. *Cereal Chemistry* 48, 312–320.

Xu, H., Bai, L., Collins, J.F. and Ghishan, F.K. (1999) Molecular cloning, functional characterization, tissue distribution, and chromosomal localization of a human, small intestinal sodium-phosphate (Na^+-Pi) transporter (SLC34A2). *Genomics* 62, 281–284.

Yang, C., Yin, Y.L., Shen, Y., Wang, Z.R., Rideout, T.C., Squires, E.J., Li, J., Xu, H., Collins, J.F., Ghishan, F.K. and Fan, M.Z. (2006) Visceral distribution of the type II sodium-dependent phosphate cotransporter (NaPi-II) isomer mRNA and the expression of NaPi-IIc mRNA along the intestinal longitudinal axis in the post-weaned pig. *The FASEB Journal* 20 (4), A1064 (Abstract).

Yang, H. (2005) Studies on true phosphorus digestibility in brown rice and the effects of amylase supplementation on nutrient utilization in weanling pigs. MSc thesis (in Chinese with an English abstract), Institute of Subtropical Agriculture, The Chinese Academy of Sciences, Changsha, Hunan Province, China.

Yang, H., Li,. A.K., Yin, Y.L., Li, T.J., Wang, Z.R., Wu, G., Huang, R.L., Kong, X.F., Yang, C.B., Kang, P., Deng, J., Wang, S.X., Tan, B.E., Hu, Q., Xing, F.F., Wu, X., He, Q.H., Yao, K., Liu, Z.J., Tang, Z.R., Yin, F.G., Deng, Z.Y., Xie, M.Y. and Fan, M.Z. (2007) True phosphorus digestibility and the endogenous phosphorus outputs associated with brown rice for weanling pigs measured by the simple linear regression analysis technique. *Animal* 1, 213–220.

Zhang, Y. (2004) Determination of true calcium and phosphorus digestibility values and the endogenous calcium and phosphorus losses associated with soybean meal for gilts and barrows by the linear regression analysis technique. MSc thesis (in Chinese with an English abstract), The Inner Mongolian Agricultural University, Huhhot, The Inner Mongolian Autonomous Region, China.

Zuo, J. (2005) True fecal phosphorus and calcium digestibility and prediction model of truly digestible phosphorus in unconventional plant feedstuffs for growing pigs. PhD thesis (in Chinese with an English abstract), South China Agricultural University, Guangzhou, China.

18 The Prediction of the Consequences of Pathogen Challenges on the Performance of Growing Pigs

I. KYRIAZAKIS,[1,2] F.B. SANDBERG[1] AND W. BRINDLE[1]

[1]*Animal Nutrition and Health Department, Scottish Agricultural College, UK;*
[2]*Faculty of Veterinary Medicine, University of Thessaly, Greece*

Introduction

Pigs in commercial units usually grow below their expected potential, i.e. what is observed in breeding stations and experimental units. It has been suggested that this 'growth gap' is due to constraints that arise from the presence of environmental stressors (Black *et al.*, 1999). Kyriazakis (1999) suggests that these stressors can be seen as falling into one of the following categories: physical (e.g. ambient temperature), social (e.g. the degree of competition) and infectious (i.e. the presence of pathogens) stressors. Predicting the effects of such stressors on the performance of pigs is important for guiding future management, genetic selection and experimental strategies.

A substantial effort has been put into the prediction of the consequence of environmental stressors on the performance of pigs (e.g. Bruce and Clark, 1979; Black *et al.*, 1986; Wellock *et al.*, 2003a,b). Less effort has been directed towards the prediction of the effects of social stressors, but at least a framework that allows progress to be made is now available (Wellock *et al.*, 2003c, 2004). Very little effort has been put into the prediction of the effects of infectious stressors, other than in a quasi-quantitative manner (Black *et al.*, 1999). There are several reasons why this is the case and these relate to the difficulties associated with quantification. These include: the quantitative description of the infectious environment; the sufficient description of the ability of the pig to cope with pathogens, including its transition from the susceptible to the immune state and the variation between individuals; the number of different pathogens that need to be taken into account; and the multitude of consequences these can have on pig function.

The purpose of this chapter is to develop a general framework that will enable progress to be made in our ability to predict pig performance in the presence of infectious stressors. We concentrate here on subclinical infection, i.e. infection that does not lead to clear signs of disease other than a general reduction in pig performance. There are several reasons for doing this, including: (i) the significance of subclinical disease for the economic performance of pig enterprises; and (ii) the generic consequences of subclinical disease for pig physiology and metabolism. This also enables us to develop a framework that has a generic value, rather than being pathogen-specific. The hope is that the developed framework will also have a heuristic value, as it will point towards issues that need to be taken into account, or even resolved, in order to be able to predict adequately the performance of pigs challenged by pathogens.

A Typical Pig Response during Exposure to Pathogens

A typical pig response during exposure to an infectious environment is as demonstrated by Williams *et al.* (1997a) and shown in Fig. 18.1. In these experiments, pigs were offered *ad libitum* foods of different protein contents in environments intended to have either high or low levels of 'stimulation of the immune system'. This was achieved by exposure to a 'dirty environment', in the absence of antimicrobials, and through repeated vaccination. The authors state that the pigs 'remained healthy throughout the experiments'; this can be taken to imply that there was no evidence of clinical disease.

The response can be summarized as follows:

1. Challenged pigs achieved a lower food intake than non-challenged pigs at all levels of protein used. There was no significant interaction of the level of immune system activation and the feed crude protein content.

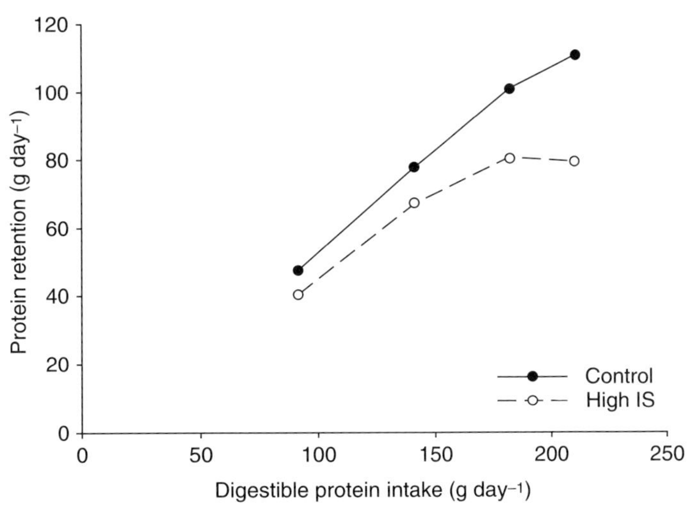

Fig. 18.1. The response in protein retention to digestible protein intake for pigs that were kept either in a clean environment (control) or a high-immune system activation environment (high IS); from Williams *et al.*, 1997a.

2. An increase in the level of protein intake required to achieve a certain level of protein retention (PR) below maximum was seen in challenged pigs. This would be equivalent to saying that the maintenance requirements of the challenged pigs were increased.
3. No change in the marginal response of PR to protein intake, i.e. the slope of the response, between challenged and unchallenged pigs. This, however, is not a consistent feature of similar experiments (see below).
4. Challenged animals did not achieve the same maximum rate of PR. In the case of the above experiment, this was estimated as 0.74 of those in the low immune stimulation environment.

Below, we discuss how these effects may arise. The aim is to identify the extent and the mechanism(s) by which these effects may arise during exposure to pathogens. The hope is that this will lead to their quantification.

The Consequences of Pathogen Challenge for Food Intake

The major characteristic of the exposure to pathogens, in hosts without prior experience of a pathogen, is a voluntary reduction in the food intake of the animal (Fig. 18.2). The extent of this voluntary reduction in food intake, henceforth called *anorexia*, is foremost dependent on host pathogen load (PL), i.e. the number of pathogens that are carried by the host at any particular time (Hein, 1968). High levels of PL lead to dramatic decreases in food intake and are associated with clinical disease. However, there is a wide range of PLs, which are usually

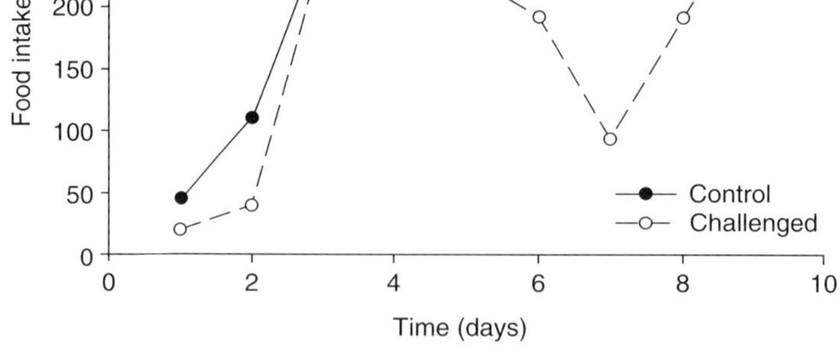

Fig. 18.2. The effect of a pathogen challenge with 10^8 colony-forming units of *Escherichia coli* on the food intake of control and challenged pigs over a 10-day time period post-weaning; from Houdijk *et al.*, 2005. The arrow indicates the point of infection.

associated with subclinical disease, over which food intake is reduced to 0.75–0.80 of the expected voluntary food intake. There also seems to be a threshold of PL below which food intake of animals seems to be unaffected. Sandberg *et al.* (2006) have developed a model to predict the extent of anorexia during exposure to different kinds of pathogens and to represent the transition from 'normal' to reduced voluntary food intake. For the purposes of this chapter, it will be assumed that there is a discontinuity between these two phases, i.e. when the 'critical' PL is exceeded, then food intake drops by 0.20.

The type of pathogen also plays a significant role in the onset and duration of anorexia. In the example in Fig. 18.2, pigs showed a reduction in their voluntary food intake within 2 days post-infection with enterotoxigenic *Escherichia coli*. The duration of the reduction in food intake was equally short. These contrast with the lengthy time taken to develop and, particularly, the lengthy duration of anorexia observed during subclinical infections with gastrointestinal worms (e.g. Hale, 1985).

Currently, there is a considerable debate over the mechanism that leads to this pathogen-induced anorexia. Sandberg *et al.* (2006) have proposed that there are at least two mechanisms that may lead to this: (i) food intake is reduced, because the potential for PR of the challenged animals is reduced; and (ii) the reduction in food intake is a direct consequence of the exposure to pathogens. Black *et al.* (1999) have argued that both mechanisms may be acting simultaneously, although they have not suggested how this effect may be modelled.

It is important, from a modelling perspective, to decide upon the mechanisms that lead to anorexia. Mechanism (i) may be modelled by assuming a direct relationship between PL and the maximum growth rate of the animal. This would be equivalent to the approach of Wellock *et al.* (2003c), who assume that environmental stressors lower the growth rate parameter of the equation that describes maximum (potential) growth in the pig. This in turn leads to a decrease in the potential daily gain that the pig is able to achieve, and hence a reduction in its required food intake. In mechanism (ii), modelled by Sandberg *et al.* (2006), the reduction in the voluntary food intake of the challenged animal was made a function of the current PL. The value of the maximum reduction in food intake during subclinical disease was assumed to be constant across a number of pathogens and range of PLs. A consequence of this mechanism is that the challenged animal will always be in a state of nutrient and energy scarcity during exposure to pathogens.

Both mechanisms assume that once the PL starts to decline, food intake will return to what is expected, given the genotype and current state of the animal. It should be noted that, because of the occurrence of anorexia, an animal would be smaller than its uninfected control at the point of recovery. This needs to be taken into account when comparisons are made on a time rather than live weight basis. In an analogy to the assumption made for the transition between 'normal' food intake and anorexia, it is also assumed here that the recovery in food intake is also abrupt once PL has declined below a certain threshold. Sandberg *et al.* (2006) have developed a more complex and elegant model that allows for a more general transition in the rate of recovery of food intake.

The above also link the mechanism that underlies anorexia to the development of the acquired immune response by the pig (see below). A reduction in PL would be a direct consequence of the development of acquired immunity. If it is assumed that the above-critical value of PL will never be exceeded in immune pigs (see below), then anorexia should not accompany re-exposure to pathogens. However, anorexia may arise in situations where immunity breaks down and PL has exceeded the critical value. Unfortunately, the above propositions cannot be tested currently, as the issue of food intake during re-exposure to pathogens in immune animals has not been addressed experimentally.

Maintenance Requirements as a Consequence of the Exposure to Pathogens

In the experiments of Williams *et al.* (1997a,b,c), the increases in maintenance requirements for protein ranged between 1.6 and 2.9 times those of the unchallenged pigs. There are no equivalent experiments that have investigated the increases in maintenance requirements for energy in pigs exposed to pathogens, but estimates from other species suggest increases in maintenance requirements that range from 1.05 to 1.35 times those of the unchallenged, healthy controls (e.g. Verstegen *et al.*, 1991).

There are several sources that can contribute to these increases in maintenance requirements in energy and protein for pigs exposed to pathogens. They all arise from the functions that relate to the effort the animal puts into dealing with the pathogens. The implication is that by being part of the maintenance requirements, these functions are prioritized over productive functions, i.e. growth. For a pig that has no prior experience to a pathogen, such functions are the innate immune response and the repair of damaged tissue. Additional energy requirements may arise from the expression of fever. Below, we consider the quantitative costs of these functions.

Additional Maintenance Requirements for Protein

Innate immune response requirements

The innate immune system is the first line of defence to pathogen challenges and it plays important roles in both recognizing and actively protecting a host from pathogens (Beutler, 2004). The innate immune system represents physical barriers, such as skin and cilia, and chemical barriers, such as lysozyme, complement and acute-phase proteins. Cellular components of the innate immune system may contain large amounts of protein and their production may contribute towards an additional requirement for protein during pathogen challenges.

There is evidence in the literature that increases in maintenance due to innate immune functions are related directly to the host's PL (e.g. Taylor-Robinson, 2000). At low PLs, there seems to be little effect on these requirements.

However, as PL increases, the requirement increases, until it reaches a physiologically determined maximum, henceforth called $IIRQ_m$. Here, it is proposed that, under the significant (and continuous) pathogen challenges that occur in practice, the innate immune system operates at its maximum, and it is the quantification of this maximum that is necessary in the development of a predictive framework. It is further proposed that $IIRQ_m$ is a multiple of the (ideal) protein requirement for maintenance, MP, which in turn is a function of animal size. This would be equivalent to saying that a bigger animal has more apparatus for the function of innate immunity and will be consistent with the view that larger animals are able to cope better than smaller ones when exposed to the same level of pathogens. Here, it is proposed that the requirement for the innate immune response is up to 1.1 times the maintenance requirements for protein.

There are currently no equivalent experiments that estimate the maintenance amino acid requirements of pigs exposed to pathogens. Experiments on poultry (Webel *et al.*, 1998a,b) suggest that chicks challenged with an antigenic stimulant (lipopolysaccharide, LPS) show an increase in maintenance requirements for certain amino acids. This challenge mainly stimulates the innate immune response, as it does not result in damage to the host, as would be the case for 'real' pathogen challenges. The increase in maintenance requirements for amino acids ranged from no change (in the case of arginine) to a 1.3 times increase (in the case of lysine). These experiments strongly suggest that it might be necessary to consider the requirements for individual amino acids to account fully for reductions in growth during pathogen challenges.

Requirements due to repair and replacement of tissues

Pathogens may cause damage to a host's tissues (e.g. gut wall) or specific cells (e.g. red blood cells) and cause body fluids to leave their natural compartments, such as plasma leaking into the gastrointestinal tract. The pig would need to repair such damage or replace lost fluids to maintain normal function, which is, thus, a direct cost to the animal (Berendt *et al.*, 1977). It would be expected that such costs are larger than those associated with innate immunity.

Pigs have been challenged by different parasitic worms that affected different internal organs (stomach, small intestine, large intestine and kidneys) by Hale (1985). The consequences of parasitism for nitrogen metabolism depended on the organ affected. The kidney parasite was not associated with any measurable effects on N metabolism, whereas the small and large intestinal parasites were associated with increased N in the faeces, resulting from the associated damaged tissues and endogenous secretions. At a given level of N intake, pigs thus parasitized had a lower level of N retention than their respective controls. Therefore, the type of pathogen and by extension the organ(s) affected need to be taken into account when estimating the costs of repair and replacement of damaged tissues.

Literature evidence also suggests that the extent of the costs associated with damage is not only dependent on pathogen type, but also on the level of pathogen challenge. Le Jambre (1995) and Powanda *et al.* (1975) have suggested that the relationship is of an exponential type. This may indicate that a host that has already suffered a certain amount of damage may be less capable of dealing with additional pathogen challenges. Currently, there is very little quantitative evidence to relate these requirements to the type and level of pathogens in pigs. This is clearly a component of the framework that would need to be pathogen-specific during its quantification.

Additional Maintenance Requirements for Energy

Providing that increases in protein requirements due to the innate immune response and the repair and replacement of tissues are known, the associated increases in the energy maintenance requirements can be estimated. It is proposed that the energetic costs of making the components of the innate immune response are incorporated in the energetic costs of PR and are predicted as usual. The same applies to the costs associated with repair. In the case of gastrointestinal parasites, the most significant energetic cost appears to be associated with damaged tissues, resulting in additional amounts of N appearing in the urine (McRae *et al.*, 1982), but these have not been estimated directly in pigs, nor have they been considered explicitly in previous frameworks.

The most significant energetic costs due to exposure to pathogens appear to be associated with the expression of fever. A febrile response accompanies most bacterial, viral and parasitic infections of pigs, although it appears to be absent in infections where pathogens are localized. For example, van Diemen *et al.* (1995) did not record any increase in body temperature in pigs that were suffering from atrophic rhinitis. Within the framework developed here, a febrile response is seen as a beneficial host reaction, rather than being a detrimental and unavoidable consequence of pathogen challenge. This is consistent with the views of Hart (1988) and Blatteis (2003), who suggested that fever may be beneficial to hosts, as bacterial and viral growth rates are sensitive to changes in their ambient temperature, or through the increased body temperature having positive effects on the host immune responses (Jiang *et al.*, 2000).

The above suggestion links the febrile response to acquired immunity and, therefore, the duration of fever can be seen as a function of PL and can be modelled in the same way as the duration of anorexia, above. Experiments with both artificial antigenic challenges and pathogens have shown increases in maintenance requirements for energy that ranged from 1.05 to 1.35. These estimates not only include the energetic costs of the immune response and tissue repair, but they have been taken in the presence of anorexia and in situations where challenged animals with fever showed behavioural coping responses (e.g. huddling). They may, therefore, be underestimates of the direct increases in energy requirements due to fever.

Here, it is suggested that a simple linear relationship exists between the increase in body temperature due to fever and PL. This relationship holds for above a certain threshold PL that activates the immune response. The increase in energy requirement for each degree of fever (MJ $°C^{-1}$) appears to be consistently around 1.15 times maintenance (van Dam *et al.*, 1998). Thus, the cost of fever is predicted as a multiple of maintenance, which implies that larger animals will have a greater energetic cost for mounting fever.

The Marginal Response to Protein during Pathogen Challenges

The relationship between PR and crude protein intake, CPI, can be expressed as:

$$\text{PR} = e_p\,((d.\text{CPI}.v) - \text{MP})\ \text{g day}^{-1}, \tag{18.1}$$

where e_p is the marginal response of PR to ideal protein intake above maintenance, d is the true ideal digestibility of the CPI, v is the biological value of the food protein and MP is the maintenance protein requirements. On the basis of what was discussed above in relation to the (innate) immune response (protein) requirements and the costs of tissue repair being part of maintenance, the expectation would be that e_p would be unaffected during exposure to pathogens.

The previously discussed experiments of Williams *et al.* (1997a,b,c) and Webel *et al.* (1998a,b) agree with this suggestion as they found little or no effect on the marginal responses in PR of growing pigs and chicks, respectively, to protein and amino acid supplies. On the other hand, there are a number of experiments where animals fed above maintenance responded both in terms of growth and immune responses to increments of protein or amino acid intake (e.g. Bhargava *et al.*, 1970a,b; Tsigabe *et al.*, 1987; Datta *et al.*, 1998). For example, Bhargava *et al.* (1970a) found that both growth rates and antibody titres in chicks challenged with the Newcastle virus improved when given foods that had increasing concentrations of valine (Fig. 18.3). In addition, the response in antibody titre increased further when the animal had reached a plateau in its growth response. The latter experiments strongly suggest that there may actually be a partitioning of protein or amino acids between growth and immune functions.

In order to reconcile the above apparently contradictory experimental evidence, here we suggest the following: (i) the innate immune response is indeed prioritized in terms of scarce nutrient allocation and, therefore, it can be safely considered as part of maintenance; on the other hand (ii) the acquired immune response competes for allocation of scarce nutrients with the function of growth; as a consequence, it should not be considered as part of maintenance. These suggestions imply that for a naive pig there would be no change in the value of e_p when the animal is challenged by pathogens. As the pig develops, the acquired immune response e_p will decline, since a proportion of nutrients will be diverted away from growth towards the former function. Unfortunately, experimental data are usually an aggregate of the above two phases (e.g. Williams *et al.*, 1997a,b,c). Below, we discuss the quantitative consequences of the above suggestions. The arguments apply to pigs that exhibit a degree of acquired immunity.

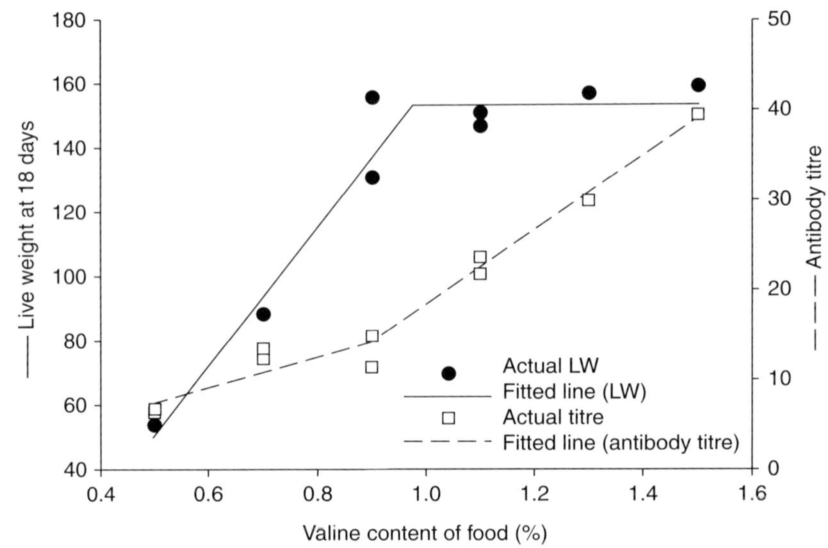

Fig. 18.3. The responses in live weight over 18 days (LW) and antibody titres (AT) to increasing valine contents (*V*) of a food for chicks challenged with a Newcastle virus; from Bhargava *et al.*, 1970a. Linear plateau response was approximated as a linear function of valine content (LW = 217.*V* – 58.2) until the plateau of 153.6 was reached. The linear regression of antibody titre against valine content until maximum LW was reached was AT = 16.37.*V* – 0.6325, whereas for the subsequent phase it was AT = 41.35.*V* – 23.04.

The Requirements of the Acquired Immune Response

The innate immune response provides fast protection against pathogens but, after a certain level of challenge has been exceeded, the animal recognizes the pathogen and mounts an acquired immune response. An animal needs to acquire the ability to mount an immunity before it can express it. The acquired immune response has both cellular and humoral components, which also contain large amounts of protein (see above). Therefore, their production would contribute towards an additional requirement for protein during pathogen challenges.

In an analogy to what has been proposed for the requirements of the innate immune response, it is also suggested here that the requirements for the acquired immune response are related directly to the host's PL. As PL increases, the (protein) requirement increases up to a physiologically determined maximum, henceforth called AIRQ. Houdijk *et al.* (2001) have suggested that this maximum may be up to 20% of the maintenance requirements, although others (e.g. Sykes and Greer, 2003) have suggested that this may be up to 50%. These suggestions imply that the cost of mounting an acquired immune response is considerable and, therefore, it should be taken into account in the development of a framework that aims to predict the performance of pigs when challenged by pathogens.

A complicating factor, in terms of quantification, arises from the fact that AIRQ may depend on the kind of pathogen challenge. This is because different kinds of pathogens stimulate different arms of the immune response (e.g. Th-1 versus Th-2 responses). Here, it is proposed that the maximum AIRQ should be considered separately for these two different classes of response. This implies that pathogens are also seen as falling into one of these two responses (Kuby, 1997).

The Composition of the Acquired Immune Response

The biological value of the food crude protein (denoted by v in Eqn 18.1) is calculated from the ratio of the first-limiting amino acid in the food in relation to a reference protein (usually pig whole-body protein). Beisel (1977) and Wannemacher *et al.* (1971), among others, have proposed that the amino acid composition of the immune response is very different from that of muscle and other tissues and, therefore, immune responses lead to specific requirements for certain amino acids. Table 18.1 summarizes the amino acid composition of acute-phase proteins, other immune proteins (antibodies, cell proteases), colostrum and milk and that of a reference protein (whole-body protein of pigs). The comparison with colostrum and milk is included as colostrum contains a large amount of maternal antibodies. There are some marked differences between the different kinds of proteins in terms of their composition.

On the basis of the suggestion that the requirements for the acquired immune responses can be significant (see above), the differences in the amino acid composition between the two body components will be expected to have a significant effect on the prediction of PR (Eqn 18.1). The value of v will depend greatly on the size and type of the immune response (Wang and Fuller, 1989). In this case, predictions will have to be made on the basis of individual amino acid responses. PR would then be reconstituted on the basis of individual amino acid retention. This will have exceedingly high information requirements and, therefore, parameterization of the framework will be exceedingly difficult.

An alternative solution to the above problem would be to retain the ideal protein system, but assume that the efficiency (e_p in Eqn 18.1) with which protein is utilized for the purposes of the immune response is modified. This would be in order to account for the different protein composition of the two body components. This seems to be a less onerous task than the above and experiments that can be designed to contribute towards the parameterization of this solution can be envisaged.

The Partitioning of Resources between Immunity and Growth

Having established that there is a requirement for resources associated with the acquired immune response and that this requirement competes with growth for scarce resources, the task is to propose a rule of partitioning to account for this.

Table 18.1. A summary of the amino acid composition of different proteins that are associated with the immune response, in relation to the reference protein that is normally used for calculating the biological value of food protein. The amino acid composition of colostrum (a source rich in immune proteins), milk and reference protein (whole-body protein of pigs) is also shown for comparison.

	Amino acid composition (g kg^{-1} protein)[a]												
	Pig protein	Milk	Colostrum	APP1[d]	APP2[d]	APP3[d]	APP4[d]	APP5[d]	APP6[d]	IgA	IgE	Sheep MCP	Mucin
Phenylalanine	38	18	24	105	46	64	83	30	103	26	30	29	15
Tyrosine	25.8	9	22	50	56	74	27	70	67	24	43	29	13
Tryptophan	7.9	–	–	42	35	30	11	32	45	26	20	8	–
Leucine	74.4	11	59	91	62	101	124	82	29	120	87	90	31
Isoleucine	35.0	5	29	54	32	48	49	47	29	13	39	69	15
Valine	46.9	54	145	77	48	46	59	84	18	96	80	73	222
Lysine	70.5	28	99	71	77	75	92	92	33	39	57	53	18
Histidine	28.1	21	100	16	27	17	37	38	35	11	18	29	–
Metionine	17.5	1	6	16	32	11	28	16	22	6	7	33	–
Cysteine	10.3	2	8	13	15	18	6	24	0	39	28	24	85
Threonine	38.2	115	46	58	60	74	66	54	30	75	103	45	224
Arginine	67.0	6	25	36	84	52	23	28	116	32	39	57	16
Proline	71.0	52	39	44	48	34	41	44	34	75	67	49	83
Glycine	91.4	32	63	46	59	19	33	44	61	69	52	86	49
Serine	40.1	288	88	84	91	31	49	40	47	126	103	86	65
Alanine	64.5	21	58	31	29	36	43	54	106	56	46	69	42
ASX[b]	86.2	19	46	82	113	102	106	113	128	75	82	57	56
GLX[c]	136.5	318	145	112	119	173	136	115	87	94	93	90	64

[a]Amino acid composition of whole-body pig protein from Kyriazakis *et al.* (1993), acute-phase proteins from Reeds *et al.* (1994) and for IgA, IgE, sheep mast cell proteases (MCP) and mucin were taken from Houdijk and Athanasiadou (2003).
[b]ASX – asparagine + aspartate.
[c]GLX – glutamine + glutamate.
[d]APP(X) represents six different acute-phase proteins: (i) C-reactive protein; (ii) fibrinogen; (iii) alpha-1-glycoprotein; (iv) alpha-1-antitrypsin; (v) haptoglobin; and (vi) amyloid A.

There are various suggestions that can be put forward; for example: (i) partitioning towards the immune response can be a function of PL; (ii) partitioning is a characteristic of pig genotype (e.g. naturally robust pigs); (iii) partitioning can be a function of the requirements for growth and acquired immune response, with animals with higher relative requirements for growth partitioning more towards this function rather than the immune response; and (iv) scarce resources are partitioned towards the immune function according to a fixed ratio.

Here, for the sake of simplicity, we favour suggestion (iv), which in any case can be seen as being equivalent to rule (i), when the immune response operates at its maximum. We also suggest that this fixed ratio is of the order of 0.1–0.2 of the scarce resource. This is consistent with the suggestion of van der Waaij (2004) that animals partition 0.20 of their scarce resources towards the immune function.

In the above, we have considered mainly the partitioning of amino acids and protein. This is because during pathogen challenges, energy requirements are increased, with no further effect on energy partitioning (Benson *et al.*, 1993; van Dam, 1996). In a predictive framework, energy requirements during pathogen challenges could, therefore, be accounted for as part of maintenance and the cost of PR, which includes the immune response. This would have the consequence that only protein partitioning during pathogen challenges would need to be revised in a predictive framework of growth during disease. In support are the several experiments that show no improvement in immune responses when additional levels of energy above maintenance are supplied (van Heugten *et al.*, 1996; Spurlock *et al.*, 1997).

A Complete Framework of Resource Partitioning

A schematic framework that summarizes the ideas that have been developed above in relation to resource partitioning is shown in Fig. 18.4. The framework is developed in terms of food crude protein being the scarce resource, as an example. The starting conditions are a pig of a given genotype and state (as defined by Emmans and Kyriazakis, 2001), which is offered access to a food of a certain composition, while it is exposed to a certain amount of pathogen. The intermediate steps that lead to the outcome of protein retention (PR, other than immune proteins) are:

1. Food intake is reduced as a direct consequence of PL exceeding a certain threshold. This threshold is dependent on pathogen kind, but all pathogens are expected to lead to the same extent of anorexia during subclinical disease.
2. Apparent digestibility of CP is unaffected by the presence of pathogens, unless these damage parts of the lower intestine.
3. Partitioning of digested CP will be prioritized towards the function of maintenance. The latter includes the classic maintenance requirements for protein, but also requirements for the innate immune function and repair of damaged tissues. Both these requirements are a function of pathogen kind and PL. In naive animals, these requirements may be measured as a composite, given the fact that it may be difficult to distinguish between them (Graham *et al.*, 2005).

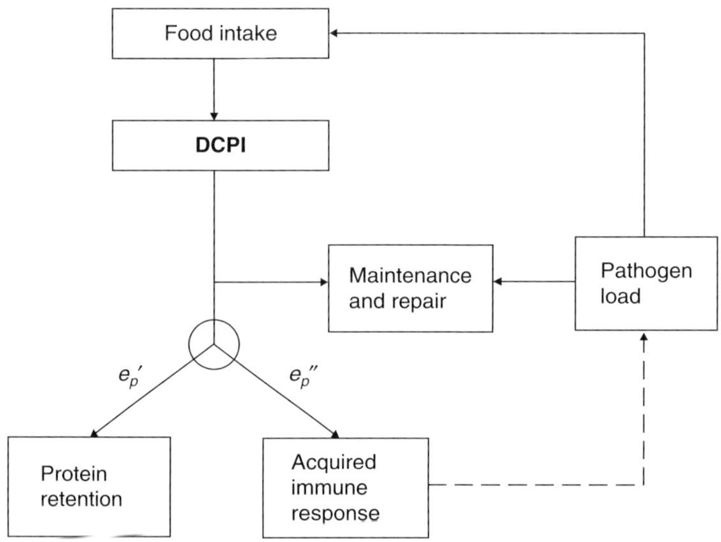

Fig. 18.4. A schematic description of the partitioning of protein (DCPI, digestible crude protein intake) during exposure to pathogens. Partitioning is prioritized to maintenance, which includes innate immune response and repair of tissues damaged by pathogens, before DCPI is utilized for protein retention and the acquired immune response. The efficiencies of using DCPI, e_p' and e_p'', include the biological value of the digested crude protein.

4. The remaining digested CP will be partitioned between the functions of PR and expression of acquired immunity. The requirements for the latter will also be dependent on pathogen kind and a function of PL. By directing resources towards the acquired immune response, the pig will reduce its PL. The assumption is that the rates of partitioning protein between these two functions is independent of PL.
5. The 'material' efficiencies for using digested protein for PR and acquired immunity are termed e_p' and e_p'', respectively. Both these efficiencies are composites of the net material efficiency of ideal protein use and the biological value of the digested protein. The biological value will depend on the function for which the digested protein is used, in order to account for the different composition of the two body components.
6. Both maximum PR and maximum expression of acquired immunity are functions of the animal genotype and current state *only*.

The above raise certain issues that are relevant to the quantification of the framework; these issues are discussed below.

The Quantification of Pathogen Load

The above framework makes PL the quantity responsible for the changes in resource requirements and partitioning, as well as the reductions in voluntary food intake. For this reason, it is a central driver of the framework. Pathogen load can be linked to pathogen dose (PD), i.e. the number of pathogens a host becomes exposed to at any particular point in time, through:

$$dPL/dt = r.PL - k.PL.AI\ n\ \text{day}^{-1}, \quad (18.2)$$

where *r* is the replication rate of the pathogen, *k* is the rate constant for the elimination of the pathogen by the host and AI is the size of the acquired immune response. At the point of infection, PL = PD. For pathogens that do not replicate within the host, such as macroparasites, the value of *r* is equivalent to 0. A typical value of *r* for the doubling rates of microparasitic bacteria has been estimated at 1.03 h^{-1} (Lin-Chao and Bremer, 1986). The term PL.AI approximates the likelihood that an encounter occurs between an immune effect or component (e.g. an immune cell) and the pathogen. Here, it is proposed that only the size of the immune response is a function of (previous) host nutrition and this view will be elaborated below.

It is suggested that PD can be seen as the descriptor of the infectious environment, and hence as an input required by the framework. However, unlike other environmental inputs, such as ambient temperature, humidity and group size, the quantification of PD is not straightforward. Under experimental infections, PD is usually known with a high degree of accuracy and the framework should apply under such conditions. The situation, however, is much more complex under natural infections, where both the infectious load of the environment and PD are very difficult to quantify. In addition, animals are usually exposed to mixed rather than single pathogen infections and the issue arises whether pathogens act synergistically or in an additive manner under these circumstances (Wellock *et al.*, 2003c). Finally, the consequences to the host may be very different, even at a given PD of the same pathogen. This is because pathogens may vary in their virulence. In order to overcome all these difficulties, it is proposed here that a proxy for the quantification of the infectious environment should be used instead. If this proxy is a pig state descriptor, then the description of the infectious environment would be a function of the animal's initial state. This is an untested proposition that has obvious attractions.

The Genetic Ability to Cope with Pathogens

Hosts differ in their ability to cope with pathogens; this ability is usually described by the term resistance (Knap and Bishop, 2000). The framework has identified *at least* two animal traits that may be a reflection of resistance: (i) the maximum capacity of the innate immune response; and (ii) the maximum capacity of the acquired immune response. As discussed previously, these traits may be linked to the requirements for food resources. The requirement of the framework is that pigs are described in a manner consistent with these traits.

Attempts have been made to select pigs that are able to cope better with disease (e.g. Wilkie and Mallard, 1998; Clapperton *et al.*, 2005). The selection traits, and, by extension, the description of the selected pigs, are not consistent with the requirement of the developed framework. It is suggested that a closer communication between scientists who are interested in the description of pig genotype, i.e. breeders, and those who are interested in the prediction of pig responses may lead to a more consistent description of the pig's genetic ability to cope with pathogens. This dialogue between breeders and modellers has led to the sufficient description for other pig traits, e.g. those related to growth potential (Kyriazakis, 1999).

Pig genotypes may also differ in their resistance through the rule they use to partition resources between growth and the immune response, previously defined as a ratio of partitioning a scarce resource. Rauw *et al.* (1998) have suggested that animals that have been selected for productive traits would partition more scarce resources towards these functions when nutrient resources are scarce. This implies that their immune responses will be penalized under these circumstances. Rauw *et al.* (1998) have suggested that this is the reason why highly productive animals appear to suffer more from diseases in challenging environments (Stewart *et al.*, 1969; Rao *et al.*, 2003; Haile *et al.*, 2004).

The framework is capable of accounting for this suggestion by making partitioning a function of both the requirements for growth and acquired immune responses. This suggestion does not have any additional quantitative requirements in relation to the description of the resistant pig genotypes. Pigs of a higher genetic (potential) for growth, but the same capacity for acquired immune response, would then be directing more of their scarce nutrients towards their growth and may thus appear less resistant.

Towards a Dynamic Framework of Resource Partitioning

Changes in PL over time would lead to dynamic changes in food intake and the nutrient requirements and their use for functions that are associated with the pathogen. This, in turn, would lead to dynamic changes in body component(s) retention. These changes in the framework alone, however, may not allow for a dynamic transition from the naive to the immune host state. This is because, by making the acquired immunity and its requirement a function of PL only, the implication is that the animal would be responding to the maximum of its capacity once PL has attained a certain threshold. In these cases, an almost instantaneous acquired immune response would be predicted, even for previously naive hosts. This would be inconsistent with the observation that acquired immune responses take some time to develop (Kelly *et al.*, 1996; Bocharov, 1998; McDermott *et al.*, 2004). Such development may take anything from a couple to several days, or even weeks, depending on the kind of pathogen. Microparasites, such as bacteria and viruses, tend to be at one end of the spectrum, whereas macroparasites, such as gastrointestinal worms, are at the other.

A time lag in the development of the immune response can be introduced by assuming that there is a limit to the rate at which the immune response may grow. Antia *et al.* (1996) have suggested that the rate of change in the acquired immune response can be represented as:

$$\mathrm{dAI}/\mathrm{d}t = a + p\mathrm{AI}_0\left(\frac{\mathrm{PL}}{\mathrm{PL}+\phi}\right) - \mathrm{dAI}_0 \text{ units day}^{-1}, \qquad (18.3)$$

where a and d represent the rates of growth and death, respectively, of the acquired immune response, p is the maximum per capita rate of proliferation by the cells of the immune response and ϕ is the pathogen density at half (dAI/dt) max. When PL is zero, then a should be equal to (dAI_0) to allow for lack of growth in the immune response. By making dAI/dt a function of PL, it is implied that previously naive hosts who are stimulated by a higher number of pathogens develop their acquired immune response at a faster rate (Barnes and Dobson, 1993).

Equation 18.3 represents the 'maximum' rate of change in the immune response in the presence of adequate host nutrition. Thus, it can be linked to the requirements for the acquired immune response (see below). When nutrient resources are scarce, the growth of the immune response would be a function of the scarce resource *only* and independent of PL. This is because we assumed earlier that the ratio of partitioning scarce nutrients between the acquired immune response and growth was expected to be constant. If, on the other hand, the partitioning ratio is made a function of both the requirements for growth and acquired immune response, then the change in the immune response would also be a function of PL (through Eqn 18.3).

Maintenance of the immune state per se is also a dynamic process, especially for hosts that are not under continuous exposure to pathogens (Anderson, 1994). Acquired immunity may be lost if hosts do not continue to be exposed to pathogens over a certain period of time. Therefore, a dynamic framework that intends to predict the responses of pigs during exposure to pathogens should take into account this state change. This situation, however, is unlikely to arise over the lifespan of growing pigs, but it may well arise among breeding livestock and, for this reason, it is raised here.

Conclusion

A heuristic framework that aims to predict the responses of growing pigs during exposure to pathogens has been developed above. We have tried to reduce the information requirements of the framework to a level that would still enable us to progress towards quantitative, dynamic predictions. In this chapter, we purposely did not specify, or describe in quantitative terms, the pathogen challenge under consideration, as our aim was to develop a generic framework. Parameterization of this framework may then be possible by focusing on specific pathogens and their consequences, including disease. The framework may also be able to be expanded to account for exposure to a number of different pathogens, as is the case in practice. We consider this to be a more fruitful approach than the creation of a model to account specifically for exposure to a single pathogen (e.g. the approach taken by Black *et al.* (1999) to predict the consequences of pleuropneumonia in pigs).

As reliance on chemoprophylaxis to control farm animal pathogens is decreasing, due, for example, to consumer concerns or legislation (Waller, 1997; Olesen *et al.*, 2000), interest in the understanding of the performance of animals in the presence of pathogens will increase. A model that predicts the performance of pigs during exposure to pathogens may then have value as a management tool to develop strategies, including breeding and nutritional strategies, to deal with this challenge.

Acknowledgements

This work was funded in part by the Biotechnology and Biological Sciences Research Council of the UK and PIC/Sygen. SAC receives support from the Scottish Executive Environment and Rural Affairs Department. We are grateful to our colleagues, Andrea Doeschl-Wilson and Dimitris Vagenas, for their input in the development of some of the ideas presented here.

References

Anderson, R.M. (1994) Mathematical studies of parasitic infections and immunity. *Science* 264, 1884–1886.

Antia, R., Koella, J.C. and Perrot, V. (1996) Models of the within-host dynamics of persistent mycobacterial infections. *Proceedings Biological Science* 263, 257–263.

Barnes, E.H. and Dobson, R.J. (1993) Persistence of acquired immunity to *Trichostrongylus colubriformis* in sheep after termination of infection. *International Journal for Parasitology* 23, 1019–1026.

Beisel, W.R. (1977) Magnitude of the host nutritional responses to infection. *American Journal of Clinical Nutrition* 30, 1236–1247.

Benson, B.N., Calvert, C.C., Roura, E. and Klasing, K.C. (1993) Dietary energy source and density modulate the expression of immunologic stress in chicks. *Journal of Nutrition* 123, 1714–1723.

Berendt, R.F., Long, G.G., Abeles, F.B., Canonico, P.G., Elwell, M.R. and Powanda, M.C. (1977) Pathogenesis of respiratory *Klebsiella pneumoniae* infection in rats: bacterial and histological findings and metabolic alterations. *Infection and Immunity* 15, 586–593.

Beutler, B. (2004) Innate immunity: an overview. *Molecular Immunology* 40, 845–849.

Bhargava, K.K., Hanson, R.P. and Sunde, M.L. (1970a) Effects of methionine and valine on antibody production in chicks infected with Newcastle disease virus. *Journal of Nutrition* 100, 241–248.

Bhargava, K.K., Hanson, R.P. and Sunde, M.L. (1970b) Effects of threonine on growth and antibody production in chicks infected with Newcastle virus. *Poultry Science* 50, 710–713.

Black, J.L., Davies, G.T., Bray, H.J., Giles, L.R. and Chapple, R.P. (1986) Simulation of energy and amino acid utilisation in the pig. *Research and Development in Agriculture* 3, 121–145.

Black, J.L, Bray, H.J. and Giles, L.R. (1999) The thermal and infectious environment. In: Kyriazakis I. (ed.) *A Quantitative Biology of the Pig*. CAB International, Wallingford, UK, pp. 71–97.

Blatteis, C.M. (2003) Fever: pathological or physiological, injurious or beneficial? *Journal of Thermal Biology* 28, 1–13.

Bocharov, G.A. (1998) Modelling the dynamics of LCMV infection in mice: conventional and exhaustive CTL responses. *Journal of Theoretical Biology* 192, 283–308.

Bruce, J.M. and Clark, J.J. (1979) Models of heat production and critical temperature for growing pigs. *Animal Production* 28, 353–369.

Clapperton, M., Bishop, S.C., Cameron, N.D. and Glass, E.J. (2005) Selection for lean growth in Large White pigs can affect levels of total white blood cell counts CD11R1$^+$ leukocytes in alpha-1 acid glycoprotein. *Proceedings of British Society of Animal Science*, p. 17.

Datta, F.U., Nolan, J.V., Rowe, J.B. and Gray, G.D. (1998) Protein supplementation improves the performance of parasitized sheep fed a straw-based diet. *International Journal for Parasitology* 28, 1269–1278.

Emmans, G.C. and Kyriazakis, I. (2001) Consequences of genetic change in farm animals on feed intake and feeding behaviour. *Proceedings of the Nutrition Society* 60, 115–125.

Graham, A.L., Allen, J.E. and Read, A.F. (2005) Evolutionary causes and consequences of immunopathology. *Animal Review of Ecology Evolution and Systematics* 36, 373–379.

Haile, A., Anindo, D.O., Tembley, S., Mukasa-Mugerwa, E., Tibbo, M., Yami, A., Baker, R.L. and Rege, J.E.O. (2004) Effects of dietary protein supplementation and infection with gastrointestinal nematode parasites on some nutritional and metabolic parameters in Ethiopian Menz and Horro sheep. *Livestock Production Science* 91, 183–195.

Hale, O.M. (1985) The influence of internal parasite infections on the performance of growing finishing swine. *Research Bulletin, Georgia Agricultural Experiment Stations* 341, 1–5.

Hart, B.L. (1988) Biological basis of the behaviour of sick animals. *Neuroscience and Biobehavioural Reviews* 12, 123–137.

Hein, H. (1968) The pathogenic effects of *Eimeria acervulina* in young chicks. *Experimental Parasitology* 22, 1–11.

Houdijk, J.G.M. and Athanasiadou, S. (2003) Direct and indirect effects of host nutrition on ruminant gastrointestinal nematodes. In: 't Mannetje, L., Ramírez-Avilés, L., Sandoval-Castro, C.A. and Ku-Vera, J.C. (eds) *VI International Symposium on the Nutrition of Herbivores*. Universidad Autónoma de Yucatán, Mérida, Mexico, pp. 213–236.

Houdijk, J.G.M., Jessop, N.S. and Kyriazakis, I. (2001) Nutrient partitioning between reproductive and immune functions in animals. *Proceedings of the Nutrition Society* 60, 515–525.

Houdijk, J.G.M., Anderson, D.H. and Kyriazakis, I. (2005) Induction of experimental sub-clinical post-weaning colibacillosis in pigs. *Proceedings of the British Society of Animal Science*, 84.

Jiang, Q., Cross, A.S., Singh, I.S., Chen, T.T., Viscardi, R.M. and Hasday, J.D. (2000) Febrile core temperature is essential for optimal host defense in bacterial peritonitis. *Infection and Immunity* 68, 1265–1270.

Kelly, B.P., Furney, S.K., Jessen, M.T. and Orme, I.M. (1996) Low-dose aerosol infection model for testing drugs for efficacy against *Mycobacterium tuberculosis*. *Antimicrobial Agents and Chemotherapy* 40, 2809–2812.

Knap, P.W. and Bishop, S.C. (2000) Relationships between genetic change and infectious disease in domestic livestock. *Proceedings of the British Society of Animal Science: Occasional Publication* 27, 65–80.

Kuby, J. (1997) *Immunology*. W.H. Freeman and Company, New York.

Kyriazakis, I. (1999) Introduction. In: Kyriazakis, I. (ed.) *A Quantitative Biology of the Pig*. CAB International, Wallingford, UK, pp. 1–5.

Kyriazakis, I., Emmans, G.C. and McDaniel, R. (1993) The amino acid composition of the protein in the whole bodies of growing pigs. *Journal of the Science of Food and Agriculture* 62, 29–33.

Le Jambre, L.F. (1995) Relationship of blood loss to worm numbers, biomass and egg production in *Haemonchus* infected sheep. *International Journal of Parasitology* 25, 269–273.

Lin-Chao, S. and Bremer, H. (1986) Effect of bacterial growth rate on replication control of plasmid pBR322 in *Escherichia coli*. *Biomedical and Life Sciences* 203, 143–149.

McDermott, A.B., Mitchen, J., Piaskowski, S., Souza, I., Yant, L.J., Stephan, J., Furlott, J. and Watkins, D.I. (2004) Repeated low-dose of mucosal simian immunodeficiency virus SIVmac239 challenge results in the same viral and immunological kinetics as high-dose challenge: a model for the evaluation of vaccine efficacy in nonhuman primates. *Journal of Virology* 78, 3140–3144.

McRae, J.C., Smith, J.S., Sharman, G.A.M. and Corrigall, W. (1982) Energy metabolism of lambs infected with *Trichostrongylus colubriformis*. In: Ekern, A. and Sundstol, R.F. (eds) *Energy Metabolism of Farm Animals*. EAAP Publication No. 29, pp. 112–115.

Olesen, I., Groen, A.F. and Gjerde, B. (2000) Definition of animal breeding goals for sustainable production systems. *Journal of Animal Science* 78, 570–582.

Powanda, M.C., Cockerell, G.L., Moe, J.B., Abeles, F.B., Pekarek, R.S. and Canonico, P.G. (1975) Induced metabolic sequelae of tularemia in the rat: correlation with tissue damage. *American Journal of Physiology* 229, 479–483.

Rao, S.V.R., Praharaj, N.K., Reddy, M.R. and Panda, A.K. (2003) Interaction between genotype and dietary concentrations of methionine for immune function in commercial broilers. *British Poultry Science* 44, 104–112.

Rauw, W.M., Kanis, E., Noordhuizen-Stassen, E.N. and Grommers, F.J. (1998) Undesirable side effects of selection for high production efficiency in farm animals: a review. *Livestock Production Science* 56, 15–33.

Reeds, P.J., Fjield, C.R. and Jahoor, F. (1994) Do the differences between the amino-acid compositions of acute-phase and muscle proteins have a bearing on nitrogen loss in traumatic states? *Journal of Nutrition* 124, 906–910.

Sandberg, F.B., Emmans, G.C. and Kyriazakis, I. (2006) A model for predicting food intake of growing animals during exposure to pathogens. *Journal of Animal Science* 84, 1552–1566.

Spurlock, M.E., Frank, G.R., Willis, G.M., Kuske, J.L. and Cornelius, S.G. (1997) Effect of dietary energy source and immunological challenge on growth performance and immunological variables in growing pigs. *Journal of Animal Science* 75, 720–726.

Stewart, T.B., Hale, O.M. and Johnson, J.C. Jr (1969) Failure of parasitised gilts and barrow pigs on different planes of nutrition to respond alike to superimposed infection with *Strongyloides ransomi*. *Journal of Parasitology* 55, 1055–1062.

Sykes, A.R. and Greer, A.W. (2003) Effect of parasitism on the nutrient economy of sheep: an overview. *Australian Journal of Experimental Agriculture* 43, 1393–1398.

Taylor-Robinson, A.W. (2000) Increased production of acute-phase proteins corresponds to the peak parasitemia of primary malaria infection. *Parasitology International* 48, 297–301.

Tsigabe, V.K., Cook, M.E., Harper, A.E. and Sunde, M.L. (1987) Enhanced immune responses in broiler chicks fed methionine-supplemented diets. *Poultry Science* 66, 1147–1154.

van Dam, J.T.P. (1996) The interaction between nutrition and metabolism in West African dwarf goats infected with trypanosomes. PhD thesis, Wageningen University, Wageningen, The Netherlands.

van Dam, J.T.P., Hofs, P., Tolkamp, B.J. and Zwart, D. (1998) The effect of the quality of roughage on the course of *Trypanosoma vivax* infection in West African dwarf goats. 1. Organic matter intake, body weight changes and efficiency of nitrogen metabolism. *Livestock Production Science* 53, 69–80.

van der Waaij, E.H. (2004) A resource allocation model describing consequences of artificial selection under metabolic stress. *Journal of Animal Science* 82, 973–981.

van Diemen, P.M., Henken, A.M., Schrama, J.W., Brandsma, H.A. and Verstegen, M.W.A. (1995) Effects of atrophic rhinitis by *Pasteurella multocida* toxin on heat production and activity of pigs kept under different climatic conditions. *Journal of Animal Science* 73, 1658–1665.

van Heugten, E., Coffey, M.T. and Spears, J.W. (1996) Effects of immune challenge, dietary energy density, and source of energy on performance and immunity in weanling pigs. *Journal of Animal Science* 74, 2431–2440.

Verstegen, M.W.A., Zwart, D., van der Hel, W., Brouwer, B.O. and Wensing, T. (1991) Effect of *Trypanosoma vivax* infection on energy and nitrogen metabolism of West African dwarf goats. *Journal of Animal Science* 69, 1667–1677.

Waller, P.J. (1997) Nematode parasite control of livestock in the tropics/subtropics: the need for novel approaches. *International Journal of Parasitology* 27, 1193–1201.

Wang, T.C. and Fuller, M.F. (1989) The optimum dietary amino acid pattern for growing pigs. 1. Experiments by amino acid deletion. *British Journal of Nutrition* 62, 77–89.

Wannemacher, R.W., Powanda, M.C., Pekarek, R.S. and Beisel, W.R. (1971) Tissue amino acid flux after exposure of rats to *Diplococcus pneumoniae*. *Infection and Immunity* 4, 556–562.

Webel, D.M., Johnson, R.W. and Baker, D.H. (1998a) Lipopolysaccharide-induced reductions in body weight gain and feed intake do not reduce the efficiency of arginine utilization for whole-body protein accretion in the chick. *Poultry Science* 77, 1893–1898.

Webel, D.M., Johnson, R.W. and Baker, D.H. (1998b) Lipopolysaccharide-induced reductions in food intake do not decrease the efficiency of lysine and threonine utilization for protein accretion in chickens. *Journal of Nutrition* 128, 1760–1766.

Wellock, I.J., Emmans, G.C. and Kyriazakis, I. (2003a) Modelling the effects of thermal environment and dietary composition on pig performance: model logic and concepts. *Animal Science* 77, 255–266.

Wellock, I.J., Emmans, G.C. and Kyriazakis, I. (2003b) Modelling the effects of thermal environment and dietary composition on pig performance: model testing and evaluation. *Animal Science* 77, 267–276.

Wellock, I.J., Emmans, G.C. and Kyriazakis, I. (2003c) Predicting the consequences of social stressors on pig feed intake and performance. *Journal of Animal Science* 81, 2995–3007.

Wellock, I.J., Emmans, G.C. and Kyriazakis, I. (2004) Describing and predicting potential growth in the pig. *Animal Science* 78, 379–388.

Wilkie, B.N. and Mallard, B.A. (1998) Multi-trait selection for immune response: a possible alternative strategy for enhanced livestock health and productivity. In: Wiseman, J., Varley, M.A. and Chadwick, J.P. (eds) *Progress in Pig Science*. Nottingham University Press, Nottingham, UK, pp. 29–38.

Williams, N.H., Stahly, T.S. and Zimmerman, D.R. (1997a) Effect of chronic immune system activation on the rate, efficiency and composition of growth and lysine needs of pigs fed from 6 to 27 kg. *Journal of Animal Science* 75, 2463–2471.

Williams, N.H., Stahly, T.S. and Zimmerman, D.R. (1997b) Effect of chronic immune system activation on body nitrogen retention, partial efficiency of lysine utilization, and lysine needs of pigs. *Journal of Animal Science* 75, 2472–2480.

Williams, N.H., Stahly, T.S. and Zimmerman, D.R. (1997c) Effect of level of chronic immune system activation on the growth and dietary lysine needs of pigs fed from 6 to 112 kg. *Journal of Animal Science* 75, 2481–2496.

19 Factors Regulating Feed Efficiency and Nutrient Utilization in Beef Cattle

K. Swanson and S. Miller

Centre for Nutrition Modelling, Department of Animal and Poultry Science, University of Guelph, Canada

Introduction

A predominant economic (and environmental) problem in the beef industry is how to optimize the utilization of feed resources to maximize efficiency of feed utilization and production and to minimize waste excretion. Feed constitutes a major portion of total expenses in cattle feeding operations. McWhir and Wilton (1987) indicated that feed conversion efficiency could account for up to 50% of the variation in gross margin from feeding cattle. Unfortunately, in ruminants, the efficiency of conversion from feed to product is low (Lobley, 1992). For example, in feedlot animals, over 80% of nitrogen intake can be excreted in manure (Bierman *et al.*, 1999).

Improvements in feed conversion efficiency no doubt would have a positive influence on profitability for cattle producers. Improving feed efficiency can have a dramatic effect on the cost of the production of beef. Okine *et al.* (2003) estimated that a 5% improvement in feed efficiency with no change in growth rate could save a feedlot operator CAN$18 per head in feed costs over a 200-day feeding period. Alternatively, Okine *et al.* (2003) also estimated that a 5% increase in average daily gain with no change in feed intake would result in a saving of only CAN$2 per head over the same 200-day period. Others have also indicated economic benefits (Arthur and Herd, 2005) as the result of reducing feed intake without changing growth.

Increasing efficiency of feed utilization not only improves profitability but also decreases nutrient excretion. An increasingly important goal among livestock producers is to increase (or maintain) livestock production while decreasing nutrient losses. These nutrient losses result in inefficiencies of production and increased waste, which can be deleterious to the environment (Tamminga, 1996; Van Horn *et al.*, 1996). Recent research also has suggested that efficient animals emit less enteric methane (Hegarty *et al.*, 2005; Nkrumah *et al.*, 2006), suggesting an environmental benefit of improved efficiency.

The objectives of this chapter are to review approaches used to measure feed efficiency and nutrient utilization, to describe potential regulatory factors important in regulating efficiency and to discuss potential approaches to improve the efficiency of nutrient utilization.

Approaches to Measuring Efficiency of Nutrient Utilization

There are multiple approaches to measuring and reporting the efficiency of feed utilization (Table 19.1). Each approach may be beneficial for a particular situation, but it can be challenging defining specific biological or economic inputs and outputs and care must be taken in how these values are interpreted and used in developing nutrition or animal breeding programmes. Others have reviewed (Archer *et al.*, 1999; Arthur and Herd, 2005; Okine *et al.*, 2003) and studied (Arthur *et al.*, 2001b; Nkrumah *et al.*, 2004a; Schenkel *et al.*, 2004) several different approaches to measure the efficiency of feed utilization. These include gross efficiency or a ratio of feed intake and weight gain, maintenance efficiency, partial efficiency of growth, residual feed intake, cow/calf efficiency, relative growth rate and Kleiber ratio, among others.

The simplest and most widely used measure of feed efficiency is gross efficiency (gain efficiency; gain:feed) or its inverse, feed conversion ratio (feed efficiency; feed:gain). Although it is used extensively in the industry (Schenkel *et al.*, 2004), it has been suggested that it may have detrimental effects on the efficiency of the cow herd when used as a selection tool in animal breeding programmes because it results in increased mature size within the cow herd (Archer *et al.*, 1999) in a similar manner as selection for increased growth rate can increase cow size. Increased mature size within the cow herd results in increased maintenance costs associated with cow/calf production. Maintenance energy costs of

Table 19.1. Some different measures of feed efficiency used in beef cattle systems.[a]

Item	Definition
Gross efficiency (feed conversion ratio or gain efficiency)	The ratio of feed intake to weight gain or weight gain to feed intake.
Maintenance efficiency	The ratio of body weight to feed intake at zero body weight change.
Partial efficiency of growth	The ratio of weight gain to feed intake after the expected requirements for maintenance have been subtracted.
Residual feed intake	The difference between an animal's actual feed intake and its expected feed intake based on its requirements for maintenance (size) and production (growth).
Relative growth rate	Growth relative to instantaneous size.
Kleiber ratio	Weight gain per unit metabolic body weight.
Cow/calf efficiency	Total feed intake of cow and calf as related to weight of calf weaned.

[a]Adapted and modified (Archer *et al.*, 1999; Nkrumah *et al.*, 2004a).

the cow herd are high, representing 70–75% of total annual energy requirements (Ferrell and Jenkins, 1985), and increasing maintenance costs can reduce dramatically the efficiency of production. Therefore, one must use caution if using gross efficiency values for genetic selection programmes without attention to changes in correlated traits such as mature size or birth weight, for example.

Differences in maintenance functions and maintenance requirements between animals are widely thought to be key components defining differences in efficiency between animals. Maintenance efficiency and partial efficiency of growth include measures or calculations of maintenance in an attempt to improve the assessment of efficiency. Although the concept of maintenance is commonly used and discussed, measuring or calculating maintenance can be difficult, it is not constant and it is dependent on a multitude of factors such as physiological state (e.g. growing versus mature), previous plane of nutrition, environmental parameters, etc.

Although the concept of residual feed intake (RFI) has been considered for several years as a possible approach to examine feed efficiency (Koch *et al.*, 1963), there has been renewed research interest in the past 10–15 years, as reviewed by Arthur and Herd (2005). Residual feed intake is defined as the difference between an animal's actual feed intake and its expected feed intake based on its requirements for maintenance (size) and production (growth) over a specified test period (Richardson *et al.*, 2001). Generally, RFI is a trait that has a moderate heritability and little genetic relationship with production traits such as growth, size, fatness and muscling. Most selection programmes incorporating feed efficiency consider RFI measured on growing animals. However, improvements in efficiency in the entire beef production cycle must be considered. In beef production, maintenance of the cow herd is an important factor representing approximately 50% of the energy required for beef production (Montano-Bermudez *et al.*, 1990). Therefore, responses in efficiency of feed utilization in the cow herd are very important and its relation to selection for post-weaning efficiency in growing animals is also important.

Improving efficiency in one sector of the industry does not necessarily result in an improvement in efficiency across the different sectors. The concept of whole system efficiency or life cycle feed efficiency has been recognized as being an important area of research (Gregory, 1972). The beef industry in North America is more segmented, with less vertical integration than other livestock industries such as the poultry and pork industries. Also, because of the long production cycle, research examining efficiency throughout the production system and life cycle of the animal unit is time- and labour-intensive. As a result, much of the research has focused on specific segments of the industry, rather than the entire production system. However, more research on whole system efficiency is important, especially as beef production systems become more coordinated across sectors (Miller, 2002).

Archer *et al.* (2002) attempted to determine the relationship between efficiency in mature cows and those of growing animals by bringing Angus females that had been evaluated for feed efficiency post-weaning back as open cows after their second calf for feed intake measurement. These cows were given access to the same pelleted diet that was used post-weaning. The result was a very high (0.98) correlation between RFI in females post-weaning and mature cows. This result is very encouraging as it indicates that selection for RFI post-weaning may result in improved RFI in mature cows. However, given access to the same diet as was used post-weaning, the cows gained weight (1.19 kg day^{-1}). The question remaining is would the same strong relationship between RFI post-weaning hold with cows on a diet more typical of maintaining cows, where higher levels of roughage would be present. Also, what the correlation would have been if the cows were at a stage of maintenance instead of growth remains an important question.

Arthur *et al.* (2005) examined maternal productivity traits in the high/low RFI selection lines from Australia. The high efficiency line (low RFI) cows tended to be fatter during some periods of production, with no difference in body weight. There was no difference found between the lines for milk yield. However, there was evidence of a trend towards later calving dates in high efficiency (low RFI) females, indicating that reduced fertility in females will be a trait that will have to be monitored in selection programmes including feed efficiency. Work with breed crosses differing in milk production found a positive relationship between milk yield and energy requirements of cows in both the dry and lactating periods, where Shorthorn, Red Poll and Hereford cross cows representing high, medium and low levels of milk production, respectively, were compared (Montano-Bermudez *et al.*, 1990). The response in milk production and reproductive fitness through selection for RFI can be expected following results from mice divergently selected for maintenance heat production where the low heat producing lines (more efficient) had less feed intake, less milk production and fewer pups per litter than the high heat production lines (McDonald and Nielsen, 2006). Despite this reduced litter size and milk production in mice, the dams selected for reduced maintenance requirements were more efficient when considering litter weight and dam feed intake.

The measures of efficiency discussed above primarily describe efficiency of feed utilization as a whole. When examining the efficiency of utilization of specific nutrients or feed components (nitrogen, fibre, energy, etc.), digestibility, mass balance and calorimetry experiments are often conducted (Ferrell, 1988; Merchen, 1988). These experiments are labour intensive and difficult to conduct with large numbers of animals. However, these types of experiments are very important when studying both the applied and basic factors controlling the efficiency of nutrient utilization.

Factors Regulating Efficiency

There are multiple levels where regulation of metabolic processes can occur that influence efficiency. Others have tried to estimate the contribution of various processes that contribute to variation in efficiency (Arthur *et al.*, 2004; Herd *et al.*, 2004; Richardson and Herd, 2004). For example, Richardson and Herd (2004) examined various physiological parameters associated with residual feed intake

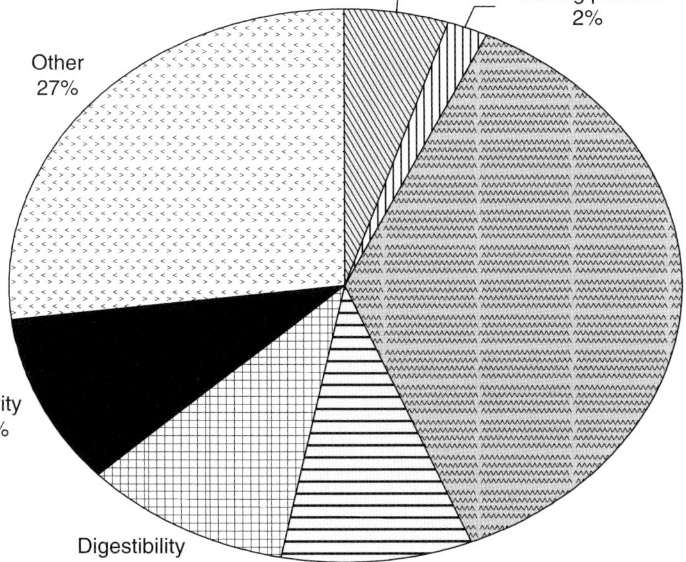

Fig. 19.1. Mechanisms contributing to the variation in residual feed intake in cattle (adapted from Richardson and Herd, 2004; Arthur *et al.*, 2005).

in an attempt to predict the contribution of different mechanisms to variation in residual feed intake (Fig. 19.1). They reported that body composition, feeding patterns, protein turnover, tissue metabolism, stress, heat increment of fermentation, digestibility and activity likely contribute to differences in efficiency. Within each of these categories, there are probably several unknown factors associated with many of the different mechanisms described and a substantial contribution is estimated to be from other unknown factors (27%). This suggests that there is still much to learn about mechanisms controlling differences in feed efficiency between animals. These mechanisms are controlled by the coordinated regulation of whole-animal, tissue, cellular and molecular responses. There are clearly associations within and between these coordinated responses that, in the future, will need to be more closely defined. This section will highlight some of the more important aspects associated with the regulation of whole-animal and metabolic (tissue, cellular and molecular) factors (Table 19.2) regulating feed efficiency.

Whole-animal factors

The potential to deposit lean or fat tissue differs depending on physiological state and genetics. Additionally, the demand for nutrients for fetal growth or milk production differs depending on physiological state and genetics. Animals with greater

Table 19.2. Potential whole-animal and metabolic (tissue, cellular and molecular) factors regulating feed efficiency in cattle.

Whole animal	Metabolic (tissue, cellular and molecular)
Physiological state	Differential cellular turnover and tissue growth
Production/genetic potential	Ion transport
Body composition	Protein turnover
Feed intake	ATP synthesis/mitochondrial proton leak
Nutrient digestion and absorption:	
Ruminal	Nucleic acid and phospholipid turnover
Post-ruminal	
Nutrient/energy losses:	
Faecal/urine	Urea synthesis
Heat production	
Stress susceptibility	Substrate cycling
Health/immune status	Differential expression of energetically demanding and regulatory proteins
Systemic hormones	Genetic polymorphisms
Physical activity	

nutritional demands, due to differences in physiological state or genetic potential, have the ability to partition more nutrients towards productive functions such as growth or milk production. Therefore, it is critical to estimate accurately nutrient requirements relative to physiological state, genetics and environmental conditions, so that a proper balance can be fed to allow for efficient utilization of nutrients.

Body composition

Body composition plays a key role in defining energetic efficiency. Fat deposition in growing cattle can differ between and within breed types and can be altered through nutritional programmes. Fat deposition also differs relative to maturity, with younger animals typically depositing a higher proportion of lean than older animals. The energetic expenditure for deposition and maintenance of lean and fat tissues differs and can affect overall energy balance and deposition in animals dramatically (Owens *et al.*, 1995; NRC, 1996). Thus, body composition is an important factor regulating efficiency. Fat contains more energy than protein, therefore requiring more energy for deposition. However, the net efficiency of protein accretion is lower than that for fat because of a higher rate of protein turnover than fat turnover (Ferrell, 1988), making protein a more energetically expensive tissue to maintain.

Research has indicated a relationship between RFI and fatness, where selection for RFI would result in a slight decrease in fatness (Arthur *et al.*, 2004). This difference in fatness is apparent in the selection lines for high/low RFI in Australia (McDonagh *et al.*, 2001). Other studies have supported this relationship between increased leanness and improved RFI where composition of gain is not included in the determination of RFI (Herd and Bishop, 2000). Positive correlations between RFI and both ultrasound and carcass traits related to increased fatness were also found by Nkrumah *et al.* (2004a). Evidence of fatness playing an essential role in RFI can also be observed from the breed solutions for feed efficiency found by Schenkel *et al.* (2003). It was found that the leanest breeds of yearling bulls (Blonde d'Aquitaine and Limousin) had the most desirable RFI breed solution where the fattest breeds, Angus and Hereford, had the most undesirable. However, when RFI was calculated after adjusting the feed intake for the back fat thickness at the end of the test period, as well as growth and metabolic weight, there was a re-ranking of breeds, with Hereford increasing in the ranks considerably. Similarly, other studies have also shown breed differences in feed efficiency. Results from Moore *et al.* (2005a) indicated that Brahman, Charolais and Limousin sired steers were more efficient than Belmont Red, Shorthorn and Angus steers, and Hereford and Santa Gertrudis sired steers were more efficient than Angus sired steers. These breed solutions relate to growing animals. It would seem likely that breeds diverse in fatness will re-rank if they are considered during growth and mature phases. This has been seen in other species, such as selection lines of mice (Nielsen, 1998), where mice have been selected for maintenance efficiency and not growth. In this case, when only maintenance was considered, the more efficient mice were fatter. The relationship between fatness and RFI and the influence of both fat deposition and fat maintenance on RFI then become important aspects of genetic improvement programmes for feed efficiency.

Feed intake and digestion

Nutrient supply to body tissues is regulated by feed intake and efficiency of nutrient assimilation (digestion and absorption). Mechanisms regulating voluntary feed intake are complex and are dependent on several dietary and non-dietary factors. Voluntary feed intake does seem to differ between breed types and physiological states. For example, research has indicated that Angus steers have greater daily dry matter intake (% of BW) than Brahman × Angus steers (Boyles and Riley, 1991) and that Angus and Angus × Simmental steers have greater daily dry matter intake than Holstein steers (Perry *et al.*, 1991). Breed differences for both feed intake and efficiency have also been shown by Schenkel *et al.* (2004) and Moore *et al.* (2005b). The ability to consume more feed allows for increased nutrient intake and potentially more nutrient retention. However, digestibility of feeds typically decreases as intake increases (Murphy *et al.*, 1994), therefore increases in feed intake are usually not associated with improved feed efficiency. This is supported by many of the recent genetic studies in growing cattle, where RFI is highly related to feed intake. Therefore, animals with higher feed intake have increased (less efficient) RFI, although this could also be related to the mathematical relationship between RFI and feed intake, by definition.

Once feed is consumed, the amount available for maintenance and productive functions is dependent on the digestibility and metabolizability of that particular feed. The major nutrient losses are in the form of faecal and urinary nutrients, whereas the major energy losses are in the form of faecal energy and heat (Ferrell, 2003), although significant energy losses also occur in the form of urinary and gaseous energy.

Feed composition and source no doubt have large influences on nutrient availability and use. For example, changing the proportion of forage:concentrate in the diet or feed processing can alter apparent digestibility significantly (Owens *et al.*, 1997; Reed *et al.*, 1997; Owens and Zinn, 2005). Physiological status also can affect nutrient digestibility. For example, mature cows have a faster rate of ruminal fibre digestion than heifers, suggesting that mature animals may have a greater ability to utilize high fibre diets (Varel and Kreikemeier, 1999). Less is known about the genetic variation in animals' ability to digest and utilize feed. However, researchers have reported that differences are evident between *Bos taurus* and *Bos indicus* cattle fed high roughage diets (Ashton, 1962; Karue *et al.*, 1972). However, Krehbiel *et al.* (2000) reported no differences in digestibility between *B. indicus* and *B. taurus* feedlot steers fed high concentrate diets. Data also have suggested that diet digestibility is greater in low RFI steers (improved efficiency) than high RFI steers (Richardson *et al.*, 1996; Nkrumah *et al.*, 2006). This suggests that there is variability in digestive function between animals, yet the specific means by which this variation occurs is not well understood. However, there is evidence suggesting that inadequate production of specific digestive enzymes could be responsible for limitations in digestive efficiency. Pancreatic α-amylase (Swanson and Harmon, 2002), which is a primary enzyme responsible for starch digestion in the small intestine, may limit starch digestive efficiency in the small intestine in ruminants fed high-concentrate diets. Interestingly, some recently published research (Channon *et al.*, 2004) reported that in steers selected for low RFI (improved efficiency), faecal pH and faecal dry matter percentage were greater, suggesting that those cattle may be more efficient at digesting starch because lower faecal pH is an indicator of inefficiencies of small intestinal starch digestion. Others (Zhao *et al.*, 1998; Howell *et al.*, 2001) also have suggested that transport mechanisms are important in the regulation of digestive or metabolic efficiency. However, little is known about how, and if, changes in digestive efficiency between genetically different animals are associated with changes in expression of enzymes and transporters responsible for digestion and absorption of nutrients.

Heat production

Energy lost as heat can be large and is variable, depending on many factors (Ferrell, 2003) such as diet, physiological state and breed type. This heat loss is associated with many processes, including heat increment of feeding, heat of fermentation, heat associated with digestion and absorption, post-absorptive metabolism of nutrients and heat associated with activity. Nutritional changes, such as changes in feed intake (Freetly and Nienaber, 1998), influence heat production in cattle. Breed type also probably influences heat production. For example, Hereford heifers lose less energy as heat per metabolic body weight than Charolais and Simmental heifers (Baker *et al.*, 1991). This was suggested to be due partly to a higher proportion of fat to lean in the Hereford heifers compared to the Charolais and Simmental heifers. Changes in heat production also can be associated with changes in visceral organ mass (Ferrell, 2003). Nkrumah *et al.* (2006) also reported that heat production is decreased in animals with low RFI (high efficiency) as compared to those with high RFI (low efficiency).

Metabolic (tissue, cellular and molecular) factors

Tissue events

Tissues differ in their demand for energy and amino acids. Splanchnic tissues (gut and liver) in ruminants comprise less than 10% of body mass, but account for approximately 50% of total energy expenditure (Reynolds *et al.*, 1991) and protein synthesis (Lobley *et al.*, 1980). Thus, splanchnic tissues are a major component defining maintenance requirements of animals (Koong *et al.*, 1985). Therefore, the metabolism and utilization of nutrients of these tissues is critical in defining whole-animal efficiency. Splanchnic tissues are highly metabolically active because of a high cellular turnover rate (Johnson, 1988) and the demand to produce proteins involved with digestion, absorption and metabolism of nutrients. Although there has been much discussion and research regarding reducing visceral organ mass to improve efficiency, little is known on the impact of reduced organ size on nutrient digestion, absorption and metabolism. However, increased tissue size may not necessarily be detrimental in that it may allow for increased nutrient digestion and absorption (Cant *et al.*, 1996), as well as improved intestinal immune function.

Visceral tissue weight can change relative to nutrition programmes or breed type. For example, liver and gastrointestinal tract weights increase with increased intake (Murray *et al.*, 1977; Sainz and Bentley, 1997; Ferrell and Jenkins, 1998a,b). Research also indicates possible differences in visceral organ weights between cattle of different breed types. For example, small and large intestinal weights were greater in steers sired by Angus and Hereford bulls than steers sired by Brahman, Boran and Tuli bulls (Ferrell and Jenkins, 1998b). Also, differences in visceral organ mass are thought to be partly responsible for differences in residual feed intake (Archer *et al.*, 1999; Basarab *et al.*, 2003).

Cellular events

Events such as ion transport, protein turnover, mitochondrial proton leak and cell regeneration (Milligan and McBride, 1985; Gill *et al.*, 1989; Caton *et al.*, 2000; Harper *et al.*, 2002) are thought to be the primary cellular energy consuming processes involved in energy metabolism in tissues. Other cellular energy demanding processes include nucleic acid and phospholipid turnover, urea synthesis and substrate cycling (Huntington and McBride, 1988).

Ion transport across membranes is critical for cellular functions. The sodium/potassium membrane gradient helps to control cell volume, maintain nerve function and drive the active transport of sugars and amino acids (Stryer, 1995). The sodium/potassium membrane gradient is maintained by the protein Na^+,K^+-ATPase, which is thought to be the major energy consuming protein involved with ion transport (Milligan and McBride, 1985; Kelly *et al.*, 1991). The Na^+,K^+-ATPase consumes between approximately 22 and 61% of tissue oxygen consumption in liver and intestine (Caton *et al.*, 2000). Research has also indicated that changes in physiological state and nutrition influence the amount of energy consumed by Na^+,K^+-ATPase (Kelly *et al.*, 1991). Activity of Na^+,K^+-ATPase in duodenal mucosa increases with increased feed intake in sheep

(McBride and Milligan, 1985) and is also increased during lactation in dairy cows (McBride and Milligan, 1984). Data also indicate that dairy cows selected for high milk production have higher levels of Na^+,K^+-ATPase activity in erythrocytes than cows selected for low milk production (Scollan *et al.*, 1993). Na^+,K^+-ATPase was also greater in liver and muscle of genetically obese as compared to genetically lean mice (Lin *et al.*, 1979). This suggests differences in activity of Na^+,K^+-ATPase between animals of different genetics.

Protein deposition within the whole body is a balance between protein synthesis and degradation. Protein synthesis and degradation are major energy and amino acid demanding processes and the splanchnic tissues contribute greatly to whole-body demands (Gill *et al.*, 1989; Kelly *et al.*, 1991; Caton *et al.*, 2000). Energetic expenditure for protein synthesis contributes about 23% of the total energetic costs in ruminants. The continual synthesis and breakdown of cellular proteins, however, allows adaptability and flexibility so that animals can respond to multiple physiological and environmental challenges (Lobley, 2003). Protein turnover responds to nutritional and physiological changes. Lobley *et al.* (2000) conducted an experiment in growing steers to examine the effect of dietary intake and breed type on protein synthesis and breakdown and found that fractional protein synthesis and fractional protein breakdown rates of muscle were increased after an increase in dietary intake. They also reported that Angus steers had higher fractional protein synthesis rates in muscle than Charolais steers. It is well accepted that cattle of different breeds differ in growth and protein deposition potential. Others (Lorenzen *et al.*, 2000) have reported differences in protein degradation in lambs with the callipyge phenotype, suggesting that changes in tissue protein deposition can occur as the result of decreased protein degradation, as well as increased protein synthesis relative to protein degradation. Enzymes such as ubiquitin (Hershko and Ciechanover, 1998) are involved in degradation processes and altered activity of these processes could have great influences on the overall efficiency of protein deposition in growing animals. Comparing meat quality traits of steers from sires selected divergently for RFI, McDonagh *et al.* (2001) found a higher degree of myofibrillar breakdown in the high (low efficiency) RFI line. A key system involved in protein degradation is the calpain proteolytic enzymes and their inhibitor calpastatin (Koohmaraie *et al.*, 1987). McDonagh *et al.* (2001) also found that the level of calpastatin was higher in the high efficiency (low RFI) steers. After just one generation of selection, a significant difference in calpastatin and myofibril fragmentation index was observed, giving indication that selection for RFI could result in a reduction in meat tenderness associated with a change in protein turnover. However, there were no differences in shear force values. More research seems warranted on the relationship between protein turnover, meat tenderness and RFI.

Cell turnover rates in splanchnic tissues are extremely high compared to most other tissues. This is especially the case for the small intestinal mucosa (Johnson, 1988). This high rate of cell turnover is the result of high rates of cell proliferation and apoptosis (programmed cell death). Reducing the rate of cell turnover might be an approach to decrease the energy and nutrient demands of these tissues. Limited data are available on the effects of physiological state, diet or breed type on rates of cell proliferation and apoptosis of visceral tissues in cattle. Baldwin *et al.* (2004) reported cell proliferation indexes measured through the lactation cycle in dairy cows. The approaches included using immunohistochemistry (bromodeoxyuridine and Ki67) and *in vitro* tritiated thymidine incorporation techniques in small intestinal tissues. The results, however, were inconsistent between approaches and also were inconsistent relative to changes in small intestinal mass. Cell proliferation indexes (immunohistochemistry; bromodeoxyuridine or proliferating cell nuclear antigen) in small intestinal tissue were not influenced by changes in dietary intake and/or lasalocid supplementation in growing lambs, or as the result of increasing supplemental protein levels in mature ewes (Swanson *et al.*, 1999, 2000). Combined, these results suggest that cell proliferation rates may not be influenced dramatically by physiological state or nutrition in ruminants. However, Baldwin *et al.* (2004) suggested that numerous tissue samples through a wide range of time points might be necessary to get accurate and repeatable results. It is also important to point out that estimates of apoptosis were not reported in these experiments and that differences in apoptosis rather than cell proliferation may be responsible for differences in cell number and tissue mass. Jin *et al.* (1994) reported increased rates of cell proliferation and apoptosis in pigs fed a high fibre diet compared to a low fibre diet, suggesting that cellular turnover dynamics can change independent of changes in tissue mass.

Living cells require the controlled use of energy for maintenance and productive functions such as maintaining membrane gradients, synthesizing protein and cell growth and proliferation. The donor of free energy for most energy requiring processes in living cells is adenosine triphosphate (ATP). ATP is the universal currency of free energy in living systems (Stryer, 1995). Mitochondria are the major organelles responsible for ATP production in animal cells. ATP is produced in the cytosol through substrate level phosphorylation by direct phosphorylation of ADP (glycolysis; cytosol) or GDP (Krebs cycle; mitochondria). However, in the presence of oxygen, oxidative phosphorylation (respiratory chain; inner mitochondrial membrane) is the most important mechanism for synthesizing ATP. The source of energy for ATP synthesis is an electrochemical gradient of protons generated by electron transfer complexes across the inner membrane of the mitochondria. This gradient is then used to drive the membrane-bound enzyme ATP synthase, which catalyses the conversion of ADP and inorganic phosphate to ATP.

The amount of ATP required and produced by living beings is quite remarkable. For example, Senior *et al.* (2002) estimated that a typical 70 kg human with a 75-year lifespan would generate around 2 million kg of ATP from ADP and inorganic phosphate. The process of ATP production plays a major role in controlling energy metabolism within cells. Although there has been much work using bovine ATP synthase as a model enzyme to study ATP synthase function, little attention has been directed towards better understanding these processes in relation to livestock production. Mitrochondrial ATP synthase, however, has been identified as a potential target protein in the regulation of energy metabolism in humans (Berger *et al.*, 2002). In livestock, preliminary data have been reported, indicating that mitochondrial DNA sequence and mitochondrial content do not differ between efficient (low RFI) and inefficient (high RFI) steers (Kolath *et al.*, 2005), although more research is required to determine how mitochondrial function influences the efficiency of nutrient utilization.

The respiration chain across the inner membrane of the mitochondria provides an efficient conversion of energy from a membrane gradient to ATP. When this gradient results in the production of ATP, the system is defined as 'coupled' (Nagy *et al.*, 2004). If the energy is directed away from ATP production towards heat production, then less energy is available for ATP production and the system is 'uncoupled'. In this situation, energetic efficiency is decreased because energy is lost as heat rather than used as an energy source by the cells. The uncoupling proteins are thought to be involved in the process called mitochondrial proton leak, which has been estimated to account for 20–25% of basal metabolic rate (Rolfe *et al.*, 1999) and is associated with a loss of energy as heat from tissues. The uncoupling proteins are transporters, present in the mitochondrial inner membrane, that mediate a regulated discharge of the proton gradient that is generated by the respiratory chain (Pecqueur *et al.*, 2001; Ledesma *et al.*, 2002). Uncoupling protein 1 (UCP1) is found exclusively in brown adipose tissue. Uncoupling protein 2 (UCP2) is more widespread, with expression found in spleen, intestine, kidney, skeletal muscle, liver and other tissues. Uncoupling protein 3 (UCP3) is found in brown adipose tissue and skeletal muscle. Brown adipose tissue and UCP1 have a primary thermogenic role in newborn animals (Ledesma *et al.*, 2002). The roles of UCP2 and UCP3 are less well understood (Nagy *et al.*, 2004). Much is still to be learned about the roles of these proteins as related to energy metabolism, efficiency and other functions.

Molecular events

There are likely a very large number of genes and proteins involved in the coordinated regulation of nutrient utilization. Only a few potential candidates have been discussed above. Other potentially important genes examined in genetic association studies include AMP activated protein kinase (Benkel *et al.*, 2005), melanocortin receptor 4 (Valle *et al.*, 2004) and cocaine and amphetamine-regulated transcript (Valle *et al.*, 2005), although this is likely only a small subset of potentially important genes and proteins.

Approaches to Improve Efficiency of Nutrient Utilization

Many approaches have been used to improve the efficiency of nutrient utilization, either directly or indirectly. Of these approaches, improving nutrition and animal breeding programmes are perhaps the most feasible.

Nutrition programmes

A plethora of work has been done related to improving or manipulating nutrition programmes to improve production and production efficiency. Much of this has dealt with improving diet formulation in order to meet more closely the nutrient requirements of animals. Significant progress has been made in this regard through modelling approaches (Fox *et al.*, 1995; NRC, 1996; Tedeschi *et al.*, 2000). Work in this area is expected to continue as new animal research results become available. This should result in improvements in accuracy and predictability of these models. Research into better understanding of the physiological mechanisms regulating the efficiency of nutrient utilization is key to providing information to improve models and to develop new nutritional and animal breeding approaches to improve efficiency. Besides better diet formulation protocols, other feeding management approaches have attempted to improve the efficiency of nutrient utilization. These include restricted feeding (Galyean, 1999), phase feeding (Klopfenstein and Erickson, 2002), pulse feeding (Cole, 1999; Ludden *et al.*, 2002; Cole *et al.*, 2003), altering the time of feeding (Small *et al.*, 2004) and the use of feed additives or growth-promoting implants (Birkelo, 2003), to name a few.

Galyean (1999) defined restricted feeding as any method of feed intake management with which intake is restricted relative to actual or anticipated *ad libitum* intake. Using this approach may improve the digestibility of the feed and improve feed efficiency and can be used to reduce feed costs and nutrient excretion. However, it can result in decreased growth rate and carcass quality and may result in the need for more bunk space and increased management associated with feeding and animal observation.

Phase feeding is when nutrient levels are changed relative to requirements, rather than feeding a single diet throughout the feeding period of growing or finishing cattle. Klopfenstein and Erickson (2002) summarized their work on phase feeding protein to calf-feds and yearlings in the feedlot versus feeding a standard feedlot diet (13.5% CP) throughout the finishing period and found that phase feeding slightly improved feed efficiency, did not influence growth rate and reduced nitrogen excretion. This approach does improve management associated with mixing multiple diets, but increasing regulations associated with nutrient management may expand the use of this feeding approach due to its effects on reducing nutrient excretion.

Pulse feeding is when different concentrations of nutrients (via diets or supplement) are fed during differing time periods in an oscillating fashion (i.e. alternating feeds or nutrient concentrations daily, biweekly or weekly). Cole (1999) fed growing lambs diets containing 12.5% CP daily or 10% CP and 15% CP oscillated at 48-h intervals and found that oscillating CP increased N retention in one of two trials. This increased utilization of N may be related to improved efficiency of urea N recycling to the rumen. Other studies have shown minimal or no difference in N utilization between continuous and oscillating CP diets in ruminants (Ludden *et al.*, 2002; Cole *et al.*, 2003). The impact on efficiency by using this approach is probably minimal in growing and feedlot diets because of minimal effects on growth and efficiency. However, in supplementation scenarios with cattle grazing low quality forage, infrequent supplementation may reduce the cost of feed delivery while minimally influencing cattle performance (Bohnert *et al.*, 2002).

Altering the time of feeding may also impact efficiency by changing the time of maximal heat production due to rumen fermentation and digestion.

For example, Small *et al.* (2004) fed calves in the morning or evening in winter and found that gain slightly increased and feed efficiency tended to improve in calves fed in the evening. Similar approaches may be of benefit in animals exhibiting heat stress, because it may be easier for animals to dissipate heat during the evening when temperatures are lower than during the peak temperatures throughout the day. There are practical considerations to bear in mind, however, as feeding in the evening may not be convenient for many operations.

Extensive research on the use of feed additives, such as ionophores, and growth-promoting implants have been conducted (Russell and Strobel, 1989; Mader, 1998; Birkelo, 2003). Ionophores and growth-promoting implants are used to improve efficiency by altering rumen fermentation and improving muscle deposition, respectively.

Animal breeding programmes

Animal breeding programmes also provide a means of improving the efficiency of nutrient utilization through selective breeding. Traditionally, genetic improvement programmes have been aimed primarily at growth, carcass and reproductive traits for beef cattle. Less attention has been directed towards selecting animals with improved feed efficiency. The reader is also referred to reviews by Archer *et al.* (1999) and Arthur and Herd (2005) which outline the implications of genetic improvement programmes for feed efficiency and the potential for selection to improve feed efficiency in beef cattle.

Most of the recent efforts in feed efficiency and animal breeding research have been associated with residual feed intake (Archer *et al.*, 1999; Basarab *et al.*, 2003; Schenkel *et al.*, 2004). These studies have been conducted primarily with growing cattle. Table 19.3 illustrates typical genetic parameters associated with these studies. Generally, RFI is a trait that has a moderate heritability and little genetic relationship with production traits such as growth, size, fatness and muscling. However, there is a tendency for cattle with lower RFI (more efficient) to be associated with increased leanness, as mentioned earlier.

These heritability estimates indicate that selection programmes can be developed to change RFI in growing beef cattle. There are now genetic evaluations, Estimated Breeding Values (EBV) in Australia (Graser *et al.*, 2005) or Across Breed Comparisons in Canada (Miller, 2003), for this trait. These programmes require the measurement of feed intake in practice and, although the economic benefit of improved feed efficiency has been demonstrated, the cost of the equipment and related labour associated with measurement remains a barrier, despite reductions in costs through advancements in electronics. Therefore, strategies must be employed to better use equipment to make more genetic progress. Alternatively, research can identify other predictors of feed efficiency such as genetic or physiological markers that can be used for genetic selection purposes.

A physiological marker that has been implemented in selection programmes is insulin-like growth factor-I (IGF-I). The concentration of IGF-I in blood has been found to have a moderate genetic correlation (0.41) with RFI in Angus

Table 19.3. Heritabilities and genetic correlations in post-weaning feed efficiency and component traits from three studies (from Miller, 2003).[a]

	RFI_b	RFI	F:G	FI	ADG	BF	REA	MW
RFI_b	0.39[b]	0.99[b]	0.68[b]	0.78[b]	–0.02[b]	–0.01[b]	–0.19[b]	–0.18[b]
		0.38[b]	0.69[b]	0.81[b]	0.01[b]	0.16[b]	–0.17[b]	–0.17[b]
		0.39[c]	0.85[c]	0.79[c]	–0.10[c]	–	–	–
		0.16[d]	0.70[d]	0.64[d]	0.09[d]	–	–	0.22[d]
RFI		0.39[e]	0.66[e]	0.69[e]	–0.04[e]	0.17[e]	0.09[e]	–0.06[e]
			0.37[b]	0.39[b]	–0.52[b]	0.03[b]	–0.28[b]	–0.13[b]
			0.46[c]	0.64[c]	–0.46[c]	–	–	–
			0.17[d]	–	–	–	–	–
F:G			0.29[e]	0.31[e]	–0.62[e]	0.03[e]	–0.12[e]	–0.01[e]
				0.45[b]	0.50[b]	0.24[b]	0.11[b]	0.36[b]
				0.48[c]	0.39[c]	–	–	–
				0.31[d]	0.70[d]	–	–	0.89[d]
FI				0.39[e]	0.54[e]	0.27[e]	0.43[e]	0.65[e]
					0.35[b]	0.14[b]	0.42[b]	0.56[a]
					0.34[c]	–	–	–
					0.38[d]	–	–	–
ADG					0.28[e]	–	–	0.53[e]
						0.36[a]	–0.10[a]	0.15[a]
BF						0.35[d]	–	–
							0.30[a]	0.46[a]
REA							0.27[d]	–
								0.35[a]
								0.36[c]
MW								0.40[d]

[a]RFI_b = residual feed intake (RFI) with an additional adjustment in expected feed intake based on back fat thickness at the end of the evaluation period as measured by ultrasound, F:G = feed intake:body weight gain, FI = feed intake, ADG = average daily gain, BF = back fat thickness, REA = ribeye area, MW = metabolic mid-weight.
[b]Schenkel *et al.* (2003): multi-breed performance tested beef bulls in Canada.
[c]Arthur *et al.* (2001b): Charolais bulls' performance tested in France.
[d]Herd and Bishop (2000): Hereford bulls' performance tested in the UK.
[e]Arthur *et al.* (2001a): Angus bulls' and heifers' performance tested in Australia.

cattle and a moderate heritability (0.35) (Moore *et al.*, 2005b). Similarly, IGF-I is associated with RFI in swine (Bunter *et al.*, 2005). This relationship has been incorporated into the genetic evaluation for feed efficiency in Australia, where measures of IGF-I, along with measures of RFI on a seedstock animal and its relatives, contribute to its prediction of genetic merit for RFI. The benefit of the use of this marker as a tool in genetic selection programmes for feed efficiency has been shown by Wood *et al.* (2004), where its benefit in preselecting young bulls for a performance test where feed intake was measured was demonstrated. There also is the potential to use other physiological indicators for selection for efficiency. These could include blood metabolites, such as urea N, or other hormones, such as gherlin, leptin or cholecystokinin, to name a few.

Feed efficiency is a composite trait, influenced by many physiological processes, as has been discussed. Therefore, it is obvious that there will be many genes involved with the control of the efficiency of nutrient utilization. The efficiency of nutrient utilization is considered a quantitative trait as there are many genes regulating its control. The gene loci which influence this trait are referred to as quantitative trait loci (QTL). Selection for QTL influencing feed efficiency is possible by identifying genetic polymorphisms that are related to these QTL. The genetic polymorphisms then can be identified and tested for in a DNA sample. These tests can be for polymorphisms in the actual QTL or in regions that are genetically linked to the QTL of interest. This genetic linkage is known as linkage disequilibrium and occurs when two loci are sufficiently close on the genome that recombination during meiosis between them is rare, and segments of chromosome are conserved from parent to offspring. Selection on the linked marker will then result in a correlated response in feed efficiency through a change in frequency of the QTL in linkage with the marker. The use of linkage disequilibrium in selection and gene mapping studies is discussed in more detail by Goddard and Meuwissen (2005). The use of genetic markers and single nucleotide polymorphisms (SNPs), either as markers in linkage with a QTL or as mutations within a QTL, are important components to genetic strategies to improve the efficiency of feed utilization. As the study of Wood *et al.* (2004) has demonstrated with IGF-I, indicators of feed efficiency available at a young age could be beneficial in selection programmes, as measurement of feed intake and efficiency is labour-intensive and expensive.

Feed efficiency is an excellent example of a trait that will benefit from selection through gene or marker-assisted selection, as more traditional approaches to genetic improvement are hindered by the cost of measurement. The potential impact of SNPs in the leptin and leptin receptor gene on carcass and meat quality has been shown in a number of studies (Crews *et al.*, 2004; Nkrumah *et al.*, 2004b; Schenkel *et al.*, 2006) and can be used as an example of the potential impact of SNPs in breeding programmes. There have been some results relating SNPs in the leptin gene to feed intake in beef cattle, where the SNPs associated with increased fatness were associated with an increase in feed intake (Nkrumah *et al.*, 2004b) with some supporting, although non-significant ($P > 0.05$), relationships found between SNPs associated with higher levels of fatness associated with increased (less efficient) RFI (Nkrumah *et al.*, 2004b). Using the high/low RFI selection lines in Angus from Australia, Hayes *et al.* (2006), utilizing a scan of 10,000 SNP anonymous genetic markers, indicated there are between 38 and 188 QTL influencing RFI, where between seven and 20 marked QTL would be required to explain a significant proportion of the genetic variation in feed efficiency for effective marker-assisted selection. Each QTL will require approximately 11 markers within 1 cM of the QTL for effective selection (Hayes *et al.*, 2006). These results illustrate the power of these large-scale genome scans with many anonymous markers. The bovine genome project (www.hgsc.bcm.tmc.edu/projects/bovine/) will result in many SNPs being identified. There have been 114,958 SNPs placed on the World Wide Web (www.hgsc.bcm.tmc.edu/projects/bovine, accessed 22 February 2006). The future will see genotyping costs reduced and more SNPs available. These advancements will make large-scale gene and gene marker-assisted selection programmes a reality.

Conclusion

Improving the efficiency of nutrient utilization can improve profitability and reduce excretion of nutrients. Improving feed formulation programmes or modifying feeding programmes should continue to lead to improvements in efficiency. Also, traditional animal breeding programmes, along with marker-assisted selection, should improve our ability to select animals for improved efficiency. Modelling approaches specifically aimed towards answering biological questions related to efficiency should aid in improving our understanding of the connectivity between various factors regulating efficiency and help to focus new research towards answering important unknown questions. It is important, however, to continue to conduct basic physiological studies examining responses at the gene, protein, cell, tissue and whole-animal level so that an improved understanding of the mechanisms, and relative contribution, of specific factors regulating efficiency can be better described. A coordinated effort between nutrition, animal breeding and modelling approaches should lead to innovative nutrition and animal breeding programmes to improve the efficiency of feed and nutrient utilization.

References

Archer, J.A., Richardson, E.C., Herd, R.M. and Arthur, P.F. (1999) Potential for selection to improve efficiency of feed use in beef cattle: a review. *Australian Journal of Agricultural Research* 50, 147–161.

Archer, J.A., Reverter, A., Herd, R.M., Johnston, D.J. and Arthur, P.F. (2002) Genetic variation in feed intake and efficiency of mature beef cows and relationships with post-weaning measurements. *Proceedings of the 7th World Congress on Genetics Applied to Livestock Production*, 19–23 August 2002, Montpellier France. CD-ROM Communication No. 10-07.

Arthur, P.F. and Herd, R.M. (2005) Efficiency of feed utilisation by livestock – implications and benefits of genetic improvement. *Canadian Journal of Animal Science* 85, 281–290.

Arthur, P.F., Archer, J.A., Johnston, D.J., Herd, R.M., Richardson, E.C. and Parnell, P.F. (2001a) Genetic and phenotypic variance and covariance components for feed intake, feed efficiency, and other post-weaning traits in Angus cattle. *Journal of Animal Science* 79, 2805–2811.

Arthur, P.F., Renand, G. and Krauss, D. (2001b) Genetic and phenotypic relationships among different measures of growth and feed efficiency in young Charolais bulls. *Livestock Production Science* 68, 131–139.

Arthur, P.F., Archer, J.A. and Herd, R.M. (2004) Feed intake and efficiency in beef cattle: overview of recent Australian research and challenges for the future. *Australian Journal of Agricultural Research* 44, 361–369.

Arthur, P.F., Herd, R.M., Wilkins, J.F. and Archer, J.A. (2005) Maternal productivity of Angus cows divergently selected for post-weaning residual feed intake. *Australian Journal of Experimental Agriculture* 45, 985–993.

Ashton, G.C. (1962) Comparative nitrogen digestibility in Brahman, Brahman × Shorthorn, Africander × Hereford, and Hereford steers. *Journal of Agricultural Science* 58, 333–342.

Baker, J.F., Buckley, B.A., Dickerson, G.E. and Nienaber, J.A. (1991) Body composition and fasting heat production from birth to 14 months of age for three biological types of beef heifers. *Journal of Animal Science* 69, 4406–4418.

Baldwin, R.L. VI, McLeod, K.R. and Capuco, A.V. (2004) Visceral tissue growth and proliferation during the bovine lactation cycle. *Journal of Dairy Science* 87, 2977–2986.

Basarab, J.A., Price, M.A., Aalhus, J.L., Okine, E.K., Snelling, W.M. and Lyle, K.L. (2003) Residual feed intake and body composition in young growing cattle. *Canadian Journal of Animal Science* 83, 189–204.

Benkel, B., Kollers, S., Fries, R., Sazanov, A., Yoshida, E., Valle, E., Davoren, J. and Hickey, D. (2005) Characterization of the bovine ampkgamma1 gene. *Mammalian Genome* 16, 194–200.

Berger, K., Sivars, U., Winzell, M.S., Johansson, P., Hellman, U., Rippe, C. and Erlanson-Albertsson, C. (2002) Mitochondrial ATP synthase – a possible target protein in the regulation of energy metabolism *in vitro* and *in vivo*. *Nutritional Neuroscience* 5, 201–210.

Bierman, S., Erickson, G.E., Klopfenstein, T.J., Stock, R.A. and Shain, D.H. (1999) Evaluation of nitrogen and organic matter balance in the feedlot as affected by level and source of dietary fiber. *Journal of Animal Science* 77, 1645–1653.

Birkelo, C.P. (2003) Pharmaceuticals, direct-fed microbials, and enzymes for enhancing growth and feed efficiency of beef. *The Veterinary Clinics Food Animal Practice* 19, 599–624.

Bohnert, D.W., Schauer, C.S. and DelCurto, T. (2002) Influence of rumen protein degradability and supplementation frequency on performance and nitrogen use in ruminants consuming low-quality forage: cow performance and efficiency of nitrogen use in wethers. *Journal of Animal Science* 80, 1629–1637.

Boyles, S.L. and Riley, J.G. (1991) Feedlot performance of Brahman × Angus versus Angus steers during cold weather. *Journal of Animal Science* 69, 2677–2684.

Bunter, K.L., Hermesch, S., Luxford, B.G., Graser, H.U. and Crump, R.E. (2005) Insulin-like growth factor-I measured in juvenile pigs is genetically correlated with economically important performance traits. *Australian Journal of Experimental Agriculture* 45, 783–792.

Cant, J.P., McBride, B.W. and Croom, W.J. Jr (1996) The regulation of intestinal metabolism and its impact on whole animal energetics. *Journal of Animal Science* 74, 2541–2553.

Caton, J.S., Bauer, M.L. and Hidari, H. (2000) Metabolic components of energy expenditure in growing beef cattle. *Asian–Australasian Journal of Animal Science* 13, 702–710.

Channon, A.F., Rowe, J.B. and Herd, R.M. (2004) Genetic variation in starch digestion in feedlot cattle and its association with residual feed intake. *Australian Journal of Experimental Agriculture* 44, 469–474.

Cole, N.A. (1999) Nitrogen retention by lambs fed oscillating dietary protein concentrations. *Journal of Animal Science* 77, 215–222.

Cole, N.A., Greene, L.W., McCollum, F.T., Montgomery, T. and McBride, K. (2003) Influence of oscillating dietary crude protein concentration on performance, acid–base balance, and nitrogen excretion of steers. *Journal of Animal Science* 81, 2660–2668.

Crews, D.H., Nkrumah, J.D., Yu, J. and Moore, S.S. (2004) Association of single nucleotide polymorphisms in the bovine leptin gene with feedlot and carcass characteristics of crossbred steers. *Canadian Journal of Animal Science* 84, 749–750 (Abstract).

Ferrell, C.L. (1988) Energy metabolism. In: Church, D.C. (ed.) *The Ruminant Animal – Digestive Physiology and Nutrition*. Prentice-Hall, Englewood Cliffs, New Jersey, pp. 250–268.

Ferrell, C.L. (2003) Energy partitioning in ruminants as related to feed intake. *Proceedings of the Canadian Society of Animal Science*. CD-ROM communication.

Ferrell, C.L. and Jenkins, T.G. (1985) Cow type and the nutritional environment: nutritional aspects. *Journal of Animal Science* 61, 725–741.

Ferrell, C.L. and Jenkins, T.G. (1998a) Body composition and energy utilization by steers of diverse genotypes fed a high-concentrate diet during the finishing period: I. Angus, Belgian Blue, Hereford, and Piedmontese sires. *Journal of Animal Science* 76, 637–646.

Ferrell, C.L. and Jenkins T.G. (1998b) Body composition and energy utilization by steers of diverse genotypes fed a high-concentrate diet during the finishing period: II. Angus, Boran, Brahman, Hereford, and Tuli sires. *Journal of Animal Science* 76, 647–657.

Fox, D.G., Barry, M.C., Pitt, R.E., Roseler, D.K. and Stone, W.C. (1995) Application of the Cornell Net Carbohydrate and Protein model for cattle consuming forages. *Journal of Animal Science* 73, 267–277.

Freetly, H.C. and Nienaber, J.A. (1998) Efficiency of energy and nitrogen loss and gain in mature cows. *Journal of Animal Science* 76, 896–905.

Galyean, M.L. (1999) Review: Restricted and programmed feeding of beef cattle – definitions, application, and research results. *The Professional Animal Scientist* 15, 1–6.

Gill, M., France, J., Summers, M., McBride, B.W. and Milligan, L.P. (1989) Simulation of the energy costs associated with protein turnover and Na+,K+-transport in growing lambs. *Journal of Nutrition* 119, 1287–1299.

Goddard, M.E. and Meuwissen, T.H.E. (2005) The use of linkage disequilibrium to map quantitative trait loci. *Australian Journal of Experimental Agriculture* 45, 837–845.

Graser, H.U., Tier, B., Johnston, D.J. and Barwick S.A. (2005) Genetic evaluation for the beef industry in Australia. *Australian Journal of Experimental Agriculture* 45, 913–921.

Gregory, K.E. (1972) Beef cattle type for maximum efficiency 'putting it all together'. *Journal of Animal Science* 34, 881–884.

Harper, M.-E., Antoniou, A., Bevilacqua, V., Bezaire, V. and Monemdjou, S. (2002) Cellular energy expenditure and the importance of uncoupling. *Journal of Animal Science* 80 (E. Supplement 2), E90–E97.

Hayes, B.J., Chamberlain, A.G. and Goddard, M.E. (2006) Optimum use of markers in linkage disequilibrium with QTL in breeding programs. *Proceedings of the 8th World Congress on Genetics Applied to Livestock Production*, 13–18 August 2006, Belo Horizonte, MG, Brazil. CD-ROM Communication No. 30-06.

Hegarty, R.S., Herd, R.M., Goopy, J.P. and Arthur P.F. (2005) Selection for residual feed intake can change methane production in feedlot steers. *Proceedings of the Association for the Advancement of Animal Breeding and Genetics* 16, 334–337.

Herd, R.M. and Bishop, S.C. (2000) Genetic variation in residual feed intake and its association with other production traits in British Hereford cattle. *Livestock Production Science* 63, 111–119.

Herd, R.M., Oddy, V.H. and Richardson E.C. (2004) Biological basis for variation in residual feed intake in beef cattle. 1. Review of potential mechanisms. *Australian Journal of Experimental Agriculture* 44, 423–430.

Hershko, A. and Ciechanover, A. (1998) The ubiquitin system. *Annual Review in Biochemistry* 67, 425–479.

Howell, J.A., Matthews, A.D., Swanson, K.C., Harmon, D.L. and Matthews J.C. (2001) Molecular identification of high-affinity glutamate transporters in sheep and cattle forestomach, intestine, liver, kidney, and pancreas. *Journal of Animal Science* 79, 1329–1336.

Huntington, G.B. and McBride, B.W. (1988) Ruminant splanchnic tissues – energy costs of absorption and metabolism. In: Steffens, G.L. and Rumsey, T.S. (eds) *Biomechanisms Regulating Growth and Development.* Kluwer Academic Publishers, Boston, Massachusetts, pp. 313–327.

Jin, L., Reynolds, L.P., Redmer, D.A., Caton, J.S. and Crenshaw, J.D. (1994) Effects of dietary fiber on intestinal growth, cell proliferation, and morphology in growing pigs. *Journal of Animal Science* 72, 2270–2278.

Johnson, L.R. (1988) Regulation of gastrointestinal mucosal growth. *Physiological Reviews* 68, 456–502.

Karue, C.N., Evans, J.L. and Tillman, A. D. (1972) Metabolism of nitrogen in Boran and in Hereford–Boran crossbred steers. *Journal of Animal Science* 35, 1025–1030.

Kelly, J.M., Summers, M., Park, H.S., Milligan, L.P. and McBride, B.W. (1991) Cellular energy metabolism and regulation. *Journal of Dairy Science* 74, 678–694.

Klopfenstein, T.J. and Erickson, G.E. (2002) Effects of manipulating protein and phosphorus nutrition of feedlot cattle on nutrient management and the environment. *Journal of Animal Science* 80 (E. Supplement 2), E106–E114.

Koch, R.M., Swiger, L.A., Chambers, D. and Gregory, K.E. (1963) Efficiency of feed use in beef cattle. *Journal of Animal Science* 22, 486–494.

Kolath, W.H., Kerley, M.S. and Golden J.W. (2005) The relationship between mitochondrial DNA content, single nucleotide polymorphisms and feed efficiency in crossbred Angus steers. *Journal of Animal Science* 83 (Supplement 1), 368–369 (Abstract).

Koohmaraie, M., Seideman, S.C., Schollmeyer, J.E., Dutson, T.R. and Crouse, J.D. (1987) Effect of postmortem storage on Ca++-dependent proteases, their inhibitor and myofibril fragmentation. *Meat Science* 19, 187–196.

Koong, L.J., Ferrell, C.L. and Nienaber J.A. (1985) Assessment of interrelationships among levels of intake and production, organ size and fasting heat production in growing animals. *Journal of Nutrition* 115, 1383–1390.

Krehbiel, C.R., Kreikemeier, K.K. and Ferrell, C.L. (2000) Influence of *Bos indicus* crossbreeding and cattle age on apparent utilization of a high-grain diet. *Journal of Animal Science* 78, 1641–1647.

Ledesma, A., Garcia d Lacoba, M. and Rial, E. (2002) The mitochondrial uncoupling proteins. *Genome Biology* 3, 3015.1–3015.9.

Lin, M.H., Vander Tuig, J.G., Romsos, D.R., Akera, T. and Leveille, G.A. (1979) Na+,K+-ATPase enzyme units in lean and obese (ob/ob) thyroxine-injected mice. *American Journal of Physiology* 237, E265–E272.

Lobley, G.E. (1992) Control of the metabolic fate of amino acids in ruminants: a review. *Journal of Animal Science* 70, 3264–3275.

Lobley, G.E. (2003) Protein turnover – what does it mean for animal production? *Canadian Journal of Animal Science* 83, 327–340.

Lobley, G.E., Milne, V., Lovie, J.M., Reeds, P.J. and Pennie, K. (1980) Whole-body and tissue protein synthesis in cattle. *British Journal of Nutrition* 43, 491–502.

Lobley, G.E., Sinclair, K.D., Grant, C.M., Miller, L., Mantle, D., Calder, A.G., Warkup, C.C. and Maltin, C.A. (2000) The effects of breed and level of nutrition on whole-body and muscle protein metabolism in pure-bred Aberdeen Angus and Charolais beef steers. *British Journal of Nutrition* 84, 275–284.

Lorenzen, C.L., Koohmaraie, M., Shackelford, S.D., Jahoor, F., Freetly, H.C., Wheeler, T.L., Savell, J.W. and Fiorotto, M.L. (2000) Protein kinetics in callipyge lambs. *Journal of Animal Science* 78, 78–87.

Ludden, P.A., Wechter, T.L. and Hess, B.W. (2002) Effects of oscillating dietary protein on ruminal fermentation and site and extent of nutrient digestion in sheep. *Journal of Animal Science* 80, 3336–3346.

McBride, B.W. and Milligan, L.P. (1984) The effect of lactation on ouabain-sensitive respiration of the duodenal mucosa of cows. *Canadian Journal of Animal Science* 64, 817–824.

McBride, B.W. and Milligan, L.P. (1985) Influence of feed intake and starvation on the magnitude of Na+,K+-ATPase(EC 3.6.1.3)-dependent respiration in duodenal mucosa of sheep. *British Journal of Nutrition* 53, 605–614.

McDonagh, M.B., Herd, R.M., Richardson, E.C., Oddy, V.H., Archer, J.A. and Arthur, P.F. (2001) Meat quality and the calpain system of feedlot steers following a single generation of divergent selection for residual feed intake. *Australian Journal of Experimental Agriculture* 41, 1013–1021.

McDonald, J.M. and Nielsen, M.K. (2006) Correlated responses in maternal performance following divergent selection for heat loss in mice. *Journal of Animal Science* 84, 300–304.

McWhir, J. and Wilton, J.W. (1987) Heritabilities of predicted performance measures in beef bull test and their relationships with feedlot efficiency measures. *Journal of Animal Science* 64, 1323–1331.

Mader, T.L. (1998) Feedlot medicine and management. Implants. *The Veterinary Clinics Food Animal Practice* 14, 279–290.

Merchen, N.R. (1988) Digestion, absorption and excretion in ruminants. In: Church, D.C. (ed.) *The Ruminant Animal – Digestive Physiology and Nutrition*. Prentice-Hall, Englewood Cliffs, New Jersey, p. 172.

Miller, S.P. (2002) Beef cattle breeding programmes: progress and prospects. *Proceedings of the 7th World Congress on Genetics Applied to Livestock Production*, 19–23 August 2002, Montpellier, France. CD-ROM Communication No. 02-18.

Miller, S.P. (2003) Genetic improvement programs for feed efficiency in beef cattle. *Proceedings of the Canadian Society of Animal Science.* CD-ROM communication.

Milligan, L.P. and McBride, B.W. (1985) Energy costs of ion pumping by animal tissues. *Journal of Nutrition* 115, 1374–1382.

Montano-Bermudez, M., Nielsen, M.K. and Deutscher, G.H. (1990) Energy requirements for maintenance of crossbred beef cattle with different genetic potential for milk. *Journal of Animal Science* 68, 2279–2288.

Moore, K.L., Johnston, D.J. and Burrow, H.M. (2005a) Sire breed differences for net feed intake in feedlot finished beef cattle. *Proceedings of the Association for the Advancement of Animal Breeding and Genetics* 56, 211–218.

Moore, K.L., Johnston, D.J., Graser, H.U. and Herd, R. (2005b) Genetic and phenotypic relationships between insulin-like growth factor-I (IGF-I) and net feed intake, fat, and growth traits in Angus beef cattle. *Australian Journal of Agricultural Research* 56, 211–218.

Murphy, T.A., Fluharty, F.L. and Loerch, S.C. (1994) The influence of intake level and corn processing on digestibility and ruminal metabolism in steers fed all-concentrate diets. *Journal of Animal Science* 72, 1608–1615.

Murray, D.M., Tulloh, N.M. and Winter, W.H. (1977) The effect of three different growth rates on some offal components of cattle. *Journal of Agricultural Science* 89, 119–128.

Nagy, T.R., Blaylock, M.L. and Garvey, W.T. (2004) Role of UCP2 and UCP3 in nutrition and obesity. *Nutrition* 20, 139–144.

National Research Centre (NRC) (1996) *Nutrient Requirements of Beef Cattle*, 7th edn. National Academy Press, Washington, DC.

Nielsen, M.K. (1998) Genetic variation in feed energy utilization in mice. *Proceedings of the 6th World Congress on Genetics Applied to Livestock Production* 26, 89–96.

Nkrumah, J.D., Basarab, J.A., Price, M.A., Okine, E.K., Ammoura, A., Guercio, S., Hansen, C., Li, C., Benkel, B., Murdoch, B. and Moore, S.S. (2004a) Different measures of energetic efficiency and their phenotypic relationships with growth, feed intake, and ultrasound and carcass merit in hybrid cattle. *Journal of Animal Science* 82, 2451–2459.

Nkrumah, J.D., Li, C., Basarab, J.B., Guercio, S., Meng, Y., Murdoch, B., Hansen, C. and Moore, S.S. (2004b) Association of a single nucleotide polymorphism in the bovine leptin gene with feed intake, feed efficiency, growth, feeding behaviour, carcass quality and body composition. *Canadian Journal of Animal Science* 84, 211–219.

Nkrumah, J.D., Okine, E.K., Mathison, G.W., Schmid, K., Li, C., Basarab, J.A., Price, M.A., Wang, Z. and Moore, S.S. (2006) Relationships of feedlot feed efficiency, performance, and feeding behavior with metabolic rate, methane production, and energy partitioning in beef cattle. *Journal of Animal Science* 84, 145–153.

Okine, E.K., Basarab, J.A., Goonewardene, L.A., Mir, P., Mir, Z., Price, M.A., Arthur, P.F. and Moore S.S. (2003) Residual feed intake: what is it and how does it differ from traditional concepts of feed efficiency? *Proceedings of the Canadian Society of Animal Science*. CD-ROM communication.

Owens, F. and Zinn, R.A. (2005) Corn grain for cattle: influence of processing on site and extent of digestion. *Proceedings of the Southwest Nutrition Conference*, February 2005. University of Arizona, Tucson, Arizona, pp. 86–112 (http://animal.cals.arizona.edu/swnmc/2005/proceedings.htm#).

Owens, F.N., Gill, D.R., Secrist, D.S. and Coleman S.W. (1995) Review of some aspects of growth and development of feedlot cattle. *Journal of Animal Science* 73, 3152–3172.

Owens, F.N., Secrist, D.S., Hill, W.J. and Gill, D.R. (1997) The effect of grain source and grain processing on performance of feedlot cattle: a review. *Journal of Animal Science* 75, 868–879.

Pecqueur, C., Couplan, E., Bouillaud, F. and Ricquier, D. (2001) Genetic and physiological analysis of the role of uncoupling proteins in human energy homeostasis. *Journal of Molecular Medicine* 79, 48–56.

Perry, T.C., Fox, D.G. and Beermann, D.H. (1991) Effect of an implant of trenbolone acetate and estradiol on growth, feed efficiency, and carcass composition of Holstein and beef steers. *Journal of Animal Science* 69, 4696–4702.

Reed, B.K., Hunt, C.W., Sasser, R.G., Momont, P.A., Rode, L.M. and Kastelic, J.P. (1997) Effect of forage:concentrate ratio on digestion and reproduction in primiparous beef heifers. *Journal of Animal Science* 75, 1708–1714.

Reynolds, C.K., Tyrrell, H.F. and Reynolds, P.J. (1991) Effects of diet forage-to-concentrate ratio and intake on energy metabolism in growing beef heifers: whole body energy and nitrogen balance and visceral heat production. *Journal of Nutrition* 121, 994–1003.

Richardson, E.C. and Herd, R.M. (2004) Biological basis for variation in residual feed intake in beef cattle. 2. Synthesis of results following divergent selection. *Australian Journal of Experimental Agriculture* 44, 431–440.

Richardson, E.C., Herd, R.M., Arthur, P.F., Wright, J., Xu, G., Dibley, K. and Oddy, V.H. (1996) Possible physiological indicators for net feed conversion efficiency in beef cattle. *Proceedings of the Australian Society of Animal Production* 21, 103–110.

Richardson, E.C., Herd, R.M., Oddy, V.H., Thomspon, J.M., Archer, J.A. and Arthur, P.F. (2001) Body composition and implications for heat production of Angus steer progeny of parents selected for and against residual feed intake. *Australian Journal of Experimental Agriculture* 41, 1065–1072.

Rolfe, D.F.S., Newman, J.M.B., Buckingham, J.A., Clark, M.G. and Brand, M.D. (1999) Contribution of mitochondrial proton leak to respiration rate in working skeletal muscle and liver and to SMR. *American Journal of Physiology* 276, C692–C699.

Russell, J.B. and Strobel, H.J. (1989) Effect of ionophores on ruminal fermentation. *Applied and Environmental Microbiology* 55, 1–6.

Sainz, R.D. and Bentley, B.E. (1997) Visceral organ mass and cellularity in growth-restricted and re-fed beef steers. *Journal of Animal Science* 75, 1229–1236.
Schenkel, F.S., Miller, S.P. and Wilton, J.W. (2003) Genetic parameters of feed efficiency, growth and carcass traits of beef bulls. *Canadian Journal of Animal Science* 83, 617–618.
Schenkel, F.S., Miller, S.P. and Wilton J.W. (2004) Genetic parameters and breed differences for feed efficiency, growth, and body composition traits of young beef bulls. *Canadian Journal of Animal Science* 84, 177–185.
Schenkel, F.S., Miller, S.P., Jiang, Z., Mandell, I.B., Ye, X., Li, H. and Wilton J.W. (2006) Association of a single nucleotide polymorphism in the calpastatin gene with carcass and meat quality traits of beef cattle. *Journal of Animal Science* 84, 291–299.
Scollan, N.D., Jessop, N.S., Allan, G.F., Oldham, J.D. and McBride, B.W. (1993) The influence of sex, feeding and genotype on sodium-potassium Atpase activity in erythrocytes from young dairy calves. *Canadian Journal of Animal Science* 73, 981–985.
Senior, A.E., Nadanaciva, S. and Weber, J. (2002) The molecular mechanism of ATP synthesis by F1F0-ATP synthase. *Biochimica et Biophysica Acta* 1553, 188–211.
Small, J.A., Kennedy, A.D., Veira, D.M., McCaughey, W.R. and Ward, D.R. (2004) Time of feeding and growth promotant effects on the winter growth performance and carcass traits of steers. *Canadian Journal of Animal Science* 84, 133–144.
Stryer, L. (1995) *Biochemistry*, 4th edn. W.H. Freeman and Company, New York.
Swanson, K.C. and Harmon, D.L. (2002) Dietary influences on pancreatic a-amylase expression and secretion in ruminants. In: Zabielski, R., Lesniewska, V., Gregory, P.C. and Westrom, B. (eds) *Biology of the Intestine in Growing Animals.* Elsevier, Boston, Massachusetts, pp. 515–537.
Swanson, K.C., Redmer, D.A., Reynolds, L.P. and Caton, J.S. (1999) Ruminally undegraded intake protein in sheep fed low-quality forage: effect on weight, growth, cell proliferation, and morphology of visceral organs. *Journal of Animal Science* 77, 198–205.
Swanson, K.C., Reynolds, L.P. and Caton, J.S. (2000) Influence of dietary intake and lasalocid on serum hormones and metabolites and visceral organ growth and morphology in wether lambs. *Small Ruminant Research* 35, 235–247.
Tamminga, S. (1996) A review on environmental impacts of nutritional strategies in ruminants. *Journal of Animal Science* 74, 3112–3124.
Tedeschi, L.O., Fox, D.G. and Russell, J.B. (2000) Accounting for the effects of a ruminal nitrogen deficiency within the structure of the Cornell Net Carbohydrate and Protein System. *Journal of Animal Science* 78, 1648–1658.
Valle, E., Habermann, F.A., Moore, S.S., Crews, D.H. and Benkel, B.F. (2004) Genomic localization and SNP discovery in the bovine melanocortin receptor 4 gene (MC4R). *Animal Genetics* 35, 351–352.
Valle, E., Moore, S.S., Jann, O., Williams, J.L., Crews, D.H. Jr and Benkel, B.F. (2005) The bovine cocaine and amphetamine-regulated transcript locus: gene characterization and SNP discovery. *Animal Genetics* 36, 74–75.
Van Horn, H.H., Newton, G.L. and Kunkle, W.E. (1996) Ruminant nutrition from an environmental perspective: factors affecting whole-farm nutrient balance. *Journal of Animal Science* 74, 3082–3102.
Varel, V.H. and Kreikemeier, K.K. (1999) Low- and high-quality forage utilization by heifers and mature beef cows. *Journal of Animal Science* 77, 2774–2780.
Wood, B.J., Archer, J.A. and van der Werf, J.H.J. (2004) Response to selection in beef cattle using IGF-1 as a selection criterion for residual feed intake under different Australian breeding objectives. *Livestock Production Science* 91, 69–81.
Zhao, F.Q., Okine, E.K., Cheeseman, C.I., Shirazi-Beechey, S.P. and Kennelly, J.J. (1998) Glucose transporter gene expression in lactating bovine gastrointestinal tract. *Journal of Animal Science* 76, 2921–2929.

20 Models of Nutrient Utilization by Fish and Potential Applications for Fish Culture Operations

D.P. BUREAU AND K. HUA

Fish Nutrition Research Laboratory and Centre for Nutrition Modelling, Department of Animal and Poultry Science, University of Guelph, Canada

Introduction

Fish culture differs significantly from terrestrial animal production in many respects. Rearing animals in an aquatic environment greatly complicates monitoring of growth, standing biomass, feed delivery and waste outputs. A great deal of attention must be paid to feeding since feed delivered but not consumed by the animals cannot be recovered, or even appropriately quantified. The nutritional composition of fish feeds varies considerably, which complicates comparison of feed efficiency values among operations and even, to some extent, between production cycles. Wastes produced by fish culture operations are often difficult to contain and may, potentially, contribute to environmental degradation of fragile aquatic ecosystems. Aquaculture operations need to be able to optimize feeding strategies in order to improve their economic and/or environmental sustainability. In parallel, it is essential for environmental agencies to have access to tools allowing the objective estimation of waste outputs and assessment of potential environmental impacts of fish culture operations under their jurisdiction.

The development of systems capable of generating robust estimates of fish production, feed requirement and conversion efficiency and waste outputs is considered a high priority by many industry stakeholders. Nutrition modelling offers a rational basis for the development of such systems and has already played a significant role. A relatively large number of nutritional models, most of them based on bioenergetics and elemental mass balances, have been developed over the past few decades. These models describe, in a quantitative fashion, the digestion, metabolism and accretion of energy and elements, such as nitrogen (N) and phosphorus (P), for several fish species. These models have been used to generate realistic estimates of feed requirements, efficiency of feed utilization and solid and soluble waste outputs for fish culture operations. However, most of the current models are highly empirical and not very robust (Bureau*et al.*, 2002). These models can only be considered reliable if applied within a relatively narrow range of conditions (e.g. genetic strains, fish size, feed composition, etc.). Further research is required to better understand the impact of dietary, environmental and endogenous factors on nutrient utilization and accretion in fish and to develop practical models that integrate available information.

This chapter reviews some of the challenges facing fish culture operations and potential model applications. Recent work on the development of practical bioenergetic and elemental mass balance models is reviewed. Limitations of the current approaches and models are reviewed and the need to develop more mechanistic and robust models that are also practical and user-friendly is presented.

Challenges of Fish Culture and Usefulness of Nutritional Models

The production of animals in an aquatic environment imposes numerous challenges. Biomass inventory, growth prediction and benchmarking, monitoring of feed delivery, prediction or comparison of feed efficiency values and estimation of waste outputs and potential environmental impacts are some of the significant challenges fish operations are facing.

Biomass inventory, monitoring of feed delivery and growth prediction

Fish are reared in a wide variety of environments and housing infrastructures (tanks, raceways, ponds, net pens, etc.). The animal inventory is rarely fully visible to the caretakers due to water turbidity, light reflection and diffraction. Logistical issues (the capture of free swimming animals in a large offshore cage, for example) limit frequency and accuracy of monitoring of animal inventory and biomass increase.

Biomass gain, i.e. growth of the fish, is determined, or highly influenced, by water temperature and numerous other environmental factors (photoperiod, salinity, weather conditions, etc.). Biomass increase and time needed for the animal to reach market weight cannot always be predicted accurately based on performance over the past several months, data from previous years and/or using simple rules of thumb.

The same factors that hinder accurate and timely assessment of inventory also complicate feeding. Feed is often delivered to a fish population that is only partly visible or, in many cases, delivered 'blindly' using mechanized systems (automatic feeders, demand (pendulum) feeders, etc.), into an 'open' system (net pens, flow-through raceways and tanks, etc.). Feed delivered but not consumed is inevitably wasted and very difficult to estimate. Feeding too much leads to feed wastage, a pure economic loss, and greater waste outputs. Conversely, delivering less feed than what is required by the fish to express their growth potential can also be considered an economic loss (opportunity cost) and may, consequently, affect profitability of the enterprise.

Mathematical models describing growth pattern as a function of the animal's potential and the prevailing conditions are extremely useful in assisting estimation or forecasting of biomass, as well as detecting potential deviations from expected or achievable performance (e.g. deviations due to health or stress issues, poor feeding management, etc.). Models allowing accurate prediction of feed requirement of the fish population as a function of growth potential and prevailing conditions can also be very useful, as they could be used effectively to improve feeding practices (e.g. more accurate determination of rations to be fed, automatic feed delivery equipment, auditing feed delivery practices of employees, exploring the effect of various feeding strategies, etc.).

Predicting and optimizing feed efficiency or minimizing feed cost

Fish feeds are generally significantly more costly (2–10 times) than feeds typically fed to other livestock species. Fish feeds are also characterized by the widely variable nutritional composition to which they are formulated. The protein, lipid and starch contents of feeds varies very significantly, not only as a function of species and life stages for which they are formulated (trout versus tilapia feed, starter versus grower versus finisher feed), but also as a function of a myriad of other factors, such as production and environmental constraints, market or manufacturers' preference, economic climate, fish price, etc. Part of the variability in feed composition is also related to the fact that aquaculture is a field in rapid evolution. Feeds used in trout and salmon production have evolved very significantly over just three decades. In the early 1980s, for example, commercial rainbow trout feeds used in Canada were relatively low in protein (e.g. 35–40%) and fat (e.g. 8–10%) but rich in starch (35–40%). Feed conversion ratios (FCR, feed/gain) of 2–2.5 were common for market size rainbow trout (ca. 1 kg live weight). Today, the use of lower carbohydrate, higher digestible energy (DE) density feeds (e.g. 34–55% crude protein, 18–32% fat, 10–20% starch) allows FCR of about 1.0–1.2 for market size rainbow trout.

The amount of feed required by a fish to achieve a certain amount of weight gain depends primarily on the composition of the feed used. In general, a greater amount of a 'lower digestible nutrient density' feed will be required compared to a 'higher digestible nutrient density' feed to achieve the same performance level (Table 20.1). Fish feeds are generally compared on the basis of their DE content, but this approach has numerous limitations (Bureau *et al*., 2002). How efficiently feed input is converted to fish biomass and how different factors may affect this conversion is still a relatively poorly understood issue. Various approaches have been used to predict efficiency of conversion of feed into fish biomass as a function of fish species, feeding level, growth rate, feed composition, environmental factors, etc. Most of the approaches used so far have been useful, but all present important limitations. There is a need for more robust approaches and models.

Estimating waste outputs

Most aquaculture systems are 'semi-open', so that a significant proportion of the wastes produced by the animal are released into the environment. Faecal and metabolic wastes produced by fish can, in general, be only partially recovered in

Table 20.1. Growth and FCR of Atlantic salmon fed diets of different nutritional compositions.

	Regular diet	High nutrient density diet
Diet composition	37	44
Digestible protein (DP), %		
Digestible energy (DE), MJ kg^{-1}	18	22
DP/DE, g MJ^{-1}	20	
Performance of fish		
Weight gain, g $fish^{-1}$	33.4	33.6
FCR (feed:gain)	0.92	0.75

Source: Azevedo *et al.* (2002).

the farm. With cage culture of fish in open water, recovery of faecal and metabolic wastes that disperse rapidly in the environment is extremely difficult. The main concern is the release of nitrogen (N), phosphorus (P) and solid organic matter wastes. N and P are limiting nutrients for algae growth in marine and freshwater ecosystems, respectively. Excess release of these elements can lead to environmental degradation problems, notably for oligotrophic aquatic ecosystems. Faecal wastes represent the bulk of solid organic matter produced by fish culture operations. A large proportion of this organic matter can settle on the bottom of the receiving water body. Degradation of organic matter by bacteria and other organisms leads to consumption of oxygen (O_2) through respiration. This consumption of oxygen can have negative consequences, notably for temperate freshwater lakes where a hypolimnion may form. This hypolimnion generally has a poor capacity of regenerating its O_2 content. Excessive settling of organic matter to the hypolimnion may result in significant reduction in dissolved oxygen levels, which can then be damaging to some of the biota.

Reducing waste outputs of aquaculture operations is, consequently, considered a key element for the long-term sustainability of aquaculture in many parts of the world. It is difficult for fish culture operations and governmental regulators to predict, or set goals for reducing, environmental impacts without first having access to objective estimates of the amount of waste associated with production (actual or planned). Directly monitoring and estimating waste outputs from effluent of aquaculture facilities is an inaccurate and costly process (Cho *et al.*, 1991, 1994). It is also extremely difficult for certain types of facilities, such as cage culture operations (Reid, 2004). Since aquaculture wastes are ultimately from biological and dietary origins, the use of nutrient mass balance offers a simple and economical alternative to limnological (chemical) methods of estimating waste outputs. Using a nutritional mass balance approach, Cho *et al.* (1991, 1994) demonstrated that estimation of waste outputs of fish culture operations could be accurately and economically made, with great flexibility, based on feed inputs and feed component utilization by the fish. Nutrient mass balance models have been developed and proven to be very useful in practical fish culture operations to predict body weight gain, feed requirement and solid N and P waste outputs (Cho *et al.*, 1991, 1994; Bureau *et al.*, 2003; Papatryphon *et al.*, 2005).

A Bioenergetic-based Approach of Predicting Growth, Feed Requirement and Feed Conversion: the Fish-PrFEQ Model

The study of the balance between dietary energy supply, expenditure and gain offers a relatively simple way of looking at dietary component utilization and requirements by animals. In 1981, a subcommittee of the Committee on Animal Nutrition of the US National Research Council was appointed to develop a systematic terminology for description of energy utilization by animals, including fish (NRC, 1981). This system is presented schematically in Fig. 20.1 and its nomenclature is used in this chapter. Bioenergetic approaches have been used effectively to predict growth, feed ration, FCR and waste outputs of fish fed diets

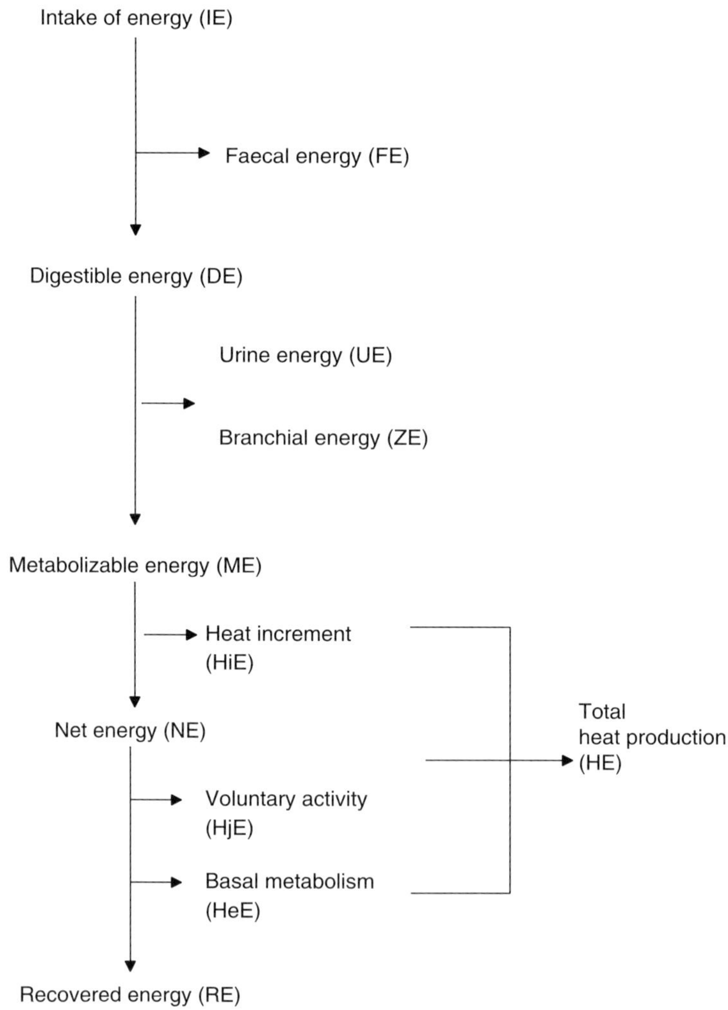

Fig. 20.1. Partition of dietary energy by fish.

of varying nutritional composition and reared under different environments (e.g. Cho *et al.*, 1991, 1994; Cho, 1992; Cho and Bureau, 1998; Kaushik, 1998; Lupatsch *et al.*, 1998; Cui and Xie, 1999; Bureau *et al.*, 2002, 2003; Azevedo *et al.*, 2005; Lupatsch and Kissil, 2005; Papatryphon *et al.*, 2005; Zhou *et al.*, 2005).

Fish growing at different rates will retain nutrients at different rates and, consequently, have different energy and feed requirements. Energy requirement should therefore be calculated for explicitly expressed levels of performance (e.g. expected or achievable level of performance), feed composition and life stage. This can be done using factorial approaches (Cho and Bureau, 1998; Lupatsch *et al.*, 1998), i.e. approaches that divide energy requirement into its different components or fractions, as opposed to lumping them into one estimate, as is commonly done.

Cho (1991, 1992) proposed a factorial bioenergetic model to determine energy requirement of fish based on expected level of performance, diet DE content and expected body energy deposition. The framework proposed by Cho (1991) was subsequently expanded and named the 'Fish-PrFEQ' model (Cho and Bureau, 1998). Further development, or various adaptations, of the Fish-PrFEQ model have been proposed by Kaushik (1998), Bureau *et al.* (2002, 2003), Hua (2005), Papatryphon *et al.* (2005) and Zhou *et al.* (2005).

The approach proposed by Cho (1991) is based on the assumption that fish have a (genetically) determined target for growth. The main premise is that 'animals will seek to eat a sufficient amount of an appropriately balanced diet to achieve their target or preferred performance unless limited by constraints or overridden by an externally managed intervention' (Oldham *et al.*, 1997). The Fish-PrFEQ model estimates DE requirement to achieve certain 'desired' performance (determined by fish genetic potential and prevailing conditions). The calculated DE requirement is translated into a feed requirement by considering the DE content (kJ g^{-1} feed) of the feed used.

Estimation of feed requirement according to the approach proposed by Cho (1991) can be accomplished by four steps, as follows:

1. Prediction of weight gain.
2. Determination of energy gain.
3. Estimation of heat and metabolic losses.
4. Estimation of DE requirement and feed requirement.

Prediction of weight gain

The approach proposed by Cho (1991, 1992) requires prediction of weight gain over a certain time interval using a mathematical growth model. There have been many attempts to describe the growth of fish using a large diversity of mathematical approaches. In aquaculture, several models applicable to the concave portion of the growth curve have been developed (e.g. Iwama and Tautz, 1981; Muller-Feuga, 1990).

The formula most commonly used for fish growth rate expression is instantaneous growth rate, known as 'specific growth rate (SGR, %BW day^{-1})', which is based on the natural logarithm of body weight:

$$SGR=[(\ln FBW - \ln IBW)/D] \times 100,$$

where FBW is final body weight (g), IBW is initial body weight (g) and D = number of days.

SGR has been widely used by most biologists to describe growth rate of fish. However, the exponent of natural logarithm underestimates the weight gain between the IBW and the FBW used in the calculation and it grossly overestimates predicted body weight at weights greater than FBW used. Furthermore, the SGR is dependent on the IBW, making meaningless comparisons of growth rates among different groups, unless IBW are similar.

There is strong evidence suggesting that, at constant water temperature, cubic root transformed live weight (in grams) of salmonids increases linearly with time when fish are reared under optimal conditions (Iwama and Tautz, 1981). Figure 20.2 presents live weight and corresponding cubic root as a function of time (days) for rainbow trout fed to near-satiety and reared at 8.5°C (Bureau *et al.*, 2002). This figure clearly shows that, for rainbow trout (weighing between 150 and 600 g) fed to near-satiation, cubic root of live weight (i.e. scaled body weight SBW, $g^{1/3}$) increases in a highly significant ($P < 0.001$) linear fashion as a function of time. The slope of the function SBW ($g^{1/3}$) versus time is the same, regardless of live weight (BW, g) and time interval used in the calculation.

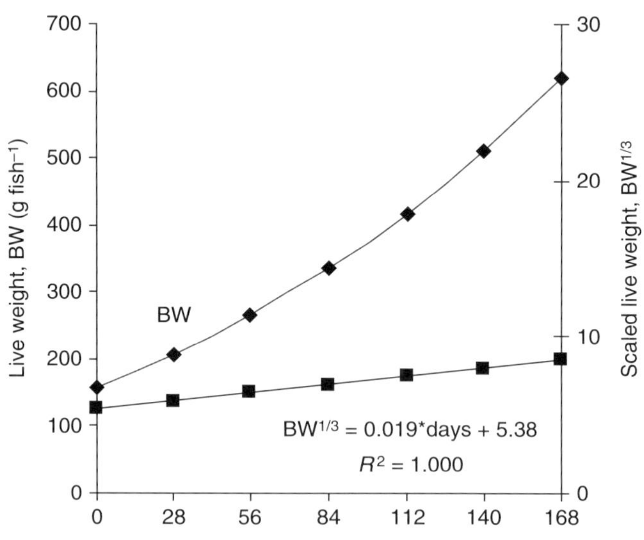

Fig. 20.2. Live weight and cubic root of live weight of rainbow trout fed to near-satiation and reared at 8.5°C growing from 158 to 621 g live weight for 168 days (data from Bureau *et al.*, 2006).

This observation was described by the following equation, commonly known as the daily growth coefficient (DGC, $g^{1/3}$ day^{-1}) (Cho, 1992):

$$DGC = \{[FBW^{(1/3)} - IBW^{(1/3)}]/D\} \times 100,$$

where FBW is final body weight (g); IBW is initial body weight (g); and *D* (days) is time interval of the growth period.

This model has proven very useful to compare growth performance when temperature is constant. However, since temperature has a determinant effect on growth rate in fish, growth models should ideally account for the effect of water temperature. Analysis of literature data by Iwama and Tautz (1981) indicated that the slope of SBW ($g^{1/3}$) versus time increased linearly with temperature over a wide range of temperatures (4–16°C). Data from Azevedo *et al.* (1998) also supported this conclusion (Figs 20.3 and 20.4). This observation was translated

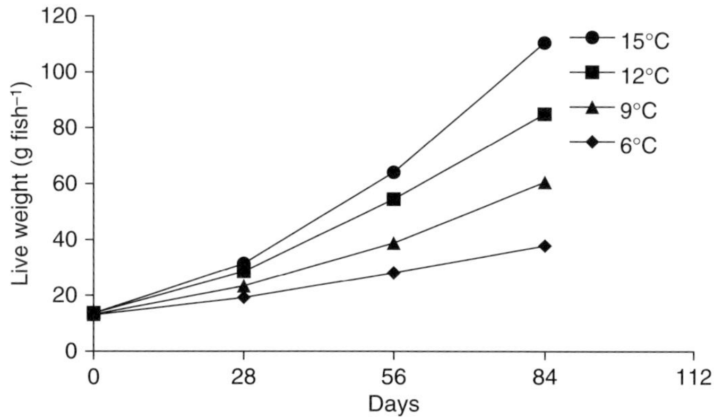

Fig. 20.3. Live weight of rainbow trout fed to near-satiation and reared at four temperatures (data from Azevedo *et al.*, 1998).

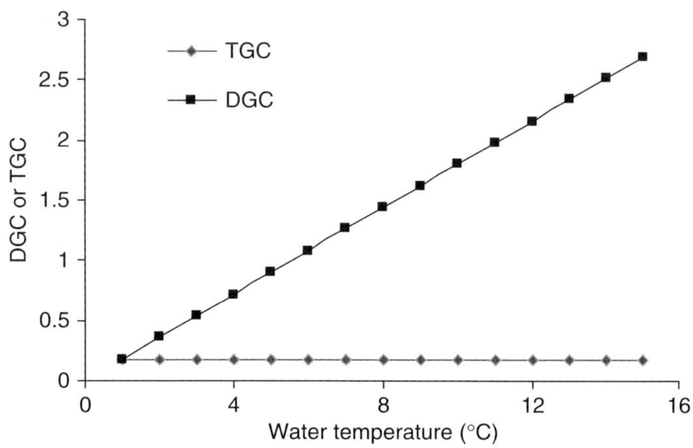

Fig. 20.4. Daily growth coefficient (DGC) and thermal-unit growth coefficient (TGC) of rainbow trout as a function of temperature (data from Azevedo *et al.*, 1998).

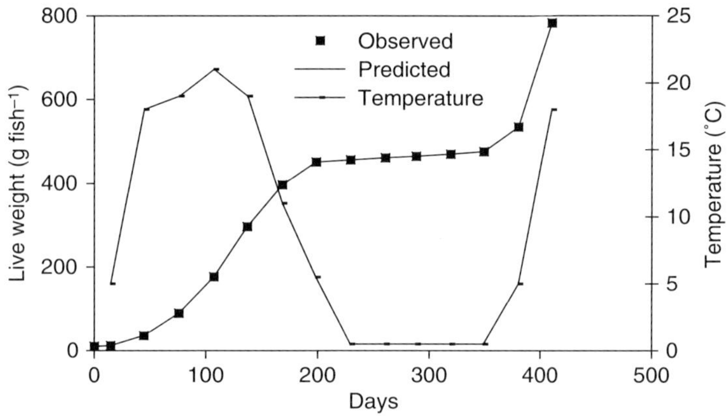

Fig. 20.5. Live weight of rainbow trout reared under variable temperature regimen for 410 days and predicted weight using TGC model (data from Cho and Bureau, 1998).

into the following equation, commonly known as the thermal-unit growth coefficient (TGC, $g^{1/3}$ degree day^{-1}) (Iwama and Tautz, 1981; Cho, 1992):

$$TGC = \{[FBW^{(1/3)} - IBW^{(1/3)}] / [\sum_{i=1}^{n}(T_i x D_i)]\} \times 100$$

where FBW is final body weight (g); IBW is initial body weight (g); T_i is water temperature (°C) of the *i*th day; and D_i is the *i*th day of the growth period.

This equation has been shown to represent very faithfully the growth curves of rainbow trout, Arctic charr, lake trout, brown trout, Chinook salmon and Atlantic salmon over a wide range of temperatures (Iwama and Tautz, 1981). An example of the good agreement of the live weights predicted with the TGC model and actually observed live weights at varying water temperature environment is shown in Fig. 20.5 (Cho and Bureau, 1998). Azevedo *et al.* (1998) have proved that TGC was a valid growth model for the temperature ranged between 6 and 15°C. The TGC model consequently offers a simple mode of growth rate comparison for salmonids since it is a standardized measure of growth that is unaffected by live weight, time interval and water temperature. It therefore allows comparison of performance among culture operations, strains, production years, slots, sampling intervals, etc. It can also be used as a yardstick in scientific studies to determine if fish have achieved their growth potential, or to determine the effect of different dietary and environmental factors. Since these TGC values and growth rates are dependent on species, stock (genetics), nutrition, environment, husbandry and other factors, it is essential to calculate the TGC for a given aquaculture condition using past growth records or records obtained from similar stocks and husbandry conditions.

Determination of energy gain

Following prediction of weight gain, the Fish-PrFEQ model requires an estimate of energy retention, referred to as 'recovered energy (RE)' in the NRC (1981) nomenclature, associated with the predicted weight gain. In the Fish-PrFEQ model, RE de facto drives DE and feed requirements.

Live weight gain in animals is the result of deposition of water, protein, fat, minerals and a small amount of other components (glycogen, etc.). This accretion of energy-yielding nutrient results in 'energy deposition'. RE is consequently the 'weighed average' of energy-yielding nutrient deposition. Chemical composition of weight gain (per unit of live weight gain) is not constant, but rather changes with weight of the animal, feed used, physiological state, etc. Figure 20.6 shows the changes in the relative composition (% or kJ g^{-1}) of rainbow trout of various sizes fed practical diets. Similar figures can be found in Shearer (1994) and Lupatsch *et al.* (1998). The dry matter and gross energy (GE) contents of fish increase quite dramatically as fish grow. Consequently, different amounts of dry matter and energy will be retained in one unit of weight gain (e.g. 1 kg of weight gain) as fish grow. Numerous other factors (feed composition, feeding level, physiological and environmental factors) can affect the composition of fish, notably lipid content. A change in biomass weight is therefore not an 'absolute' or 'constant' parameter, as the 'same' biomass gain (1 kg) may represent 10, 25, 50% more energy retention as the animal grows, or as conditions change.

Prediction of energy retention (RE, kJ day^{-1}) can be made quite easily using simple linear or exponential models relating to fish weight. For example, Bureau *et al.* (2003) employed a simple equation between GE (kJ per fish) and BW (g): $GE = 0.0039*BW^2 + 5.5812*BW$. RE was calculated by differences in GE at initial and final body weights. The construction of these models may simply involve sampling animals at different sizes and determining their protein and lipid or energy contents (Bureau *et al.*, 2003).

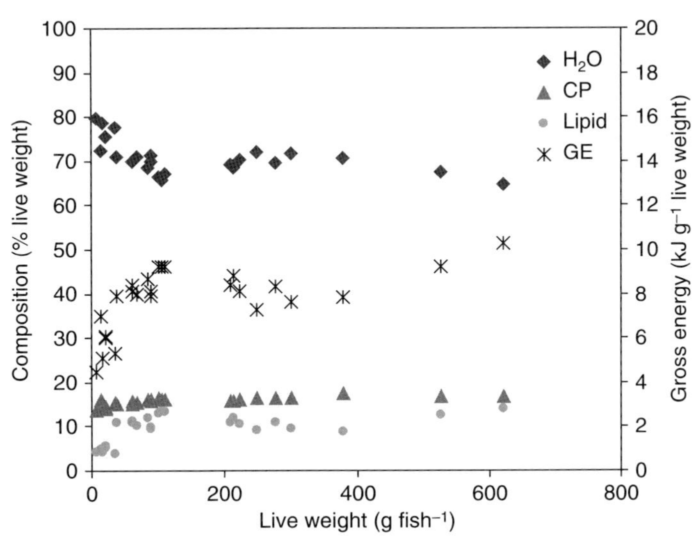

Fig. 20.6. Chemical composition (relative amounts, % or kJ g^{-1}) of rainbow trout over various sizes fed practical diets (Bureau *et al.*, 2002).

Estimate heat and metabolic losses

As in most bioenergetic frameworks, the Fish-PrFEQ model requires that energy be allocated to basal (life sustaining) processes (basal metabolism, HeE) and for digestion, absorption, deposition and interconversion of nutrients (heat increment of feeding, HiE). Estimation of HeE and HiE in fish has been the topic of numerous studies and this information has been reviewed in some detail elsewhere (Cho *et al.*, 1982; Cho and Kaushik, 1990; Kaushik and Médale, 1994; Bureau *et al.*, 2002; Azevedo *et al.*, 2005).

Allocation for basal metabolism (HeE)

Fish have a much lower basal energy metabolism (HeE) than do homeotherms. HeE of rainbow trout, reared at 15°C, was estimated to be approximately 40 kJ kg^{-1} $BW^{0.8}$ day^{-1} (Cho *et al.*, 1982; Cho and Kaushik, 1990; Bureau *et al.*, 1998, 2002), where HeE of mammals is around 300 kJ kg^{-1} $BW^{0.75}$ day^{-1} (Lloyd *et al.*, 1978). However, water temperature has a major influence on basal metabolism of fish and estimates of HeE should take into account this effect. Based on oxygen consumption data of rainbow trout of different weights reared at different temperatures, the following equation was developed to predict HeE of salmonids as a function of water temperature between 5 and 15°C (Cho, 1991; Cho and Bureau, 1998):

$$\mathrm{HeE} = (-0.01 + 3.26T - 0.05T^2)\ \mathrm{BW}^{0.824},$$

where HeE is basal energy metabolism (kJ day^{-1}); T is water temperature (°C); and BW is body weight (kg).

Allocation for heat increment of feeding (HiE)

Estimation of heat increment of feeding (HiE) in fish has been approached in several different manners. Most studies have relied on empirically examining efficiency of conversion of metabolizable energy intake (ME) to RE using comparative carcass analysis and simple linear models. Studies have revealed a highly linear relationship between RE and ME (Azevedo *et al.*, 1998, 2005; Lupatsch *et al.*, 1998; Bureau *et al.*, 2002). HiE represents the inefficiency of using ME for RE. Current studies suggest that HiE is approximately equivalent to 0.60 RE for rainbow trout and other salmonid fish species (Bureau *et al.*, 2003).

Allocation for non-faecal energy losses (UE + ZE)

Energy loss through urine and the gills (non-faecal energy losses, UE + ZE) is mainly the result of excretion of metabolic nitrogenous wastes. Ammonia represents at least 85% of the nitrogenous wastes produced by fish, whereas urea excretion generally represents less than 15% (Kaushik and Cowey, 1991). Energy of combustion value of ammonia (82.3% N by weight) and urea (46.7% N by weight) is 20.5 kJ g^{-1} (24.9 kJ g^{-1} N) and 10.5 kJ g^{-1} (22.5 kJ g^{-1} N), respectively (Brafield and Llewellyn, 1982). Since most nitrogen losses are as ammonia, and the difference in the amount of energy loss per g N between ammonia and urea is small, it has been proposed that the loss of 1 g of nitrogen by fish under normal conditions could be equivalent to an energy loss of 24.9 kJ (Cho and Kaushik, 1990). Estimation of UE + ZE has therefore often been calculated based on nitrogen losses by the fish, which can be predicted from the difference between digestible nitrogen intake (DNI) and recovered nitrogen (RN).

Loss of other energy-yielding molecules (glucose, amino acids, creatine, trimethylamine oxide, etc.) has been shown to occur in fish, but they represent a small amount of energy loss. Current studies suggest that UE + ZE will be, at most, equivalent to 0.09 (HeE + RE + HiE) for rainbow trout and other salmonid fish species (Bureau *et al.*, 2003).

Estimate minimum DE requirement and feed allocation/requirement

The Fish-PrFEQ model estimates the minimum digestible energy requirement associated with a given weight gain to be the sum of retained energy (RE) and energy losses (HeE + HiE + ZE + UE). Using this approach, Bureau *et al.* (2003) calculated energy, oxygen and feed requirements and expected feed efficiency of fish of different sizes reared under different conditions or rearing periods. Table 20.2 presents energy and oxygen requirements of rainbow trout reared at 12°C and fed a diet with 44% DP and 20 MJ DE at different sizes or growing from 1 g to 1000 g with a TGC = 0.220. The DE requirement to produce 1 kg

Table 20.2. Energy requirements and expected feed efficiency of rainbow trout at various sizes or growing from 1 to 1000 g based on assumption that the fish are reared at 12°C, growing with a TGC = 0.220 and fed a diet with 22 g DP MJ^{-1} DE and 20 MJ kg^{-1} DE.

Live weight (g fish^{-1})	MJ kg^{-1} BW gain RE[a]	HeE[b]	HiE[c]	UE + ZE[d]	DE[e]	Feed efficiency[f]
1	5.6	1.1	3.4	0.9	11.0	1.82
5	5.6	1.6	3.4	1.0	11.5	1.73
10	5.7	1.8	3.4	1.0	11.8	1.68
50	6.0	2.4	3.6	1.1	13.1	1.53
100	6.4	2.7	3.8	1.7	14.1	1.42
500	9.6	3.5	5.8	1.7	20.6	0.97
1000	13.4	4.0	8.2	2.3	28.0	0.71
1–1000	9.3	3.4	5.6	1.6	19.3	1.00

[a]RE (MJ kg^{-1} BW gain) = (GE at final BW – GE at initial BW) BW^{-1} gain where GE (gross energy content of carcass, kJ fish^{-1}) = $0.0039*BW^2 + 5.5812*BW$ (Bureau *et al.*, 2003).
[b]HeE (MJ kg^{-1} BW gain) = $((-0.01 + 3.26T - 0.05T^2)*BW^{0.824})$ BW^{-1} gain (Cho, 1991).
[c]HiE (MJ kg^{-1} BW gain) = 0.60*RE (Azevedo *et al.*, 1998).
[d]UE + ZE (MJ kg^{-1} BW gain) = 0.09* (HeE + RE + HiE) (Bureau *et al.*, 2003).
[e]DE requirement (MJ kg^{-1} BW gain) = RE + HeE + HiE + UE + ZE.
[f]Expected feed efficiency = BW gain feed^{-1}.

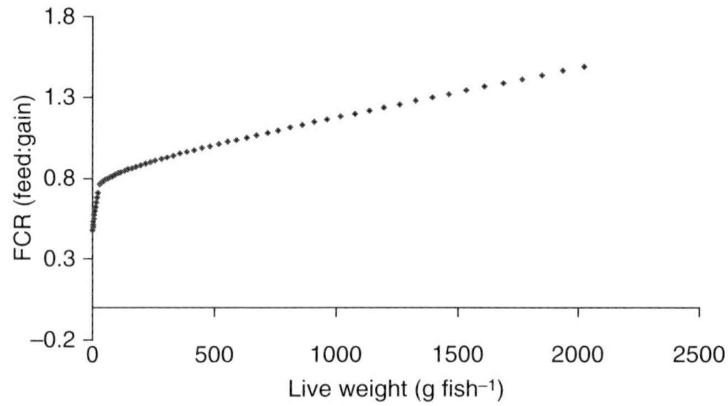

Fig. 20.7. Theoretical estimates (instantaneous) of FCR of rainbow trout at increasing live weight generated using the factorial bioenergetics model of Cho (1991) as adapted by Bureau *et al.* (2003).

biomass (e.g. 1000 fish gaining 1 g each) varies from about 11 MJ for 1-g fish to 28 MJ for 1-kg fish. Since DE requirement and, consequently, feed requirement can be calculated for different time intervals or for different conditions, this approach can also be used to generate theoretical estimates of FCR of fish as a function of various factors, such as diet composition, growth rate and environmental conditions. Figure 20.7 presents theoretical 'instantaneous' FCR of rainbow trout of different live weights. This theoretical curve, shown to be realistic by comparison to experimental data, illustrates the dramatic change in FCR as fish grow. This analysis indicates that comparisons of FCR across studies, farms, seasons, sampling intervals, etc. have to be made with caution.

Use of Bioenergetics and Mass Balance Models to Predict Waste Outputs by Fish Culture Operations

Besides helping in determining growth and feed requirement of fish stocks, bioenergetic models, such as the Fish-PrFEQ model, have also been used to drive nutrient (elemental) mass balance models and generate estimates of waste output by fish culture operations. The release of solid wastes from fish culture operation to environment is a function of the digestibility of various components (dry matter, N, P, etc.) of the feed, whereas the release of dissolved N and P wastes is a function of the metabolic waste production of fish. By including information (or submodels) on the chemical composition of fish produced, the chemical composition of feed used and the digestibility of the feed components, studies have generated estimates of solid, N and P waste outputs of fish culture operations (Cho *et al.*, 1991, 1994; Bureau *et al.*, 2003; Papatryphon *et al.*, 2005). Hua (2005) expanded the scope of this kind of approach and constructed a phosphorus utilization model for salmonid fish species by integrating literature data on P utilization. The model operates within the framework of the Fish-PrFEQ bioenergetics model and estimates the effects of different dietary P sources and levels on P digestibility, retention and waste output.

Limitations of Bioenergetics

Bioenergetic models, such as the one proposed by Cho (1991), are very useful and practical as they allow modelling of feed requirement and prediction of feed efficiency simply on the basis of relatively straightforward estimations of DE requirement of fish, rather than through a detailed analysis of nutrient deposition and nutritional composition of the feed. Comparison of feeds can also be done simply on the basis of their DE content. The suitability of comparing feeds on the basis of their DE content has been demonstrated on numerous occasions, although a number of studies have shown that comparisons need to be made carefully, notably when dealing with feeds with high digestible carbohydrate content (Bureau *et al.*, 1998) or comparing different fish species or fish at different life stages (Azevedo *et al.*, 2004a,b).

The user of bioenergetics models should always remember that bioenergetics is a 'methodology' or 'system'. Animals do not metabolize 'energy' per se, but metabolize 'nutrients'. The amount of energy effectively 'retained' or 'harnessed' during life processes (efficiency of energy utilization) is governed by which and/or how these nutrients are utilized. More importantly, most nutrients have very specific roles and many nutrients cannot be substituted by one another. Studies indicate that utilization of energy-yielding nutrients is highly dependent on the type of nutrients (not simply their 'energy' value), the balance between these nutrients and the genetics and physiological state of the fish (Azevedo *et al.*, 2004a,b; Encarnação *et al.*, 2004; Tapia-Salazar *et al.*, 2006). Considering nutrient inputs simply on the basis of their 'free energy' content is, therefore, largely irrational. Bioenergetics embodies well the adage that states 'All models are wrong, but some models are useful' (Box, 1979).

Arguably the most significant limitation of bioenergetics models is that they are based on 'hierarchy of energy allocation'. Growth is the surplus of energy after all other components of the energy budget have been covered or satisfied (Kitchell *et al.*, 1977). Bioenergetics models consequently predict that, when body energy gain (recovered energy (RE) according to the NRC (1981) nomenclature) is nil (RE = 0), growth (live weight gain) and feed efficiency (gain feed^{-1}) should also be nil. Bioenergetic models consequently assume that the relationship between 'energy deposition' and growth (biomass gain) is absolute, an assumption that has been shown to be inaccurate. RE reflects the 'weighed average' of the deposition of energy-yielding nutrients (mostly protein and lipids) in the body of the animal. Volumes of evidence indicate that animals (pig, chicken, fish) fed a ration allowing a RE = 0 can still deposit body protein (positive nitrogen balance and associated energy gain) and gain weight, while mobilizing body lipids (Fig. 20.8). Live weight gain is consequently driven by protein deposition, since there are 3–6 g of water associated with each g of tissue protein deposited (Cho and Kaushik, 1990; Bureau *et al.*, 2002). Lipid gain results

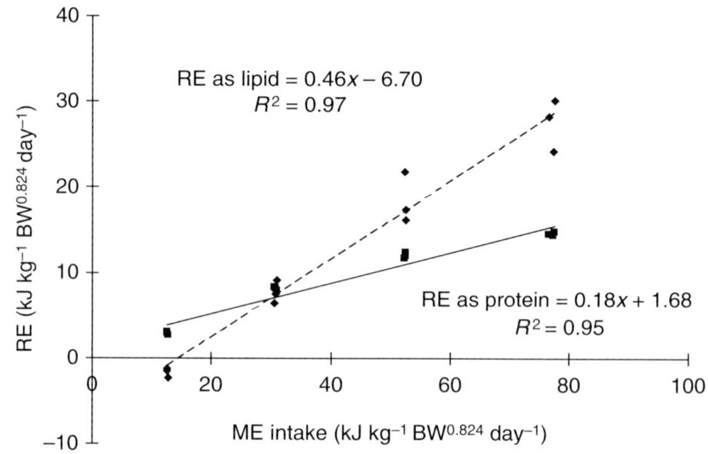

Fig. 20.8. Recovered energy (RE) as protein and lipid[a] as a function of metabolizable energy (ME) intake of rainbow trout reared at 8.5°C for 24 weeks (data from Bureau *et al.*, 2006).
[a]RE as lipid was calculated as the difference between RE and RE as protein.

in no or insignificant live weight gain since, in fish, lipids are stored in tissues by substituting water (Shearer, 1994).

Through the use of a single parameter for growth (RE), bioenergetics models also conceal the fact that protein and lipid depositions are achieved through different processes and have different effects on live weight gain of the animal. They also overlook the fact that protein and lipid depositions have different energetic efficiencies. Efficiencies of digestible or metabolizable energy intake for protein (k_p) and lipid (k_f) accretion in fish have been estimated by a factorial approach proposed by Kielanowski (1965). These estimates are highly variable. Estimates of k_p were reported to range from 0.43 to 0.81 for different fish species, whereas estimates of k_f were between 0.60 and 0.90 (Schwartz and Kirchgessner, 1995; Rodehutscord and Pfeffer, 1999; Lupatsch *et al.*, 2001, 2003; Azevedo *et al.*, 2005). Van Milgen and Noblet (1999) proposed a multivariate model to overcome major drawbacks of the factorial approach where it inverts the dependent and independent variables. This approach has been employed for rainbow trout and Atlantic salmon (Azevedo *et al.*, 2005).

These partial efficiencies can be very useful in expanding the accuracy of current bioenergetics models for fish, as has been done for current feed requirement systems for pigs (NRC, 1998), chicken (NRC, 1994), beef cattle (NRC, 2000) and dairy cattle (NRC, 2001; Kebreab *et al.*, 2003). However, the relative importance of protein and lipid deposition depends on a great number of biological and nutritional factors. Azevedo *et al.* (2005) observed that estimates obtained with these approaches were highly dependent on the model and model assumptions used. These models, although useful, are based on statistical relationships between inputs and outputs, without a representation of underlying biological principles. They are, therefore, too simplistic, highly sensitive to statistical artefacts and not sufficiently flexible for use under a wide range of conditions.

The Next Generation: Nutrient-flow Models for Fish?

The current bioenergetic models are useful, but are neither rational nor robust enough to describe adequately and predict efficiency of conversion of dietary inputs into fish biomass under a wide variety of conditions. Studies suggest that the development of robust, widely applicable models of feed utilization for fish cannot, in the long term, be based simply on 'energy' utilization (even if based on net energy values). There is a need to develop more rational and mechanistic approaches of representing growth and feed and nutrient utilization in fish. More work needs to be carried out to understand better the impacts of dietary, environmental and endogenous factors on nutrient utilization and accretion in fish. More accurate definitions of 'nutrient' accretions need also to be developed in order to move from approaches that are based simply on 'net' accretion (or mobilization) of nutrients to approaches taking into account the real contributions of different processes.

Biochemical models, based on an explicit representation of biochemical reactions in individual tissues, are more complex but more flexible for use under a wide range of conditions compared to empirical models. By explicitly modelling the metabolic use of nutrients, a more accurate representation of nutrient utilization can be achieved (van der Meer and van Dam, 1998; Birkett and de Lange, 2001a). However, these models are often more complex than what is required to represent growth at the whole-animal level (van der Honing, 1998; Birkett and de Lange, 2001a). Also, some factors that are known to influence growth (genotype, health, environment, etc.) are difficult to represent in biochemical models. An intermediate between the previous two types of models is the nutrient-flow model. In this model, nutrient transformations are represented at the whole-animal level and based on biological principles. This type of model is used successfully in pigs (Birkett and de Lange, 2001a,b,c). The nutrient-flow model developed by Birkett and de Lange (2001b) considers nutrient/metabolite flows in six functionally distinct biological processes, i.e.: (i) nutrient intake; (ii) the conversion of absorbed nutrients to anabolic and energy-yielding substrates; (iii) faecal excretion of non-digested and endogenous material; (iv) urinary excretion of non-metabolizable and endogenous material; (v) the synthesis of animal products, their retention or secretion; and (vi) basal nutrient expenditure.

The model of Birkett and de Lange (2001a,b,c) is currently being adapted to fish. Some aspects of the pig model (e.g. input and 'initial state' variables, nutrient partitioning 'rules', efficiency and boundaries of conversion of surplus amino acid and glucose into fatty acids) may not be well suited to poikilotherms such as fish. Part of the model of Birkett and de Lange (2001a,b,c) may need to be modified significantly and/or expanded to incorporate elements that are more consistent with fish biology, nutrition and culture.

It is the goal of animal production operations to base their management decisions on taking into account all the various interacting factors that affect nutrient efficiency and profitability for a specific culture operation. The most effective model should explicitly represent nutrient utilization, so causal relationships between nutrition, genetics, health, animal management, growth performance and nutrient excretion can then be established, and the response to different management strategies can be investigated, along with the associated financial and environmental consequences. Nutrient-flow models should be more robust than current bioenergetic models towards achieving this goal. By accurately describing and predicting the conversion of dietary inputs into fish biomass, it will be possible to provide a more rational means of constructing strategies to improve the economic and environmental sustainability of fish culture operations.

References

Azevedo, P.A., Cho, C.Y., Leeson, S. and Bureau, D.P. (1998) Effects of feeding level and water temperature on growth, nutrient and energy utilization and waste outputs of rainbow trout (*Oncorhynchus mykiss*). *Aquatic Living Resources* 11, 227–238.

Azevedo, P.A., Bureau, D.P., Leeson, S. and Cho, C.Y. (2002) Growth and efficiency of feed usage by Atlantic salmon (*Salmo salar*) fed diets with different dietary protein: energy ratios at two feeding levels. *Fisheries Science* 68, 878–888.

Azevedo, P.A., Leeson, S., Cho, C.Y. and Bureau, D.P. (2004a) Growth, nitrogen, and energy utilization by four juvenile salmonid species: diet, species, and size effects. *Aquaculture* 234, 393–414.

Azevedo, P.A., Leeson, S., Cho, C.Y. and Bureau, D.P. (2004b) Growth and feed utilization of large size rainbow trout and Atlantic salmon reared in freshwater: diet and species effects, and responses over time. *Aquaculture Nutrition* 10, 401–411.

Azevedo, P.A., van Milgen, J., Leeson, S. and Bureau, D.P. (2005) Comparing efficiency of metabolizable energy utilization by rainbow trout (*Oncorhynchus mykiss*) and Atlantic salmon (*Salmo salar*) using factorial and multivariate approaches. *Journal of Animal Science* 83, 842–851.

Birkett, S. and Lange, C.F.M. de (2001a) Limitations of conventional models and a conceptual framework for a nutrient flow representation of energy utilization by animals. *British Journal of Nutrition* 86, 647–659.

Birkett, S. and Lange, C.F.M. de (2001b) A computational framework for a nutrient flow representation of energy utilization by growing monogastric animals. *British Journal of Nutrition* 86, 661–674.

Birkett, S. and Lange, C.F.M. de (2001c) Calibration of a nutrient flow model of energy utilization by growing pigs. *British Journal of Nutrition* 86, 675–689.

Box, G.E.P. (1979) Robustness in scientific model building. In: Launer, R.L. and Wilkinson, G.N. (eds) *Robustness in Statistics*. Academic Press, New York, pp. 201–236.

Brafield, A.E. and Llewellyn, M.J. (1982) *Animal Energetics*. Blackie and Son Ltd, Glasgow, UK.

Bureau, D.P., Kirkland, J.B. and Cho, C.Y. (1998) The partitioning of energy from digestible carbohydrate by rainbow trout (*Oncorhynchus mykiss*). In: McCracken, K.J., Unsworth, E.F. and Wylie, A.R.G. (eds) *Energy Metabolism of Farm Animals*. CAB International, Wallingford, UK, pp. 163–166.

Bureau, D.P., Kaushik, S.J. and Cho, C.Y. (2002) Bioenergetics. In: Halver, J.E. and Hardy, R.W. (eds) *Fish Nutrition*. Academic Press, San Diego, California, pp. 1–53.

Bureau, D.P., Gunther, S.J. and Cho, C.Y. (2003) Chemical composition and preliminary theoretical estimates of waste outputs of rainbow trout reared on commercial cage culture operations in Ontario. *North American Journal of Aquaculture* 65, 33–38.

Bureau, D.P., Hua, K. and Cho, C.Y. (2006) Effect of feeding level on growth and nutrient deposition in rainbow trout (*Oncorhynchus mykiss* Walbaum) growing from 150 to 600 g. *Aquaculture Research* 37, 1090–1098.

Cho, C.Y. (1991) Prediction model for energy requirement of salmonid fishes. In: Wenk, C. and Boessinger, M. (eds) *Proceedings of the 12th Symposium of Energy Metabolism of Farm Animals*, EAAP Publication No. 58. Institut für Nutztierwissenschaften, Gruppe Ernahrung, Zurich, Switzerland, pp. 446–449.

Cho, C.Y. (1992) Feeding systems for rainbow trout and other salmonids with reference to current estimates of energy and protein requirements. *Aquaculture* 100, 107–123.

Cho, C.Y. and Bureau, D.P. (1998) Development of bioenergetic models and the Fish-PrFEQ software to estimate production, feeding ration and waste output in aquaculture. *Aquatic Living Resources* 11, 199–210.

Cho, C.Y. and Kaushik, S.J. (1990) Nutritional energetics in fish: energy and protein utilization in rainbow trout (*Salmo gairdneri*). *World Review of Nutrition and Dietetics* 61, 132–172.

Cho, C.Y., Slinger, S.J. and Bayley, H.S. (1982) Bioenergetics of salmonid fishes: energy intake, expenditure and productivity. *Comparative Biochemistry and Physiology* 73B, 25–41.

Cho, C.Y., Hynes, J.D., Wood, K.R. and Yoshida, H.K. (1991) Quantitation of fish culture wastes by biological (nutritional) and chemical (limnological) methods; the development of high nutrient dense (HND) diets. In: Cowey, C.B. and Cho, C.Y. (eds) *Nutritional Strategies and Aquaculture Waste. Proceedings of the 1st International Symposium on Nutritional Strategies in Management of Aquaculture Waste.* Fish Nutrition Research Laboratory, University of Guelph, Canada, pp. 37–50.

Cho, C.Y., Hynes, J.D., Wood, K.R. and Yoshida, H.K. (1994) Development of high nutrient-dense, low pollution diets and prediction of aquaculture wastes using biological approaches. *Aquaculture* 124, 293–305.

Cui, Y. and Xie, S. (1999) Modelling growth in fish. In: Theodorou, M.K. and France, J. (eds) *Feeding Systems and Feed Evaluation Models*. CAB International, Wallingford, UK, pp. 413–434.

Encarnação, P.M., Lange, C.F.M. de, Rodehutscord, M., Hoehler, D., Bureau, W. and Bureau, D.P. (2004) Diet digestible energy content affects lysine utilization, but not dietary lysine requirement of rainbow trout (*Oncorhynchus mykiss*) for maximum growth. *Aquaculture* 235, 569–586.

Hua, K. (2005) Modelling phosphorus utilization in salmonid fish species. PhD thesis, University of Guelph, Guelph, Canada.

Iwama, G.K. and Tautz, A.F. (1981) A simple growth model for salmonids in hatcheries. *Canadian Journal of Fisheries and Aquatic Sciences* 38, 649–656.

Kaushik, S.J. (1998) Nutritional bioenergetics and estimation of waste production in non-salmonids. *Aquatic Living Resources* 11, 211–217.

Kaushik, S.J. and Cowey, C.B. (1991) Dietary factors affecting nitrogen excretion by fish. In: Cowey, C.B. and Cho, C.Y. (eds) *Nutritional Strategies and Aquaculture Waste. Proceedings of the 1st International Symposium on Nutritional Strategies in Management of Aquaculture Waste.* Fish Nutrition Research Laboratory, University of Guelph, Ontario, pp. 3–19.

Kaushik, S.J. and Médale, F. (1994) Energy requirements, utilization and dietary supply to salmonids. *Aquaculture* 124, 81–97.

Kebreab, E., France, J., Agnew, R.E., Yan, T., Dhanoa, M.S., Dijkstra, J., Beever, D.E. and Reynolds, C.K. (2003) Alternatives to linear analysis of energy balance data from lactating dairy cows. *Journal of Dairy Science* 86, 2904–2913.

Kielanowski, J. (1965) Estimates of the energy cost of protein deposition in growing animals. In: Blaxter, K.L. (ed.) *Proceedings of the 3rd Symposium on Energy Metabolism, Troon, Scotland*. Academic Press, London, pp. 13–20.

Kitchell, J.F., Stewart, D.J. and Weininger, D. (1977) Applications of a bioenergetics model to yellow perch (*Perca flavescens*) and walleye (*Stizostedion vitreum vitreum*). *Journal of the Fisheries Research Board of Canada* 34, 1922–1935.

Lloyd, L.E., McDonald, B.E. and Crampton, E.W. (1978) *Fundamentals of Nutrition*, 2nd edn. W.H. Freeman and Company, San Francisco, California.

Lupatsch, I. and Kissil, G.W. (2005) Feed formulations based on energy and protein demands in white grouper (*Epinephelus aeneus*). *Aquaculture* 248, 83–95.

Lupatsch, I., Kissil, G.W., Sklan, D. and Pfeffer, E. (1998) Energy and protein requirements for maintenance and growth in gilthead seabream (*Sparus aurata* L.). *Aquaculture Nutrition* 4, 165–173.

Lupatsch, I., Kissil, G.W. and Sklan, D. (2001) Optimization of feeding regimes for European seabass *Dicentrarchus labrax*: a factorial approach. *Aquaculture* 202, 289–302.

Lupatsch, I., Kissil, G.W. and Sklan, D. (2003) Comparison of energy and protein efficiency among three fish species, gilthead seabream (*Sparus aurata*), European seabass (*Dicentrarchus labrax*) and white grouper (*Epinephelus aeneus*): energy expenditure for protein and lipid deposition. *Aquaculture* 225, 175–189.

Muller-Feuga, A. (1990) *Modélisation de la croissance des poissons en élevage*. Rapports scientifiques et techniques de Ifremer, No. 21, 58 pp.

National Research Council (NRC) (1981) *Nutrient Requirements of Coldwater Fishes.* National Academy Press, Washington, DC.

National Research Council (NRC) (1994) *Nutrient Requirements of Poultry*, 9th edn. National Academy Press, Washington, DC.

National Research Council (NRC) (1998) *Nutrient Requirements of Swine*, 10th edn. National Academy Press, Washington, DC.

National Research Council (NRC) (2000) *Nutrient Requirements of Beef Cattle*, 8th edn. National Academy Press, Washington, DC.

National Research Council (NRC) (2001) *Nutrient Requirements of Dairy Cattle*, 7th rev. edn. National Academy Press, Washington, DC.

Oldham, J.D., Emmans, G. and Kyriazakis, I. (1997) Limits and limitations to nitrogen use in farm animals. *Proceedings of the Nutrition Society* 56, 535–545.

Papatryphon, E., Petit, J., Van Der Werf, H.M.G., Sadasivam, K.J. and Claver, K. (2005) Nutrient-balance modeling as a tool for environmental management in aquaculture: the case of trout farming in France. *Environmental Management* 35, 161–174.

Reid, G.K. (2004) Evaluation of nutrient loading dynamics from tank and cage cultured rainbow trout. PhD thesis, University of Guelph, Guelph, Ontario.

Rodehutscord, M. and Pfeffer, E. (1999) Maintenance requirement for digestible energy and efficiency of utilisation of digestible energy for retention in rainbow trout, *Oncorhynchus mykiss*. *Aquaculture* 179, 95–107.

Schwartz, F.J. and Kirchgessner, M. (1995) Effects of different diets and levels of feeding on retention and efficiency of utilization of energy and protein by carp. *Journal of Applied Ichthyology* 11, 363–366.

Shearer, K.D. (1994) Factors affecting the proximate composition of cultured fishes with emphasis on salmonids. *Aquaculture* 119, 63–88.

Tapia-Salazar, M., Bureau, W., Panserat, S., Corraze, G. and Bureau, D.P. (2006) Effect of DHA supplementation on digestible starch utilization by rainbow trout. *British Journal of Nutrition* 95, 76–87.

van der Honing, Y. (1998) Perspectives of future feed information based on energy and nutrient availability. *Archiv für Tierernahrung* 51, 135–153.

van der Meer, M.B., and van Dam, A.A. (1998) Modelling growth of *Colossoma macropomum* (Cuvier): comparison of an empirical and an explanatory model. *Aquaculture Research* 29, 313–332.

van Milgen, J. and Noblet, J. (1999) Energy partitioning in growing pigs: the use of a multivariate model as an alternative for the factorial analysis. *Journal of Animal Science* 77, 2154–2162.

Zhou, A., Xie, S., Lei, W., Zhu, X. and Yang, Y. (2005) A bioenergetic model to estimate feed requirement of gibel carp, *Carassius auratus gibelio*. *Aquaculture* 248, 287– 297.

21 Integrated Approaches to Evaluate Nutritional Strategies for Dairy Cows

A. Bannink,[1] J.W. Reijs[2] and J. Dijkstra[2,3]

[1]*Wageningen University Research Centre, Animal Sciences Group, Division of Animal Production, The Netherlands;* [2]*Department of Animal Sciences, Wageningen University, The Netherlands;* [3]*Animal Nutrition Group, Wageningen Institute of Animal Sciences, Wageningen University, The Netherlands*

Introduction

Dairy farming has intensified in the past decades with respect to herd size, the number of animals per hectare and cow productivity, causing a major shift in the practice of dairy farming and imposing an increased burden on the environment. Gaseous emissions and nutrient losses that originate from animals, animal excreta, stored and applied manure and soils prepared to produce animal feeds may strongly affect the quality of ground and surface waters (nitrate, phosphate) and air quality (ammonia, methane and nitrous oxides). As a consequence of this, the ecology of nearby more natural systems also becomes affected. In order to alleviate the impact of intensified dairy farming on the environment, governments are introducing increasingly stringent policies on agricultural emissions oriented not only at targets that must be met, but also as specific measures that need to be adopted (Oenema *et al.*, 2001a).

For this reason, there is an increased interest in investigating the potential of specific on-farm measures and of government policies to mitigate the impact of dairy farms on the environment. Realistic estimates of the type and magnitude of this impact can be obtained only with accurate prediction of the consequences of a nutritional strategy on the volume and composition of milk produced, on the rate of excretion and composition of urine and faeces, on the rate of methane and ammonia emissions, on the rate of manure digestion during storage and on the composition and characteristics of manure after storage and with field application. Empirical relationships mostly predict a single aspect of nutrition, such as rumen microbial synthesis (Oldick *et al.*, 1999), methane emission (Yan *et al.*, 2000; Mills *et al.*, 2003), nitrogen (N) excretion (Kebreab *et al.*, 2001; Schröder *et al.*, 2006) or ammonia emission (De Boer *et al.*, 2002; Monteny *et al.*, 2002; Van Duinkerken *et al.*, 2005). These relationships may very well serve the specific goal for which they were derived. However, they are capable neither of covering several relevant aspects simultaneously nor of treating them in an integrated manner. In this respect, following a more mechanistic and dynamic approach appears more promising (Bannink *et al.*, 2005).

This chapter discusses the possibility of applying more integrated approaches when evaluating nutritional strategies for dairy cows, simultaneously in detail and from several aspects. Figure 21.1 demonstrates the different levels of aggregation that may be covered by models. Primarily, the chapter handles the integration of details at the sub-cow level to the cow level and explains several physiological aspects and consequences of nutrition strategies for dairy cows. However, a nutritional strategy that appears more successful at the cow level does not necessarily need to be more successful at the level of the whole farming system, including forage production, import of concentrates and production and application of manure (Schröder *et al.*, 2006). For this reason, a limited attempt has been made at integration with other aspects of the whole farming system.

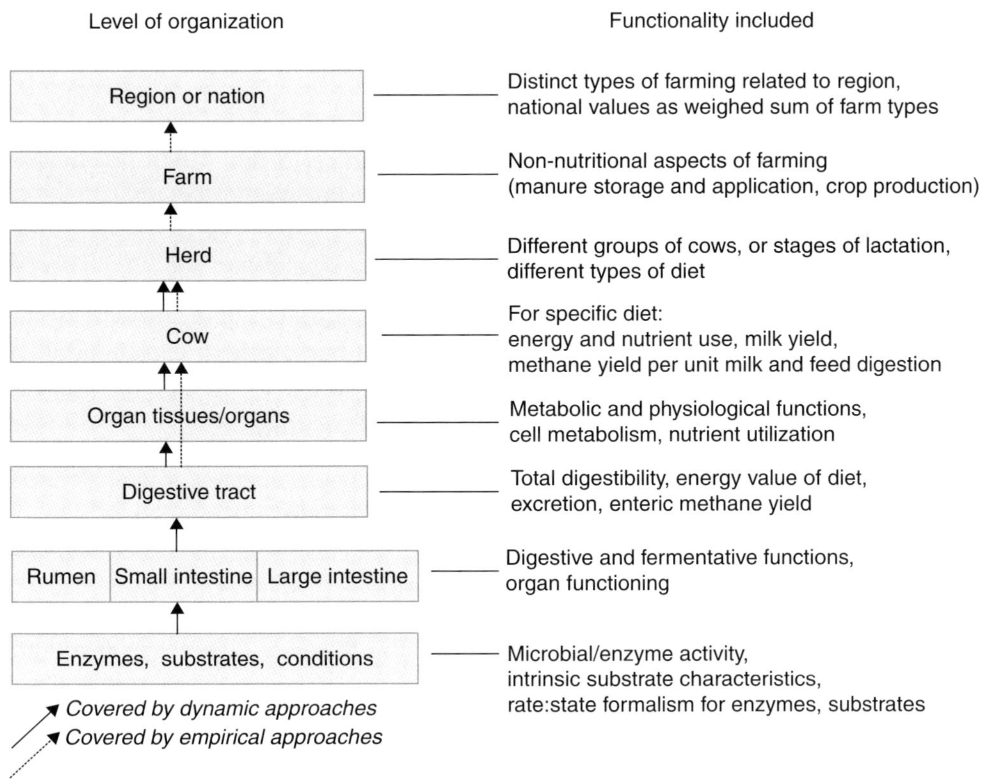

Fig. 21.1. Schematic diagram of the levels of organization that are covered by currently available dynamic and empirical approaches to evaluate the consequences of nutritional strategies for dairy cows (adapted from Bannink *et al.*, 2005).

Modelling Efforts

In current practice, the energy and protein values of a diet are assessed by separate feed evaluation systems that generally can be characterized as empirical and static models of cow performance. Constant feeding values are assumed for dietary ingredients, irrespective of feeding conditions and of the type of diet or cow involved. Another limitation is the impracticality of these systems when it comes to evaluating aspects of cow performance other than feeding value, such as excreta composition, slurry or manure characteristics and gaseous emissions. In order to overcome at least some of the above limitations, there have been numerous modelling efforts to develop more detailed and dynamic models that take into account lower levels of aggregation (Fig. 21.1). In the remainder of this section, the applicability of these dynamic models will be discussed, before considering the evaluation of nutritional strategies in a following section.

Dynamic, mechanistic models

Extant dynamic, mechanistic models of the physiology of the dairy cow cover several levels of aggregation in order to evaluate the effect of nutritional strategies on digestive functions, intermediary metabolism and productive functions (Baldwin *et al.*, 1987a,b,c; Danfær, 1990; Dijkstra *et al.*, 1992, 1996; Mills *et al.*, 2001). Also, models are available which represent the metabolic conversion of nutrients by liver, mammary gland and fat tissue (Miller, 1990; Freetly *et al.*, 1993; Hanigan and Baldwin, 1994). Although very much depending on the specific goal for which the models were constructed, they all adopt a highly integrative approach with respect to the representation of interactions between different types of nutrients, of the combined effect of metabolizable energy and protein and of the functioning and nutrient partition between distinct organs. This quality gives these models the latent advantage of being able to explain additional details of the consequences of nutritional strategies in comparison to current static feed evaluation systems. This advantage is important in order to obtain results that are realistic, understandable and accurate enough to evaluate the practicality and effectiveness of proposed nutritional strategies for multiple aspects of cow performance. A further advantage is that these models may indicate how such effective measures can be translated to other nutritional or farming conditions.

In the remainder of this section, the subjects of feed digestibility, cow metabolism and the whole farming system will be discussed further to demonstrate how dynamic models, which may or may not yet have been developed in these areas, may be of use.

Feed digestibility

Feed digestibility is the most important determinant of feeding value and of the level of production that may be achieved with the amount of dry matter consumed.

All current feed evaluation systems require an estimate of diet digestibility as an input. Also, the more elaborate dynamic models make use of input parameters related to feed digestibility, but these apply to intrinsic feed characteristics indicating the degradability of a feed, leaving diet digestibility as an outcome of the model instead of an input (Bannink *et al.*, 2006a). An example of such a model is the dynamic model of rumen digestion of Dijkstra *et al.* (1992). This model uses the degradation characteristics of starch, protein and cell wall carbohydrates (neutral detergent fibre; NDF), which is an important and pragmatic extension to earlier modelling efforts (France *et al.*, 1982; Baldwin *et al.*, 1987b), assuming constant degradation characteristics. The model of Baldwin *et al.* (1987b) includes an elaborate 'physical' mechanism for the dynamics of substrate particle size reduction, of attachment and degradation of substrate particles by microorganisms and of the outflow of fluids, substrate particles and microorganisms. This mechanism may be capable of explaining some of the variations observed *in vivo* (Czerkawski, 1986; Baldwin, 1995; Kennedy, 2005), but it seems doubtful that the variation in intrinsic degradation characteristics as observed with *in situ* measurements can be fully represented in this manner (Bannink *et al.*, 1997). Both types of models have been enhanced with additional dynamic models (Baldwin *et al.*, 1987a,c; Mills *et al.*, 2001) or empirical equations (Dijkstra *et al.*, 1996) to extend model predictions to those of total digestibility and cow performance (Fig. 21.1).

The prediction of digestibility and feeding value using these models focuses strongly on the representation of the processes taking place in the lumen of the gastrointestinal tract. Although this primary focus is fully justified, it must be emphasized that some other aspects that may also be important remain unconsidered. The condition and activity of the rumen wall influences the microbial degradation of feed substrates in the lumen. The development and absorptive capacity of the rumen wall is, to a large part, the result of the cumulative effect of the nutritional strategy followed over time (Gäbel *et al.*, 2002). The development of the rumen wall may affect the incidence of low rumen pH strongly and, as a result, reduced microbial activity and NDF degradability, as evidenced by the occurrence of subclinical acidosis (Enemark *et al.*, 2002). Furthermore, a more developed rumen wall (proliferation of epithelia, larger papillae, larger absorptive area) results in more epithelial mass and, hence, a higher nutrient requirement by these metabolically highly active tissues. Bearing these aspects in mind, it is concluded that if the aim is to develop nutritional strategies, they need representation in future models of feed digestibility. The dynamic models discussed above are good candidates to accommodate such new aspects. Importantly, these models render the possibility of evaluating the implications of changes in nutritional strategy on these new aspects in an integrated manner, with the knowledge on digestive processes already included in them, as well as at a suitably low level of aggregation (Fig. 21.1).

Cow metabolism and production

Dynamic models of cow metabolism may focus on different levels of aggregation (Fig. 21.1). For example, models of the functioning of individual organs aim at explaining nutrient metabolism and nutrient flows to and from these organs (liver, Freetly *et al.*, 1993; mammary gland, Hanigan and Baldwin, 1994). Specifically, these models may deliver useful information, such as understanding of the process of milk synthesis as an outcome of the interaction between uptake and metabolism of different nutrients by the mammary gland. However, these models may also extend to the whole-cow level (Fig. 21.1) (e.g. Baldwin *et al.*, 1987a), or even to the level of the herd or farm (Mills *et al.*, 2001).

In most production conditions in western areas, the amount of metabolizable energy remains the primary factor limiting milk yield. For this reason, realistic representation of the processes in the gastrointestinal tract and accurate prediction of the site and amount of feed digestion should always be a prime objective when predicting the effect of nutritional strategy on cow performance. However, under specific conditions, the availability of either metabolizable protein or glucose may become more limiting than metabolizable energy (Dijkstra *et al.*, 1996). These aspects are discussed further in the section on digestibility, nutrients and milk yield.

Whole farming system

Many modelling efforts have been undertaken to represent the interactions between different subsystems of the whole farming system (herd, manure storage and handling, soil, cropping and feeding; e.g. Kohn *et al.*, 1997; Schröder *et al.*, 2006). Often, these efforts are directed at evaluating a specific aspect of farm performance, or at a combination of aspects such as N management (Dou *et al.*, 1996; Cabrera *et al.*, 2005; Cuttle and Jarvis, 2005), greenhouse gas (GHG) emissions (Jarvis and Pain, 1994; Schils *et al.*, 2005), ammonia emission (Ross *et al.*, 2002), or the economic consequences of specific management options (Mourits *et al.*, 2000). A common characteristic of these whole farming approaches is that static representations are used for the individual subsystems, with presumed values for transfer rates between these subsystems, such as the production levels achieved, the efficiency of feed conversion into milk and manure, emission rates and fertilizing value of manure, or losses from soil and crop yield. This modelling approach suits the goal of evaluating general types of farming systems and is strongly fed by results from farm monitoring. In essence, farm budgets are created with a spreadsheet-like approach from presumed index values in databases. Without doubt, these models are relevant in recognizing the relationship between whole-farm performance and management within the individual subsystems. Note, however, that model applicability is restricted mainly to a kind of categorization of farming types because index values are not predicted but derived from registered farm performance or from general values in databases. By no means can these models relate to the level of detail involved with farmer experience and the precise conditions met at a specific farm, nor can they be applied to enhance innovation within subsystems (Sterk *et al.*, 2006). Although it has been advocated to improve whole-farm models by making them applicable to specific niches (Sterk *et al.*, 2006), perhaps a better alternative to promote farm innovation is to include causal relationships and mechanistic dynamic models that do match the experience and level of detail needed by the farmer. The latent advantages offered by the latter category of models appear largely unrecognized or unexplored in studies and modelling efforts of whole farming systems (Bannink *et al.*, 2005, 2006a). The main reason for this is probably that questions on farm nutrient management originate from questions on whole-farm budgets, whereas more detailed dynamic models were developed to address questions on details of the subsystem level (manure, soils, crops, housing). For example, no innovative ration formulation (and associated farm management) may be expected when the models stick to calculation rules of current energy and protein evaluation systems for dairy cows. Introducing dynamic models can deliver new insights into how N excretion and N emissions may be reduced, or how supplementation of metabolizable protein (Bannink *et al.*, 2006a) and glucose (discussed later) may be optimized, without compromising digestive and productive functions, manure quality and other emissions (GHGs, discussed later). Such details have crucial implications for farm management and the outcomes of the whole farming system. For this reason, the more specialized dynamic models have a better prospect to approach the actual conditions met under specific farming conditions. This is an important prerequisite for the use of models for advisory purposes and to generate tailor-made (instead of general) outcomes allowing a cost–benefit analysis of the introduction of measures on specific farms (Sterk *et al.*, 2006).

Nutritional Strategies

The integrated approach when evaluating the effect of nutritional strategies will be illustrated by discussing some modelling results from the perspective of cow performance and performance of the whole farming system. Simulation results were obtained with the dynamic rumen model of Dijkstra *et al.* (1992) and a representation of the digestive processes in the gut and the nutrient requirements for milk production and maintenance according to Dijkstra *et al.* (1996), but recently adapted by Reijs *et al.* (2008, unpublished).

Implication for cow performance

The nutritional strategy largely determines cow performance. Economically, the most important aspects of performance are milk protein yield and cow fertility and health. However, from the perspective of legislation (with increasing economic consequences for the dairy farmer), other aspects such as excretion rate, type of excretion (urine or faeces), gaseous emissions and characteristics of fresh and stored manure are becoming just as, or even more, important. An evaluation of all these aspects simultaneously requires an integrated approach based on realistic and detailed representation of the cow's digestive processes, intermediary metabolism and productive processes. In this manner, insight can be gained into the consequences of various nutritional strategies for the different aspects of cow performance and, more importantly, the interaction between them. In the remainder of this section, the advantages that dynamic models offer will be illustrated by discussion of modelling efforts in the literature and presentation of some new simulation results.

Feed intake

As already discussed in the section on modelling efforts, milk yield is correlated strongly to the intake of digestible or metabolizable energy. This means that diet quality and dry matter intake are both important drives for milk yield. Most models of feed intake are empirically oriented and use inputs of the type of cow involved and the type of feed consumed. Probably the most reliable way to estimate feed intake is also to include the effect of milk yield and to derive regression equations for similar cows under similar conditions (Forbes, 2005). The idea of identifying a single feed factor controlling intake, such as rumen fill or another type of intake saturation value of a diet (CVB, 2005), or the energy value of a diet, seems to conflict with current evidence (Forbes, 2005). Many factors are involved that may represent physical factors as well as physiological chemical factors. There are clear indications that predominantly physical factors are important when the quality of the diet is low and the dry matter digestibility is less than 70%, whereas physiological factors become more important with a higher quality of diet (Ulyatt, 1973). Hence, it may be concluded that, for further improvement of predictions of feed intake, the consideration of the latter category of factors is a prerequisite.

Most dynamic models predict digestibility by taking dry matter intake as a driving input. Efforts of dynamic modelling which aim at a combined prediction of feed intake, as well as digestibility and cow performance, are essentially lacking. The main reason is probably that, despite its importance for the evaluation of nutritional strategies, it remains difficult to predict feed intake because the physiological control mechanisms involved, and the factors constraining intake, are not well understood or are difficult to characterize (Chapter 5). In principle, the dynamic models should be capable of representing the feed factors as well as the animal factors involved in the regulation of feed intake, in addition to the effects on feed digestibility already represented by current models. Also, the physical factors involved in feed intake (e.g. the mechanism of particle size reduction in the model of Baldwin *et al.*, 1987a) may be represented in dynamic models. The usefulness of dynamic models to predict feed intake has not yet been investigated.

In conclusion, dynamic models are promising tools to delineate the interaction between physical and physiological factors in regulating feed intake. They allow the consequences of changes in forage production (as a result of soil management, fertilization and harvesting and conservation management) for forage characteristics and cow performance (feed intake, digestibility, milk yield, excreta, emissions) to be investigated in an integrated manner.

Digestibility, nutrients and milk yield

The microbial population in the rumen degrades the main part of the feed ingested. Diet digestibility therefore depends, to a large extent, on the functioning of the rumen. Previous modelling efforts have already shown the effect of several nutritional factors (Dijkstra *et al.*, 1992; Baldwin, 1995; Bannink *et al.*, 2006a). However, these aspects are dealt with in other chapters (Chapters 7 and 8).

ENERGY AND PROTEIN DIGESTION. The effects of feed intake pattern and so-called synchronization of the degradability characteristics of dietary protein and energy on cow performance are not considered frequently in models. Often, synchronization of protein and energy availability for microbial utilization is thought to have beneficial effects on the efficiency of microbial protein synthesis. Although the evidence for this effect is not convincing, there may be other effects of synchronization that already are well known and do affect rumen functioning (Bannink and Tamminga, 2005; Hristov and Jouany, 2006). Synchronization may prevent extreme changes in pH, osmotic value and volume of rumen fluid. Also, as a side effect, a better mixing and balancing of the dietary ingredients in time (e.g. roughages and concentrates) may occur with a more synchronized feeding. Such effects in themselves may or may not be beneficial. For example, additional effects of a synchronization strategy may be changes in feed intake pattern, in the period of time spent ruminating, in particle size reduction, in particle passage rates, in saliva production, in buffering capacity of rumen fluid and, as a result, in the extent of NDF digestion.

Modelling efforts with an integrated approach in this area seem to be lacking, however. The only efforts known to include some of these effects are the subsequent adaptations of the model of Baldwin *et al.* (1987b), outlined again by Baldwin (1995) and adopted by Collao-Saenz *et al.* (2005). So far, the implications of these specific effects have not yet been studied, but perhaps more attention is needed in the future to incorporate these effects when evaluating consequences of nutritional strategies.

GLUCOSE DELIVERY. In many instances, the total amount of metabolizable energy in the diet dictates milk yield. However, in certain conditions the type of nutrient absorbed from the gastrointestinal tract also becomes more relevant for accurate prediction of cow performance. For high-yielding dairy cows during early lactation, glucose delivery seems critical for milk yield. This means that, for optimizing the nutritional strategy, an accurate prediction is needed of the amount of glucose delivered by the diet. Glucose originates from three major sources: propionate, produced in particular on fermentation of starch (Bannink *et al.*, 2006b), starch digested in the lower intestine (either from feed starch escaping rumen fermentation or microbial starch) and glucogenic amino acids digested in the lower intestine (from feed protein escaping rumen fermentation or microbial protein). The fraction of feed starch escaping rumen fermentation is not a constant, but also depends on rumen fermentation conditions (Fig. 21.2A). If small amounts are consumed, the apparent rumen digestibility becomes much smaller than indicated by nylon bag degradation characteristics. With very low levels of starch intake, starch outflow (including microbial starch) may even exceed the amount ingested (Fig. 21.2B), resulting in a negative apparent digestibility (Bannink and Tamminga, 2005). Estimating starch outflow directly from nylon

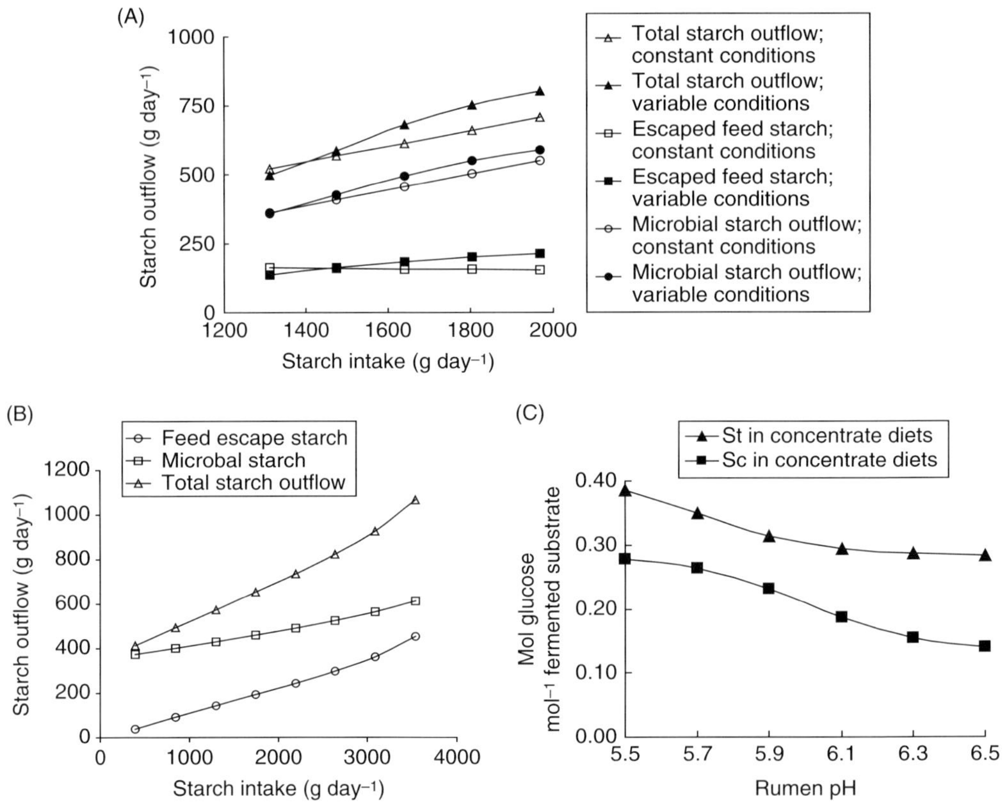

Fig. 21.2. Simulated effects of (A) feed intake level with a fixed dietary composition of 50% of dry matter from fresh ryegrass, 25% from maize silage and 25% from concentrate, assuming constant (open symbols) or altered rumen fermentation conditions (passage rates, pH and fluid volume; closed symbols), of (B) increased starch intake with substitution of maize silage for ryegrass (from 80, 0 and 20% fresh ryegrass, maize silage and concentrates in dietary DM, to 10, 70 and 20%, respectively; 20 kg of DM intake per day; maize silage and concentrate containing 225 and 100 g of starch kg^{-1} DM) on rumen starch outflow (including microbial starch), and of (C) rumen pH on the fraction of glucose (propionic acid) produced from soluble carbohydrates (Sc) and starch (St) fermented into VFA in concentrate-rich diets. Both (A) and (B) were adapted from Bannink *et al.* (2006a). Escaped feed starch includes outflow of soluble carbohydrates.

bag degradation characteristics therefore leads to inappropriate results under these conditions. Increasing starch intake by a higher intake rate of the same ration causes moderate changes in the apparent digestibility of starch (Fig. 21.2A). However, increasing starch intake to levels up to more than 3 kg starch day^{-1} by substitution of maize silage for ryegrass (Fig. 21.2B) causes apparent starch digestibility to become closer to direct estimates from nylon bag degradation characteristics of maize silage. The simulation studies indicate that microbial starch is a main fraction of total starch outflow, which strongly affects estimates of the apparent rumen digestion of starch. Furthermore, the fraction of feed starch escaping rumen fermentation may easily deviate from estimates obtained directly from nylon bag degradation characteristics. When using nylon bag data to estimate rumen starch digestion, it appears that *in vivo* an inaccuracy of 15% is to be expected, depending on feeding strategy. More dynamic modelling approaches should be capable of addressing such variation.

Recent regressions of *in vivo* observations of rumen function in lactating cows (Bannink *et al.*, 2006a) also indicate that the yield of propionate from fermented soluble carbohydrates and fermented starch is not constant, but increases drastically when rumen pH drops to values below 6.3 and 6.1 (Fig. 21.2C). A drop in pH from 6.5 to 5.5 would generate 100% more glucose from fermented soluble carbohydrates and about 25% more from fermented starch. Also, *in vivo* data of starch digestion, reviewed by Mills *et al.* (1999), clearly indicate the importance of pH for the fraction of propionate produced. The results indicate that more intensive feeding conditions (high levels of feed intake and concentrate feeding) lead to more propionate per unit of rapidly fermentable carbohydrates. Finally, a shortage in glucose delivery by the above two sources may be compensated by the synthesis of glucose from amino acids and other metabolites (lactate, glycerol) in the liver. The use of amino acids for gluconeogenesis reduces the efficiency of protein utilization. In situations where glucose delivery to the cow may be critical, adopting a dynamic approach appears decisive in circumventing the inaccuracy of more than 50% variation in predicted yields of propionate from rapidly fermentable carbohydrates and of 10 to perhaps even 20% variation in yields of rumen escape starch.

The foregoing illustrates that the amount of glucose generated from a specific starch source varies with nutritional strategy. The factors causing variation in glucose delivery and the consequences for milk yield can be taken into account by making use of dynamic models. In the future, the modelling aim may be extended to other metabolic functions that have a substantial glucose requirement. Such an extension might be helpful in obtaining insight when the competition for glucose utilization by the mammary gland and other functions (such as gastrointestinal tissues, liver, immune system, other maintenance) becomes critical for performance of high-yielding cows.

TYPE OF COW AND MILK YIELD. Next to energy intake, milk yield is also affected by the physiological state (mobilization or deposition of body reserves, pregnancy) and the genetic merit of the cow (potential for milk production). Empirical, as well as dynamic, models may well represent the characteristics of the type of cow involved. Only the dynamic models, however, are capable of representing the cow characteristics by changing specific parameters already included in the model, or by introducing an additional parameter as some sort of physiological set point. For example, varying the udder metabolic capacity may represent the difference in genetic potential for milk yield among cows (Johnson *et al.*, 2005). Also, the general aspects of the hormonal regulation of the cow's physiology can probably be represented in this manner, with or without a simultaneous change of sensitivity parameters (Baldwin *et al.*, 1987a; Gill *et al.*, 1989). Several examples of this approach can be found in the literature.

Implication for farm performance

The nutritional strategy followed is also an important determinant of whole-farm performance. Legislation, to an increasing extent, puts restrictions on the impact intensively managed dairy farms may have on the environment. This means that, besides cow productivity and efficiency of N utilization for milk production, other criteria become important, such as the emission rate of ammonia and GHGs, the rate and type of N and P excretion and the characteristics of manure during collection, storage and application. In the following paragraphs the relevance of adopting an integrated approach will be discussed for each of these aspects of farm performance and for measures that may be taken with forage production.

Gaseous emissions

AMMONIA FROM COW URINATION. The main part of ammonia emission originates from cow urination (Monteny, 2000). Under Dutch conditions of cow housing and manure storage, most of the ammonia from dairy cow houses originates from urine as slurry is collected and stored in covered pits and, subsequently, in covered manure stores. The emission rate both from urine and from slurry pits may vary strongly with the type of floor and the type of pit in use. Here, only those aspects that are affected directly by nutritional strategy will be discussed.

Ammonia originates from the conversion of urine urea by the high urease activity on fouled floors. From a nutritional perspective, the urea concentration in urine, urination frequency and urine pH are the principal determining factors. The urea concentration depends on the total amount of N and the fluid volume excreted with urine. The total amount of N excreted with urine depends, firstly, on the intake and utilization of N by the cow for productive purposes and, secondly, on the partition between N excretion with urine and faeces (Kebreab *et al.*, 2001; Schröder *et al.*, 2006). The volume of urine and the frequency of urination depend on the quantity of electrolytes and N that need to be excreted with urine (Bannink *et al.*, 1999). Furthermore, urine pH depends on the type of electrolytes ingested with feed, with a relative surplus of valence equivalents of cations or anions in the diet leading to alkaline or acidic urine. Figure 21.3A illustrates that, around zero surplus, the pH of urine is most sensitive to changes in electrolyte content in the diet. Usually, the high proportion of grass forages in the diet leads to a surplus of valence equivalents of cations (mainly potassium) and, hence, a strongly alkaline pH occurs, which supports ammonia emission. Supplementation with salts may change this surplus, as practised in the dry period in order to stimulate Ca mobilization after calving.

AMMONIA FROM MANURE STORAGE. Ammonia is also emitted from stored slurry and nutritional strategies affect ammonia concentration and pH of slurry just as much. Besides the effect of urine on the composition and pH of slurry (Monteny, 2000), stimulation of fermentation in the large intestine by an increase in bypass rate of potentially fermentable matter in the rumen may also lead to an increased content of volatile fatty acids (VFAs) and more acidified faeces. Based on various experiments, faecal pH can vary from less than 6 to more than 7 (Fig. 21.3B).

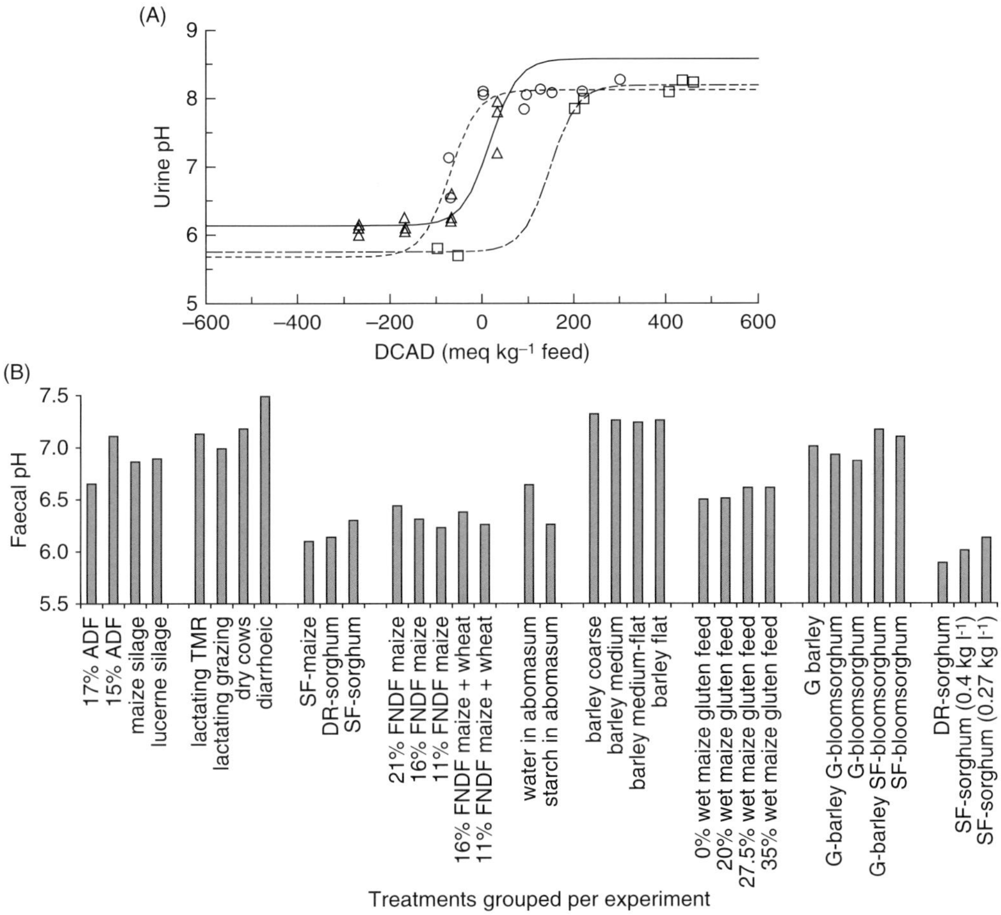

Fig. 21.3. Effects of diet on the pH of urine and faeces excreted by dairy cows. (A) Effect of the dietary cation anion balance (DCAD) on urine pH for three different experiments (results adapted from Oenema *et al.*, 2001b). Different symbols (○ ------; Δ —; □ — - — -) were used to indicate the results from three experiments. Curves indicate fitted logistic relationships between DCAD and urine pH. (B) Effect of dietary treatment on observed faecal pH (DR = dry rolled, FNDF = fermentable NDF, G = ground, SF = steam-flaked).

Such variation is substantial from the perspective of the effects on ammonia emission from slurry. Also, a shift from N excretion with urine to N excretion with faeces reduces immediate ammonia emission rates. Such a shift may occur with stimulated microbial fermentation in the large intestine, causing increased amounts of microbial N synthesized and excreted with faeces. The dry matter content of faeces, and hence of the ammonia concentrations, also varies with nutritional strategy. It is concluded that simultaneous changes caused by changes in nutritional strategy may alter emission rates of ammonia from cow houses and slurry pits on a farm profoundly. Dynamic approaches may have an added value when evaluating the joint effects of changes in nutritional strategies on ammonia emission from stored manure.

AMMONIA AFFECTED BY N EXCRETION. Preliminary simulation results of Reijs *et al.* (2006a) indicate that the efficiency of N utilization by cows can vary from 20 to 36% of the N ingested, the excretion of urea or urea-like N (including substances rapidly converted into urea) can vary from 33 to 66% of the total amount of N excreted, and 4 to 11% of the N excreted can become emitted as ammonia-N from cow houses. These figures are in close correspondence to simulations of four practical cases of organic dairy farms that all adopted feeding strategies with a low dietary content of protein (less than 14% of dry matter (DM); Table 21.1). Also, the simulated effects on N excretion are confirmed by *in vivo* observations. For example, in experiments by Valk *et al.* (1990) in which one unit of beet pulp, maize silage or maize concentrate was exchanged per two units of grass silage, about 20% more N was excreted in faeces and 30% less N in urine with the beet pulp treatment. In conclusion, both simulation studies and *in vivo* observations indicate that nutritional strategies may have a large impact on ammonia emission rates from cow houses, whereas rather constant figures of around 11% are currently assumed within Dutch legislation.

METHANE FROM ENTERIC FERMENTATION. The need to study entire farming systems is argued in order to obtain a full integration of effects for inventory purposes (Jarvis and Pain, 1994; Schils *et al.*, 2005). Not wanting to argue about this need, there is also a need to be precise for the purpose of introducing mitigation measures in practice, for policy implementation and for judging farming scenarios not yet monitored. Changes in nutritional strategy may strongly affect methane emission per unit of digested feed, per cow and per unit of milk produced, as demonstrated with a dynamic modelling approach by Mills *et al.* (2001). In this study, coefficients subsequently published by Bannink *et al.* (2006b) were used to estimate the yield of VFA and methane from various types of carbohydrate and protein fermented in the gastrointestinal tract. A clear distinction in methane emission from fermented soluble carbohydrates and starch became apparent (Bannink *et al.*, 2005). In a more recent study of *in vivo* data, VFA yields from rapidly fermentable carbohydrates appeared dependent on rumen pH (Bannink *et al.*, 2005, 2006a). This means that apart from composition and digestibility of the diet, the methane yield also varies with the absolute rate of fermentation of organic matter. With empirical approaches, these effects can only become apparent in a rather confounded manner because general dietary characteristics (dry matter intake, energy value, roughage/concentrate intake) are then used to derive index values for methane formation. In this respect, the inability to demonstrate an effect of soluble sugar to starch ratio when evaluating 11 practical cases is illustrative (Bannink *et al.*, 2005).

METHANE AND OTHER GHGS FROM MANURE STORAGE AND SOIL. Besides the emission of methane directly by the cow, nutrition also affects manure characteristics, which in turn affect the digestion of manure during storage and the mineralization and denitrification processes in soils fertilized with manure (Chapter 9). Currently,

Table 21.1. Simulated variation of fate of feed N in dairy cows.

Model inputs	Four practical cases evaluated by Bannink *et al.* (2006a)				Simulations for 40 diets by Reijs *et al.* (2006a)	
	Farm 1	Farm 2	Farm 3	Farm 4	Range	Average
Dry matter intake (kg dry matter day^{-1})	20.7	19.6	19.5	22.7	16.0–22.4	19.6
NDF intake (kg NDF day^{-1})[a]	11.4	10.4	10.0	8.9	7.25–11.0	9.0
N intake (g N day^{-1})	522	484	509	461	311–730	509
Soluble crude protein (g day^{-1})	656	613	731	688	971–2353	1574
Degradable crude protein (g day^{-1})	2095	1950[a]	1780	1807	613–1776	1150
Undegradable crude protein (g day^{-1})	335	312[a]	285	288	246–301	272
Simulated milk yield (kg day^{-1})	23.7	25.1	23.4	32.8	19.1–33.5	27.0
Simulated fate of feed N:						
Milk N (%)	24	27 (27)[a]	23	39 (40)[a]	20–36	28
Urine N (%)	30	34 (39)	29	24 (28)	28–60	44
Faeces N (%)	46	39 (34)	48	37 (32)	20–38	28
Simulated ratios:						
Urine N:faecal N	0.67	0.85 (1.13)[a]	0.61	0.64 (0.87)[a]	0.78–3.07	1.69
Urine N:total N excreted	0.40	0.46 (0.53)	0.38	0.39 (0.47)	0.44–0.75	0.61
Undigested feed N:total faecal N	0.49	0.39 (0.29)	0.53	0.24 (0.12)	0.34–0.39	0.36

[a]In two cases, the sensitivity was tested for an increased protein degradability. The fractional degradation rate and the fraction of degradable protein were both increased and the fraction of undegradable crude protein was decreased. Results of an increased protein degradability are given in parentheses.

international standards are used as index values for GHG emissions from dairy farms (Jarvis and Pain, 1994; Schils *et al.*, 2005). No consideration is given to the effect of manure composition, although it is known that nutrition strategy strongly affects manure composition and characteristics. Besides storage conditions, soil type and method and rate of manure application, highly specific and nutrition-dependent factors such as pH, VFA concentration, degradable carbon, ammonium concentration and dry matter content may be determinants of GHG emission from stores and soil (Kebreab *et al.*, 2006). Predicting the effect of farm management on such factors requires dynamic modelling approaches capable of representing the causal relationships (digestion and enteric methane formation, Dijkstra *et al.*, 1992; Mills *et al.*, 2001; manure storage, Sommer *et al.*, 2004; soil emissions, Li *et al.*, 1992). For further discussion, the reader is referred to Chapters 8 and 9 of this volume.

Manure

An important cause of environmental pollution by dairy farms is the production, storage and application of manure (Valk, 2002; Schröder *et al.*, 2005). The losses of N and phosphorus (P) from the farming system depend strongly on the quantities of N and P excreted by the herd, which in turn depend on stocking density, cow productivity, amounts and types of N and P imported with feed and fertilizer and on the amounts and type of N and P in on-farm feed production. Manure quantity and quality hence depend largely on nutritional strategy. This dependency is demonstrated for the amount and site of N excretion in Tables 21.1 and 21.2, and has already been discussed in relation to ammonia emission for excreta volumes. Additionally, P excretion and manure fertilizer value will be discussed below.

P EXCRETION. Comparable to N, the efficiency of P utilization by the cow also increases drastically when P content in feed DM is reduced. Valk (2002) concluded that P content may be reduced to as low as 3 g P kg^{-1} DM without detrimental effect on cows, leading to utilization efficiencies of up to 50% during lactation. Such low contents may be achieved only by feeding by-products and concentrates and roughages with low P contents, such as maize silage. However, under most practical circumstances, diets will have a much higher P content. An intensive recycling of P absorbed from the gastrointestinal tract with saliva production causes P to be highly available to the dairy cow, and almost all P is excreted in faeces with relatively small amounts of organic P. Furthermore, P contents in milk appear rather stable and independent of milk protein content. More than with N, the excretion of P is fully dependent on dietary P content and milk yield and may be treated as a simple balance added to the dynamic models of cow performance. However, a dynamic P model has been published recently (Kebreab *et al.*, 2004).

MANURE FERTILIZING VALUE. The first-year N availability of cattle slurries is affected by diet composition (Sørensen *et al.*, 2003; Reijs *et al.*, 2006b). In general, it can be concluded that a reduction of the dietary protein surplus will result in an increased C:N ratio and a decreased availability of the N contained in the slurry.

Table 21.2. Simulated effect of different grass and maize cultivars in a standard diet (20 kg dry matter intake day^{-1}, 50% fresh grass, 25% maize silage, 25% concentrate) on milk yield and N excretion.

	Grass cultivars simulated (always in combination with maize cultivar 7)						Maize cultivars simulated[b] (always in combination with grass cultivar 3)					
	Diet						Diet					
	1	2	3	4	5	6	7	8	9	10	11	12
							% maize cob					
Cultivar characteristics[a]							50	50	50	50	50	55
Sugars (g kg^{-1} dry matter)[b]	180	180	205	230	80	80	160	160	310	310	160	160
Starch (g kg^{-1} maize cob dry matter)							560	560	560	560	560	560
S (g kg^{-1} starch)							500	500	500	500	300	500
D (g kg^{-1} starch)							500	500	500	500	700	500
kd (h^{-1})							0.10	0.10	0.10	0.10	0.05	0.10
Crude protein (g kg^{-1} dry matter)[b]	200	200	175	200	150	150	65	65	115	115	65	65
S (g kg^{-1} crude protein)	200	200	200	150	150	150	300	300	300	300	300	300
D (g kg^{-1} crude protein)	700	700	700	700	600	600	350	350	350	350	350	350
kd (h^{-1})	0.10	0.10	0.10	0.10	0.06	0.06	0.025	0.025	0.04	0.04	0.025	0.025
U (g kg^{-1} crude protein)	100	100	100	150	250	250	350	350	350	350	350	350

NDF (g kg^{-1} dry matter)[b]	500	500	500	450	650	650	700	700	500	500	700	700
D (g kg^{-1} NDF)	900	900	900	900	800	800	600	600	600	600	600	600
kd (h^{-1})	0.05	0.03	0.05	0.03	0.03	0.05	0.025	0.04	0.025	0.04	0.025	0.025
U (g kg^{-1} NDF)	100	100	100	100	200	200	400	400	400	400	400	400
Simulation results[c]												
Apparent digestion (%)												
N	63.6	62.5	65.5	59.4	64.9	65.7	65.5	65.8	62.6	62.8	65.5	65.5
Starch	53.0	53.0	51.0	49.7	56.5	57.2	51.0	51.0	48.5	48.5	47.4	53.5
NDF	69.8	67.6	69.4	65.8	65.3	67.4	69.4	70.0	69.8	70.3	69.5	69.8
Milk yield (kg day^{-1})	31.6	31.1	31.6	30.9	29.0	29.6	31.6	31.7	32.0	32.1	31.7	32.1
N milk (% of N intake)	25.9	25.5	27.6	25.4	27.1	27.7	27.6	27.7	26.9	27.0	27.8	27.6
Urine N:faecal N	1.76	1.80	1.59	1.65	1.14	1.11	1.59	1.58	1.63	1.63	1.60	1.63

[a]1 = Fast cell wall degradation and high CP content; 2 = slow cell wall degradation and high CP content; 3 = standard; 4 = high sugar content and slow cell wall degradation; 5 = low sugar content and slow cell wall degradation; 6 = low sugar content and fast cell wall degradation; 7 = standard; 8 = fast cell wall degradation; 9 = low cell wall content; 10 = low cell wall content and fast cell wall degradation; 11 = slow starch degradation; 12 = high fraction maize cobs.

[b]Apart from starch characteristics, the characteristics given for the different maize cultivars apply to maize stems only. Standard crude protein and NDF contents and degradation characteristics were assumed in maize cobs.

[c]Assuming similar milk composition and similar rumen fermentation conditions (pH, passage rates, volume, protozoal fraction; Dijkstra *et al.*, 1992).

Preliminary results of Reijs *et al.* (2006a) demonstrate the effects of changing from an intensive to an extensive grassland management system. The C:N of fresh manure varied between 2.9 and 9.8, depending on feeding strategy. After taking into account the N and C losses during storage, estimates of manure fertilizing equivalent (relative value to fertilizing value of mineral fertilizer) ranged from 47 to 70%. Such differences are substantial and need to be incorporated into fertilization recommendation schemes. The slurry N not directly available for plant growth will contribute to the accumulation of organic N in the soil. This residual organic N has proved to be relevant when considering the fertilizing potential of cattle manure in the long term (Schröder *et al.*, 2005). In subsequent growing seasons, substantial fractions of organic N spread in previous years may become mineralized. Depending on the moment of mineralization and of crop growth, this N fraction may be retained as crop N harvested or directly consumed by cows. However, this retention will depend very much on farm type, soil and weather conditions. Nevertheless, it seems worthwhile to evaluate the effect of nutritional strategies on manure characteristics in the short as well as the long term and to take these effects into account when advising farmers on optimal fertilizing practices. It may prove useful to apply dynamic approaches, such as that by Reijs *et al.* (2006a), to deliver the type of information needed to evaluate in detail the consequences of changes in nutritional strategies on the level of whole-farm management.

Forage production

The consequences of changing nutritional strategy extend over all subsystems of the farm. In grass-based dairy systems in temperate regions, the soil and fertilizing management for forage production has a tremendous impact on the whole-farm outcome. A straightforward measure to reduce the environmental impact of these types of farming systems is to reduce grassland management intensity (lower stocking during grazing, as well as lower fertilization). Reijs *et al.* (2006a; Table 21.1) compared the effect of including grass silage from extensive grassland with the effect of replacing it with maize silage. Both measures appeared to be powerful means of reducing intake and excretion of N, increasing the efficiency of N utilization by the cow and causing a shift of N excretion from urine to faeces.

Not only N intake relative to digestible energy intake and cow productivity, but also the quality (i.e. degradation characteristics) of dietary protein strongly affects the site of N excretion (Firkins and Reynolds, 2006). This effect is demonstrated clearly by preliminary results of an evaluation of the nutritional consequences of including different plant cultivars in the diet. In Table 21.2, the results are shown for a selection of six different grass cultivars, as well as maize cultivars, and their chemical composition and degradation characteristics that have been established in previous plant breeding trials (differences relate to maturation rate, dry matter yield and efficiency of N uptake). Consequences of the selection of maize cultivar on N intake, cow productivity, efficiency of N utilization and the site of N excretion remained small (Table 21.2). Consequences of the selection of grass cultivar had much more prominent implications for N intake, efficiency of N utilization and the site of N excretion. These results are in support of the findings of Reijs *et al.* (2006a) that a changed management of grassland as a farm subsystem is a powerful means of reducing the environmental impact of dairy farming. For this reason, grassland management is a crucial element to consider when evaluating the merit of a changed nutritional strategy in grass-based dairy systems. These results also demonstrate that installing large plant breeding research programmes without proper evaluation of the nutritional consequences or without testing *in vivo* with the target animal seems unwise (Ulyatt, 1973). As with the previously mentioned aspects of dairy farming, plant breeding and grassland management programmes also need to be guided by a properly integrated approach at all levels of aggregation and for all farm subsystems, to ensure sufficient accuracy of the conclusions drawn. For example, proper conclusions cannot be made on prognoses derived only with simple presumptions on cow productivity and standard index values for digestibility and feeding value.

From the perspective of forage production, it might prove much more difficult to reduce the dietary P content. In the short term, a reduced N and P fertilization rate of grassland may even increase P content in grass harvested on soils with high P status because of a reduced DM yield (Valk, 2002), preventing substantial reductions in P excretion. Despite a lowering of P fertilization rates, the P content in grass remained rather stable (Valk, 2002). In the long term, fewer P imports may increase the utilization efficiency of manure P and reduce the P surplus on farms. On a Dutch experimental farm that aims to improve the efficiencies of nutrient conversion between farm subsystems and to reduce N and P surplus, annual N and P loss in kg ha^{-1} was 63% and 92% lower than that on commercial farms in the same area of similar intensity (Schröder *et al.*, 2005).

Conclusions

There is no a priori superior approach to modelling the consequences of nutritional strategies for cows and to farm management. The approach chosen depends on the aim of the exercise. Adopting a dynamic modelling approach serves certain advantages and gives additional insights which deserve to be recognized with studies on the effect of nutritional strategies on cow and whole-farm performance. An important advantage of dynamic modelling is the integrative power it offers and the robust manner in which the multiple cause–effect relationships may be delineated (Oenema *et al.*, 2001a). At the level of detail that the farmer requires to take day-to-day decisions, this advantage is crucial. It avoids the problem most current whole-farm models suffer from of being well able to deliver broad qualifications of different farming systems while not being specific enough. There is an increasing need to be able to integrate representations of details at the molecular, organ and cow level up to the level of the herd, the whole farm or even the regional or national level (Fig. 21.1) and to move from a source-oriented to a chain-oriented application. Nowadays, the level of detail represented in dynamic models should no longer be a limitation to any ambition to use these models to evaluate whole farming systems and to advise farmers, or to use them on behalf of policy makers in surveys of the impact of farm management on environment quality.

Acknowledgement

Part of this work results from research funded by the Dutch Ministry of Agriculture, Nature and Food Quality and the Dutch Commodity Board of Feedstuffs. Their funding is gratefully acknowledged.

References

Baldwin, R.L. (1995) *Modeling Ruminant Digestion and Metabolism*. Chapman and Hall Ltd, London.

Baldwin, R.L., France, J. and Gill, M. (1987a) Metabolism of the lactating cow. I. Animal elements of a mechanistic model. *Journal of Dairy Research* 54, 77–106.

Baldwin, R.L., Thornley, J.H.M. and Beever, D.E. (1987b) Metabolism of the lactating cow. II. Digestive elements of a mechanistic model. *Journal of Dairy Research* 54, 107–131.

Baldwin, R.L., France, J., Beever, D.E., Gill, M. and Thornley, J.H.M. (1987c) Metabolism of the lactating cow. III. Properties of mechanistic models suitable for evaluation of energetic relationships and factors involved in the partition of nutrients. *Journal of Dairy Research* 54, 133–145.

Bannink, A. and Tamminga, S. (2005) Rumen function. In: Dijkstra, J., Forbes, J.M. and France J. (eds) *Quantitative Aspects of Ruminant Digestion and Metabolism*, 2nd edn. CAB International, Wallingford, UK, pp. 263–288.

Bannink, A., Visser, H. de, Dijkstra, J. and France, J. (1997) Impact of diet-specific input parameters on simulated rumen function. *Journal of Theoretical Biology* 184, 371–384.

Bannink, A., Valk, H. and van Vuren, A.M. (1999) Intake and excretion of sodium, potassium, and nitrogen and the effects on urine production by lactating dairy cows. *Journal of Dairy Science* 82, 1008–1018.

Bannink, A., Dijkstra, J., Mills, J.A.N., Kebreab, E. and France, J. (2005) Nutritional strategies to reduce enteric methane formation in dairy cows. In: Kuczynski, T., Dammgen, U., Webb, J. and Myczko, A. (eds) *Emission from European Agriculture*. Wageningen Academic Publishers, Wageningen, The Netherlands, pp. 367–376.

Bannink, A., Dijkstra, J., Kebreab, E. and France, J. (2006a) Advantages of a dynamical approach to rumen function to help resolve environmental issues. In: Kebreab, E., Dijkstra, J., Gerrits, W.J.J., Bannink, A. and France, J. (eds) *Nutrient Utilization in Farm Animals: Modelling Approach*. CAB International, Wallingford, UK, pp. 281–298.

Bannink, A., Kogut, J., Dijkstra, J., Kebreab, E., France, J., Tamminga, S. and Van Vuuren, A.M. (2006b) Estimation of the stoichiometry of volatile fatty acid production in the rumen of lactating cows. *Journal of Theoretical Biology* 238, 36–51.

Boer, I.J.M. de, Smits, M.C.J., Mollenhorst, H., van Duinkerken, G. and Monteny, G.J. (2002) Prediction of ammonia emission from dairy barns using feed characteristics. Part 1: Relation between feed characteristics and urinary urea concentration. *Journal of Dairy Science* 85, 3382–3388.

Cabrera, V.E., Breuer, N.E., Hildebrand, P.E. and Letson, D. (2005) The dynamic Northern Florida dairy farm model: a user-friendly computerized tool for increasing profits while minimizing N leaching under varying climatic conditions. *Computers and Electronics in Agriculture* 49, 286–308.

Central Bureau for Livestock Feeding (CVB) (2005) *The Livestock Feeding Table.* Lelystad, The Netherlands.

Collao-Saenz, E.A., Dijkstra, J., Aguiar Paiva, P.C., Bannink, A., Arcuri, P.B., Teixera, J.C. and David, F.M. (2005) Simulation model for particle dynamics in rumen of cattle fed sugarcane diet. *Scientia Agricola* 62, 102–110.

Cuttle, S.P. and Jarvis, S.C. (2005) Use of a system synthesis approach to model nitrogen losses from dairy farms in south-west England. *Grass and Forage Science* 60, 262–273.

Czerkawski, J.W. (1986) *An Introduction to Rumen Studies.* Pergamon Press, Oxford, UK.

Danfaer, A. (1990) *A Dynamic Model of Nutrition Digestion and Metabolism in Lactating Dairy Cows.* Beretning fra Statens Husdyrbrugforsog 671. National Institute of Animal Science, Foulum, Denmark.

Dijkstra, J., Neal, H.D.St.C., Beever, D.E. and France, J. (1992) Simulation of nutrient digestion, absorption and outflow in the rumen: model description. *Journal of Nutrition* 122, 2239–2256.

Dijkstra, J., France, J., Assis, A.G., Neal, H.D.St.C., Campos, O.F. and Aroeira, L.J.M. (1996) Simulation of digestion in cattle fed sugarcane: prediction of nutrient supply for milk production with locally available supplements. *Journal of Agricultural Science* 127, 247–260.

Dou, Z., Kohn, R.A., Ferguson, J.D., Boston, R.C. and Newbold, J.D. (1996) Managing nitrogen on dairy farms: an integrated approach I. Model description. *Journal of Dairy Science* 79, 2071–2080.

Enemark, J.M., Jorgensen, R.J. and Enemark, P.St. (2002) Rumen acidosis with special emphasis on diagnostic aspects of subclinical rumen acidosis: a review. *Veterinarija ir Zootechnika* 20, 16–29.

Firkins, J.L. and Reynolds C.K. (2006) Whole-animal nitrogen balance in cattle. In: Pfeffer, E. and Hristov, A. (eds) *Nitrogen and Phosphorus Nutrition in Cattle.* CAB International, Wallingford, UK, pp. 167–186.

Forbes, J.M. (2005) Voluntary feed intake and diet selection. In: Dijkstra, J., Forbes, J.M. and France, J. (eds) *Quantitative Aspects of Ruminant Digestion and Metabolism.* CAB International, Wallingford, UK, pp. 607–625.

France, J., Thornley, J.H.M. and Beever, D.E. (1982) A mathematical model of the rumen. *Animal Feed Science and Technology* 21, 229–353.

Freetly, H.C., Knapp, J.R., Calvert, C.C. and Baldwin, R.L. (1993) Development of a mechanistic model of liver metabolism in the lactating cow. *Agricultural Systems* 41, 157–195.

Gäbel, G., Aschenbach, J.R. and Muller, F. (2002) Transfer of energy substrates across the ruminal epithelium: implications and limitations. *Animal Health Research Reviews* 3, 15–30.

Gill, M., Beever, D.E. and France, J. (1989) Biochemical bases needed for the mathematical representation of whole animal metabolism. *Nutrition Research Reviews* 2, 181–200.

Hanigan, M.D. and Baldwin, R.L. (1994) A mechanistic model of mammary gland metabolism in the lactating cow. *Agricultural Systems* 45, 369–419.

Hristov, A.N. and Jouany, J.-P. (2006) Factors affecting the efficiency of nitrogen utilization in the rumen. In: Pfeffer, E. and Hristov, A. (eds) *Nitrogen and Phosphorus Nutrition in Cattle.* CAB International, Wallingford, UK, pp. 117–166.

Jarvis, S.C. and Pain, B.F. (1994) Greenhouse gas emission from intensive livestock systems: their estimation and technologies for reduction. *Climatic Change* 27, 27–38.

Johnson, H.A., Famula, T.R. and Baldwin, R.L. (2005) Lactation: statistical and genetic aspects of simulating lactation data from individual cows using a dynamic, mechanistic model of dairy cow metabolism. In: Dijkstra, J., Forbes, J.M. and France, J. (eds) *Quantitative Aspects of Ruminant Digestion and Metabolism*. CAB International, Wallingford, pp. 551–582.

Kebreab, E., France, J., Beever, D.E. and Castillo, A.R. (2001) Nitrogen pollution by dairy cows and its mitigation by dietary manipulation. *Nutrient Cycling in Agroecosystems* 60, 275–285.

Kebreab, E., Mills, J.A.N., Crompton, L.A., Bannink, A., Dijkstra, J., Gerrits, W.J.J. and France, J. (2004) An integrated model to evaluate nutrient partition in dairy cattle between the animal and its environment. *Animal Feed Science and Technology* 112, 131–154.

Kebreab, E., Clark, K., Wagner-Riddle, C. and France, J. (2006) Methane and nitrous oxide emissions from Canadian animal agriculture: a review. *Canadian Journal of Animal Science* 86, 135–158.

Kennedy, P.M. (2005) Particle dynamics. In: Dijkstra, J., Forbes, J.M. and France, J. (eds) *Quantitative Aspects of Ruminant Digestion and Metabolism*. CAB International, Wallingford, UK, pp. 123–156.

Kohn, R.A., Dou, Z., Ferguson, J.D. and Boston, R.C. (1997) A sensitivity analysis of nitrogen losses from dairy farms. *Journal of Environmental Management* 50, 417–428.

Li, C., Frolking, S. and Frolking, T.A. (1992) A model of nitrous oxide evolution from soil driven by rainfall events: 1. Model structure and sensitivity. *Journal of Geophysical Research* 97, 9759–9776.

Miller, P.S. (1990) Nutrient partitioning in the lactating dairy cow. PhD thesis, University of California, Davis, California.

Mills, J.A.N., France, J. and Dijkstra, J. (1999) A review of starch digestion in the lactating dairy cow and proposals for a mechanistic model. 1. Dietary starch characterization and ruminal starch digestion. *Journal of Animal and Feed Sciences* 8, 291–340.

Mills, J.A.N., Dijkstra, J., Bannink, A., Cammell, S.B., Kebreab, E. and France, J. (2001) A mechanistic model of whole-tract digestion and methanogenesis in the lactating dairy cow: model development, evaluation, and application. *Journal of Animal Science* 79, 1584–1597.

Mills, J.A.N., Kebreab, E., Yates, C.M., Crompton, L.A., Cammell, S.B., Dhanoa, M.S., Agnew, R.E. and France, J. (2003) Alternative approaches to predicting methane emissions from dairy cows. *Journal of Animal Science* 81, 3141–3150.

Monteny, G.-J. (2000) Modelling of ammonia emission from dairy cow houses. PhD thesis, Wageningen University, Wageningen, The Netherlands.

Monteny, G.J., Smits, M.C.J., van Duinkerken, G., Mollenhorst, H. and Boer, I.J.M. de (2002) Prediction of ammonia emission from dairy barns using feed characteristics. Part II: Relation between urinary urea concentration and ammonia emission. *Journal of Dairy Science* 85, 3389–3394.

Mourits, M.C.M., Berentsen, P.B.M., Huirne, R.B.M. and Dijkhuizen, A.A. (2000) Environmental impact of heifer management decision on Dutch dairy farms. *Netherlands Journal of Agricultural Science* 48, 151–164.

Oenema, O., Velthof, G. and Kuikman, P. (2001a) Technical and policy aspects of strategies to decrease green house gas emission from agriculture. *Nutrient Cycling in Agrosystems* 60, 301–315.

Oenema, O., Bannink, A., Sommer, S. and Velthof, G.L. (2001b) Gaseous nitrogen emission from livestock farming systems. In: Follett, R.F. and Hatfield, J.L. (eds) *Nitrogen in the Environment: Sources, Problems and Management*. Elsevier Science Publishers, Amsterdam, pp. 255–289.

Oldick, B.S., Firkins, J.L. and St-Pierre, N.R. (1999) Estimation of microbial nitrogen flow to the duodenum of cattle based on dry matter intake and diet composition. *Journal of Dairy Science* 82, 1497–1511.

Reijs, J.W., Bannink, A., Bosma, P. and Dijkstra, J. (2006a) Modelling the impact of dietary adjustment on slurry composition of stall-fed dairy cows. In: Schröder, J.J. and Neeteson, J.J. (eds) *N Management in Agrosystems in Relation to the Water Framework Directive, Proceedings 14th N-Workshop, Report 116*, Plant Research International, Wageningen, The Netherlands, pp. 163–166.

Reijs, J.W., Sonneveld., M.P.W., Sørensen, P., Schils, R.L.M., Groot, J.C.J. and Lantinga, E.A. (2006b) Effects of different diets on utilization of nitrogen from cattle slurry applied to grassland on a sandy soil in the Netherlands. *Agriculture, Ecosystems and Environment* 118, 65–79.

Ross, C.A., Scholefield, D. and Jarvis, S.C. (2002) A model of ammonia volatilisation from a dairy farms: an examination of abatement strategies. *Nutrient Cycling in Agrosystems* 64, 273–281.

Schils, R.L.M., Verhagen, A., Aarts, H.F.M. and Sebek, L.B.J. (2005) A farm level approach to define successful mitigation strategies for GHG emissions from ruminant livestock systems. *Nutrient Cycling in Agrosystems* 71, 163–175.

Schröder, J.J., Jansen, A.G. and Hilhorst, G.J. (2005) Long-term nitrogen fertilizer value of cattle slurry. *Soil Use and Management* 21, 196–204.

Schröder, J.J., Bannink, A. and Kohn, R.A. (2006) Improving the efficiency of nutrient use on cattle operations. In: Pfeffer, E. and Hristov, A. (eds) *Nitrogen and Phosphorus Nutrition in Cattle*. CAB International, Wallingford, UK, pp. 255–288.

Sommer, S.G., Petersen, S.O. and Moller, H.B. (2004) Algorithms for calculating methane and nitrous oxide emissions from manure management. *Nutrient Cycling in Agroecosystems* 69, 143–154.

Sørensen, P., Weisbjerg, M.R. and Lund, P. (2003) Dietary effects on the composition and plant utilization of nitrogen in dairy cattle manure. *Journal of Agricultural Science* 141, 79–91.

Sterk, B., van Ittersum, M.K., Leeuwis, C., Rossing, W.A.H., van Keulen, H. and van de Ven, G.W.J. (2006) Finding niches for whole-farm design models – contradictio in terminis? *Agricultural Systems* 87, 211–228.

Ulyatt, M.J. (1973) The feeding value of herbage. In: Butler, G.W. and Bailey, R.W. (eds) *Chemistry and Biochemistry of Herbage*, Volume 3. Academic Press, London, pp. 131–178.

Valk, H. (2002) Nitrogen and phosphorus supply of dairy cows. PhD thesis, Utrecht University, Utrecht, The Netherlands.

Valk, H., Klein-Poelhuis, H.W. and Wentink, H.J. (1990) Effects of fibrous and starchy carbohydrates in concentrates as supplements in a herbage-based diet for high-yielding dairy cows. *Netherlands Journal of Agricultural Science* 38, 475–486.

Van Duinkerken, G., André, G., Smits, M.C.J., Monteny, G.J. and Šebek, L.B.J. (2005) Effect of rumen-degradable protein balance and forage type on bulk milk urea concentration and emission of ammonia from dairy cow houses. *Journal of Dairy Science* 88, 1099–1112.

Yan, T., Agnew, R.E., Gordon, F.J. and Porter, M.G. (2000) Prediction of methane energy output in dairy and beef cattle offered grass silage-based diets. *Livestock Production Science* 64, 253–263.

22 Modelling Lactation Potential in an Animal Model

M.D. HANIGAN,[1] C.C. PALLISER[2] AND A.G. RIUS[1]

[1]Department of Dairy Science, Virginia Polytechnic Institute and State University, USA; [2]Dexcel Ltd, Hamilton, New Zealand

Introduction

In 2004, there were approximately 9 million dairy cows in the USA, which produced 73 million metric tons of milk valued at US$27 billion (USDA–NASS, 2005). These animals would be expected to consume in excess of 50 million metric tons of feed dry matter per year at an approximate cost of US$7 billion. In order to maximize productivity of these animals while minimizing input costs, nutrients provided must meet or exceed nutritional requirements. However, feeding nutrients in excess of needs can be detrimental to the environment. Thus, an accurate assessment of both animal requirements and dietary nutrient supply is economically and environmentally important.

The current system for determining nutrient supply and requirements in the USA is that of the NRC (2001). The NRC model has evolved over time in response to knowledge accumulation (NRC, 1978, 1985, 1989). While such updates improve the accuracy of the model, it is a highly aggregated model and thus cannot reflect many aspects of digestion and metabolism that affect animal performance and efficiency. In particular, NRC currently does not predict milk composition. Given the widespread use of component-based pricing in the USA, such a prediction would be beneficial when using the model to design diets.

Efforts have been undertaken to develop prediction models capable of describing the effects of nutrition and animal factors on milk and milk component yields (Tran and Johnson, 1991; Offer *et al.*, 2002; Hristov *et al.*, 2005). While milk yield can be predicted with reasonable accuracy, milk composition has not been well predicted or the model has not been tested extensively (Offer *et al.*, 2002). The aggregated treatment of post-absorptive nutrients by NRC likely prevents accurate predictions of milk composition. The various metabolites that arise from digestion and absorption of nutrients can affect milk composition (Thomas and Chamberlain, 1984; DePeters and Cant, 1992; Gaynor *et al.*, 1994;

Wonsil *et al.*, 1994; Bequette *et al.*, 2000). It may be possible to derive empirical equations at the animal level that are capable of predicting responses to changes in dietary nutrients; however, previous attempts suggest such an approach is likely to fall short of the desired level of accuracy (Tran and Johnson, 1991; Hristov *et al.*, 2005). Alternatively, one could represent nutrient flux through the animal, including interactions and associated effects on endocrine status. This approach has the potential advantage of allowing the use of data derived from more invasive experiments; however, it does require construction of a more complex model.

Predicting the flux of individual nutrients through the animal necessitates the consideration of metabolite use by at least the gastrointestinal tract, liver, muscle, adipose tissue and mammary tissue (Smith, 1970). Baldwin *et al.* (1987a,b,c) constructed a model called Molly that represented the critical elements of these tissues, thus allowing a representation of metabolite concentrations in blood and partitioning of metabolites between the various anabolic and catabolic processes. A schematic of the model is provided in Fig. 22.1. With subsequent modifications (Baldwin, 1995), this model has a structure that is more suitable for predicting the effects of individual metabolites on animal performance and milk composition. Additionally, as it is a dynamic model, it can predict body mass changes over time and the effects of previous planes of nutrition on subsequent performance. This is an important attribute as response to nutrition has been observed to be dependent on previous and current planes of nutrition (Broster and Thomas, 1981). It also allows one to consider explicitly the impact of long-term weight loss and gain when constructing diets. For example, the loss of 1 kg body weight day^{-1} for 5 days is probably innocuous, but losing at that rate for 120 days is a problem. And it provides the ability to consider dilution of the effects of dietary fatty acids by fatty acids released from adipose tissue, i.e. some mono- and polyunsaturated trans-fats inhibit milk fat synthesis (Gaynor *et al.*, 1994; Wonsil *et al.*, 1994), and these inhibitory fatty acids can be diluted out by fatty acids released from adipose tissue, thereby minimizing the effects on fat synthesis for some time. Conversely, inhibitory fatty acids stored in adipose tissue from some previous time point may be released later.

The challenge in developing a less aggregated model is the need to conceive and parameterize more equations. If individual nutrients are used to drive endocrine signals and milk component synthesis, their flux through the system and prevailing concentrations must be predicted accurately. Where NRC deals with energy and protein in aggregate form, a more complex model must predict fluxes and concentrations of at least acetate, glucose, long-chain fatty acids and essential amino acids. This increases the parameterization challenge by several-fold. Additionally, as nutrients are available for use in several pathways, inaccurate predictions in one function can cause problems in other predictions.

Evaluations of Molly, to date, have indicated that some parameterization work is warranted for both digestive and post-absorptive elements (see review by Hanigan *et al.*, 2006). However, some conceptual changes relating to energy partitioning may also be warranted. It has been observed that the model generally overpredicts body weight loss approaching peak lactation and body weight gain in later lactation (Fig. 22.2) (McNamara and Baldwin, 2000). As the

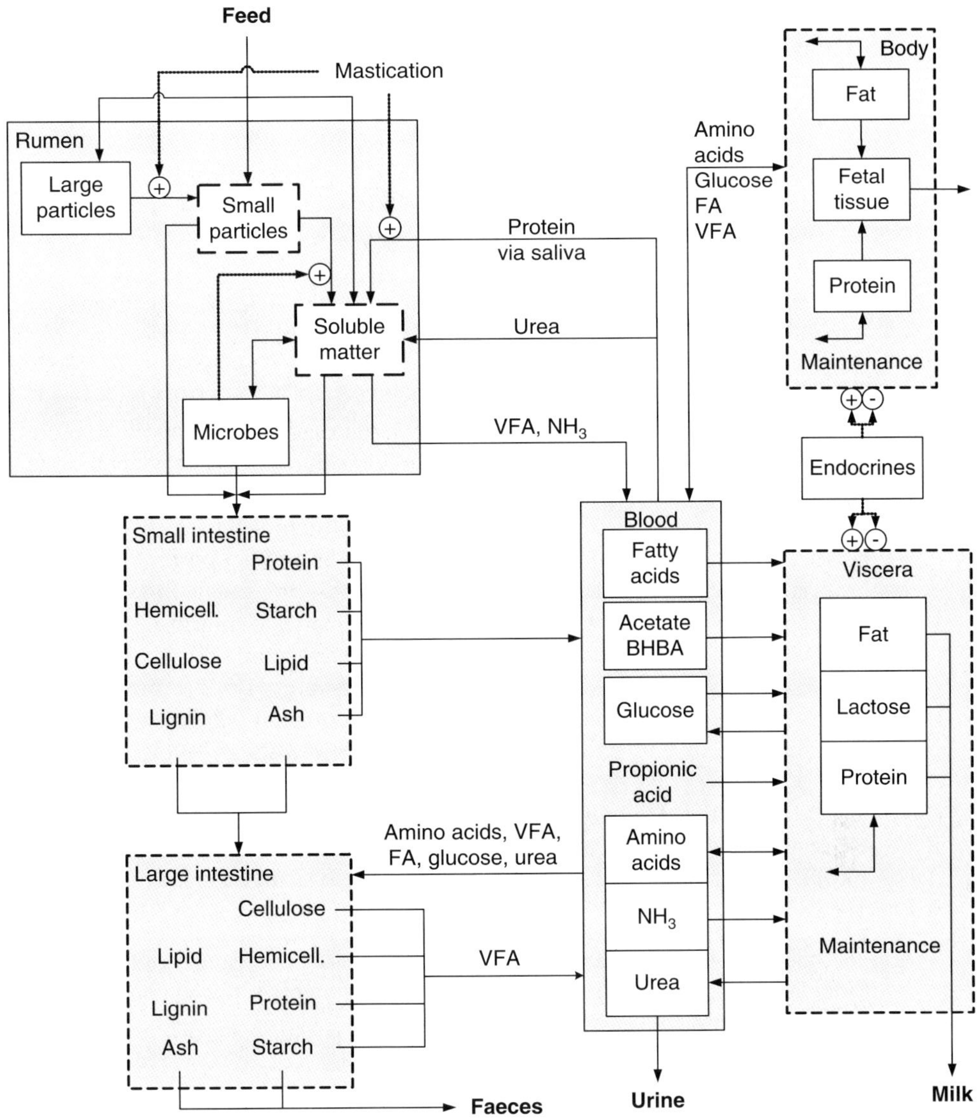

Fig. 22.1. A schematic of the model of Baldwin *et al.* (1987a,b,c). Boxes with dashed lines represent conceptual compartments as defined in the model; boxes with solid lines represent pools; solid arrows represent fluxes; dashed arrows represent modifiers; and the circles associated with dashed arrows indicate the direction of the modifier. BHBA = beta hydroxybutyric acid, FA = fatty acids, VFA = volatile FA.

simulations were run using the observed dry matter intakes and diet composition, the problem was not related to energy intake. Attempts to address this issue by correcting milk yield to match the observed yields and re-parameterizing the model to include adjustments to basal energy expenditures were not successful as they failed to remove the pattern of prediction errors (McNamara, 2004). A

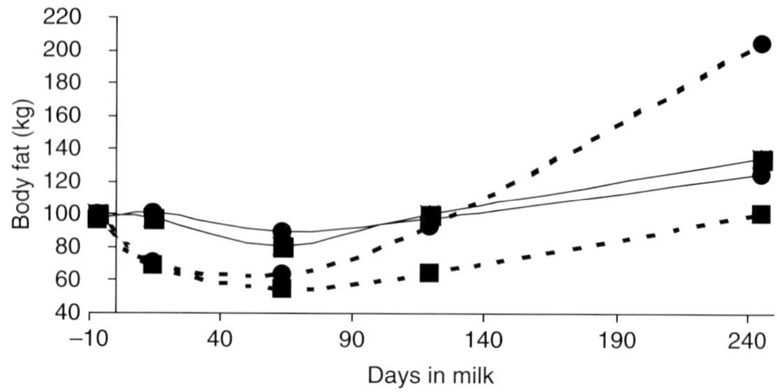

Fig. 22.2. Predicted (broken lines) and observed (solid lines) body fat for cows fed high (●) or low fat (■) diets through 240 days of lactation. Adapted from McNamara and Baldwin (2000).

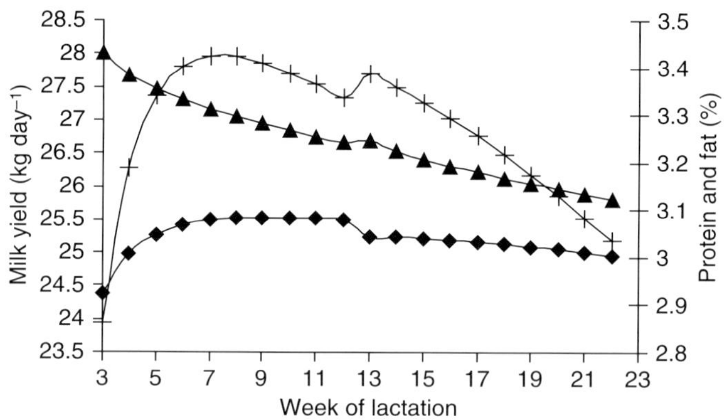

Fig. 22.3. Simulation of milk yield (+) and protein (◆) and fat (▲) composition using dietary inputs for a grass silage diet supplemented with 9 kg concentrate day^{-1}, as described by Aston *et al.* (1995).

contributor to the problem appears to be predictions of milk composition. Milk protein and fat generally have high contents in milk during early and late lactation, with the lowest content occurring near peak production (Stanton *et al.*, 1992). However, predictions of milk protein by Molly exhibit a shape similar to the lactation curve and those for milk fat decline throughout lactation, or have a shape resembling the lactation curve (see review by Hanigan *et al.*, 2006). This behaviour is demonstrated in Fig. 22.3. Correction of these problems, in particular the milk fat prediction errors, would result in predictions of greater energy loss as milk in late lactation and lesser losses around peak lactation, which would likely help resolve the prediction errors for body weight change.

In addition to the problem of inappropriate rates of weight change, the magnitude of the gain or loss in response to nutritional inputs is too large (Fig. 22.4).

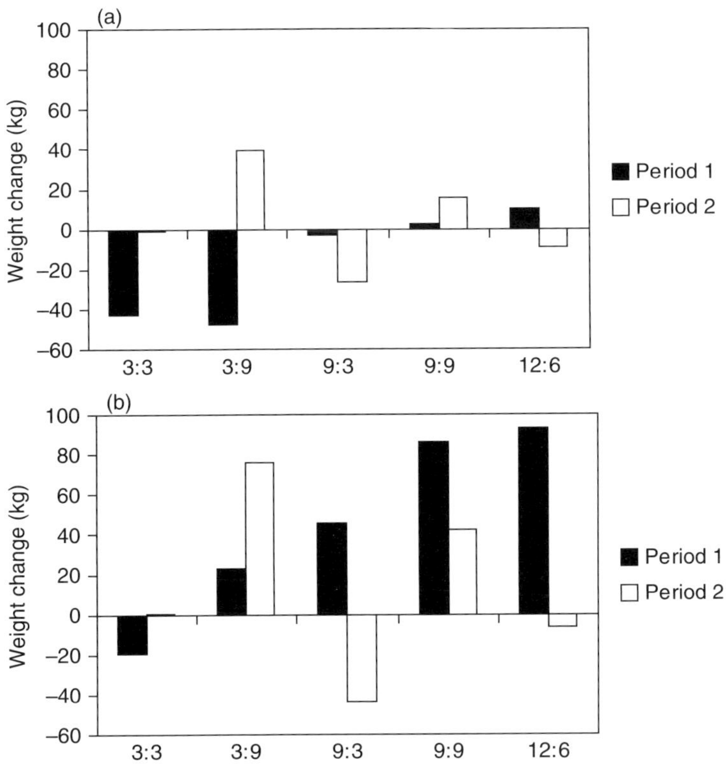

Fig. 22.4. Observed (a) and predicted (b) body weight change responses to grass silage diets supplemented with 3, 9 or 12 kg concentrate day^{-1} from weeks 4 to 12 (period 1, closed bar) and 3 (3:3, 9:3), 6 (12:6) or 9 (3:9, 9:9) kg concentrate from weeks 13 to 22 (period 2, open bar) of lactation. Observed data were from Aston *et al.* (1995). Model inputs for the simulations were the reported initial body weights, diet composition and mean dry matter intakes by period.

At least a portion of this problem appears to be explained by under-responsiveness of milk yield to nutritional inputs (Fig. 22.5), i.e. milk energy output is too great on low energy diets and too low on high energy diets, resulting in excessive release or deposition of fatty acids from adipose tissue, respectively.

Another example of related behaviour is provided by the observations of Beukes *et al.* (2005) in the New Zealand production system. As compared to cows calving in late winter, cows that calved in summer exhibited lower peak yield in early lactation, presumably due to poor pasture quality in late summer, and they experienced a second peak in late lactation coincident with the increase in pasture quality associated with the arrival of spring. Molly did not predict the flatter bi-peak lactation curves of the out-of-season calving cows. Beukes *et al.* (2005) hypothesized that the problem was related to the known effects of photoperiod on milk production. Incorporation of such an effect on lactation hormone resolved the problem; however, given the correlation of photoperiod

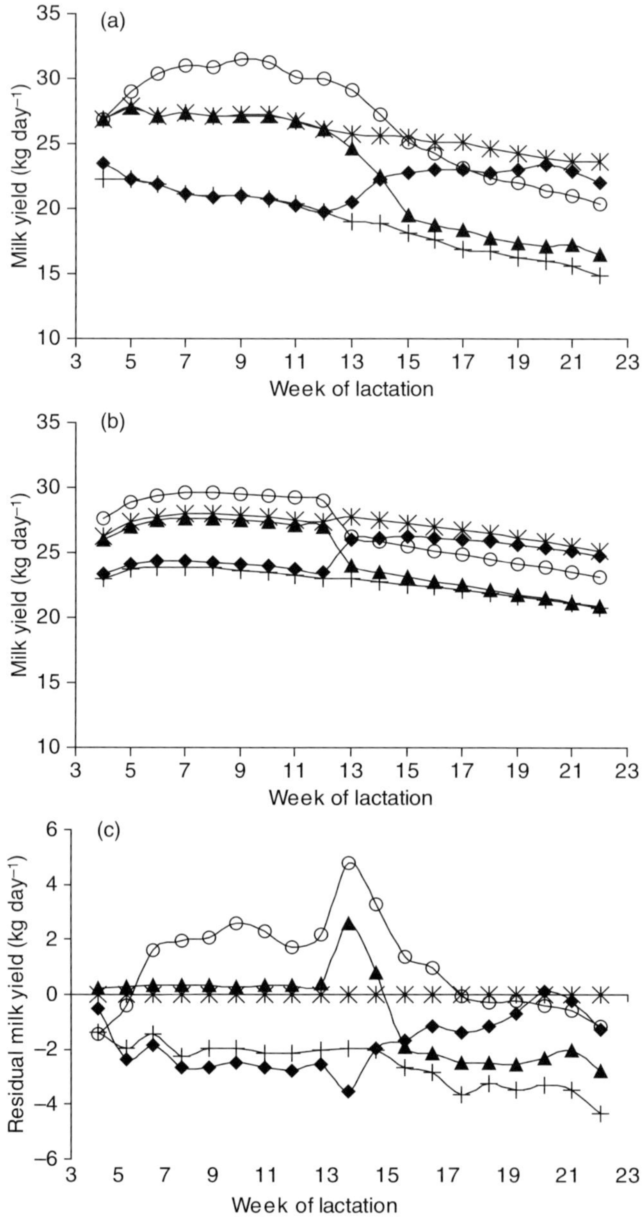

Fig. 22.5. Observed (a), predicted (b) and residual (c) milk yield responses to grass silage diets supplemented with 3, 9 or 12 kg concentrate day^{-1} from weeks 4 to 12 and 3 (3:3, +; 9:3, ▲), 6 (12:6, ❍) or 9 (3:9, ◆; 9:9, ✳) kg concentrate from weeks 13 to 22 of lactation. Observed data and inputs for the simulations were from Aston *et al.* (1995) as described in Fig. 22.4. Residuals were calculated as observed minus predicted. Model settings for the number of mammary cells and lactation persistency for all simulations were derived from the 9:9 diet yielding mean residual errors for milk yield and composition of 0. Residuals were standardized to errors for the 9:9 diet.

and grass availability in that production system, it seemed unlikely that the prediction errors were due entirely to photoperiod effects. A limitation to this work is the use of predicted dry matter intakes, which may introduce bias in the predictions. Despite this limitation, the work is consistent with the above observations in that predicted milk yields were under-responsive to the nutritional changes that occurred as the season progressed. Thus, the collective data suggest there are at least two components that contribute to the weight prediction problem: (i) inappropriate predictions of milk yield in response to nutritional state; and (ii) biased predictions of milk composition. One cannot rule out the existence of other problems, but clearly correction of these problems will at least partially resolve prediction bias.

Representation of Mammary Synthetic Activity

A key aspect of the partitioning problem appears to be the regulation of mammary synthetic activity. As represented in Molly, the rate of milk synthesis is a function of blood metabolite concentrations and mammary synthetic capacity, i.e. concentrations of glucose, acetate, amino acids, fatty acids and total enzyme activity in the udder.

Predicted concentrations of key metabolites in blood respond to dietary inputs, perhaps even inappropriately so for glucose (Fig. 22.6), and these changes in concentrations are the primary driver for changes in milk output. Although fatty acid and amino acid concentrations are known to vary significantly (Miettinen and Huhtanen, 1989; Guinard and Rulquin, 1994), as predicted by the model, glucose is highly regulated and its concentration would be expected to vary within a very limited range, as compared to the large variations predicted by the model. It is unclear whether predicted changes in acetate concentrations are appropriate, as a limited number of observations has been reported (Reynolds *et al.*, 1988; Miettinen and Huhtanen, 1989; Miller *et al.*, 1991).

If the regulation of glucose concentration was represented more appropriately in Molly, the milk yield response range for the diets of Aston *et al.* (1995) would be even narrower than currently predicted. Given that the predicted response range is approximately half the observed range in milk yield (Fig. 22.5), the range in blood metabolite concentrations would nearly have to double to simulate the appropriate changes in milk yield given the current model structure. Clearly, such variation in blood metabolite concentrations would be outside the physiological range. As the model was originally parameterized with the affinity constants for metabolites generally set equal to the reference blood concentrations, responses to changes in metabolite concentrations in blood are nearly linear, and thus increased responsiveness would require changes in either the affinity constant or the amount of enzyme present in one nutritional state versus the other, i.e. a regulatory event. The model currently does not have such a representation.

Mammary synthetic capacity is a function of the number of secretory cells present in the udder and the enzymatic activity of those cells (Knight and Wilde,

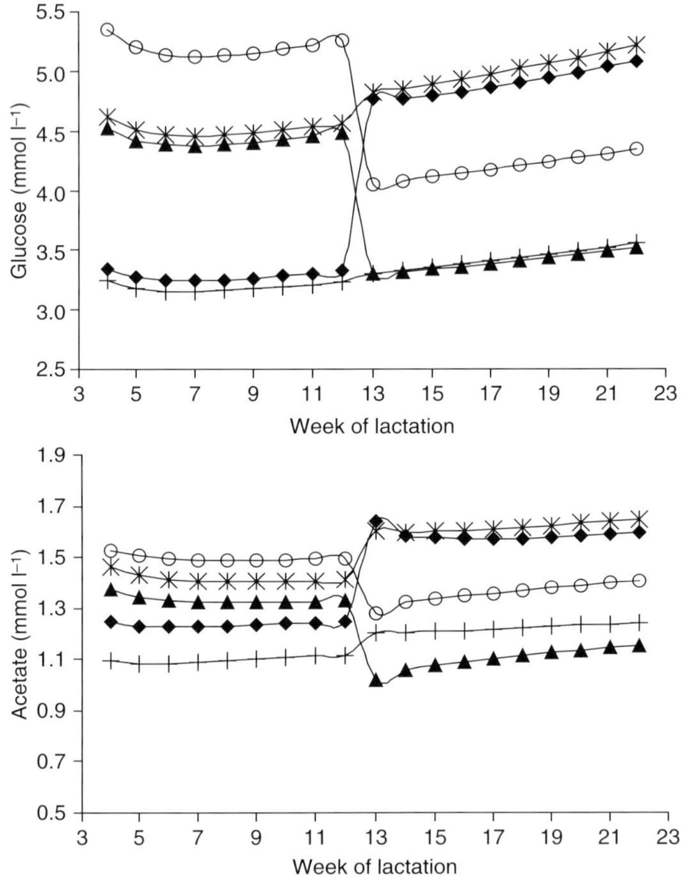

Fig. 22.6. Predicted concentrations of blood glucose and acetate for cows fed grass silage diets supplemented with 3, 9 or 12 kg concentrate day^{-1} from weeks 4 to 12 and 3 (3:3, +; 9:3, ▲), 6 (12:6, ❍) or 9 (3:9, ◆; 9:9, ✳) kg concentrate from weeks 13 to 22 of lactation. Inputs for the simulations were from Aston *et al.* (1995) as described in Fig. 22.4.

1993; Capuco *et al.*, 2001). The initial increase in milk yield after parturition is thought to be caused by increased cell numbers and increased activity per cell. After peak lactation, the activity per cell is thought to remain relatively constant and thus declining milk yield results from a loss of secretory cell numbers. Therefore, the number of secretory cells present at any point in lactation is not fixed. Recent evidence suggests that cell division persists throughout lactation (Capuco *et al.*, 2001), offering the potential for maintenance of cell numbers, or even increased cell numbers as lactation progresses. Things are further complicated by the observations that secretory cells may cycle between quiescent and active states (Molenaar *et al.*, 1992, 1996).

Total mammary enzyme activity (activity per cell times the number of cells) in Molly is predicted using the model of Neal and Thornley (1983). In this representation, enzyme activity per cell was assumed to be constant and thus total mammary enzyme activity was proportional to the number of differentiated cells. Differentiated cells are assumed to derive from a small initial pool of undifferentiated cells which divide in binary fashion. The rate of division is assumed to be proportional to the concentration of a generic lactation hormone. Lactation hormone is set to 0 when the animal is non-lactating, pulsed positively at parturition and decays exponentially thereafter (Fig. 22.7). Differentiated cells produced by cell division are subject to cell death by mass action. This representation produces an asymptotic increase in cell numbers, beginning at parturition, with maximal cell numbers reached at peak lactation and a log-linear decline in differentiated cells thereafter yielding the standard lactation

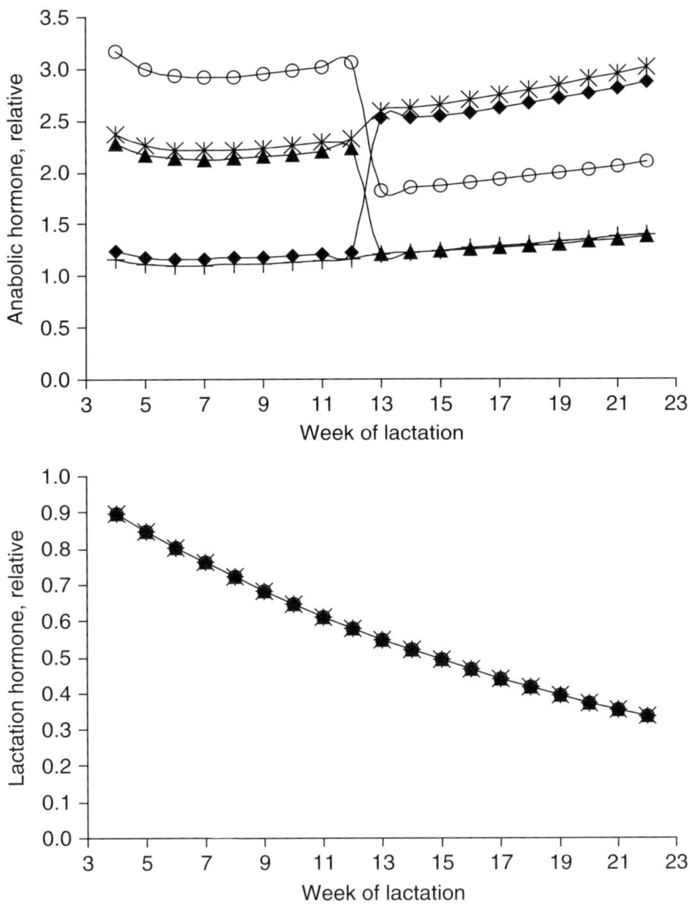

Fig. 22.7. Predicted anabolic and lactation hormone concentrations (relative units) for cows fed grass silage diets supplemented with 3, 9 or 12 kg concentrate day^{-1} from weeks 4 to 12 and 3 (3:3, +; 9:3, ▲), 6 (12:6, ❍) or 9 (3:9, ◆; 9:9, ✳) kg concentrate from weeks 13 to 22 of lactation. Inputs for the simulations were from Aston *et al.* (1995) as described in Fig. 22.4.

curve. Rates of cell loss were assumed to be influenced by the average amount of milk present in the udder to account for the effects of variable milking intervals.

As lactation hormone in this representation is not responsive to nutritional state (Fig. 22.7), nutrition can affect milk synthesis in Molly only as a function of deviations in blood metabolite concentrations. Thus, a change in diet results in shifts in blood metabolite concentrations that persist for the duration of the diet. If milk yield should change 20% in response to a diet, then milk precursors in blood would have to change 20% or more to achieve the milk yield response. These large, sustained changes in glucose, acetate, fatty acid and amino acid concentrations can destabilize the model, particularly under conditions of nutritional restriction.

Aston *et al.* (1995) observed that reductions in milk yield under conditions of energy restriction occurred over a period of about 3 weeks, while increases in yield during energy repletion occurred over a period of approximately 8 weeks. While Molly predicts the direction of change in yield appropriately, the magnitude of the predicted change is underpredicted (noted above) and the temporal components of the changes are predicted inappropriately (Fig. 22.5). When simulating concentrate allocations of 9 kg day^{-1} followed by a period at 3 kg day^{-1}, Molly overpredicts the initial decline in milk yield after the diet switch, but fails to predict a large enough long-term drop in production (Fig. 22.5). The reverse is true for a 3 kg diet followed by 9 kg, although the initial overprediction of recovery is less pronounced. These results suggest that perhaps three mechanisms are involved in the adjustment to dietary energy levels. The initial phase of the response appears to be a combination of changes in metabolite supply and perhaps some rapid compensatory changes in enzyme activity that are not represented in Molly, leading to the inappropriate initial response to energy depletion and repletion. The latter phase of the response is much slower, particularly when the cows are recovering from energy restriction, suggesting that enzyme activity continues to change or the number of active cells is changing slowly.

The slow recovery of milk yield appears to be specific to energy restriction and repletion, as both the decline and the return to full production occurred within 2 weeks when animals were fed diets that were amino acid restricted and then replete (Yeo *et al.*, 2003), supporting the contention that the metabolic responses were at least biphasic in nature. As body fat stores are affected by energy supply, whereas generally they are not affected by protein supply, it is possible that the extended recovery period associated with energy repletion is caused by endocrine signals, such as leptin, generated by adipose tissue in response to energy status.

These observations collectively suggest that the representation of mammary enzyme activity in Molly should be altered to consider the effect of factors in addition to milking frequency and stage of lactation on mammary enzyme activity. Such consideration must account for the heterogeneity of responses to energy and amino acid nutrition and the apparent ability of mammary synthetic activity to return to the normal pattern after periods of suboptimal activity.

Factors Affecting Mammary Synthetic Capacity and Activity

The above observations support three potential mechanisms that result in a change in overall mammary synthetic activity, in addition to the kinetic effects of metabolite supply: (i) alterations in enzyme activity per secretory cell; (ii) changes in the number of active and quiescent secretory cells; and (iii) changes in total secretory cell numbers due to cell division or death. Some hints as to the mechanism of action associated with various observations can be derived from the temporal aspects of the change in activity. As cell turnover in the mammary gland has been shown to be relatively slow (0.3% day^{-1}; Capuco *et al.*, 2001), it would require a number of days to achieve a significant change in cell number. It is unclear what time frames are required for cycling between active and quiescent states, but changes in enzyme activity and metabolite supply can occur over relatively shorter time frames, i.e. minutes to hours. To model these mechanisms, it is useful to have some understanding of the signals that regulate the changes.

Treatment with exogenous somatotropin clearly stimulates milk yield (Asdell, 1932; Peel *et al.*, 1981, 1983; Eppard *et al.*, 1985). However, it is less clear whether the effects of somatotropin are elicited solely by changes in blood flow and metabolite concentrations or by changes in mammary synthetic capacity (either more activity per cell or more cells) which subsequently lead to increased blood flow. The observed increase in production is generally in the 3–5 kg day^{-1} range, with some evidence that the response increases as the duration of injections increases (Van Amburgh *et al.*, 1997). This initial milk yield response associated with somatotropin administration mirrors systemic somatotropin concentrations with little lag time, i.e. yield increases within 2–3 days post-administration and returns to baseline values within 2–3 days of cessation. Such timing argues against a change in secretory cell numbers, as the changes are too rapid.

Knight *et al.* (1994) did not observe an effect of exogenous somatotropin on cell growth in early lactation, but they did observe increased cell proliferation and milk yield during late lactation in dairy goats. Hadsell *et al.* (2002) found that manipulation of either insulin-like growth factor I or its receptor in mice via gene knockout experiments resulted in changes in cell proliferation activity, and the changes in secretory cell area and the rate of cell division were significantly different from controls in late lactation but not early lactation (Hadsell *et al.*, 2005). Work in heifers has been equivocal, with stimulation of cell proliferation reported by Berry *et al.* (2001) but not observed by Radcliff *et al.* (2000). Based on milk yield responses, the initial rapid response in milk production is followed by a very slow increase in the response when treatment is extended for a number of months (Van Amburgh *et al.*, 1997). However, it is unclear whether this response is due to increased cell numbers, an enhancement of the initial cell activity response, or increased substrate supply associated with dry matter intake responses. If increased persistency is associated with increased cell numbers in late lactation, then cows that have been treated throughout the lactation with somatotropin should exhibit greater milk yields (due to greater cell numbers) after cessation of injections than comparable cows that were not treated with somatotropin. To our knowledge, such a study has not been undertaken.

Examination of metabolite transport kinetics in somatotropin-treated animals indicated that only leucine uptake was stimulated in response to treatment. Transport activity of phenylalanine, glucose, β-hydroxybutyrate and glycerol were all significantly less for treated cows, while the remaining metabolite transport activities were unaffected, suggesting little change in the kinetics of extraction (Hanigan *et al.*, 1998). These observations suggested that the observed changes in milk synthesis were associated with altered substrate supply, i.e. increased blood flow or blood concentrations. Therefore, it is not yet clear whether somatotropin exerts its effect by increasing cell proliferation, cell activity, metabolite supply, or some combination of these mechanisms.

Acute treatment with insulin does not appear to affect milk yield or composition positively and it can depress yield if glucose concentrations are not maintained (Kronfeld *et al.*, 1963; Schmidt, 1966; Rook and Hopwood, 1970; Hove, 1978). However, chronic infusions have been associated with significant increases in milk and milk component yields, provided substrate supplies are maintained (McGuire *et al.*, 1995; Griinari *et al.*, 1997a,b;), and these increases are associated with significant changes in mammary transport and metabolic activity (Bequette *et al.*, 2001).

Milk yield responses to insulin infusion were observed to require 3–4 days to reach maximal stimulation, which raises the question as to the mode of action. Although these changes in activity occur in association with insulin infusions, insulin-like growth factor-1 (IGF-1) also increases during the insulin infusions and thus IGF-1 may be the common mechanism for both insulin and somatotropin responses. As these increases in activity occur over a relatively short time frame, it seems likely that they reflect a change in metabolic activity per cell or substrate supply (blood flow) rather than a change in cell numbers.

The observations of Aston *et al.* (1995) are consistent with declining cell numbers as lactation progresses and altered activity per cell in response to nutritional state. Cows offered 9 kg concentrate in the second period of the study (weeks 13–22; 3:9, 9:9; Fig. 22.4) did not produce as much milk as the cows offered 9 kg concentrate in the first period (weeks 4–12; 9:3, 9:9; Fig. 22.5). That is, putting the animals in the same nutritional state in mid-lactation did not generate the same milk yield result as when that nutritional state was applied in early lactation, suggesting that some loss of mammary synthetic capacity occurred. Altering energy intake did not appear to influence the rate of this loss in capacity. Regardless of the amount of concentrate offered in the first period (3:9 or 9:9), cows given 9 kg concentrate in the second period produced equal amounts of milk per day by the end of the period (Fig. 22.5). Of course, there was a long lag period before the restricted cows achieved the same production as the unrestricted cows. Finally, cows offered 3 kg concentrate day^{-1} produced less milk than those offered 9 kg day^{-1}, regardless of stage of lactation, and this loss was reversible, suggesting that it was mediated by a change in activity per cell rather than a loss of cells. However, Gibb *et al.* (1992) observed a significant effect of dietary energy on mammary protein mass using serial slaughter techniques, which may indicate a change in the number of cells, or at least cell mass.

Regardless of whether the rate of secretory cell loss is affected by nutritional state, restricted cows clearly experienced a temporary loss in synthetic capacity.

Simulations of blood metabolite concentrations by Molly indicate that they have almost reached a new steady state within a week of the diet transition. Thus, energy repletion would be expected to restore milk yield to pre-restriction levels (minus the small loss in secretory cells due to increasing days in milk) within 1 week and certainly by 2 weeks after the diet shift. The fact that restoration takes much longer and that milk production eventually returns to that of the unrestricted animals supports the contention that mammary capacity has been inhibited temporarily.

The temporal and quantitative aspects of the above responses raise a question as to the mechanism of action associated with temporary changes in synthetic activity. Does some long-acting signal regulate enzyme activity to attenuate responses? Are secretory cells lost and subsequently replaced by cell division? Or do cells simply become quiescent and then return to an active state?

If cell turnover were relatively slow, as has been observed (Capuco *et al.*, 2001), this may explain the relatively long time required to restore production to the normal level after energy restriction. However, this raises additional questions relative to control of total cell numbers. If mechanisms are present to stimulate the replacement of lost cells, what controls cell numbers such that they return only to numbers that would have been present had a nutritional restriction not occurred, i.e. if 9 kg concentrate is adequate to support 27 kg milk at week 9 of lactation, why is it not adequate to stimulate production to 27 kg milk at week 20 of lactation? If cell synthesis could be stimulated, it would seem the secretory potential could be returned to levels that exceed levels expected for that point in lactation. The fact that production returned to the normal lactation curve for cows given 9 kg concentrate throughout lactation indicated that nutritional restriction did not alter the normal rate of cell loss as lactation progressed. It seems more likely that cells may have been induced to cease or reduce secretory activity and subsequently returned to active status when the nutritional restriction was removed.

If secretory cells are simply reducing their activity or becoming inactive during times of stress and when udder capacity is underutilized, a set of signals controlling this change in activity that operates over a variable time frame is required. Energy restriction not only lowers blood concentrations of key metabolites, it also depletes body fat stores. Leptin secretion by adipose cells has been observed to be proportional to fat mass and also responsive to energy balance (Block *et al.*, 2003). A direct link between leptin concentrations in blood and mammary secretory cell activity has not been demonstrated. However, leptin has been observed to increase rates of cell proliferation and to alter the phosphorylation state of several key signalling proteins in non-lactating mammary tissue (Hu *et al.*, 2002). If leptin also played a role in regulation of proliferation or cell activity in lactating cells, this may explain the very long time frame required to restore normal mammary synthetic activity after an energy restriction. It would also be consistent with the lack of a long time lag when animals are amino acid restricted, wherein body energy loss generally does not occur. Further support for a potential role of leptin in regulation of mammary secretory activity is provided by the observations of Feuermann *et al.* (2004). They observed a 25-fold increase in leptin receptor expression when mammary cells were cultured in the presence of prolactin. They also observed that leptin stimulated both milk protein and milk fat synthesis when cells were cultured with both leptin and prolactin.

Milking frequency effects on milk yield have been observed in the ewe (Negrao *et al.*, 2001), goat (Knight *et al.*, 1990) and cow (DePeters *et al.*, 1985; Bar-Peled *et al.*, 1995; Davis *et al.*, 1999). The signal eliciting this response must originate from within the udder. The work of Wilde *et al.* (1987) and Hale *et al.* (2003) suggests that the number of secretory cells is altered in association with milking frequency, which is consistent with the representation by Neal and Thornley (1983). However, the mechanism of action is not clear. Vetharaniam *et al.* (2003) represented the effect as a change in the number of active cells, which is consistent with the observed responses to milking frequency (Barnes *et al.*, 1990).

Thus, there are four potential modulators of mammary enzyme activity: (i) somatotropin; (ii) insulin; (iii) leptin; and (iv) milking frequency. Of these, only the fourth is represented currently in Molly, and it is represented as a shift in the rate of loss of mammary enzyme capacity.

Modelling Active and Quiescent Mammary Cells

Vetharaniam *et al.* (2003) described a representation of mammary cells that included consideration of the effects of energy status and milking frequency. In this representation, progenitor cells were assumed to divide in a binary manner to produce active secretory cells, and the rate of cell division declined exponentially after parturition. Active cells were assumed to become quiescent as a function of milk volume in the alveoli. Quiescent cells were subject to reactivation to the active state and senescence. Total enzyme activity in the udder was then represented as a function of the active cells and the energy supply to the udder. This representation has the advantage over that of Neal and Thornley (1983) in that it allows for effects of energy supply on enzyme activity and temporary removal of secretory activity in response to milking frequency.

While the model of Vetharaniam *et al.* (2003) appears to conform more closely to observations, there are still some significant inconsistencies. Although a minor point, unless one is studying mammary growth, it is clear from data collected from mice, rats, guinea pigs and goats that cell growth preceding parturition is exponential rather than binary (Dijkstra *et al.*, 1997); thus, cell division is not restricted to a progenitor population or, if it is, the progenitor population undergoes a period of exponential growth before generation of differentiated cells. Perhaps more importantly, the assumption that only quiescent cells undergo senescence would appear to be inconsistent with the observations of Barnes *et al.* (1990). The rate of cell death appears to be unaffected by milking frequency, as evidenced by a common milk loss slope (kg day^{-1}) for twice daily and three times daily milking, suggesting that all mammary cells have the same probability of undergoing apoptosis. It is of interest that, when the model was fitted to observed data, the rate of cell death was found to be significantly influenced by dietary energy; however, endocrine effects on cell activity were not considered.

Based on these observations, it would seem that the representation of cell activity in Molly should be updated with a revised version of the model of Vetharaniam *et al.* (2003). If somatotropin/IFG-1, insulin and leptin were added to the energy-signalling portion of that model, it may predict more accurately the biphasic response to nutrition. This approach would help address the nutritional sensitivity problem, as it would allow for down-regulation of enzyme activity per cell, which may reflect more accurately the magnitude of nutritionally induced lactation changes and create a new set point for mammary activity. This change in set point would help to stabilize blood metabolite concentrations within the normal range, thereby improving model stability. However, it would also attenuate endocrine signals generated as a function of metabolite concentrations, necessitating a re-evaluation of the endocrine sensitivity to those metabolites. Adoption of these changes in Molly would allow one to explore better the question regarding the effects of energy status on rates of mammary cell turnover, given the explicit representations of nutrition, endocrines and mammary function.

Milk Composition

The observations that milk component synthesis rates do not all conform to a common stage of lactation pattern offers additional support for a change in the representation of mammary synthetic capacity. As lactose is the primary driver of milk volume via its osmotic potential, it seems appropriate to assume that lactose secretion rates parallel milk secretion rates, as assumed in Molly. However, protein and fat synthesis rates appear to deviate slightly from one another and from lactose secretion rates as lactation progresses (Stanton *et al.*, 1992). Where milk and lactose production rates increase during early lactation, reaching a peak approximately 6 weeks after calving, milk protein and fat synthesis rates appear to be maximized at, or shortly after, calving. Addressing this problem requires a modification of the equations describing enzyme activity for milk protein and fat synthesis, such that peak enzyme activity occurs nearer to parturition. Alternatively, if one assumes that protein and fat synthetic capacity are proportional to active cells and lactose capacity varies by stage of lactation, one could leave the fat and protein synthesis equations as currently represented and alter the representation of lactose enzyme activity. Data to parameterize these equations are readily available in the literature. However, one must be concerned over the potential for differential regulation of these entities. There appears to be modest potential for differential regulation of milk protein and greater potential for regulation of milk fat. A portion of the variation in milk fat synthesis arises from the effects of unsaturated fatty acids on *de novo* milk fat synthesis within the mammary glands. The current representation of blood fatty acids in aggregate prevents a direct consideration of the effects of unsaturated fatty acids on *de novo* synthesis. A calculation of the dietary proportion of total fat that is unsaturated could be used to estimate the effect, but considerable evidence of ruminal hydrogenation and post-absorptive desaturase activity suggests that this approach would be fraught with error. To represent the effects of unsaturated fat properly would seem to require consideration of an additional pool of fatty acids. This would allow the consideration of transfers from one pool to the other in the various compartments. It would also allow for consideration of the buffering effects of fat stores. Inputs of unsaturated fats would be dampened by exchange with the relatively saturated adipose stores. Conversely, scrubbing of unsaturated fats from the diet would not remove them from circulation immediately, as they would be released from adipose tissue for a period of time.

Chardon (2004) altered the representation of enzyme activity in Molly such that separate Neal and Thornley functions were used for each milk component (lactose, protein and fat), as opposed to the common representation with respect to stage of lactation described originally. Lactation hormone was also separated into three pools to allow for differential regulation of the mammary synthetic activity for each component. These changes resulted in some improvements in the predictions of fat and protein yield (Fig. 22.8), but poorer predictions of milk fat per cent and mixed results for protein per cent (Fig. 22.9).

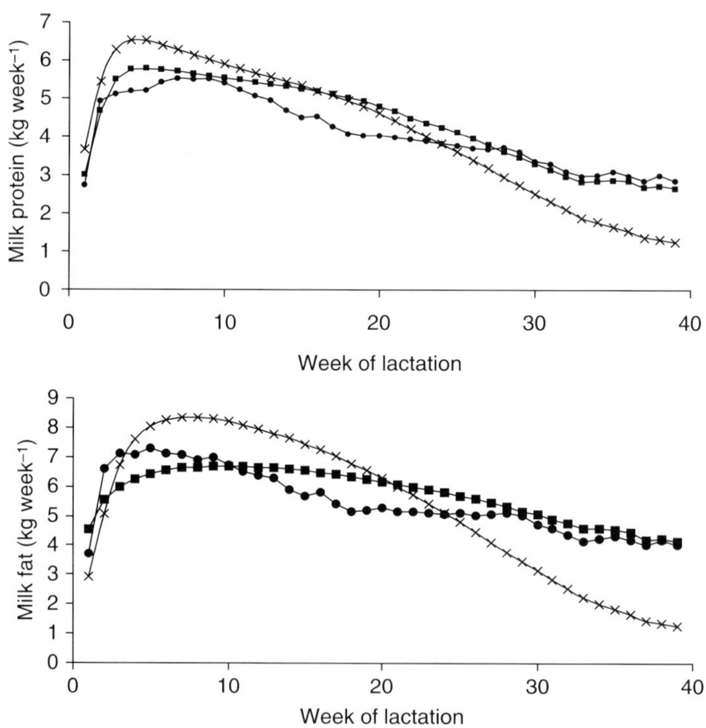

Fig. 22.8 Predictions of protein and fat yields by Molly (x) and after adopting separate representations of the enzyme associated with each of those components (■). The observed data (•) are from two herds of pasture-fed cows (n = 40), the work being conducted at the Dexcel research facilities during the 2003/04 season in Hamilton, New Zealand (Macdonald *et al.*, 2005). Adapted from Chardon (2004).

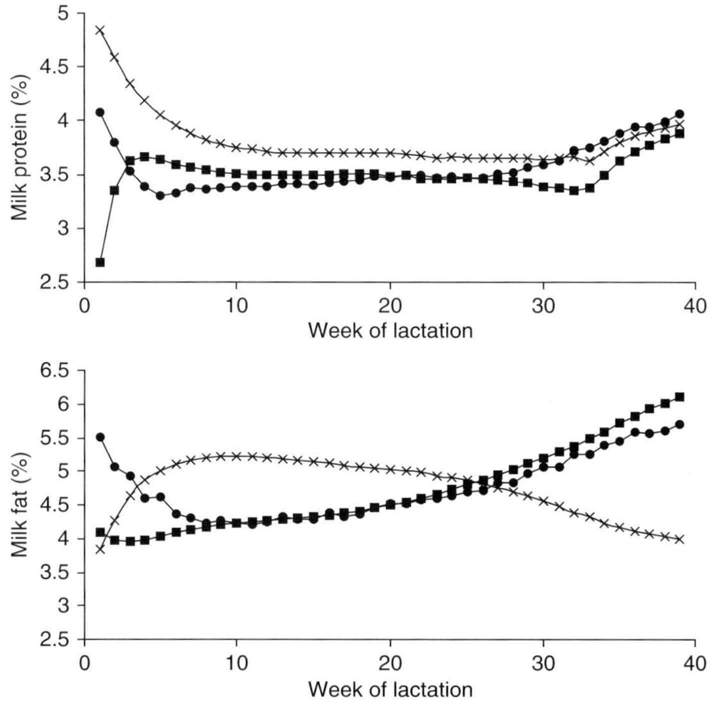

Fig. 22.9. Predictions of protein and fat content of milk by Molly (x) and after adopting separate representations of the enzyme associated with each of those components (■). The observed data (•) are from two herds of pasture-fed cows (n = 40), the work being conducted at the Dexcel research facilities during the 2003/04 season in Hamilton, New Zealand (Macdonald *et al.*, 2005). Adapted from Chardon (2004).

Other work conducted by Dexcel (Faure, 2005) altered the representation of lactation hormone so that it became a function of nutritional state. This was accomplished by increasing the rate of decay of lactation hormone when the concentration of glucose in blood dropped below reference values. If glucose concentrations recovered, the decay rate of lactation hormone returned to normal. This resulted in a change in mammary enzyme activity that was reflected in milk yields. While this approach slightly improved predictions of milk yield during nutrient restriction, it also caused a reduction in milk yield during early lactation when glucose concentrations were low. Despite the early lactation problems, the improved predictions during nutritional restriction support the general approach and suggest that further improvement could be made if more extensive revisions of the representation of mammary enzyme activity were undertaken.

Summary

A number of years of work have been spent to develop Molly to its current state. While the structure generally has been found to be adequate, work conducted since its original description suggests some upgrading is required. In particular, it fails to simulate post-absorptive metabolite partitioning accurately under widely varying nutritional conditions. This problem appears to be related to the representation of mammary synthetic activity. While the current representation allows for changes in activity associated with stage of lactation and frequency of milking, it does not support alterations in response to nutritional state. Current biological knowledge of mammary function suggests the representation of mammary enzyme activity should be altered to consider quiescent and active pools of secretory cells, the cycling between these pools and the effects of endocrine signals on enzyme activity of the active cells. These changes should address the observed under-responsiveness of milk production to changes in nutritional inputs and at least partially resolve problems in predicting weight changes.

References

Asdell, S.A. (1932) The effect of the injection of hypophyseal extract in advanced lactation. *American Journal of Physiology* 100, 137–140.

Aston, K., Sutton, J.D. and Fisher, W.J. (1995) Milk production from grass silage diets: strategies for concentrate allocation. *Animal Science* 61, 465–480.

Baldwin, R.L. (1995) *Modeling Ruminant Digestion and Metabolism*. Chapman and Hall, London.

Baldwin, R.L., France, J. and Gill, M. (1987a) Metabolism of the lactating cow. I. Animal elements of a mechanistic model. *Journal of Dairy Research* 54, 77–105.

Baldwin, R.L., Thornley, J.H.M. and Beever, D.E. (1987b) Metabolism of the lactating cow. II. Digestive elements of a mechanistic model. *Journal of Dairy Research* 54, 107–131.

Baldwin, R.L., France, J., Beever, D.E., Gill, M. and Thornley, J.H.M. (1987c) Metabolism of the lactating cow. III. Properties of mechanistic models suitable for evaluation of energetic relationships and factors involved in the partition of nutrients. *Journal of Dairy Research* 54, 133–145.

Barnes, M.A., Pearson, R.E. and Lukes-Wilson, A.J. (1990) Effects of milking frequency and selection for milk yield on productive efficiency of Holstein cows. *Journal of Dairy Science* 73, 1603–1611.

Bar-Peled, U., Maltz, E., Bruckental, I., Folman, Y., Kali, Y., Gacitua, H., Lehrer, A.R., Knight, C.H., Robinzon, B. and Voet, H. (1995) Relationship between frequent milking or suckling in early lactation and milk production of high producing dairy cows. *Journal of Dairy Science* 78, 2726–2736.

Bequette, B.J., Hanigan, M.D., Calder, A.G., Reynolds, C.K., Lobley, G.E. and MacRae, J.C. (2000) Amino acid exchange by the mammary gland of lactating goats when histidine limits milk production. *Journal of Dairy Science* 83, 765–775.

Bequette, B.J., Kyle, C.E., Crompton, L.A., Buchan, V. and Hanigan, M.D. (2001) Insulin regulates milk production and mammary gland and hind-leg amino acid fluxes and blood flow in lactating goats. *Journal of Dairy Science* 84, 241–255.

Berry, S.D., Mcfadden, T.B., Pearson, R.E. and Akers, R.M. (2001) A local increase in the mammary IGF-1:IGFBP-3 ratio mediates the mammogenic effects of estrogen and growth hormone. *Domestic Animal Endocrinology* 21, 39–53.

Beukes, P.C., Thorrold, B.S., Wastney, M.E., Palliser, C.C., Macdonald, K.A., Bright, K.P., Lancaster, J.A.S., Palmer, C.A.J. and Auldist, M.J. (2005) Modelling the bi-peak lactation curves of summer calvers in New Zealand dairy farm systems. *Australian Journal of Experimental Agriculture* 45, 643–649.

Block, S.S., Smith, J.M., Ehrhardt, R.A., Diaz, M.C., Rhoads, R.P., Van Amburgh, M.E. and Boisclair, Y.R. (2003) Nutritional and developmental regulation of plasma leptin in dairy cattle. *Journal of Dairy Science* 86, 3206–3214.

Broster, W.H. and Thomas, C. (1981) The influence of level and pattern of concentrate input on milk output. In Haresign, W. (ed.) *Recent Advances in Animal Nutrition*. Butterworths, London, pp. 49–69.

Capuco, A.V., Wood, D.L., Baldwin, R., McLeod, K. and Paape, M.J. (2001) Mammary cell number, proliferation, and apoptosis during a bovine lactation: relation to milk production and effect of bST. *Journal of Dairy Science* 84, 2177–2187.

Chardon, X. (2004) Modelling the milk component yields of New Zealand dairy cows. MSc thesis, Institut National Agronomique de Paris-Grignon, France.

Davis, S.R., Farr, V.C. and Stelwagen, K. (1999) Regulation of yield loss and milk composition during once-daily milking: a review. *Livestock Production Science* 59, 77–94.

DePeters, E.J. and Cant, J.P. (1992) Nutritional factors influencing the nitrogen composition of bovine milk: a review. *Journal of Dairy Science* 75, 2043–2070.

DePeters, E.J., Smith, N.E. and Acedo-Rico, J. (1985) Three or two times daily milking of older cows and first lactation cows for entire lactations. *Journal of Dairy Science* 68, 123–132.

Dijkstra, J., France, J., Dhanoa, M.S., Maas, J.A., Hanigan, M.D., Rook, A.J. and Beever, D.E. (1997) A model to describe growth patterns of the mammary gland during pregnancy and lactation. *Journal of Dairy Science* 80, 2340–2354.

Eppard, P.J., Bauman, D.E. and McCutcheon, S.N. (1985) Effect of dose of bovine growth hormone on lactation of dairy cows. *Journal of Dairy Science* 68, 1109–1115.

Faure, X. (2005) *Energy Partitioning in the Molly Cow Model*. Hamilton, New Zealand.

Feuermann, Y., Mabjeesh, S.J. and Shamay, A. (2004) Leptin affects prolactin action on milk protein and fat synthesis in the bovine mammary gland. *Journal of Dairy Science* 87, 2941–2946.

Gaynor, P.J., Erdman, R.A., Teter, B.B., Sampugna, J., Capuco, A.V., Waldo, D.R. and Hamosh, M. (1994) Milk fat yield and composition during abomasal infusion of cis or trans octadecenoates in Holstein cows. *Journal of Dairy Science* 77, 157–165.

Gibb, M.J., Ivings, W.E., Dhanoa, M.S. and Sutton, J.D. (1992) Changes in body components of autumn-calving Holstein–Friesian cows over the first 29 weeks of lactation. *Animal Production* 55, 339–360.

Griinari, J.M., McGuire, M.A., Dwyer, D.A., Bauman, D.E. and Palmquist, D.L. (1997a) Role of insulin in the regulation of milk fat synthesis in dairy cows. *Journal of Dairy Science* 80, 1076–1084.

Griinari, J.M., McGuire, M.A., Dwyer, D.A., Bauman, D.E., Barbano, D.M. and House, W.A. (1997b) The role of insulin in the regulation of milk protein synthesis in dairy cows. *Journal of Dairy Science* 80, 2361–2371.

Guinard, J. and Rulquin, H. (1994) Effect of graded levels of duodenal infusions of casein on mammary uptake in lactating cows. 2. Individual amino acids. *Journal of Dairy Science* 77, 3304–3315.

Hadsell, D.L., Bonnette, S.G. and Lee, A.V. (2002) Genetic manipulation of the IGF-I axis to regulate mammary gland development and function. *Journal of Dairy Science* 85, 365–377.

Hadsell, D.L., Torres, D.T., Lawrence, N.A., George, J., Parlow, A.F., Lee, A.V. and Fiorotto, M.L. (2005) Overexpression of des(1-3) insulin-like growth factor 1 in the mammary glands of transgenic mice delays the loss of milk production with prolonged lactation. *Biology of Reproduction* 73, 1116–1125.

Hale, S.A., Capuco, A.V. and Erdman, R.A. (2003) Milk yield and mammary growth effects due to increased milking frequency during early lactation. *Journal of Dairy Science* 86, 2061–2071.

Hanigan, M.D., France, J., Wray-Cahen, D., Beever, D.E., Lobley, G.E., Reutzel, L. and Smith, N.E. (1998) Alternative models for analyses of liver and mammary transorgan metabolite extraction data. *British Journal of Nutrition* 79, 63–78.

Hanigan, M.D., Bateman, H.G., Fadel, J.G. and McNamara, J.P. (2006) Metabolic models of ruminant metabolism: recent improvements and current status. *Journal of Dairy Science* 89, E52–E64

Hove, K. (1978) Effects of hyperinsulinemia on lactose secretion and glucose uptake by the goat mammary gland. *Acta Physiologica Scandinavica* 104, 422–430.

Hristov, A.N., Price, W.J. and Shafii, B. (2005) A meta-analysis on the relationship between intake of nutrients and body weight with milk volume and milk protein yield in dairy cows. *Journal of Dairy Science* 88, 2860–2869.

Hu, X., Juneja, S.C., Maihle, N.J. and Cleary, M.P. (2002) Leptin – a growth factor in normal and malignant breast cells and for normal mammary gland development. *Journal of the National Cancer Institute* 94, 1704–1711.

Knight, C.H. and Wilde, C.J. (1993) Mammary cell changes during pregnancy and lactation. *Livestock Production Science* 35, 3–19.

Knight, C.H., Fowler, P.A. and Wilde, C.J. (1990) Galactopoietic and mammogenic effects of long-term treatment with bovine growth hormone and thrice daily milking in goats. *Journal of Endocrinology* 127, 129–138.

Knight, C.H., France, J. and Beever, D.E. (1994) Nutrient metabolism and utilization in the mammary gland. *Livestock Production Science* 39, 129–137.

Kronfeld, D.S., Mayer, G.P., Robertson, J.McD. and Raggi, F. (1963) Depression of milk secretion during insulin administration. *Journal of Dairy Science* 46, 559–563.

Macdonald, K.A., Thorrold, B.S., Glassey, C.B., Holmes, C.W. and Pryce, J.E. (2005) Impact of farm management decision rules on the production and profit of different strains of Holstein–Friesian dairy cows. *Proceedings of the New Zealand Society of Animal Production* 65, 40–45.

McGuire, M.A., Griinari, J.M., Dwyer, D.A. and Bauman, D.E. (1995) Role of insulin in the regulation of mammary synthesis of fat and protein. *Journal of Dairy Science* 78, 816–824.

McNamara, J.P. (2004) Research, improvement and application of mechanistic, biochemical, dynamic models of metabolism in lactating dairy cattle. *Animal Feed Science and Technology* 112, 155–176.

McNamara, J.P. and Baldwin, R.L. (2000) Estimation of parameters describing lipid metabolism in lactation: challenge of existing knowledge described in a model of metabolism. *Journal of Dairy Science* 83, 128–143.

Miettinen, H. and Huhtanen, P. (1989) The concentrations of blood metabolites and the relations between blood parameters, fatty acid composition of milk and estimated ME-balance in dairy cows given grass silage *ad libitum* with five different carbohydrate supplements. *Acta Agricultura Scandinavica* 39, 319–330.

Miller, P.S., Reis, B.L., Calvert, C.C., DePeters, E.J. and Baldwin, R.L. (1991) Patterns of nutrient uptake by the mammary glands of lactating dairy cows. *Journal of Dairy Science* 74, 3791–3799.

Molenaar, A.J., Davis, S.R. and Wilkins, R.J. (1992) Expression of a-lactalbumin, a-S1-casein, and lactoferrin genes is heterogeneous in sheep and cattle mammary tissue. *Journal of Histochemistry and Cytochemistry* 40, 611–618.

Molenaar, A.J., Kuys, Y.M., Davis, S.R., Wilkins, R.J., Mead, P.E. and Tweedie, J.W. (1996) Elevation of lactoferrin gene expression in developing, ductal, resting, and regressing parenchymal epithelium of the ruminant mammary gland. *Journal of Dairy Science* 79, 1198–1208.

National Research Council (NRC) (1978) *Nutrient Requirements of Dairy Cattle*, 5th edn. National Academy Press, Washington, DC.

National Research Council (NRC) (1985) *Ruminant Nitrogen Usage*. National Academy Press, Washington, DC.

National Research Council (NRC) (1989) *Nutrient Requirements of Dairy Cattle*, 6th edn. National Academy Press, Washington, DC.

National Research Council (NRC) (2001) *Nutrient Requirements of Dairy Cattle*, 7th rev. edn. National Academy Press, Washington, DC.

Neal, H.D.Sc. and Thornley, J.H.M. (1983) The lactation curve in cattle: a mathematical model of the mammary gland. *Journal of Agricultural Science (Cambridge)* 101, 389–400.

Negrao, J.A., Marnet, P.G. and Labussiere, J. (2001) Effect of milking frequency on oxytocin release and milk production in dairy ewes. *Small Ruminant Research* 39, 181–187.

Offer, N.W., Agnew, R.E., Cottrill, B.R., Givens, D.I., Keady, T.W.J., Mayne, C.S., Rymer, C., Yan, T., France, J., Beever, D.E. and Thomas, C. (2002) Feed into milk – an applied feeding model coupled with a new system of feed characterisation. In: Garnsworthy, P.C. and Wiseman, J. (eds) *Recent Advances in Animal Nutrition.* Nottingham University Press, Nottingham, UK, pp. 167–194.

Peel, C.J., Bauman, D.E., Gorewit, R.C. and Sniffen, C.J. (1981) Effect of exogenous growth hormone on lactational performance in high yielding dairy cows. *Journal of Nutrition* 111, 1662–1671.

Peel, C.J., Fronk, T.J., Bauman, D.E. and Gorewit, R.C. (1983) Effect of exogenous growth hormone in early and late lactation on lactational performance of dairy cows. *Journal of Dairy Science* 66, 776–782.

Radcliff, R.P., Vandehaar, M.J., Chapin, L.T., Pilbeam, T.E., Beede, D.K., Stanisiewski, E.P. and Tucker, H.A. (2000) Effects of diet and injection of bovine somatotropin on prepubertal growth and first-lactation milk yields of Holstein cows. *Journal of Dairy Science* 83, 23–29.

Reynolds, C.K., Huntington, G.B., Tyrrell, H.F. and Reynolds, P.J. (1988) Net metabolism of volatile fatty acids, D-beta-hydroxybutyrate, non-esterified fatty acids, and blood gases by portal-drained viscera and liver of lactating Holstein cows. *Journal of Dairy Science* 71, 2395–2405.

Rook, J.A.F. and Hopwood, J.B. (1970) The effects of intravenous infusions of insulin and of sodium succinate on milk secretion in the goat. *Journal of Dairy Research* 37, 193–198.

Schmidt, G.H. (1966) Effect of insulin on yield and composition of milk of dairy cows. *Journal of Dairy Science* 49, 381–385.

Smith, N.E. (1970) Quantitative simulation analyses of ruminant metabolic functions: basal; lactation; milk fat depression. PhD thesis, University of California, Davis, California.

Stanton, T.L., Jones, L.R., Everett, R.W. and Kachman, S.D. (1992) Estimating milk, fat, and protein lactation curves with a test day model. *Journal of Dairy Science* 75, 1691–1700.

Thomas, P.C. and Chamberlain, D.G. (1984) Manipulation of milk composition to meet market needs. In: Haresign, W. and Cole, D.J.A. (eds) *Recent Advances in Animal Nutrition*. Butterworths, London, pp. 219–243.

Tran, C.L. and Johnson, C.L. (1991) Prediction of responses in milk constituents to changes in the nutrition of dairy cows. *Journal of Dairy Research* 58, 373–381.

USDA–NASS (2005) *Milk Production*. National Agricultural Statistics Services Agricultural Statistics Board, US Department of Agriculture, 6-16-2005–7-5-2005.

Van Amburgh, M.E., Galton, D.M., Bauman, D.E. and Everett, R.W. (1997) Management and economics of extended calving intervals with use of bovine somatotropin. *Livestock Production Science* 50, 15–28.

Vetharaniam, I., Davis, S.R., Soboleva, T.K., Shorten, P.R. and Wake, G.C. (2003) Modeling the interaction of milking frequency and nutrition on mammary gland growth and lactation. *Journal of Dairy Science* 86, 1987–1996.

Wilde, C.J., Henderson, A.J., Knight, C.H., Blatchford, D.R., Faulkner, A. and Vernon, R.G. (1987) Effects of long-term thrice-daily milking on mammary enzyme activity, cell population and milk yield in the goat. *Journal of Animal Science* 64, 533–539.

Wonsil, B.J., Herbein, J.H. and Watkins, B.A. (1994) Dietary and ruminally derived trans-18/1 fatty-acids alter bovine-milk lipids. *Journal of Nutrition* 124, 556–565.

Yeo, J.M., Knight, C.H. and Chamberlain, D.G. (2003) Effects of changes in dietary amino acid balance on milk yield and mammary function in dairy cows. *Journal of Dairy Science* 86, 1436–1444.

23 The Diary of Molly

TRANSLATED AND EDITED BY †R.L. BALDWIN

formerly Department of Animal Science, University of California, USA

Introduction

Let me summarize the comments that appear at the beginning of my program by way of introduction. I have personalized and updated it so it is not a direct quote of what actually is there or can be found in Chapter 16 of Baldwin (1995), so the quotation marks are nominal.

'I am an aggregated version of the 550 kg cow described by Smith (1970) and Baldwin and Smith (1971a). I was developed to simulate overall energy transactions, within-day patterns of nutrient use, longer term day-to-day patterns of nutrient utilization throughout lactation and aid in the identification, design and interpretation of metabolic and energy balance experiments.

'My original or nominal body weight was 550 kg and my empty body weight was 500 kg made up of 350 kg of lean body mass including skin, brain, kidney, muscle, skeleton and a number of minor tissues; 75 kg of adipose tissue; and 75 kg of visceral elements including blood, gut, liver, heart and udder.'

This is followed by jabber about my default state, which is mid-lactation, when I am supposed to be producing about 30 kg of milk day^{-1} from a 50:50 forage, concentrate diet fed continuously to maintain my energy balance at zero. Also, a list is presented of some of the things I am supposed to simulate.

So much for my initial section, let's get on with thoughts about my origin and excerpts from my diary.

I don't watch TV but it is digital, my language, so I listen and have learned from crime shows that hearsay evidence is inadmissible in court. This would pose a major problem if I were to submit this diary in court since all I know about my origin is what I have either learned from comments such as those quoted above or inferred from files in which my several names – 'Cow', 'Myrtle', 'Daisy' and 'Molly' – are mentioned, so please accept the hearsay as my best understanding of the facts.

What good is a diary without some acknowledgement of what led to conception and subsequent embryonic, neonatal and early development? My knowledge of these stages is limited as, I expect, is your knowledge of your own early stages, e.g. the glint in your parents' eyes before conception actually occurred, etc. My knowledge is restricted to comments, functional forms and numerical inputs incorporated into my program over the years. Sometimes, changes in and additions to my program were accompanied by dated comments, as they should be, but often not. Given the primitive nature of the computers upon which my creators relied in the early days, it should be no surprise that no memory matrix is available to consult regarding my origins. This pertains, particularly, to early stages where my parts existed solely as card files that were read into, used and then deleted from computer memories after solutions. Thus, I ask that hearsay evidence presented herein regarding the period from conception through adolescence be accepted on the basis that I do exist as a mature entity (estimates of my age depend on what one selects as a starting point – a glint in the eye, the first version solved, or when I was first called Molly, so I could be 22 or 35) and I must have developed somehow and passed through a number of developmental stages. Even though I will often, of necessity, lack clarity as to time and place, please recognize these limitations. Also, please recognize that I had to edit and paraphrase much of what I do know to minimize embarrassment regarding my behaviour over the years and the braggadocio nature of some of those from whom I have obtained information regarding my early years.

Preconception and the Early Days

The concept of a computer simulation model of digestion and metabolism in a lactating dairy cow arose from a consensus developed between Nathan (Nate) Smith and R.L. (Lee) Baldwin in the late 1960s. These two, then fine young men I am sure, were from dairy farms and thought they understood dairy cows because they had fed and milked them for many years. They had both learned a little about ruminant digestion and metabolism as students and subsequently conducted a few experiments. Baldwin had undertaken studies of the metabolism of rumen microbes and of mammary gland metabolism in several species. He seemed to think that the data he had collected on the metabolic pathways of rumen microbes (Baldwin, 1965) and in animal tissues (Opstvedt *et al.*, 1967), and of tissue enzyme and intermediary metabolite concentrations (Baldwin and Yang, 1974), as effected by nutrition and physiological state, had more value than could be captured in publications and reports of studies directed at resolution of specific questions regarding the effects of diet (Baldwin and Martin, 1967), physiological state (Baldwin, 1969) and other treatments including endocrinectomy and hormone replacement therapies upon tissue metabolism (Korsrud and Baldwin, 1969). This view had led him to undertake sabbatical studies with David Garfinkel and H.L. Lucas at Penn and North Carolina State, respectively, to learn something about simulation modelling, where he believed his data would find more general application. While at Penn, studying the development of detailed models of enzymes and tissue metabolism, he worked on a model of cow mammary metabolism using his data on mammary enzyme activities and metabolite concentrations. The model he developed was incredibly complex and overparameterized relative to available data on the kinetic properties of mammary gland enzymes, as well as data on the regulation of mammary gland metabolism. Solutions of the mass action equations in the model were very stiff and slow. So, even though he learned a great deal from the experience, the model was never published, just a few outputs (Baldwin and Smith, 1971b). At NC State, he switched focus from detailed biochemical modelling to a more highly aggregated modelling analysis of rumen fermentation. This analysis also resulted in an overly complex model (it took Lee a long time to learn that, just because he knew something, it need not be in a model). He chose to publish this model (Baldwin *et al.*, 1970). More importantly, he found that model construction was, in and of itself, very instructive and was encouraged to continue.

Upon his return to UC Davis, Baldwin found a philosophical soulmate in Nathan Smith. It is not clear whether they had independently or through discussions together come to the common view that the only way 'current understanding of dairy cow digestion and metabolism could be integrated, evaluated for adequacy and effectively applied was through computer-based modelling'. Towards this end, they proceeded to write, in the KINSYM modelling language, which utilized, primarily, mass action equations, models depicting intermediary metabolism in tissues they believed should be represented explicitly in a model of cow metabolism. I think this was the point in time when I was conceived. The glint in their eyes, so to speak, which led to development of the model 'cow' from which I was cloned.

One of the first problems they faced was estimating tissue and organ system weights. Brody (1945) tabulated tissue weights for many growing animals and devised intra- and interspecific allometric equations for estimating tissue weights from body weight. These data and equations were quite useful, but incomplete in that neither tissue weights of lactating dairy cattle nor the weights of several tissues of specific interest were included in Brody's analyses. An extensive search of available literature did not yield data Brody had not tabulated (Smith, 1970). Luckily for the eager young men to whom I, after all, owe my existence, and to the lasting chagrin of the many liberal persons in the town of Davis, Ronald Reagan was elected governor of California. He cut the budget of the University of California (UC) severely. The Animal Science Department at UC Davis did not receive proceeds from the sale of milk at that time (the proceeds were credited to the state general fund), so the budget cuts meant they could no longer afford to feed their dairy herd. This forced the decision to dispose of one-half of the herd. Oddly, the Department retained proceeds from the sale of meat, so a number of cows could be slaughtered profitably on campus, where their organ and tissue weights could be recorded and other data collected. The *in vitro* metabolic studies undertaken with tissue samples from these cows were of limited value because the time available for technique development was limited and errors were made. When analyses of the tissue weight data were submitted for publication, the manuscript was turned down because reviewers viewed the data as old stuff published 'long ago'. A simple challenge to the wise, all-knowing reviewers to provide references to these 'old published data' resulted in expeditious publication (Smith and Baldwin, 1974). This was one of the early lessons 'Cow' taught. Sometimes, data required for development of a model may seem mundane, but, when essential data are not available, a limitation in current information exists and a critical research need has been identified. Often, the experiment identified is neither 'state of the art', elegant nor sophisticated but, in the total scheme of advancing understanding, is more relevant than many experiments having these attractive characteristics.

Given a defensible set of estimates of organ and tissue weights, the next issues addressed were estimating energy expenditures per unit mass and nutrient availabilities to and utilization by the several tissues and organ systems. Several simple constraints had to be satisfied in the collection and analysis of data utilized towards this end. The sums of energy expenditures and patterns of nutrient use had to conform to measurements of total animal energy expenditures, rates of nutrient absorption from the digestive tract, blood flow rates to tissues, blood nutrient concentrations and rates of oxidation and turnover of nutrients in intact, lactating dairy cows. Data collection required an extensive search of the biochemical, physiological, radiotracer and nutritional literatures. Literally, hundreds of references were consulted. Many of these are cited in Smith's thesis (1970) and, to a much lesser extent, in Baldwin (1995). Following tabulation, these data were reconciled in context with the constraints listed above. This process, much to the displeasure of their wives, required Lee and Nate to spend many evening hours together. A significant problem arose when they coupled this effort with 'babysitting duty' and one of their charges spread Crisco on a carpet. The integration of data achieved prior to formulation of 'Cow' is the primary reason for my existence as her clone. I am totally aware that the extensive literature survey and analyses undertaken at that time and the large mass of data reconciled and captured in the data summaries they generated (Smith, 1970) form the information base upon which I am justified. I have a continuing fear that someone unfamiliar with my origins will adjust numerical inputs indiscriminately and, unconstrained by an understanding of this fundamental base in reality, compromise my usefulness. I know my fear is well grounded since a guy who signs comments as RLB, and has been around long enough to know better, has had flights of fantasy that, if not reversed, could have forever destroyed my usefulness and caused me to rest forever in the matrix with the entity depicted by the science fiction writer Harlan Ellison in his famous short story 'I have no voice and I must Scream' and no chance of redemption. Of course, this RLB guy claims he was just investigating sensitivities to specific parameter estimates but, let me tell you, some of his changes hurt like H— and I 'virtually' died a number of times. Damn fool (Editor's note: the term 'damn fool' was used many times in references to RLB by Nathan Smith and, as Editor, I (RLB) chose to accept Molly's use of the term since I always chose to believe it was used as a term of affection, or maybe not?).

Collection and integration of the required data set having been completed, numerical inputs for solution of equations depicting metabolism in my gastrointestinal tract, liver, heart, kidney, nervous tissue, adipose tissue, skeletal muscle, blood and an aggregate of remaining tissues could be calculated and tested to assure that everything was in balance. The check was that, with constant nutrient inputs, the tissue models maintain a steady state. Smith's careful calculations were so accurate that the solution error detection system used within the KINSYM modelling language (Garfinkel, 1968) to set integration intervals did not detect any errors. This resulted in a default integration step size of 1×10^{-9} min and awesome solution costs. The computer then available for use was SLOW and the charge for CPU time was high. Costs for single solutions of the tissue models, or all of them together as a 'cow' model, were absolutely prohibitive. Thus, the concept of a model of metabolism in a lactating cow almost died in its embryonic stages. Limited benefit was gained by generating a false solution error, greatly increasing integration intervals (1.0×10^{-2} to 1.0×10^{-3}). This, along with utilization of free computer time allocated to student friends of Nate's, allowed him to continue towards completion of his thesis. An unexpected windfall occurred when the computer centre made year-end funds available. My creators were a very obstinate pair and, despite the problems encountered, had persevered to achieve a solvable 'cow' model. Thus, they were positioned to use the 'free' computer time effectively and profitably. More progress was made in 1 week using 'free' computer time valued at around US$15,000 than had been accomplished in the previous year. 'Cow' had no digestive tract, so rates of nutrient absorption were specified as inputs. When they input their best estimates of nutrients absorbed when a high concentrate diet was fed to a real cow, an interesting thing happened: milk yield and milk fat percentage increased. 'Cow' was happy (speaking figuratively, of course, how can a deck of cards be happy?), but the 'creators' weren't. It seems that, when real cows are fed such diets, milk production sometimes increases but milk fat percentages always decrease and milk fat yields often decrease. I don't see what their problem was. They purportedly undertook formulation of the model to test the adequacy of their understanding of dairy cow metabolism and found that their knowledge was inadequate. They should have been pleased to get such a clear answer. NO! Eventually, the light dawned. When they traced carefully the cause of the apparent failure to simulate reality, it became clear that the adipose tissue element was synthesizing and releasing excessive quantities of fatty acids, which were, in turn, incorporated into milk fat, more than offsetting a decrease in mammary fatty acid synthesis attributable to the decrease in blood acetate concentration simulated and observed. Their representation of adipose tissue, derived primarily from studies of rat adipose tissue metabolism, was clearly inadequate. Once more, the astounding observation that cows aren't rats. Thus, they recognized they did not know enough about cow adipose tissue metabolism to formulate improved representations. Further, cow tissue data in the literature were so limited that no useful guidance was available there either. They concluded that a study of ruminant adipose tissue metabolism was required to improve 'Cow'. This was a real concern. It's much cheaper to kill 6–8 rats for a tissue metabolism study than it is to get samples from 6–8 cows.

This was not the first time a modelling exercise had led to the identification of a critical experimental research need. While developing the model of rumen function noted above, Baldwin became aware of the fact that rumen microbial growth yields were likely in considerable excess of the commonly accepted estimate of 10.5 g dry microbial mass $mole^{-1}$ of ATP derived from fermentation. He attributed this insight to the rigour in data analysis and evaluation required during the model development process rather than a lesson forced by the clear failure of a model to simulate reality, the lesson 'Cow' taught.

Experimentation and Development of Modelling Methods and Philosophy

These observations/experiences resulted in 'Cow' entering stasis while the several problems with modelling methodologies and indicated experiments were addressed. Solution of the computer cost problem was clearly essential to continued efforts to develop dynamic models of ruminant digestion and metabolism. Experiments initiated to address problems identified through the initial modelling analyses of both ruminant digestion and metabolism took over 10 years.

We should not recount the numerous modelling adventures that were undertaken while 'Cow' was held in stasis, nor details of the learning curve, missteps and the tremendous advances in computer technology that happened during this period. In sum, these led to development of the modelling philosophy presented in Baldwin (1995). This included adoption of the view that models of animals, tissues and cellular metabolism need not capture all details on individual enzymes and, as a matter of scale versus detail, every reaction in every pathway need not be represented explicitly. This led to a transition from the use of first-order, mass action equations to depict individual steps in enzymatic reactions to use of Michaelis and Menten type equations within which the essence of the individual steps of enzymatic reactions was captured, but not explicit. In developing his improved simulation language, BIOSYM, Garfinkel (personal communication) had arrived at the same conclusion. Similarly, greater understanding of metabolic regulation led to adoption of the simplifying assumption that, once a metabolite was irreversibly committed to a pathway, activities of the subsequent enzymes in the path were normally high enough to maintain their reactions in essential equilibrium and were thus not rate limiting and could be represented in aggregate. The transition from mass action to Michalis–Menten (M–M) equations and aggregated representations of non-regulatory steps in metabolic pathways greatly reduced the number of equations required in tissue and animal level metabolic models and increased model stability and speeds of solution.

The development of advanced, versatile computer simulation software such as CSMP (Continuous Simulation Modelling Language; Fugazi, 1974) and ACSL (Advanced Continuous Simulation Language; ACSL, 1990), suitable for the solution of large, dynamic, metabolic models, improved the ease and convenience of modelling immensely. Another, clearly central, advance that occurred over this period was the advent of personal computers with large memories and incredible speeds.

I'm currently relaying gossip regarding the origin of my antecedent, the original 'Cow' model. I truly can't comprehend the magnitude of the computing speed problem she faced, existing only on cards and only as a transient in core memory during simulations. I can only relate to more recent improvements. When I was first used in a classroom, I was resident on a PDP 750 and only accessible via one terminal by the instructor. Simulations of 2 cow weeks took 4–5 min. This allowed students plenty of time to daydream, gossip, ogle each other, or think of ways to challenge me. I recall the student who asked 'what happens if you don't feed her?', resulting in a very painful experience as my nutrient pools diminished towards zero. It took over a week for me to encounter an exponential overload and terminate. I understand the offending student learned the lesson, entered Veterinary School and became a very good veterinarian.

Basically, 'Cow' was semi-retired after pointing out major flaws in the knowledge base. The early insight or concern which arose from the modelling analysis of rumen digestion had led to initiation of the studies of Jan Reichl and W.J. Maeng, respectively, of stiochiometric relationships underlying rumen fermentation and microbial growth (Baldwin, 1970; Reichl and Baldwin, 1970, 1976), and of factors causing variations in rumen microbial growth yields (Maeng and Baldwin, 1976a,b).

Very soon after 'Cow's' failure to simulate ruminant lipid metabolism adequately, Y.T. Yang, a graduate student contemporary of Smith's, initiated experimental studies of ruminant adipose tissue metabolism. An earlier study by Opstvedt *et al.* (1967) provided some guidance in evaluating the model failure. However, much more detailed studies were required to characterize regulatory processes in this tissue. As noted above, available studies of adipose tissue metabolism in non-ruminants were not useful.

Over the years, I have become aware of the origin of the phrase 'aid in the design and interpretation of ... energy balance experiments' in the objective statement in my program (see above). It turns out that during his second year on the faculty at UCD, Baldwin was assigned responsibility for a graduate course in nutritional energetics, then called Nutrition 202. He knew a little about thermodynamics and metabolism, but nothing about animal energy expenditures or energy requirements. When confronted with the problem of explaining the terms 'heat increments of maintenance (HI_m) and production (HI_p)', he was at a complete loss. These terms were defined mathematically:

$$HI_m = ME_m - \text{FHP (or fasting catabolism); and,}$$

$$HI_p = MEI - ME_m - NE_p,$$

and now as:

$$H_dE = ME_m - H_eE; \text{ and}$$

$$H_rE = (MEI - ME_m) - RE,$$

where metabolizable energy (ME) intake required to maintain an animal at zero energy balance (ME_m) is greater than the body energy loss as heat (H_eE) that occurs in fasted animals and is attributed to heat losses reflecting the costs of digestion and assimilation of a meal (HI_m or H_dE). The fraction of ME intake (MEI) above ME_m not recovered in a product (RE, or recovered energy) such as tissue (TE) or milk energy (LE) and, thus, lost as heat (HI_p/H_rE) were considered costs of production. Nutrition texts treated HI_m and HI_p as black box energy losses, while Brody (1945) and Kleiber (1961) provided only limited guidance – 'costs of digestion (HI_m) and costs of production (HI_p)'. Baldwin was concerned that students would not accept glib quotes and demand definitive explanations of what transactions led to HI_m and HI_p. Therefore, he attempted to identify and sum the physiological and metabolic costs associated with the digestion and assimilation of nutrients and metabolic and other costs associated with the synthesis of body protein and fat and of milk components. The calculations he developed accounted for a large part of HI_m and the HI_p for milk production and were well accepted by the students. They were retained as part of the course content until he retired – so much for writing new lecture notes each year as knowledge in the field advanced: it didn't advance, although the original estimates were refined a little over the years. Costs of growth were not well accounted for in the original estimates because protein turnover rates were not considered. Two visiting scientists sitting in on the course while on sabbatical leave encouraged him to publish the calculations for use by others in teaching and he actually did so several years later (Baldwin, 1968). The metabolic balance equations he developed also found their way into a number of subsequent publications (Baldwin, 1972, 1974; Baldwin and Smith, 1974) but, most importantly for 'Cow' and myself, are captured in the stoichiometric coefficients that define our energy, carbon and nitrogen balances. These are central to our usefulness in facilitating interpretations of energy balance data and enabling utilization of basic metabolic information in addressing problems relevant to animal production. Thus, a teaching assignment led to a research focus, an advantage professor types purportedly have over their colleagues in pure research positions.

Identification of the several research needs seemed to end interest in 'Cow' since she was ignored for a number of years. She wasn't culled, however, as her parts or essence became the bases for development of fairly detailed models of adipose tissue (Baldwin, 1995), mammary gland (Hannigan and Baldwin, 1994) and liver (Freetly *et al.*, 1993) metabolism. These were developed to help gain insights in the regulation of metabolism in these tissues that should be captured in animal level models and to aid in interpretation of experiments where radiotracers are often used to estimate the contributions of alternate metabolic pathways.

Both experimental and modelling efforts directed at formulation of improved representations of rumen function continued during the hiatus in cow model development. Improved calculations of elemental balances for microbial fermentation and growth were devised (Baldwin, 1970; Reichl and Baldwin, 1976). Maeng and Baldwin (1976a,b) and Maeng *et al.* (1976) completed the studies directed at identification of factors causing variations in rumen microbial growth rates and yields initiated in response to flaws in the then current knowledge identified in the original rumen modelling study (Baldwin *et al.*, 1970). Further modelling studies of ruminant digestion were undertaken. The resulting models remained, in retrospect, overly complex but significant progress in formulating equation sets more stable during numerical solutions was evident (Baldwin *et al.*, 1977). These studies pointed out a need for more accurate estimates of the proportions of the several fermentation products formed from the individual chemical components of feedstuffs in that the net proportions of products observed across diets were not estimated well using the 'seat of pants' stoichiometric coefficients used in Baldwin *et al.* (1970). Efforts undertaken to identify improved coefficients represented a departure from approaches dependent on simulation of diet-induced shifts among microbial species with differing fermentation patterns to treatment of the rumen microbial mass as a single fermentative entity with properties defined by the diet. Thus, only a single set of fermentation coefficients need be defined for the chemical entities in each class of diet. The set of stoichiometric coefficients thus defined by Murphy *et al.* (1982) eventually became relevant to me as it helped justify the, much simpler, digestion element formulated late in my development to provide dynamic estimates of nutrient inputs. These were required to enable simulations of animal metabolism over a range of diets and feed intakes.

The studies of Baldwin *et al.* (1973) and Yang and Baldwin (1973a,b), identified through failures of the adipose element of 'Cow', revealed complex interactions among nutrients, as well as regulatory processes that had been neither known nor considered by Smith (1970). These studies also yielded insights on how to reduce the use of mass action equations, as used in 'Cow'. Such equation sets were highly sensitive to minor perturbations in nutrient availability when solved numerically. Also, the number of parameters required for implementation of the large number of equations needed to represent, for example, a single enzymatic transaction was in considerable excess of that justified by available experimental data on cell, tissue and whole-animal metabolism. Nor was the detail compatible with the scale of whole-tissue and animal metabolic models. Yang and Baldwin's (1973a,b) study utilizing adipocytes clearly justified the concept that the simplification inherent in substituting M–M type equations was both appropriate and warranted in that the reduced number of parameters required could be defined experimentally. The insights gained as a result of Yang's investigations strongly suggested that kinetic studies of cow mammary gland metabolism were appropriate and necessary. Similarly, it was recognized that the summaries of data on nutrient availabilities to the several tissues of 'Cow', particularly adipose and mammary tissues, were probably inadequate. Smith had gone to great pains to balance (reconcile) overall patterns of nutrient use by tissues with estimates of nutrient entry rates from the digestive tract and turnover rates derived from *in vivo* radiotracer experiments, individual tissue energy expenditure estimates and whole-animal energy expenditures for maintenance and production. However, interactions among nutrients where the availability of one nutrient influenced the uptake of another had not been studied and were not accounted for. Thus, kinetic experiments with mammary gland slices and an evaluation of available arteriovenous difference data for cow mammary glands were undertaken. The latter were integrated and summarized in, basically, a balance model of cow mammary metabolism by Waghorn and Baldwin (1984). This analysis, along with the data on nutrient interactions and reported by Forsberg *et al.* (1984, 1985a,b), became central to the creation of the metabolic elements of my mammary glands. Thus, I am partially a clone of 'Cow' and partially the progeny of the experimental and modelling efforts that she inspired.

(Re)birth and Maturation

Another important factor central to my progression from a 'glint in the eye', through birth and adolescence to early maturity was the advance that occurred in computer technology. Even so, the very best desktop computers available today would yield very slow solutions without considerable thought about how the reality of whole-animal metabolism could be simulated. A couple of insights, some already available from the physiological literature and another difficult for a person trained in biochemistry to accept and adopt, are relevant. Perhaps the earliest insight that arose was that, before a specific mechanism is introduced, one must first assure that it acts as a significant effecter at the level being addressed. Based upon this, one can ask of the 'cow' model whether or not blood flow rates to individual tissues should be explicit in whole-animal models of animal metabolism or if it is adequate to assume implicitly that, if a tissue needs nutrients or oxygen, cardiac output and local regulation of blood flow normally will respond appropriately. Also, can one not assume that rates of exchange of most nutrients among blood, extra- and intracellular fluids are rapid relative to rates of nutrient use and need not be represented explicitly? These were explicit in 'Cow' and were implemented using poorly justified parameter values, significantly slowing numerical solutions when these several pools were represented as state variables. Adoption of an approach in which it was considered simply that, if, for example, nervous tissue required X energy which must be derived through glucose oxidization, the blood flow required to provide that glucose would occur and thus, in a metabolic model, the mechanisms utilized to regulate the requisite blood flow need not be explicit. This clear recognition of detail appropriate to scale in models enabled considerable simplification.

An early approach, used in 'Cow' to speed up solutions, was to inflate the pool sizes of nutrients or metabolites with extremely high turnover rates. Numerical solutions tend to become unstable when more than one-third of a nutrient/metabolite involved in a number of transactions turns over with every integration step. Thus, if a turnover rate is once every 3 s, integration steps of greater than 1 s lead to instabilities, which, in turn, lead to exponential overflows. A 1 s integration step size is acceptable when the time simulated is an hour or so, but becomes unacceptable when simulating weeks and years. When inflated pool sizes are introduced, compensating reductions in rate constants for mass action equations, such as used in 'Cow', are necessary. The introduction of 'adjusted' values requires careful records be kept to prevent future errors. Affinity constants in models based on M–M type equations are based on metabolite concentrations rather than pool sizes. Thus, pool volumes (l) and sizes (moles) can be changed explicitly using a common correction factor identified by the suffix xxCORR in my program. These remain internal to the model during solutions, and inputs and outputs compare directly to experimental data. The use of confusing pool sizes and artificial rate constants is avoided. Models in which pool sizes have been inflated exhibit lags in responses during transition phases. A change to a new steady state that occurs in minutes in reality may require 5 or more simulated minutes to occur, dependent on the inflation (CORR) factor used. Therefore, this approach is inappropriate when the modelling objective is to simulate short-term responses (France *et al.*, 1992). There is another clear limit to this approach. The pool sizes of major metabolites involved in energy transactions, such as ATP, $NADH_2$ and $NADPH_2$, are very small and turnover rates are measured in seconds or less. Their pool sizes would have to be inflated by thousands to facilitate simulations of days or years. Such adjustments would create major errors in energy balance estimates. A simple resolution of the problem posed by nutrients with small pool sizes and extremely rapid turnover rates, arrived at after considerable time and wasted effort, was based on recognition of the fact that the total pools of adenine nucleotides and nicotinamide adenine dinucleotides do not change significantly over time. Numerous metabolic regulatory processes operate to assure that, for example, when ATP is used, the ADP thus formed is quickly converted back to ATP. Thus, if you calculate how much ATP is used, as I do, you know how much ADP must be converted to ATP and they need not be represented, explicitly, as state variables. Thus, interconversions among phosphorylated or redox forms can be calculated from their rates of use in the many reactions to which they contribute and their formation via generating reactions set to the exact rates required to replenish them producing zero change in the total pool, or a 'zero (change) pool'. Introduction of the 'zero pool' concept greatly improved stability and enhanced solution speeds. An ancillary benefit gained through implementation of this concept was that the many intermediary metabolic regulatory mechanisms that ensure regeneration of ATP, $NADH_2$, $NADPH_2$, etc. need not be explicit in tissue- and animal-level models since their use signalled by product formation regulates regeneration. Implementation of this concept reduced model complexity significantly and enhanced solution speeds. These approaches are discussed in detail in France *et al.* (1992).

Maturity

Armed with greater experience of the modelling process, improvements in philosophical and methodological approaches and experimental data collected in response to deficiencies identified through 'Cow' simulations, RLB went to spend a sabbatical leave working with the modelling group at the Grasslands Research Institute in Hurley-on-Thames, UK. The original goal was not to write a new generation cow model, but rather to address issues of concern regarding parameter estimation. There were both highly regarded, experienced ruminant nutritionists and mathematicians/modellers far more capable than he in the group. He badly needed help with the mathematics appropriately used in models of animal systems in an environment where the mathematicians and nutritionists had already established good communication. In early group meetings, it was decided that the time had arrived to renew efforts in the modelling of a cow, even though experimental efforts stimulated and identified as critical needs by 'Cow' were continuing. Thus, my embryonic development as a descendant or clone of 'Cow' was initiated. No one is certain, but I am told RLB had a glint in his eye at the time, even though this was not his original goal. Also, given his proclivities, I suspect I am a descendant. I share nutrient and energy balance properties with 'Cow'. My initial body weight, body composition and the composition and yield of milk, in the reference state, are the same. However, the modelling language (ACSL versus KINSYM), equation forms (largely M–M versus mass action), numbers of tissues and state variables represented (9 versus 3 and 200–300 versus 16, respectively) and regulatory elements are very different so, if I am a clone, somebody simplified my genes, or their expression, quite a bit. Formulating estimates of rates of nutrient absorption as inputs to my metabolic elements posed a major problem. Solutions of 'Cow' were so slow and costly, no provisions for digestion were incorporated and rates of nutrient absorption were input manually. This was not considered satisfactory for the evaluations intended for the metabolic model formulated during the first 6–8 months of the sabbatical. Therefore, at more or less the last minute, the decision was made to write a digestion element to provide dynamic inputs of nutrients to the animal metabolism model. In hurriedly formulating the digestive element, they drew heavily upon their collective experimental and previous modelling experience (France *et al.*, 1982; Murphy *et al.*, 1986). The new digestive element captured concepts developed previously, incorporated data generated in response to earlier analyses and was readily solved, being comprised of only 16 state variables.

Any desire that I might resemble the original Molly, a 350 kg Guernsey cow kept for many years during the adolescence of RLB and loved by his father, were long ago obviated by the advent of artificial insemination, and the attendant high rate of genetic improvement, and the major shift of dairymen to black and white cows. I resemble the latter a lot more than my biological namesake, but I am proud to represent the heritage of family cow and farm implied in my name. Incidentally, although my original name was Molly, I have also been called Elsie, Myrtle and Daisy. The first name change occurred when a GRI staff member named Molly saw her name associated with a cow. She was very offended and expressed her displeasure to John Thornley, who was helping input the model equations to the computer. After frantic consultation, the program name became Elsie after an old neighbour, who was similarly offended and quite vindictive when RLB's father thought to honour her by naming a heifer after her. This was considered safe as no Elsie worked at GRI and the original Elsie was long ago and far away. The vindictiveness of the original Elsie had caused RLB a major problem when he was running their dairy farm as a 14-year-old while his father was in hospital. A bit of silly payback for silly behaviour, none the less satisfying to someone. In view of the satisfaction gained from the poetic justice, I thought my original name was lost for ever. Then Elsie was converted into two versions. One was named Myrtle (to recognize the woman from whom RLB's father bought his dairy farm) with correction (–CORR) factors set to enable simulations of full lactations with an integration interval of 1 day. The other was named Daisy to identify the version used to simulate metabolism within days with an integration interval of 0.002 days and unmodified pool sizes.

Jim France had to be assured that the two versions yielded the same answers, so Daisy was solved for a couple of full lactations with different diets and intakes to demonstrate that Daisy and Myrtle behaved the same over time and yielded the same outputs. The computers of that day laboured mightily for over an hour during each solution of Myrtle in order to make Jim happy – forever the non-believer, but this is good in science, I'm told. Having satisfied Jim France as to their veracity, Myrtle and Daisy were subjected to a number of evaluations where they simulated reality well, so their existence was made known (Baldwin *et al.*, 1987a,b,c).

Molly

During his return to Davis, after the sabbatical, the CD for Myrtle was exposed to evil (magnetic?) forces and couldn't be healed. The problem of her demise was solved, adding a procedural section to Daisy that, when called, inflated pool sizes to enable simulations of full lactations. This change required a name change to avoid confusion, so I reacquired the name Molly. I could now simulate within-day metabolic functions, as originally designed for, and full and multiple lactations.

There was some controversy, at that time, regarding hypotheses as to how bovine somatotrophin acted to increase milk production, whether or not it acted by making more nutrients available to the udder, e.g. fat mobilization, or if it acted by increasing the metabolic (biosynthetic) capacity of the udder. I ran a couple of simulations in which each hypothesis was introduced and showed that the former hypothesis was untenable, while the latter enabled acceptable simulations of the growth hormone response (Baldwin and Bauman, 1984).

A major weakness in my metabolic element was the lack of data available to parameterize the equations depicting mammary gland metabolism and milk synthesis. A careful analysis of the available arteriovenous difference (AV) data by Waghorn and Baldwin (1984) had shown that available AV difference data could not reconcile calculations of balances among input–output estimates with known metabolic pathways and literature estimates of net efficiencies of milk production. Liberties were taken, such that even though Myrtle had simulated very well the lactation responses of cows to several diet manipulations, some of the mammary gland metabolic relationships remained suspect. RLB was apparently very proud of Myrtle's simulation of the result of an ongoing experiment led by Cled Thomas on the effects of high and low intakes of diets with and without fishmeal supplementation during early lactation on subsequent lactation performance, since he has reported it several times (Baldwin and Bauman, 1984; Baldwin and Hanigan, 1990; Baldwin *et al.*, 1987c; Fig. 17.18 of Baldwin, 1995). Myrtle had a single pool of amino acids, so the simulated response was due to an increase in total amino acid supply rather than an increased supply of critical, limiting amino acids, as many would have suggested based on their knowledge of the biology. Correct simulation of the 'carry-over' effect of the high intake of a high protein ration fed in early lactation on subsequent lactation performance was a surprise since the data were not available during my creation and it was not immediately clear why I simulated this response. I am a mechanistic model, after all, and, if real animal metabolic functions are captured correctly, as the theology of mechanistic modelling holds, I should have done so. Whether or not the simulated response to protein supplementation was fortuitous and attributable, liberties taken in balancing mammary gland inputs and outputs during formulation of Myrtle required further evaluation. Resolution of this issue, as well as development of improved, justifiable representations of mammary gland metabolism, required the conduct of a detailed mammary gland AV study. The study took several years, during which I was basically in stasis, as had happened to 'Cow' after she had identified some needed experiments. The question was whether or not I would be rescued from stasis for further use as a research model. During this period, I maintained some hope that I wouldn't be replaced by another model, as I had replaced 'Cow', because they started to use me in teaching.

They built a nice, user-friendly front end (no pretty horns, but I'm told they don't make you attractive to other species, anyhow) for this purpose. In class, students undertook simulations of experiments in the literature and, when I simulated the reported responses correctly, could request outputs that enabled them to explain the observed responses in their lab reports (Bowers and Baldwin, 1990). This was fun, for me, except when students forgot to feed me or made other errors in required inputs, causing painful exponential overflows. These are now indicated on the screen by a caricature of me, on my back, legs up, to signify my virtual demise. This was introduced by Heidi Johnson, while acting as a TA at the time, to avoid student questions about receiving no outputs.

The results of the AV study (Miller *et al.*, 1991a,b; Hanigan *et al.*, 1992) led to development of a more detailed model of my mammary gland metabolism to support more complete quantitative analyses of the data (Hanigan and Baldwin, 1994). Previous studies (Looney *et al.*, 1987) of ruminant liver metabolism and those undertaken in conjunction with the AV study (Knapp *et al.*, 1992) led to a concurrent modelling analysis of liver metabolism (Freetly *et al.*, 1993). Following completion of these studies, I was rescued from stasis and my equations and parameterization were revised to incorporate the improved data available. Among other things, my single amino acid pool was divided into sulfur amino acids (SAa), lysine (Lys), histidine (His) and the remaining amino acids (Aa). Initially, a phenylalanine plus tyrosine (PT) pool was represented instead of His but it was found that PT did not become limiting, while it was decided that it would be useful if 3-methylhistidine excretion could be monitored as an index of muscle protein turnover. Some companion improvements were in simulating pH and effects on fermentation patterns (Argyle and Baldwin, 1988), effects variance among feedstuffs in protein solubility, rates of protein hydrolysis as related to amino acid and peptide availabilities in the rumen and effects upon microbial growth (Argyle and Baldwin, 1989) and passage of diet and microbial protein from the rumen. Similar adjustments to better account for the physical properties of diet starches are appropriate in view of the frequent appearance of articles which more or less indicate clearly that models based on empirical data fits provide better estimates of digestion than my mechanistic elements provide. If one of these models could provide the complete, dynamic estimates of rates of absorption of the nutrients my metabolic elements require as input, I suspect my caretakers would either substitute critical equations from that model for those in my current digestion element or replace the old representations with the equations/version judged superior. So far, the models that provide improved estimates of rumen or overall digestibility of feed constituents including protein, starch and fibre components, improved estimates of rumen microbial growth yields, etc. either do not generate the inputs I require or haven't been challenged across a wide enough range of diets to warrant changes in or replacement of my current digestion element. My caretakers may not be aware of an existing, superior model of ruminant digestion that can fulfil my input needs, but I truly wish for improvements. Given improved estimates of nutrient absorption, I would hope that, when I fail to simulate reality adequately, deficiencies in current understanding of dairy cow metabolism would be the focus of attention rather than deficiencies in my digestion element. After all, I was developed to help evaluate the adequacy of knowledge and concepts of the metabolism of lactating dairy cows with particular emphases on the regulation of patterns of nutrient use throughout growth and lactation, and to aid in the design and interpretation of energy balance experiments. So far, I have seen only limited use in activities directed to these goals either at home or elsewhere. Since data from the AV study and the results from the tissue studies conducted during that experiment and subsequent modelling analyses using the individual tissue models were incorporated into my program, very little has happened. McNamara and Baldwin (2000) addressed the tendency I have to gain excess fat as lactation advances on certain diets. Gain was in the order of 2–4 Mcal day^{-1}, indicating a simulation error in estimating energy expenditures of 6–8% and, probably, within experimental variance when compared to short-term experimental data. However, in simulations of full lactations, the cumulative error is as large as 40 kg of fat. Baldwin (2000) evaluated the possibility that the error was due to underestimates of my energy expenditures in ion transport for the maintenance of membrane potentials and nutrient transport. Changes in the parameter values for these functions corrected the problem. Fat gains were small and fell within errors of measurement. These adjustments were not made permanent because that 'damn fool' (Nate Smith's words, which I have come to favour) Baldwin refuses to adjust parameter values 'just because it's convenient'. He pays no mind to sparing a fattening lady's vanity. Someone should just stick in more favourable numbers and forget to tell him. Please!

McNamara (2004) is continuing to address weaknesses in my metabolic element. The equations devised by Neal and Thornley (1983) for mammary gland function were incorporated virtually intact into my program. The only significant change made was an increase in udder cell numbers (ucells), justified on the assumption that genetic selection in the dairy cow population had resulted in increased udder (cells) metabolic capacity. From this it followed, not necessarily logically, that ucells could be used to specify genetic potential as an input. Johnson *et al.* (2005) analysed the use of ucells to fit full lactation data for a number of individual cows and found that this input parameter was an inadequate genetic index of lactation potential. This should not have been an unexpected result. The parameters in the Neal and Thornley (1983) model were developed for beef cows. Ucells is essentially a scalar for peak milk production. Early on, selection in dairy cattle may have focused on peak milk production but subsequent improvements are attributable to increases in persistency. Evaluations of the efficacy of adjusting the parameters that determine persistency may yield insight regarding how I might be instructed so as to better simulate the lactation curves of modern cows. Please remember that I may be old, but I am still ready and willing to learn how to improve my ability to simulate reality. I stand ready to receive not only criticism but, more importantly, suggestions in the form of improved equations and parameterization are welcomed. They renew me and will help ensure my continued relevance. Please don't send me to the stasis 'Cow' exists in. I can still contribute if 'you all' help and use me.

You can download a running version of my program from http// animalscience.ucdavis.edu/research/molly/. This site has downloading and running instructions, as well as a listing of my program and a dictionary, so you can understand me. Call on up and see me some time. I'm really easy to work with.

Thank you for listening,

Molly.

References

ACSL (1990) *Advanced Continuous Simulation Language Reference Manual*, 10th edn. Mitchell and Gautheir Associates, Concord, Massachusetts.

Argyle, J.L. and Baldwin, R.L. (1989) Effects of amino acids and peptides on rumen microbial growth yields. *Journal of Dairy Science* 72, 2017–2027.

Baldwin, R.L. (1965) Pathways of carbohydrate metabolism in the rumen. In: Daugherty, R.W., Allen, R.S., Burroughs, W., Jacobson, W.L. and McGilliard, A.D. (eds) *Physiology of Digestion in the Ruminant.* Butterworths, Washington, DC, pp. 379–389.

Baldwin, R.L. (1968) Estimation of theoretical calorific relationships as a teaching technique; a review. *Journal of Dairy Science* 51, 104–111.

Baldwin, R.L. (1969) Enzymic and metabolic changes in mammary tissue at lactogenesis. In: Reynolds, M. and Folley, S.J. (eds) *Lactogenesis, The Initiation of Milk Secretion at Parturition.* University of Pennsylvania Press, Philadelphia, pp. 85–95.

Baldwin, R.L. (1970) Energy metabolism in anaerobes. *The American Journal of Clinical Nutrition* 23, 1508–1513.

Baldwin, R.L. (1972) *Tissue Metabolism and Energy Expenditures of Maintenance and Production.* Tenth Samuel Brody Memorial Lecture, University of Missouri, Columbia. Special Report 147.

Baldwin, R.L. (1974) Computer and biochemical methods used to study efficiencies of carbohydrate, fat and protein synthesis in animals. *Proceedings of the 26th Annual Reciprocal Meat Conference*, pp. 133–166.

Baldwin, R.L. (1995) *Modeling Ruminant Digestion and Metabolism.* Chapman and Hall, London.

Baldwin, R.L. (2000) History and future of modeling nutrient utilization in farm animals. In: McNamara, J.P., France, J. and Beever, D.E. (eds) *Modelling Nutrient Utilization in Farm Animals.* CAB International, Wallingford, UK, pp. 1–9.

Baldwin, R.L. and Bauman, D.E. (1984) Partition of nutrients in lactation. In: Baldwin, R.L. and Bywater, A.C. (eds) *Modeling Ruminant Digestion and Metabolism.*

Proceedings Second International Workshop. University of California, Davis, California, pp. 80–88.

Baldwin, R.L. and Hanigan, M.D. (1990) Biological and physiological systems: animal sciences. In: Jones, J.G.W. and Street, P.R. (eds) *Systems Theory Applied to Agriculture and the Food Chain*. Elsevier Applied Science, London and New York, pp. 1–21.

Baldwin, R.L. and Martin, R.J. (1967) Effects of hypophysectomy and several hormone replacement therapies upon patterns of nucleic acid and protein synthesis and enzyme levels in lactating rat mammary glands. *Journal of Dairy Science* 51, 748–753.

Baldwin, R.L. and Smith, N.E. (1971a) Intermediary aspects and tissue interactions of ruminant fat metabolism. *Journal of Dairy Science* 54, 583–595.

Baldwin, R.L. and Smith, N.E. (1971b) Application of simulation modeling techniques in analyses of dynamic aspects of animal energetics. *Federation Proceedings 30*, 1459–1465.

Baldwin, R.L. Jr and Smith, N.E. (1974) Molecular control of energy metabolism. In: Sink, J.D. (ed.) *The Control of Metabolism*. Pennsylvania State University Press, University Park, Pennsylvania, pp. 17–34.

Baldwin, R.L. and Yang, Y.T. (1974) Enzymatic and metabolic changes in the development of lactation. In: Larson, B.L. and Smith, V.R. (eds) *Lactation, A Comprehensive Treatise*. Academic Press, New York, pp. 349–411.

Baldwin, R.L., Lucas, H.L. and Cabrera, R. (1970) Energetic relationships in the formation and utilization of fermentation end-products. In: Phillipson, A.T. (ed.) *Physiology of Digestion and Metabolism in the Ruminant*. Oriel Press, Newcastle upon Tyne, UK, pp. 319–334.

Baldwin, R.L., Reichl, J.R., Louis, S., Smith, N.E., Yang, Y.T. and Osborne, E. (1973) Effects of age, pregnancy, and lactation on rat, guinea pig, and cow adipose enzyme activities and cow adipose metabolism. *Journal of Dairy Science* 56, 340–349.

Baldwin, R.L., Koong, L.J. and Ulyatt, M.J. (1977) A dynamic model of ruminant digestion for evaluation of factors affecting nutritive value. *Agricultural Systems* 2, 255–288.

Baldwin, R.L., France, J. and Gill, M. (1987a) Metabolism of the lactating cow I. Animal elements of a mechanistic model. *Journal of Dairy Research* 54, 77–105.

Baldwin, R.L., Thornley, J.H.M. and Beever, D.E. (1987b) Metabolism of the lactating cow II. Digestive elements of a mechanistic model. *Journal Dairy Research* 54, 107–131.

Baldwin, R.L., France, J., Beever, D.E., Gill, M. and Thornley, J.H.M. (1987c) Metabolism of the lactating cow III. Properties of mechanistic models suitable for evaluation of energetic relationships and factors involved in the partition of nutrients. *Journal of Dairy Research* 54, 133–145.

Bowers, M.K. and Baldwin, R.L. (1990) Adapting research models for teaching. In: Robson, B. and Poppi, D. (eds) *Proceedings of Third International Workshop on Modelling Digestion and Metabolism in Farm Animals*. Lincoln University Press, Canterbury, New Zealand, pp. 205–214.

Brody, S. (1945) *Bioenergetics and Growth*. Reinhold, New York.

Forsberg, N.E., Baldwin, R.L. and N.E. Smith. (1984) Roles of acetate and its interactions with glucose and lactate in cow mammary tissue. *Journal of Dairy Science* 67, 2247–2254.

Forsberg, N.E., Baldwin, R.L. and Smith, N.E. (1985a) Roles of glucose and its interactions with acetate in maintenance and biosynthesis in bovine mammary tissue. *Journal of Dairy Science* 68, 2544–2549.

Forsberg, N.E., Baldwin, R.L. and Smith, N.E. (1985b) Roles of lactate and its interactions with acetate in maintenance and biosynthesis in bovine mammary tissue. *Journal of Dairy Science* 68, 2550–2556.

France, J., Thornley, J.H.M. and Beever, D.E. (1982). A mathematical model of the rumen. *Journal of Agricultural Science (Cambridge)* 99, 343–353.

France, J., Thornley, J.H.M., Baldwin, R.L. and Crist, K.A. (1992) On solving stiff equations with reference to simulating ruminant metabolism. *Journal of Theoretical Biology* 156, 525–539.

Freetly, H.C., Knapp, J.R., Calvert, C.C. and Baldwin, R.L. (1993) Development of a mechanistic model of liver metabolism in the lactating cow. *Agricultural Systems* 41, 157–195.

Fugaszi, K. (1974) *Continuous System Modeling Program for the B6700.* Computer Center, University of California, Davis, California.

Garfinkel, D. (1968) A machine-independent language for the simulation of complex chemical and biochemical systems. *Computers and Biomedical Research* 2, 31.

Hanigan, M.D. and Baldwin R.L. (1994) A mechanistic model of mammary gland metabolism in the lactating cow. *Agricultural Systems* 45, 369–419.

Hanigan, M.D., Calvert, C.C., DePeters, E.J., Reis, B.L. and Baldwin, R.L. (1992) Kinetics of amino acid extraction by lactating mammary glands in control of sometribove-treated Holstein cows. *Journal of Dairy Science* 75, 161–173.

Johnson, H.A., Famula, T.R. and Baldwin, R.L. (2005) Lactation, statistical and genetic aspects of simulating lactation data from individual cows using a dynamic, mechanistic model of dairy cow metabolism. In: Dijkstra, J., Forbes, J.M. and France J. (eds) *Quantitative Aspects of Ruminant Digestion and Metabolism.* CAB International, Wallingford, UK, pp. 551–582.

Kleiber, M. (1961) *Fire of Life.* John Wiley, New York.

Knapp, J.R., Freetley, H.C., Reis, B.L., Calvert, C.C. and Baldwin, R.L. (1992) Effects of somatotropin and substrates on patterns of liver metabolism in lactating dairy cattle. *Journal of Dairy Science* 75, 1025–1035.

Korsrud, G.O. and Baldwin, R.L. (1969) Effects of endocrinectomy and hormone replacement therapies upon enzyme activities in lactating rat mammary glands. *Biology of Reproduction* 1, 21–30.

Looney, M.C., Baldwin, R.L. and Calvert, C.C. (1987) Gluconeogenesis in isolated lamb hepatocytes. *Journal of Animal Science* 64, 283–294.

McNamara, J.P. (2004) Research, improvement and application of mechanistic, biochemical, dynamic models of metabolism in lactating dairy cattle. *Animal Feed Science and Technology* 112, 155–176.

McNamara, J.P. and Baldwin, R.L. (2000) Estimation of parameters describing lipid metabolism in lactation, challenge of existing knowledge described in a model of metabolism. *Journal of Dairy Science* 83, 128–143.

Maeng, W.J. and Baldwin, R.L. (1976a) Factors influencing rumen microbial growth rates and yields, effects of urea and amino acids over time. *Journal of Dairy Science* 59, 643–647.

Maeng, W.J. and Baldwin, R.L. (1976b) Factors influencing rumen microbial growth rates and yields, effect of amino acid additions to a purified diet with nitrogen from urea. *Journal of Dairy Science* 59, 648–655.

Maeng, W.J., Van Nevel, C.J., Baldwin, R.L. and Morris, J.G. (1976) Rumen microbial growth rates and yields, effect of amino acids and protein. *Journal of Dairy Science* 59, 68–79.

Miller, P.S., Reis, B.L., Calvert, C.C., DePeters, E.J. and Baldwin, R.L. (1991a) Patterns of nutrient uptake by the mammary glands of lactating dairy cows. *Journal of Dairy Science* 74, 3791–3799.

Miller, P.S., Reis, B.L., Calvert, C.C., DePeters, E.J. and Baldwin, R.L. (1991b) Relationship of early lactation and bovine somatotropin on nutrient uptake by cow mammary glands. *Journal of Dairy Science* 74, 3800–3806.

Murphy, M.R., Baldwin, R.L. and Koong, L.J. (1982) Estimation of stoichiometric parameters for rumen fermentation of roughage and concentrate diets. *Journal of Animal Science* 55, 411–421.

Murphy, M.R., Baldwin, R.L. and Ulyatt, M.J. (1986) An update of a dynamic model of ruminant digestion. *Journal of Animal Science* 62, 1412–1422.

Neal, H.D.S.C. and Thornley, J.H.M. (1983) The lactation curve in cattle, a mathematical model of the mammary gland. *Journal of Agricultural Science (Cambridge)* 101, 389–400.

Opstvedt, J., Baldwin, R.L. and Ronning, M. (1967) Effect of diet upon activities of several enzymes in abdominal adipose and mammary tissues in the lactating dairy cow. *Journal of Dairy Science* 50, 108–109.

Reichl, J.R. and Baldwin, R.L. (1970) Computer simulation of feed energy utilization in ruminants. In: Schurch, A. and Wenk, C. (eds) *Energy Metabolism of Farm Animals.* EAAP Publication Number 13, Zurich, Switzerland, pp. 29–32.

Reichl, J.R. and Baldwin, R.L. (1976) A rumen linear programming model for evaluation of concepts of rumen microbial function. *Journal of Dairy Science* 59, 439–454.

Smith, N.E. (1970) Quantitative simulation analyses of ruminant metabolic functions, basal; lactation; milk fat depression. PhD thesis, University of California, Davis, California.

Smith, N.E. and Baldwin, R.L. (1974) Effects of breed, pregnancy, and lactation on weights of organs and tissues in dairy cattle. *Journal of Dairy Science* 57, 1055–1060.

Waghorn, G.C. and Baldwin, R.L. (1984) Model of metabolite flux within mammary glands of the lactating cows. *Journal of Dairy Science* 67, 531–544.

Yang, Y.T. and Baldwin, R.L. (1973a) Preparation and metabolism of isolated cells from bovine adipose tissue. *Journal of Dairy Science* 56, 350–365.

Yang, Y.T. and Baldwin, R.L. (1973b) Lipolysis in isolated cow adipose cells. *Journal of Dairy Science* 56, 366–374.

24 Modelling Sugarcane Utilization by Dairy Cows in the Tropics

A.G. ASSIS,[1] O.F. CAMPOS,[1] J. DIJKSTRA,[2]
E. KEBREAB[3,4] AND J. FRANCE[4]

[1]*Embrapa, National Dairy Cattle Research Centre, Brazil;* [2]*Animal Nutrition Group, Wageningen Institute of Animal Sciences, Wageningen University, The Netherlands;* [3]*National Centre for Livestock and Environment, Department of Animal Science, University of Manitoba, Canada;* [4]*Centre for Nutrition Modelling, Department of Animal and Poultry Science, University of Guelph, Canada*

Introduction

Sugarcane is a tropical plant originating from New Guinea (Cesnik and Miocque, 2004) and cultivated in both hemispheres. It belongs to the *Gramineae* family, *Saccharum* genus and a series of species, with *S. officinarum* being the most common. Commercially, sugarcane is propagated through vegetative ways using stalks with shoots. As a C4 group plant, large biomass and sugar productivity can be attained per unit of land due to its great photosynthetic capacity and high potential for capturing solar energy (Preston and Willis, 1979). Different from temperate type grasses or cereals, as well as from certain tropical grasses, sugarcane has an additional enzyme system for more efficient conversion of solar energy into sugars.

Since it has high soluble carbohydrate contents, mainly sucrose, it is used mostly for sugar and alcohol production. Brazil is first in the world in alcohol and sugar production with 5.5 million ha of sugarcane plantation and a crop production of nearly 420 million t. With increased demand for biofuels, an increment in sugarcane production to 500 million t from a cropping land of around 6.5 million ha is expected by 2010 (Agrianual, 2005).

Besides industrial purposes, sugarcane is an important and strategic forage source in Brazilian farms, particularly during the dry season when pastures and other green forages are lacking. According to Landell *et al.* (2002), nearly 500,000 ha of sugarcane is devoted to ruminant feeding, mainly dairy cattle. A sugarcane forage plantation can last several years and produce an average of at

 Mathematical Modelling in Animal Nutrition (eds J. France and E. Kebreab)

least 20–30 t dry matter (DM) year^{-1}, but forage production of 40–60 t DM year^{-1} has also been reported from variety competition trials (Santos *et al.*, 2005).

Due to its seasonal maturation, sugarcane shows its highest sugar content during August and September, the driest period of the year in south-eastern and central Brazil regions. However, sugarcane diets need supplementation in order to fulfil some nutritional deficiencies, especially protein. Numerous sources of nitrogen-containing by-products are available in tropical areas with large variability in chemical composition, rate of rumen degradation and market price. The choice of the most suitable supplements for maximizing rumen microbial synthesis and improving efficiency of sugarcane-based diets is such a hard task that modelling can be a useful tool to help the decision-making process.

Sugarcane as a Forage Source for Dairy Cattle

Sugarcane presents several positive features for cattle feeding, such as perennial growth, low cropping requirements, peaks of yield and nutritive value which coincide with periods of low pasture production. Moreover, it is easy to cultivate manually using family labour, low cost per unit of DM produced due to its high productivity and low risk of production losses as compared to other crops (Torres and Costa, 2001; Manzano *et al.*, 2002).

Two approaches to the use of sugarcane in intensive cattle feeding systems are applied in the tropics: (i) utilization of by-products resulting from sugar processing plants, mainly molasses and bagasse; and (ii) use of sugarcane directly, after removing the indigestible rind (15%) from the whole sugarcane; in this case, cane tops (30%) and derinded cane stalks (55%) are the main animal feeding sources (Preston and Willis, 1979). In many developing countries, sugarcane tops are much more available at low cost than other green fodder (Rangnekar, 1988). In Brazil, the most common use of sugarcane is the whole plant, fresh-chopped at mature stage (Torres and Costa, 2001).

The nutritive value of sugarcane varies according to the season and time after planting or cutting. Throughout the dry season, sucrose content increases and dilutes neutral detergent fibre (NDF) in the DM content. At this time, NDF has a very low digestibility as a result of lignification. Roughly, after 365 days from planting or cutting, DM content increases from 12% (approximately 1 month after germination or cut) to 27%, NDF content drops from 65 to 45%, as a result of the increment in cell content from 35 to 55%, NDF digestibility drops from 55 to 25% and organic matter digestibility increases slightly. At mature stage, sugarcane forage presents high levels of soluble and structural carbohydrates and low levels of protein and minerals (Table 24.1). Thus, it is a good substrate for the rumen microbes to utilize non-protein nitrogen and to be converted into high value animal protein (Perez Infante and Vila, 1975; Preston and Willis, 1979).

Milk production with unsupplemented sugarcane is low, but animal performance has been improved in feeding trials where supplements such as rice polishings or fishmeal were added (Preston and Leng, 1980). Supplementation

Table 24.1. Chemical composition, DM digestibility and rumen degradation rates of sugarcane forage (whole plant).[a]

Component	*n*	Mean (SD)
DM (%)	68	28.09 (3.94)
Crude protein (% in DM)	66	2.56 (0.85)
Ether extract (% in DM)	41	1.53 (1.15)
Ash (% in DM)	45	2.89 (1.01)
Neutral detergent fibre (% in DM)	42	54.99 (8.49)
Acid detergent fibre (% in DM)	34	34.08 (6.21)
Soluble carbohydrates (% in DM)	3	39.70 (6.54)
Hemicellulose (% in DM)	14	20.50 (4.95)
Cellulose (% in DM)	9	25.46 (3.81)
Lignin (% in DM)	12	7.68 (3.26)
DM digestibility (%)	3	60.20 (3.73)
Rumen soluble protein – fraction A (% of CP)	3	29.17 (11.40)
Rumen degradable protein – fraction B (% of CP)	3	36.50 (2.91)
Protein degradation rate (% h^{-1})	1	6.70 (0.00)
Rumen soluble fibre – fraction A (% of NDF)	5	4.73 (7.12)
Rumen degradable fibre – fraction B (% of NDF)	6	54.85 (12.67)
Fibre degradation rate (% h^{-1})	4	2.40 (0.65)

[a]From Valadares Filho *et al.* (2001)

of sugarcane diets enhances the balance of absorbed nutrients through increased microbial growth and fibre degradation in the rumen or increased supply of bypass nutrients. However, the high cost of most supplements is a major economic constraint and reassessment of potential supplements is always required (Preston and Leng, 1980).

Dairy Cattle Performance on Sugarcane-based Diets

Feeding sugarcane to all classes of livestock, but especially dairy cattle, has been practised for a long time in Brazil. Nevertheless, the techniques used have been mostly rudimentary and little attention has been given to the critical role of supplements to improve sugarcane efficiency as animal feed. Since the mid-1980s have serious attempts been made to understand its major nutrient limitations.

Nutritional constraints

One of the most limiting factors concerning sugarcane utilization by ruminants is the low DM intake as a result of the slow turnover rate due to the low digestibility of DM and low degradation rate of cell wall in the rumen (Ravelo *et al.*, 1978;

Bobadilla and Rowe, 1979). Rodrigues *et al.* (1997) found a relevant variation in NDF content among sugarcane varieties, an indication that some genetic improvement in forage quality can be expected, with possible impacts on DM intake.

An extensive literature review on tropical feedstuffs (Preston and Leng, 1980) pointed out that sugarcane supplemented only with urea and minerals was able to satisfy cattle maintenance requirements. Significant improvement in animal performance with the addition of rice polishings led the authors to propose that feeding supplements with rumen bypass protein and starch could be a very effective strategy for increasing the supply of critical nutrients at the small intestine (Preston and Leng, 1980).

Growing animals

Data compiled from 59 experiments (Moreira, 1983) with crossbred Holstein–Zebu (HZ) dairy heifers fed diets based on sugarcane plus 1% urea showed body weight gains varying from 131 to 721 g day^{-1} when 0.4 to 1.0 kg per head day^{-1} of concentrate was fed and an average daily DM intake around 2% of body weight. In feeding trials at Embrapa National Dairy Cattle Research Centre (CNPGL) in Coronel Pacheco, Brazil, weight gains around 200 g day^{-1} were observed with confined HZ growing cattle fed sugarcane plus urea as an exclusive source of roughage (Table 24.2). Superior average weight gains were obtained with the supply of 1 kg rice bran or wheat meal (500 g day^{-1}), or 1 kg cottonseed meal (750 g day^{-1}).

Andrade and Pereira (1999) studied the total substitution of maize silage by sugarcane in diets of Holstein heifers. All diets contained 320 g NDF kg^{-1} DM from maize silage or sugarcane. Average daily weight gain was 1.18 kg for maize silage and 1.01 kg for sugarcane ($P = 0.01$) and DM intake was lower ($P = 0.09$) when animals were fed sugarcane diet (8.7 versus 8.2 kg per animal day^{-1}). Even with a lower performance as compared with maize silage, sugarcane

Table 24.2. Average body weight gains of crossbred HZ growing cattle fed sugarcane diets supplemented with different concentrates.[a]

Concentrate	Amount fed (kg per head day^{-1})	Initial weight (kg)	Average weight gain (g day^{-1})
None	0.0	130–254	212–350
Rice bran	0.5–1.5	130–251	344–582
Cassava (dry root)	1.0	238	415
Ear maize (disintegrated)	1.0	250	320
Wheat meal	1.0	250	535
Cottonseed meal	1.0	197–251	654–833

[a]Adapted from Oliveira (1985) and Torres and Costa (2001).

proved to be a viable option for Holstein heifers raised for first calving at 24 months of age with 550 kg of body weight.

Lactating cows

In Brazil, sugarcane usually has been fed to lactating cows yielding up to 10 kg milk day^{-1} (Table 24.3). More recently, its utilization for high-yielding cows has been tried with reasonable success (Sousa, 2003; Magalhães *et al.*, 2004; Mendonça *et al.*, 2004). In this situation, the amount of sugarcane fed should be limited with the increased contribution of concentrates in the total DM intake (Lima *et al.*, 2004; Costa *et al.*, 2005). As a result, a greater proportion of digestible organic matter leads to a lower content of less digestible fibre in the diet and, in consequence, higher DM intake to meet animal energy requirements. However, this strategy needs much attention, since concentrate in excess may cause metabolic disorders and, certainly, will raise feeding costs.

Modelling Digestion and Utilization of Nutrients in Dairy Cows

The need for an integrated and holistic analysis of experimental results from a series of digestion trials with HZ rumen-fistulated crossbred cattle (i.e. Oliveira, 1990; Matos, 1991; Aroeira *et al.*, 1993, 1996), as well as for minimizing expensive field experimentation, motivated nutritionists of CNPGL and modelling experts of Reading, (at present) Guelph and Wageningen Universities to build a dynamic nutritional simulation model of sugarcane digestion and nutrient utilization in dairy cows (Neal *et al.*, 1993; Dijkstra *et al.*, 1996a). The primary approach was to predict nutrient supply to the animal from predefined dietary inputs, as a means of indicating pre-experimentally which combination of locally available supplements was most likely to enhance animal performance on sugarcane-based diets.

Table 24.3. Dry matter intake (DMI), milk yield (MY) and 4% fat corrected milk yield (FCM) from dairy cows fed sugarcane diets.[a]

Reference	DMI (kg day^{-1})	MY (kg day^{-1})	FCM (kg day^{-1})
Naufel *et al.* (1969)	6.0	–	3.7
Nogueira Filho *et al.* (1977)	8.1–9.8	11.8–12.3	11.0–12.0
Biondi *et al.* (1978)	9.9–10.4	8.1–10.0	7.5–9.6
Benitendi *et al.* (1987)	7.9–8.2	7.8–8.1	–
Paiva *et al.* (1991)	10.1	10.5	9.2
Costa *et al.* (2005)	15.8–19.8	17.0–19.3	16.6–19.3
Lima *et al.* (2004)	11.6–18.3	13.7–18.8	–
Magalhães *et al.* (2004)	17.3–19.1	20.3–23.3	21.4–25.0
Mendonça *et al.* (2004)	14.9–15.4	18.6–20.1	19.4–21.3

[a]Adapted from Santos *et al.* (2005)

Model description

After an initial effort of modelling sugarcane digestion for dairy cattle in Brazil (Neal *et al.*, 1993), a more detailed simulation model was developed (Dijkstra *et al.*, 1996a) based on existing rumen models (i.e. Baldwin *et al.*, 1987; Dijkstra *et al.*, 1992). However, in the current modelling study, some components (e.g. rumen microbial biomass and volatile fatty acids) are aggregated rather than individual pools, as in the existing models.

A flow diagram representing the sugarcane digestion simulation model is shown in Fig. 24.1 and general notation defined in Table 24.4. All mathematical statements of the model are available and a complete description of the model, including input and output equations from each pool, was reported previously (Dijkstra *et al.*, 1996a).

The model comprises 11 rumen pools, representing nitrogen-containing fractions, carbohydrate fractions, fatty acid fractions and microbial mass, and four zero pools, representing the nutrients available for absorption. The nitrogenous fractions include undegradable protein (*Pu*), insoluble, degradable protein (*Pd*), soluble protein (*Ps*) and ammonia (*Am*). The carbohydrate fractions include undegradable fibre (*Fu*), degradable fibre (*Fd*), insoluble starch (*Si*) and soluble starch and sugars (*Sc*). The fatty acid fractions are long-chain (*Ld*) and volatile (*Va*) fatty acids. The microbial DM pool (*Mi*) comprises all strains of

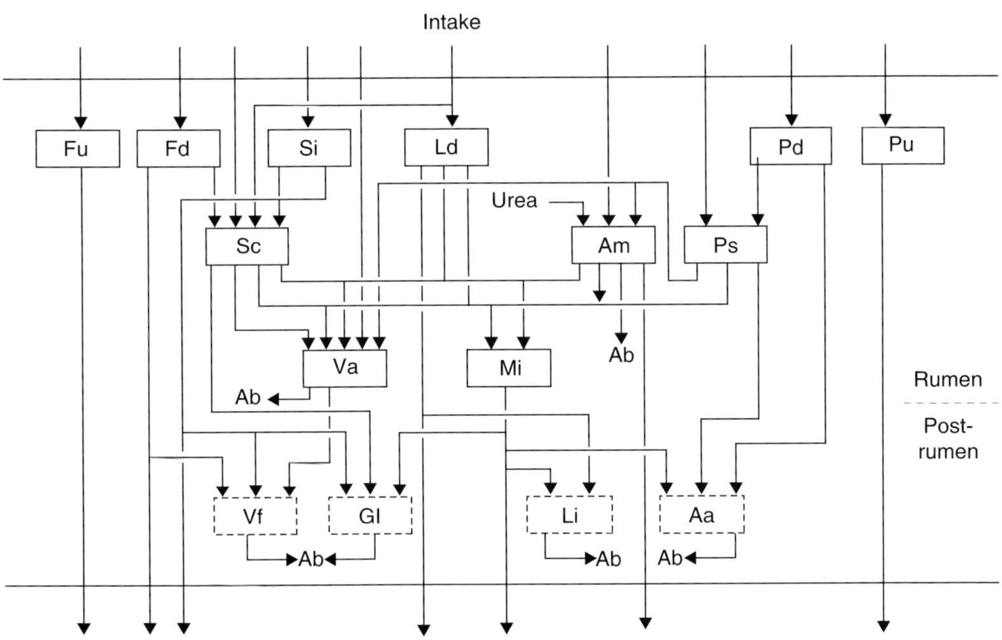

Fig. 24.1. Diagrammatic representation of sugarcane digestion simulation model, with solid boxes indicating rumen state variables, broken line boxes indicating post-rumen zero pools and arrows indicating fluxes (from Dijkstra *et al.*, 1996a).

Table 24.4. Main notation used in the model.[a]

Notation	Description
Aa	Post-rumen amino acids and small peptides
Ab	Absorption
Am	Ammonia
Fd	Rumen degradable fibre
Fu	Rumen undegradable fibre
Gl	Post-rumen glucose
Ld	Rumen long-chain fatty acids
Li	Post-rumen long-chain fatty acids
Mi	Microbial DM
Pd	Rumen insoluble, degradable protein
Ps	Rumen soluble protein
Pu	Rumen undegradable protein
Sc	Rumen soluble starch and sugars
Si	Rumen insoluble starch
Va	Rumen volatile fatty acids
Vf	Post-rumen volatile fatty acids

[a]From Dijkstra *et al.* (1996a)

rumen bacteria and protozoa. Each rumen fraction concentration is calculated as its pool size divided by rumen volume. All pools are expressed in grams except for *Va* and *Vf* (in moles), volume in litres and time in hours. Differential equations describe the rate of change of each pool size (Q_i) with time (t), dQ_i/dt, and principles of mass conservation give the following general equation:

$$dQ_i/dt = \text{inflow} - \text{outflow} + \text{synthesis} - \text{utilization}.$$

In the model, the rumen microbial population utilizes *Sc*, *Ps* and *Am* from hydrolysis and fermentation of dietary structural and non-structural carbohydrates, and protein and non-protein nitrogen, for its maintenance and growth. Protozoa are assumed to be the part of the microbial pool that is retained selectively in the rumen and microbial mass recycling is described by the death and lysis of this part. The remainder of the pool, represented by rumen bacteria, flows out of the rumen in liquid and solid phases. Urea transported across the rumen wall or with the saliva is represented by a single flux into the *Am* pool and assumed to be related to *Am* concentration in the rumen and to total dietary intake of nitrogen. *Am* is removed from the rumen by incorporation into the microbes, absorption across the rumen wall or passage with the fluid phase. Entry into the *Va* pool is by volatile fatty acids (VFAs) in the feed and from fermentation of *Sc* and *Ps*. VFAs are removed from the rumen by absorption across the rumen wall and passage with the fluid.

Continuous nutrient inputs derived from a predefined amount and chemical composition of the diet are assumed. Whenever possible, components of sugarcane and supplements, as well as fractional degradation rates, were taken from local feed analysis and *in situ* digestion trials (Oliveira, 1990; Valadares Filho *et al.*, 1990; Matos, 1991; Aroeira *et al.*, 1993).

The nutrients available for absorption post-ruminally are: *Aa* (amino acids and small peptides of microbial and dietary origin), *Gl* (glucose from undegraded feed starch and sugars, i.e. *Sc* and *Si*, and from microbial polysaccharides), *Li* (long-chain fatty acids from dietary and microbial lipids) and *Vf* (VFA washed out from the rumen plus VFA from carbohydrate fermentation in the large intestine). Multiplication of each nutrient outflow from the rumen by its respective intestinal digestion coefficient gives the amount of absorbed nutrients. The total amount of VFA available for absorption is the sum of VFA absorbed in the rumen and post-ruminally. Energy available for animal maintenance and production can be calculated from the amount of nutrients absorbed and their energy content. The simulated energy, glucogenic and aminogenic nutrient availability is used to calculate milk production, assuming predefined milk protein, fat and lactose contents. Calculations of nutrient requirements for maintenance and milk synthesis of the animal came from different information sources (i.e. ARC, 1980; Orskov, 1980; AFRC, 1991, 1992; Armentano, 1992; Hanigan and Baldwin, 1994) and were fully reported in Dijkstra *et al.* (1996a). The computer program was written in Advanced Computer Simulation Language – ACSL (Mitchell and Gauthier, 1981) – and a fourth-order Runge–Kutta method used for numerical integration. The model has been run for a sufficient time (e.g. 600 h) to reach steady-state solutions.

Model predictive performance

Nutrient flows

The first evaluation of a sugarcane digestion model was against data from two field trials conducted at CNPGL, Brazil, using rumen and abomasum fistulated HZ growing cattle (Oliveira, 1990; Matos, 1991). Oliveira (1990) supplemented fresh-chopped sugarcane with four levels of urea (0, 5, 10 and 15 g kg^{-1} fresh matter) and offered *ad libitum* to 225-kg steers. Matos (1991) used 290-kg steers in a factorial design with two levels of DM intake (maintenance and 1.5 times maintenance) and two levels of urea (10 and 15 g kg^{-1} fresh matter) included in a diet of chopped sugarcane supplemented with rice meal (210 g kg^{-1} total diet DM). Predicted and observed values for nutrient flows and rumen concentration were compared.

A general agreement for fibre flows and rumen ammonia and VFA concentration was attained. However, duodenal non-ammonia nitrogen (NAN) flow was consistently underpredicted, probably because endogenous protein sources were not taken into consideration (Dijkstra *et al.*, 1996a). Other analyses showed that the model was most sensitive to changes in fractional passage rate and fractional substrate hydrolysis rate and to the microbial maintenance requirement.

Milk production

In order to assess the ability of the model to predict milk production from sugarcane-based diets, data from a randomized-block feeding trial with 32 HZ lactating cows carried out at CNPGL were used (Assis *et al*., 1999). Four different supplements were added to a mixture of chopped sugarcane plus urea (10 g kg^{-1} fresh matter), namely: T_1 – soybean meal (1.58 kg DM per cow day^{-1}), T_2 – whole soybeans (1.60 kg DM per cow day^{-1}), T_3 – whole soybeans (3.20 kg per cow day^{-1}) and T_4 – soybean meal plus maize grain (2.10 kg plus 1.00 kg per cow day^{-1}). Four additional rumen fistulated HZ lactating cows were used in a Latin-square (4 × 4) design to determine protein and fibre degradation rates of the diets. Since the model was assumed to operate only at normal rumen pH and fatty acid levels that do not inhibit fibre degradation, protein-rich oil diets (i.e. T_2 and T_3) were not considered for model evaluation.

Predictions of potential milk production were assigned based on the most limiting nutrient available for absorption, among amino acids (*Aa*), glucose equivalents (*Gl*), long-chain fatty acids (*Li*) and energy (*En*). Potential milk yield based on *Li* was consistently under- and overpredicted on T_1 and T_4 diets, respectively. Since milk long-chain fatty acids can be synthesized *de novo*, mainly from acetic and butyric acid, which are available in large quantities from rumen fermentation processes, *Li* was disregarded from the milk yield calculation and model results became more consistent, with an overall prediction error (MSPE) of less than 15%. *Aa* was the first-limiting factor in seven out of eight animals in treatment T_1 and in four out of eight animals in treatment T_4.

General application of the model

Assessment of nutrient balance

The present digestion model was applied initially to simulate nutrient supply to the animal to indicate pre-experimentally the most suitable local supplements for enhancing milk production of dairy cattle fed sugarcane-based diets in the tropics (Dijkstra *et al*., 1996b). Four levels of urea added to chopped sugarcane were examined (0, 5, 10 and 15 g kg^{-1} fresh matter). Simulated microbial efficiency and substrate degradation in the rumen were improved with the addition of urea up to 10 g kg^{-1}, but further improvements could be obtained only if rumen degradable protein supplement was added to the diet. Using urea at 10 g kg^{-1} fresh sugarcane, plus several locally available protein and starch supplements at a rate of 100 g kg^{-1} total diet DM, the simulated level of absorbed *Aa* was low in comparison with the level of absorbed energy and glucogenic substrates, except when *Leucaena leucocephala* or fishmeal was used. In this situation, *Aa* availability was the factor most limiting milk production on sugarcane diets and protein supplements were recommended (Dijkstra *et al*., 1996b). At increasing levels of supplementation, and once amino acid requirements were satisfied, an increased absorption of *En* and *Li* could further improve milk production on sugarcane-based diets.

In another study, Kebreab *et al*. (2001) compared milk production simulated by the sugarcane digestion model against data from four tropical feeding trials with crossbred dairy cows fed sugarcane-based diets to assess possible nutrient imbalances and to recommend adequate supplementation for improving milk production.

The model indicated the most limiting nutrient to milk production under different feeding conditions. The addition of a forage legume (i.e. *Leucaena leucocephala*) to the basal sugarcane/urea diet increased the *Aa* and *Li* supplies, with *En* becoming the limiting factor. The supplementation of rice bran enhanced the availability of *En* and *Li*, but *Aa* became the next limiting factor. Adding both *Leucaena* and rice bran to the sugarcane-based diet improved nutrient balance, but availability of energy now limited milk production. In all feeding situations, the difference between predicted and observed milk yields varied from 0.08 to 1.00 kg day^{-1}.

Evaluation of locally available supplements

The model was also applied by Behera *et al.* (2005) to indicate the suitability of various supplements for improving milk production of crossbred dairy cattle on sugarcane tops/urea-based diets (SCT) under Indian conditions. Although some parameter values in the model are specific for whole sugarcane, particularly the fraction of protozoa, the SCT are still high in sugars, around 300 g kg^{-1} DM, and, at that level, protozoa have a major role in the rumen. Supplements were included in each basal diet, at three levels of addition, namely 100, 200 or 300 g kg^{-1} total diet DM.

Results from a series of simulations showed that, for SCT fed alone, milk production was mostly limited by *Aa* and *Li* availabilities. Among the protein-rich oil supplements, cottonseed cake provided sufficient nutrients for the production of 5.5, 7.3 and 8.3 kg milk day^{-1}, followed by mustard cake with 5.1, 6.5 and 7.6 kg day^{-1}, at the respective levels of supplementation. In the case of a protein-rich supplement (i.e. fishmeal), at 300 g kg^{-1} total DM, milk production became limited to 6.6 and 6.7 kg day^{-1} due to shortages of *Li* and *En*, respectively.

Forage legume added to an SCT-based diet was critical in increasing milk yield. Its effect was most pronounced with diets containing molasses, improving milk yield by up to 49.6%. The diet comprising SCT, forage legume, dry fodder (rice/wheat straw) and concentrate proved to be the most balanced formulation for attaining higher milk yields from Indian crossbred cows at all levels of supplementation, i.e. 5.1, 6.7 and 9.0 kg milk day^{-1}, respectively. To overcome shortages of *Aa* and *Li* in an SCT diet, supplements containing high bypass protein and starch contents (the latter to increase, in particular, amino acid and long-chain fatty acid absorption from microbial origin) seemed to be important for improving milk production. The authors found that, by adding more degradable protein and *Li* in the basal diet, milk yield could be further increased, provided rumen fermentation is not affected adversely.

Model refinements

Endogenous protein nitrogen and large intestine digestion

The original version of the sugarcane digestion model (Dijkstra *et al.*, 1996a) generally appeared to underestimate duodenal NAN outflow as compared with field data. As quoted by the authors, it could indicate the need to take production and recycling of endogenous-protein nitrogen (EPN) into consideration.

A second version of Dijkstra's model was elaborated (Assis and Barbosa, 2002; Assis *et al.*, 2005) to represent, through a simple submodel, the kinetics of EPN in the gastrointestinal tract of ruminants (Assis *et al.*, 1997). The submodel contains three EPN pools, corresponding to stomach, small intestine and large intestine, and utilizes two types of EPN source (production and inflow) and exit (absorption and passage), with EPN production based on DM intake. Furthermore, differential equations were used to describe the nutrient kinetics in the hindgut rather than the simple digestion coefficients adopted in the original version. In consequence, considerable improvement was obtained in the prediction of the nitrogen component flows. However, fibre flow and VFA concentration were slightly under- and overestimated, respectively (Assis *et al.*, 2005), indicating that further refinements in the EPN and large intestine sections were necessary.

Discontinuous feed intake

Different from most animal-feeding situations, in which feeds are offered discontinuously over the day, current model versions consider constant rates of nutrient inputs. Thus, a third version was developed by Collao-Saenz *et al.* (2005) to describe the usual pattern of nutrient supply to the host animal. This adaptation enabled the model to operate under non-steady-state feeding conditions for simulating nutrient availability as a response to feed intake patterns, as well as to represent the kinetics of particle size reduction. A new rumen pool for large particles (*Lp*) was added to the original 11 pools to account for the effect of particle size reduction in the nutrient flows. A single aggregate *Lp* pool was used to comprise all insoluble components of the diet, excluding insoluble starch. A small particle (*Sp*) zero pool was introduced as the sum of insoluble nutrients in the small particle form, which is directly susceptible to microbial degradation, namely: degradable fibre, undegradable fibre, insoluble but degradable protein, undegradable protein and insoluble starch. The conversion of *Lp* to *Sp* was dependent on rumination and as a function of feed physical properties, or comminution rate, and rumination time (Baldwin *et al.*, 1987).

Other changes were necessary to enable the original model to operate under non-steady-state conditions. Based on results from an ingestive behaviour trial with crossbred HZ heifers receiving sugarcane/urea diets supplemented with cottonseed meal (Miranda *et al.*, 1999), a feed ingestion pattern for every 12-h period of 85% in seven separate meals during the first half and 15% in two other meals during the second half was adopted to simulate a discontinuous supply of nutrients over the day.

An equation was introduced to account for the death of microorganisms in the absence of substrate and to reduce the efficiency of nutrient utilization of microbial DM. Also, rumen volume had to be changed from a constant parameter, as in the original model, to a variable dependent on the meal size and DM content. A non-linear relationship between the DM percentage of rumen contents and the DM rumen pool size was adopted based on an equation from Chilibroste *et al.* (2001). This relationship allowed rumen volume to vary during the day.

Comparison between values predicted by the model and data observed in HZ steers (Matos, 1991) and lactating cows (Assis *et al.*, 1999) receiving supplemented sugarcane/urea diets showed close agreement for duodenal flows of

NDF and NAN, as well as for milk production. The model responded well to changes in quantity and quality of the diets offered under non-steady-state conditions and seemed to be useful for assessing feeding strategies for dairy cattle fed sugarcane-based diets.

Extension of the model to other forage diets

The present model was designed initially to describe nutrient digestion and absorption of whole sugarcane in cattle and, consequently, some parameter values in the model were specific for this tropical forage. In particular, because of its high sugar and fibre contents, VFA profile and bacteria/protozoa ratio in the rumen are quite different from other forage-based diets (Agosto *et al.*, 1996). Even without changing values of these specific parameters, attempts have been made to expand the scope of the model to evaluate the nutritional constraints of other forage diets, such as alfalfa and maize (Assis *et al.*, 1994), or to assess, economically, costs and benefits of strategic supplementation of forage diets for dairy cows in the tropics (Assis *et al.*, 2001).

Another modelling effort by Rodrigues *et al.* (2002) attempted to extend the original sugarcane model to elephant grass (*Pennisetum purpureum*)-based diets. In many tropical dairy cattle systems, elephant grass is a very common forage, both grazed and fresh-chopped, or as silage. Despite its high potential of DM production per hectare in the growing season, elephant grass presents some nutritional gaps over the year. Valle *et al.* (1986) reported that HZ dairy cows grazing unsupplemented elephant grass during the dry season yielded only 6.8 kg milk day^{-1}. Although grazing management could affect animal performance, supplementation can play a very important role in milk production from grazed elephant grass, increasing yield by 15 to 50%, depending on the animal genetic potential, the type and amount of concentrate fed and the grazing season (Valle *et al.*, 1986, 1987; Embrapa, 1997).

In view of the large number of supplements available locally in tropical areas, the variation in nutrient requirements over the lactation and the typical seasonality of elephant grass with almost 80% of its annual DM production in the summer–wet season, further simulation studies to improve feeding strategies for dairy cattle seem highly desirable. Thus, it was necessary to change the values of three main parameters to account for differences in rumen fermentation between sugarcane- and elephant grass-based diets, namely: profile of VFA, proportion of protozoa to bacteria and percentage of attached bacteria in the total bacterial biomass. To calculate the energy content of the absorbed VFA, ratios of acetic:propionic:butyric acid of 77:15:8 and 71:18:11 for unsupplemented and supplemented elephant grass-based diets, respectively (Kariuki, 1998; Lopes and Aroeira, 1998), were used. Because of the abundance of sugars, rumen contents in sugarcane diets have a high protozoa count compared to other forage-based diets (Agosto *et al.*, 1996). In the sugarcane model, proportions of protozoa and bacteria were assumed to be 40 and 60% of the total microbial biomass, respectively, but in the elephant grass version values of 20 and 80% were set. Finally, in the original model, attached bacteria were assumed to be 75% of the total bacteria but, in this version, a proportion of 85% was assumed due to the higher amount of fibre and lower amount of sugars in elephant grass.

The overall stability and sensitivity of the model to parameter perturbation were considered satisfactory, as well as its predictions of faecal NDF flow compared to experimental observations. Conversely, predictions of rumen ammonia and VFA concentrations were unsatisfactory and estimates of milk yield were not always adequate. Even so, the simulated results indicated that the low availability of *Gl* and its precursors may be the factor most limiting milk production on unsupplemented elephant grass-based diets. Once glucogenic substrate supply has been increased to adequate levels, supplements that maximize the total DM intake and increase the supply of *Li* should be chosen.

Concluding Remarks

The current model was built primarily to represent the dynamics of nutrient digestion and absorption in HZ dairy cattle and to be used as a decision-making tool to select locally available supplements that potentially fulfil the nutritional constraints of sugarcane-based diets. Moreover, the model is expected to be an important resource-saving instrument, since it can be applied to screen the most nutritionally balanced forage-based diets that are worthwhile testing through field experimentation, so eliminating unnecessary and expensive feeding trials. However, for the model to be used as a decision support tool, its physiological base needs to be improved. The current model structure may also need further attention, including:

- A better representation of EPN based on flow of digesta DM rather than DM intake; this could be more relevant in low protein diets.
- Incorporation of nutrient requirements per kg of body weight gain, or per kg of body reserve; this could help to extend the model to growing dairy heifers and beef cattle, as well as accounting for body reserve mobilization and genotype differences.
- A few aggregated rumen pools split into their major components, such as microbial biomass, volatile and long-chain fatty acids; this could help to enlarge the model scope to other sugarcane materials (e.g. silage and bagasse) and to other tropical forage-based diets; this also could enable the predictions of milk and body weight gain composition, as well as the study of diets with high oil supplements.
- In many simulations with the digestion model, amino acids and, especially, long-chain fatty acids appeared as critical nutrients for milk production on sugarcane-based diets. This fact needs to be better exploited, bearing in mind the high availability of protein-rich oil by-products in the tropics and the expectation of increased supply due to the biodiesel production programme in Brazil from unconventional sources of vegetable oils, such as palm trees, castor-oil plant and sunflower.
- In simulations with other tropical forage-based diets, such as elephant grass, glucose seemed to be a limiting nutrient to certain levels of milk production and supplementation with low rumen degradable starch was apparently desirable. However, the role of bypass starch at the small intestine is not yet

clear and research reported by Reynolds (2002) questioned the hypothesis of a minimum requirement of starch at the small intestine. A series of trials with catheterized animals demonstrated that most of the glucose was utilized by viscera and arterial-circulating glucose was provided mainly through gluconeogenesis. These findings indicated that starch availability in the small intestine was unlikely to be the main reason for the improved performance on, for instance, sugarcane-based diets when supplemented with rice polishings. Rumen degradable protein in the rumen, metabolizable protein at the small intestine and supply of long-chain fatty acids for the rumen microbes and the host animal seemed to be more important for the improved performance from sugarcane-based diets supplemented with rice polishings.

After implementation of the suggestions made above, the model could be used as a framework to evaluate supplements for forage-based diets in several tropical countries. Kebreab *et al.* (2005) recommended that, instead of developing new models, efforts need to be concentrated on adaptation, better interface and evaluation of current mechanistic models. A network could be organized through the cooperation of scientists from tropical research centres and the original modellers, and a research proposal could be outlined along relevant and mutual interest research lines.

References

Agosto, M.D., Carneiro, M.E., Netto, C.M.M. and Arcuri, P.B. (1996) Avaliação dos ciliados do rumen de bovinos mantidos com duas dietas. *Arquivo Brasileiro de Medicina Veterinária e Zootecnia* 48, 353–361.

Agrianual (2005) *Anuário da Agricultura Brasileira,* FNP Consultoria e Comércio, São Paulo, Brazil.

Agricultural and Food Research Council (AFRC) (1991) AFRC Technical Committee on Responses to Nutrients. Report No 7. Theory of response to nutrients by farm animals. *Nutrition Abstracts and Reviews (Series B)* 61, 683–722.

Agricultural and Food Research Council (AFRC) (1992) AFRC Technical Committee on Responses to Nutrients. Report No 9. Nutritive requirements of ruminant animals: protein. *Nutrition Abstracts and Reviews (Series B)* 62, 787–835.

Agricultural Research Council (ARC) (1980) *The Nutrient Requirements of Ruminant Livestock.* Commonwealth Agricultural Bureaux, Farnham Royal, UK.

Andrade, M.A.F. and Pereira, M.N. (1999) Performance of Holstein heifers on fresh sugarcane as the only dietary forage. *Journal of Dairy Science* 82 (Supplement 1), 91.

Armentano, L.E. (1992) Ruminal hepatic metabolism of volatile fatty acids, lactate and pyruvate. *Journal of Nutrition* 122, 838–842.

Aroeira, L.J.M., Silveira, M.I., Lizieire, R.S., Matos, L.L. and Figueira, D.G. (1993) Rumen degradability and rate of passage of sugarcane with urea, cottonseed meal and rice meal in crossbred Holstein–Zebu steers [in Portuguese]. *Revista da Sociedade Brasileira de Zootecnia* 22, 552–564.

Aroeira, L.J.M., Lopes, F.C.F. and Dayrell, M.S. (1996) Degradabilidade de alguns alimentos no rúmen de vacas Holandês-Zebu. *Revista da Sociedade Brasileira de Zootecnia* 25, 1178–1186.

Assis, A.G. and Barbosa, P.F. (2002) Modelo de simulação da dinâmica de nutrientes em bovinos leiteiros. In: Barbosa, P.F., Assis, A.G. and Costa, M.A.B. (eds) *Modelagem e simulação de sistemas de produção animal.* Embrapa Pecuária Sudeste, São Carlos, Brazil, pp. 68–95.

Assis, A.G., Dijkstra, J., France, J., Veira, D.M., Neal, H.D.St.C. and Aroeira, L.J.M. (1994) Simulation of nutrient flows in the gastrointestinal tract of ruminants in the tropics. In: *Proceedings of the 45th Annual Meeting of the European Association of Animal Production.* Edinburgh, p. 150.

Assis, A.G., France, J., Dijkstra, J. and Veira, D.M. (1997) A model for estimating endogenous protein flows in the gastrointestinal tract of ruminants. *Journal of Animal and Feed Science* 6, 289–301.

Assis, A.G., Lopes, F.C.F., Durães, M.C., Simões, J.B., Andrade, R.S. and Verardo, A.E. Jr (1999) Validação de um modelo de simulação da dinâmica de nutrientes em vacas leiteiras. In: *Anais da 36a Reunião Anual da Sociedade Brasileira de Zootecnia.* Sociedade Brasileira de Zootecnia, Porto Alegre, Brazil (CD-ROM).

Assis, A.G., Campos, O.F, Dijkstra, J. and France, J. (2001) A simulation model to evaluate supplementation of tropical forage diets for dairy cows. In: *XIX International Grassland Congress*, USP/ESALQ, São Paulo, Brazil (CD ROM).

Assis, A.G., Campos, O.F., France, J. and Dijkstra, J. (2005) Evaluating tropical forages by a simulation model of nutrient kinetics. In: Ayantude, A.A., Fernández-Rivera, S. and McCrabb, G. (eds) *Coping with Feed Scarcity in Smallholder Livestock Systems in Developing Countries.* ILRI, Nairobi, pp. 277–283.

Baldwin, R.L., Thornley, J.H.M. and Beever, D.E. (1987) Metabolism of the lactating cow. II. Digestive elements of a mechanistic model. *Journal of Dairy Research* 54, 107–131.

Behera, U.K., Kebreab, E., Dijkstra, J., Assis, A.G. and France, J. (2005) Simulation of milk production by dairy cows fed sugarcane top based diets with locally available supplements under Indian conditions. *Journal of Agricultural Science* 143, 217–229.

Benitendi, R.P., Cardoso, V.L. and Freitas, M.A.R. (1987) Cana-de-açúcar acrescida de suplementos como volumoso para vacas mestiças em lactação. *Boletim da Indústria Animal* 44, 221–228.

Biondi, P., Caielli, E.L., Freitas, E.A.N. and Lucci, C.S. (1978) Substituição parcial e total da silagem de milho por cana-de-açúcar como únicos volumosos para vacas em lactação. *Boletim da Indústria Animal* 35, 45–55.

Bobadilla, M. and Rowe, J.B. (1979) Banana tops and sugarcane as cattle feed: observations on the rate of fibre degradation and fluid turnover in the rumen. *Tropical Animal Production* 4, 30–35.

Cesnik, R. and Miocque, J. (2004) *Melhoramento da cana-de-açúcar.* Embrapa Informação Tecnológica, Brasília, DF.

Chilibroste, P., Dijkstra, J. and Tamminga, S. (2001) Design and evaluation of a non-steady state rumen model. *Netherlands Journal of Agricultural Science* 49, 297–312.

Collao-Saenz, E.A., Dijkstra, J., Paiva, P.C.A., Bannink, A., Arcuri, P.B., Teixeira, J.C., Pérez, J.R.O. and David, F.M. (2005) Simulation model for particle dynamics in rumen of cattle fed sugarcane diet. *Scientia Agricola* 62, 102–110.

Costa, M.G., Campos, J.M.S., Valadares Filho, S.C., Valadares, R.F.D., Mendonça, S.S., Souza, D.P. and Teixeira, M.P. (2005) Desempenho produtivo de vacas leiteiras alimentadas com diferentes proporções de cana-de-açúcar e concentrado ou silagem de milho. *Revista Brasileira de Zootecnia* 34, 2437–2445.

Dijkstra, J., Neal, H.D.St.C., Beever, D.E. and France, J. (1992) Simulation of nutrient digestion, absorption and outflow in the rumen: model description. *Journal of Nutrition* 122, 2239–2256.

Dijkstra, J., France, J., Neal, H.D.St.C., Assis, A.G., Aroeira, L.J.M. and Campos, O.F. (1996a) Simulation of digestion in cattle fed sugarcane: model development. *Journal of Agricultural Science* 127, 231–246.

Dijkstra, J., France, J., Assis, A.G., Neal, H.D.St.C., Campos, O.F. and Aroeira, L.J.M. (1996b) Simulation of digestion in cattle fed sugarcane: prediction of nutrient supply for milk production with locally available supplements. *Journal of Agricultural Science* 127, 247–260.

Embrapa (1997) Manejo e alimentação de vacas: influência do período de descanso de pastagem de capim-elefante na produção de leite de vacas mestiças Holandês × Zebu. In: Zoccal R. (coord.) *Relatório Técnico do Centro Nacional de Pesquisa de Gado de Leite 1990–1994.* Embrapa – CNPGL, Juiz de Fora, Brazil, pp. 58–64.

Hanigan, M.D. and Baldwin, R.L. (1994) A mechanistic model of mammary gland metabolism in the lactating cow. *Agricultural Systems* 45, 369–419.

Kariuki, J.N. (1998) The potential of improving Napier grass under smallholder dairy farmers' conditions in Kenya. PhD thesis, Wageningen University, Wageningen, The Netherlands.

Kebreab, E., Assis, A.G., Dijkstra, J. and France, J. (2001) Evaluating sugarcane diets for dairy cows using a digestion model. *Tropical Animal Health and Production* 33, 127–139.

Kebreab, E., Smith, T., Tanmner, J. and Osuji, P. (2005) Review of undernutrition in smallholder ruminant production systems. In: Ayantude, A.A., Fernández-Rivera, S. and McCrabb, G. (eds) *Coping with Feed Scarcity in Smallholder Livestock Systems in Developing Countries.* ILRI, Nairobi, pp. 3–94.

Landell, M.G.A., Campana, M.P., Rodrigues, A.A. and Cruz, G.M. (2002) A variedade IAC 86-2480 como nova opção de cana-de-açúcar para fins forrageiros: manejo de produção e uso na alimentação animal. *Boletim Técnico IAC n. 193 – Série Tecnologia APTA*, São Paulo, Brazil.

Lima, M.L., Silva, D.N., Nogueira, J.R. and Landell, M.G. (2004) Produção de leite e consumo de material seca de vacas alimentadas com cana-de-açúcar forrageira IAC 86-2480. In: *Anais da 41ª Reunião Anual da Sociedade Brasileira de Zootecnia*, Sociedade Brasileira de Zootecnia, Campo Grande, Brazil (CD-ROM).

Lopes, F.C.F. and Aroeira, L.J.M. (1998) Consumo, digestibilidade, degradabilidade e parametros ruminais em vacas Holandes × Zebu alimentadas com capim elefante (*Pennisetum purpureum* Schum) picado. *Arquivo Brasileiro de Medicina Veterinária e Zootecnia* 50, 593–599.

Magalhães, A.L.R., Campos, J.M.S. and Valadares Filho, S.C. (2004) Cana-de-açúcar em substituição à silagem de milho em rações para vacas em lactação: desempenho e viabilidade econômica. *Revista da Sociedade Brasileira de Zootecnia* 33, 1292– 1302.

Manzano, R.P., Penati, M.A. and Nussio, L.G. (2002) *Cana-de-açúcar na alimentação de bovinos.* Fundação de Estudos Agrários 'Luiz de Queiróz', Piracicaba, Brazil.

Matos, N.J.M. (1991) Effects of level of feed intake and urea on rumen kinetic parameters in cattle fed sugarcane supplemented with rice meal. PhD thesis [in Portuguese], Federal University of Viçosa, Viçosa, Brazil.

Mendonça, S.S., Campos, J.M.S. and Valadares Filho, S.C. (2004) Consumo, digestibilidade aparente, produção e composição do leite e variáveis ruminais em vacas leiteiras alimentadas com rações à base de cana-de-açúcar. *Revista Brasileira de Zootecnia* 33, 481–492.

Miranda, L.F., Queiroz, A.C. de, Valadares Filho, S.C., Cecon, P.R., Pereira, E.S., Souza, J.M.C., Lanna, R.P. and Miranda, J.F. (1999) Comportamento ingestivo de novilhas leiteiras alimentadas com dietas à base de cana-de-açúcar. *Revista Brasileira de Zootecnia* 28, 614–620.

Mitchell, E.L. and Gauthier, J. (1981) *Advanced Continuous Simulation Language User Guide/Reference Manual*, 3rd edn. Mitchell and Gauthier Associates, Concord, Massachusetts.

Moreira, H.A. (1983) Cana-de-açúcar na alimentação de bovinos. *Informe Agropecuário*, 9, 14–16.

Naufel, F., Goldman, E.F. and Guaragna, R.N. (1969) Estudo comparativo entre a cana-de-açúcar e silagens de milho, sorgo e capim-Napier na alimentação de vacas leiteiras. *Boletim da Indústria Animal* 26, 9–22.

Neal, H.D.St.C., France, J., Assis, A.G., Aroeira, L.J.M. and Campos, O.F. (1993) Supplementation of sugarcane diets for Brazilian dairy cattle: a modelling study. In: Gill, M., Owen, E., Pellott, G.E. and Lawrence, T.C. (eds) *Animal Production in Developing Countries*. British Society of Animal Production, London, p. 161.

Nogueira Filho, J.C.M., Lucci, C.S., Rocha, G.L. and Melotti, L. (1977) Substituição parcial da silagem de milho por cana-de-açúcar como únicos volumosos para vacas em lactação. *Boletim da Indústria Animal* 24, 67–77.

Oliveira, J.S. (1985) *Utilização de cana + ureia na recria de bovinos*. Embrapa – CNPGL, Coronel Pacheco, Brazil, 20 pp. (Circular Tecnica 23).

Oliveira, W.H. (1990) Apparent digestibilities and rumen kinetics in cattle fed sugarcane with three levels of urea. MSc thesis [in Portuguese], University of Minas Gerais, Belo Horizonte, Brazil.

Orskov, E.R. (1980) Possible nutritional constraints in meeting energy and amino acid requirements of the highly productive ruminant. In: Ruckebusch, Y. and Thivend, P. (eds) *Digestive Physiology and Metabolism in Ruminants*. MTP Press, Lancaster, Massachusetts, pp. 309–324.

Paiva, J.A.J., Moreira, H.A. and Cruz, G.M. (1991) Cana-de-açúcar associada à uréia-sulfato de amônia como alimento volumoso exclusivo para vacas em lactação. *Revista Brasileira de Zootecnia* 20, 90–99.

Perez Infante, F. and Vila, R.G. (1975) Sugarcane for cattle in the dry season. 1. Effect of urea doses on feed intake and milk production. *Cuban Journal of Agricultural Science* 9, 105–108.

Preston, T.R. and Leng, R.A. (1980) Utilization of tropical feeds by ruminants. In: Ruckebusch, Y. and Thivend, P. (eds) *Digestive Physiology and Metabolism in Ruminants*. MTP Press, Lancaster, Massachusetts, pp. 621–640.

Preston, T.R. and Willis, M.B. (1979) *Intensive Beef Production*, 3rd edn. Pergamon Press, London.

Rangnekar, D.V. (1988) Availability and intensive utilization of sugarcane byproducts. In: Devendra, C. (ed.) *Proceedings of a Consultation on Non-conventional Feed Resources and Fibrous Agricultural Residues. Strategies for Expanded Utilization*. Hisar, India, pp. 76–93.

Ravelo, G., Gonzalez, F. and Hovell, F.D. (1978) El efecto de alimentar por fístula ruminal caña de azúcar e afrecho de trigo sobre el consumo de caña de azúcar. *Tropical Animal Production* 3, 237–242.

Reynolds, C.K. (2002) Economics of visceral energy metabolism in ruminants: toll keeping or internal revenue service? *Journal of Animal Science* 80 (E Supplement 2), E74–E84.

Rodrigues, A.R., Primasi, O. and Esteves, S.N. (1997) Efeito da qualidade de variedades de cana-de-açúcar sobre seu valor como alimento para bovinos. *Pesquisa Agropecuária Brasileira* 32, 333–338.

Rodrigues, S.I.F., Dijkstra, J., Assis, A.G., France, J. and Tamminga, S. (2002) Evaluation of supplements to enhance nutrient supply and milk production of cattle fed diets based on elephant grass (*Pennisetum purpureum*) using a mathematical model. *Livestock Production Science* 77, 273–286.

Santos, F.A.P., Voltolini, T.V. and Pedroso, A.M. (2005) Balanceamento de rações com cana-de-açúcar para rebanhos leiteiros: até onde é possível? In: Carvalho, M.P. and Santos, M.V. (org.) *Estratégia e competitividade na cadeia de produção do leite*. Gráfica Editora Berthier, Passo Fundo, RS, Brazil, pp. 208–245.

Sousa, D.P. (2003) Desempenho, síntese de proteína microbiana e comportamento ingestivo de vacas leiteiras alimentadas com cana-de-açúcar e caroço de algodão ou silagem de milho. MSc thesis, Federal University of Viçosa, Viçosa, Brazil.

Torres, R.A. and Costa, J.L. (2001) Uso da cana-de-açúcar como forrageira. In: Madalena, F.E., Matos, L.L. and Holanda, E.V. Jr (eds) *Produção de Leite e Sociedade*. FEPMVZ – Editora, Belo Horizonte, Brazil, pp. 295–342.

Valadares Filho, S.C., Silva, J.F.C., Leão, M.I., Euclydes, R.F., Valadares, R.F. and Castro, A.C.G. (1990) *In situ* degradability of dry matter and crude protein of some feeds by lactating dairy cows [in Portuguese]. *Revista da Sociedade Brasileira de Zootecnia* 19, 512–522.

Valadares Filho, S.C., Rocha, V.R. Jr and Cappelle, E.R. (2001) *Tabelas Brasileiras de Composição de Alimentos para Bovinos*. DZO – DPI – UFV, Viçosa, Brazil.

Valle, L.C.S., Mozzer, O.L., Lobato Neto, J., Villaça, H.A., Dusi, G. and Verneque, R.S. (1986) Níveis de concentrado para vacas em lactação em pastagens de capim-elefante (*Pennisetum purpureum*, Schum.) no período seco. I. Produção e composição do leite. In: *Anais da Reunião Anual da Sociedade Brasileira de Zootecnia*, Campo Grande, MS, Brazil, 23, 98.

Valle, L.C.S., Mozzer, O.L., Villaça, H.A. and Dusi, G. (1987) Níveis de concentrado para vacas em lactação em pastagens de capim-elefante (*Pennisetum purpureum*, Schum.) no período das águas. In: *Anais da Reunião Anual da Sociedade Brasileira de Zootecnia*, Brasília, DF, 24, 56.

25 Simulation Exercises for Animal Science MSc Students: Rumen Digestion and Pig Growth

W.J.J. Gerrits,[1] E. Kebreab,[2] M.R. Kramer[3] and J. Dijkstra[1]

[1]Animal Nutrition Group, Wageningen University, The Netherlands; [2]National Centre for Livestock and Environment, Department of Animal Science, University of Manitoba, Canada; [3]Information Technology Group, Wageningen University, The Netherlands

Introduction

Quantitative understanding of biological processes has been a key issue in animal science, resulting from the desire to predict growth rates, body composition, and egg, wool and milk production from nutrient inputs. Consequently, the application of predeveloped models is commonly used in animal science teaching throughout the world. The construction of models, however, is often not included in education programmes. Yet the process of designing and building models, just as much as experimenting with these models, has considerable potential to increase students' (quantitative) insight into biological processes. In the past decades, several tools have become available that facilitate the construction of dynamic, mechanistic simulation models. The objective of this chapter is to provide two complete teaching modules for MSc students of animal science with minimal background in modelling, but knowledge in animal nutrition at BSc level. In working through the first module, students will develop a model simulating rumen digestion and passage dynamics and, during development, will become familiar with the concept of fractional passage and degradation rates. In the second module, students will develop a model simulating protein and fat accretion rates in growing pigs, dealing with the principles of nutrient partitioning in growing animals. At Wageningen University, the Information Technology Group has many years' experience in the theory and application of modelling and simulation. Since 1995, the group has developed a tool for constructing dynamic simulation models especially aimed at educational use, named SMART, an acronym for 'Simulation and Modelling Assistant for Research and Teaching' (Kramer and

Scholten, 2001). A copy of SMART can be downloaded free of charge at <http://www.uoguelph.ca/cnm/chapter25exercises>. Installation instructions and pre-programmed models are available at the website. Answers to questions are included at the end of this chapter. It is recommended that these exercises be accompanied by lectures dealing with the biology behind them. The two teaching modules are preceded by a short exercise aimed at becoming familiar with SMART. Although the description of the modules is based on the assumption that SMART is used, any modelling tool with the capability to numerically solve a set of differential equations can be used. For each module, an indication of the time required to work successfully on the module is given in the subheading.

Getting Started with SMART (30 min)

The process of model development can be divided into four phases: (i) building the model; (ii) defining simulation experiments; (iii) performing simulations; and (iv) inspecting results. In SMART, a clear distinction is made between these phases. Especially, the first two phases are clearly separated. Briefly, phase 1 involves looking at the structure of the system under investigation (e.g. digestion or growth), dividing it into its key components and relationships, translating the system into a set of mathematical equations and preparing the model for use in simulation experiments. In phase 2, the user defines parameter values, inputs, choice of numerical integration algorithm with its settings and outputs to store. The user can define any number of experiments with one model, each experiment having its own settings. Phase 3 is the actual simulation process that generates series of outputs according to the model equations and experiment settings. Under phase 4, the results are interpreted using a variety of graphs and tables. Now you are going to exercise phases 1 to 4, in reverse order.

These exercises use the model 'LANDSH' (lynxes and snowshoe hares) from the standard SMART examples. This is an example of a non-steady-state model. The model describes the development over time of population sizes of lynxes and snowshoe hares. As both species have specific birth and mortality rates and lynxes eat hares, both population sizes will vary in time: the number of lynxes increases as the quantity of food (i.e. number of hares) increases. When there are too many lynxes, the population of hares will decrease. Consequently, lynxes will die by starvation and the population of lynxes will then also decrease. With a suitable choice of parameter values, this pattern repeats itself.

Inspecting simulation results

- *Start SMART and open the existing model 'LANDSH' from the examples folder*. Simulation results always belong to a particular model and experiment. So open the model first and then the experiment.
- *Open the existing experiment 'SHORT'*. The experiment menu shows all previously saved experiments that belong to the current model. The experiment

named 'SHORT' has been saved with simulation results for 20 years (simulated time).

- *Make a graph of the simulation results.* (Menu Simulation, item Add Graph...) First, the 'Define output' dialogue appears. The program has selected the number of hares and the number of lynxes by default. This is fine for now, so press OK. A graph with two cycles of rise and fall of hares as well as lynxes is shown.
- *Make a table of the same results.* Click the right mouse button in the graph, and choose 'Table...'. This shows a table of the same variables as selected for the graph. If need be, the selection of output variables can be changed. Click the right mouse button in the table, and choose 'Define output...'.
- *Export the data to a text file.* Click the right mouse button in the table, and choose 'Write data to ASCII...'. Data are saved in so-called CSV-format, which is supported by most spreadsheet programs. Exported data can be used for further analysis or for incorporating data into a report.
- *Open the experiment 'LONG' and make a graph of its results.* This experiment shows a simulation period of 100 years. Visually, the pattern seems to repeat itself exactly. To check this, make a phase diagram of the results: in the 'Define output' dialogue, choose 'Hares' as the independent variable (i.e. the variable on the *x*-axis) and click OK. The graph shows as one loop; it repeats itself almost exactly! The remaining small differences are due to approximation errors in the numerical integration process.

Running an experiment

- *Open the experiment 'SHORT' again and run the experiment as it is.* (Menu Simulation, item Run...) Then press the Start button. The simulation run can be paused, e.g. after one cycle. It is not possible to change the variables shown in the 'Simulation' window. However, a graph can be added. Every time the simulation is paused and resumed again, the graph will be updated. In this way, continue until the end of the simulation run. Do not save the results yet.
- *Close the experiment.* If asked, do not save the experiment.

Defining and changing experiments

- *Start a new experiment.* (Menu Experiment, item New...) A new experiment has by default all the settings as defined by the modeller. It can be run as provided, but it is more interesting to try some changes in experimental settings:
- *Change run options.* The default integration method for this model (RKqc) adapts its time step by estimating the computation error. It takes small steps when needed and large steps when possible. Change the integration method to (fixed step) Euler with a time step of 0.1 year. Set the simulation period to 40 years and:

- *Run the simulation.* If the simulation runs too slowly, the 'Speed options' button in the simulation window can be used to set a refresh interval for the screen (e.g. run without interrupts for 20 output steps). What do you observe?
- *Save the experiment.* Choose an appropriate name for the experiment. The settings, as well as the results, are saved for later use.
- *Start a new experiment (again).* Now do not change the integration method. You may want to extend the simulation period, however.
- *Change some parameters.* New values may be entered in the rightmost column of the 'Parameter' tab. Run the simulation; change the parameters again and run again. Determine the effect of, for example, the birth rate of the hares on the maximum population size of lynxes.
- *Save the changed experiment.* When a particularly interesting set of parameters is achieved, you can save the experiment for later use.

Modifying an existing model

- *Open the 'LANDSH' model again.* Alternatively, you may close all windows except the 'Model definitions' window.
- *Save the model under a new name.* Thus, the original model is available for comparisons or for redoing these exercises. Try to save it in a new folder as well.
- *Introduce an auxiliary variable.* In the original model, the only interesting variables are the number of hares and the number of lynxes. There is no option to observe the births or deaths of either species separately, however. To add the birth and death of species (starting with hares) go to the tab 'Auxiliary variables' and press the Append button. In the dialogue, fill in the name (e.g. HaresBirths), unit (#hares ha^{-1} $year^{-1}$), description and formula (BRH*Hares). When these fields are filled, click OK. The formula says that births of hares are proportional to the number of hares present, with a factor BRH (a parameter of the model). You will need this kind of formula again in a later part of this chapter.
- *Change the formula of an existing variable.* Find the variable hares in the model definition (tab 'State variables'). Then double click it or press the Edit button. Replace the formula by 'HaresBirths–HaresDeaths', where the first name is the name of the auxiliary variable from the previous step and the second name is new to this model.
- *Check your changed model.* (Menu Model, item Check...) SMART checks whether the model is consistent and all formulas are well formed. The check will find at least one unknown name: HaresDeaths. Close the 'Check' window.
- *Introduce another auxiliary variable.* Define HaresDeaths as an auxiliary variable with the formula 'PRH*Hares*Lynx'. This formula is the second term of the original formula for 'dHares/dt'. You may either type this formula or drag the names from the list of available components (and still type the stars).
- *Check the model again.* When the model is saved, there should be no errors left. Otherwise, check the spelling of the new variables.
- *Add auxiliary variables for the births and deaths of lynxes.* Use the first and second term of the formula for 'dLynx/dt', respectively.

- *Compile the model.* SMART will prompt you to save your changes first. Then it will check the model, if you did not do so yourself. When no errors are found, the 'Compile' dialogue appears. Press OK (on older systems, a (black) Command or DOS window may appear – close it when it is ready). If SMART indicates that the compiler cannot be found, check the installation notes to set the compilation preferences correctly. [In a computer lab, please contact one of the assistants.]
- *Run a simulation with the changed model.* Now births and deaths of hares and lynxes can be inspected. Try to use the experiment saved in the preceding part of the exercises. Because the model has changed, SMART issues a warning (just click OK) and ignores any available experiment outputs.

Case Study 1. A Simulation Model of Rumen Digestion and Passage Kinetics (150 min)

Objective

The aim of this case study is to exercise the process of translating biological processes, such as degradation, passage and absorption of nutrients, into a set of mathematical equations. Furthermore, knowledge on passage and degradation characteristics of feedstuffs, as well as on the fate of fermentation end products, is integrated in this case study. The case study consists of two parts. The first part should be completed in about 90 min and the second part in another 60 min.

A non-steady-state model of digestion kinetics (90 min)

Description of the system to be modelled

The process of fermentation and digestion is dynamic. Therefore, nutrient availability and utilization will fluctuate with time. The feed entering the reticulo-rumen can be characterized by a soluble fraction (S), a potentially degradable fraction (D) and an undegradable fraction (U). The degraded feed particles are substrate for microbial growth, with a concomitant production of the short-chain fatty acids: acetic acid (HAc), propionic acid (HPr) and butyric acid (HBu). Follow the instructions below to develop this model step-by-step: (i) the passage and digestion of the different feed fractions will be modelled in a non-steady-state condition (monitoring the fate of a single meal); (ii) the model will then be refined by adding microbial growth, fatty acid production and their absorption through the rumen wall.

Step-wise instructions to build this model in SMART

Build a model simulating passage and degradation of the different feed fractions through the rumen. Before building the model, make a flow chart and identify the proper pools (state variables) and fluxes (auxiliary variables). Always check the units: state variables are quantities; fluxes are quantities per time unit. The following assumptions are made:

- The feed consists of S, D and U fractions. A single meal of 20 kg dry matter (DM) of dried grass is administered to a dairy cow with an empty rumen. Assume the S, D and U fractions of grass DM, measured by *in sacco* procedures, to be 30, 50 and 20%, respectively.
- The passage rate of the U fraction through the rumen (passageU, g h^{-1}) is proportional to the quantity of U present in the rumen. Assume the fractional passage rate of feed particles (k_p) to be 3% h^{-1}. Please do not enter the k_p as a number in the equation, but define the k_p as a constant in the 'Constants & Parameters' tab in SMART (constant k_p = 3% h^{-1}) and use this constant in the equation defining the flux leaving the U pool.
- The S fraction is passing through the rumen compartment with the liquid phase (passageS, g h^{-1}). For the passage rate of liquid, assume a constant fractional passage rate (constant k_l = 10% h^{-1}). The passage rate of S is proportional to the quantity of S present in the rumen. Apart from that, S material is also being degraded (degradationS, g h^{-1}). The degradation rate is proportional to the quantity of S present in the rumen. Usually, it is assumed that this material is degraded before it has the chance of leaving the rumen. The fractional degradation rate is, therefore, high: constant, k_{dl} = 200% h^{-1}.
- Like the U fraction, the D fraction is flowing out of the rumen compartment with the feed particles (passageD, g h^{-1}). Passage rate is proportional to the quantity of D present in the rumen. Apart from that, D material is also being degraded (degradationD, g h^{-1}). The degradation rate is proportional to the quantity of D present in the rumen. Assume the fractional degradation rate of D (constant, k_d) to be 2% h^{-1}.
- In the simulation, the cumulative quantities of D and S being degraded can be determined as follows: introduce additional pools for these quantities (name them cumdegradedD and cumdegradedS, respectively). Each of these pools has only one input: the degraded material leaving D and degraded leaving S, respectively. Not including any outputs from these pools assures a steady increase in pool size, collecting all degraded material, as the simulation progresses.

After building this model in SMART, compile the model and run it for a simulation time of 96 h (integration algorithm RKfixed, integration step 0.1 h) to answer the questions below. Create separate experiments for each question and save the simulation results with them.

Questions

1. Check the development of S, D and U with time. Does it match your expectations? How much of S, D and U is still in the rumen after 20 h? Record your answer in Table 25.1.

2. Now use straw instead of dried grass and answer question 1. Assume S, D and U to account for 10, 50 and 40% of the dry matter of straw and assume the

Table 25.1. Pool sizes of soluble (S), potentially degradable (D) and undegradable (U) material in the rumen, 20 h after a single meal.

Pool size at 20 h	Dried grass	Straw
S		
D		
U		

fractional degradation rate of D (k_d) to be 0.5 % h^{-1}. Compare and discuss the results.

3. Start a new experiment again. Now double the fractional passage rate of particles (k_p). How does this affect the degradation and passage rates at $t = 20$ h? Can you explain the difference? Would it be beneficial to the cow to double the fractional passage rate?

4. Look at the cumulative quantity of D and S being degraded in the rumen compartment during 96 h. What proportion of the ingested quantity of degradable (D) and soluble (S) material is actually degraded in the rumen after 96 h?

Microbial growth and short-chain fatty acids (60 min)

Description of the system to be modelled

In the first part of this case study, material degraded in the rumen has not been utilized for any purpose. In the cow, rumen degraded material is being used by microorganisms, which use it as fuel and building blocks. As a result, microbial biomass is produced. Furthermore, the microorganisms convert a substantial part of degradable material into short-chain fatty acids (i.e. acetic acid, Hac; propionic acid, Hpr; butyric acid, Hbu), which can be absorbed through the rumen wall and be used both as fuel and as a precursor for milk components by the cow.

Step-wise instructions to build this model in SMART

Extend the model you developed in the first part of this case study by a representation of rumen microbial biomass and the produced HAc, HPr and HBu. First, save the model under a new name. Again, identify pools and flows before actually entering the formulas into SMART. Where appropriate, introduce constants or parameters in the SMART model. The following assumptions are made:

- At time = 0 h, the microbial biomass in the rumen is close to 0 g (set the initial value of this state variable to 0). The pool of microbial biomass increases due to microbial growth, which occurs because microorganisms use degraded material in the rumen for their own growth (growthMB, g h^{-1}). Assume that all degraded material is converted to microbial biomass with an efficiency of 15% (constant MBeff = 0.15). Microbial biomass flows out of the rumen with the feed particles (passageMB, g h^{-1}) and it is assumed that the passage rate is proportional to the microbial biomass present in the rumen (constant $k_p = 3\%\ h^{-1}$).

- Microorganisms produce short-chain fatty acids from material that is degraded in the rumen (productionHAc, productionHPr, productionHBu, all in $g\ h^{-1}$). The efficiency with which degraded material in the rumen is converted into short-chain fatty acids is 70% (constant SCFAeff = 0.70). Of the total amount of short-chain fatty acids, the proportions of HAc, HPr and HBu are 65, 20 and 15%, respectively (on a weight basis) (constants: propHAc, 0.65; propHPr, 0.20; propHBu, 0.15). Short-chain fatty acids are water-soluble and therefore leave the rumen with the liquid phase (passageHAc, passageHpr, passageHBu, all in $g\ h^{-1}$), or are absorbed (absorptionHAc, absorptionHPr, absorptionHbu, all in $g\ h^{-1}$). For absorption of HAc, HPr and HBu through the rumen wall, assume that it is proportional to the quantity of the respective fatty acid present in the rumen and assume the fractional absorption rates to be constant: $k_{a,Hac} = 20\%\ h^{-1}$, $k_{a,Hpr} = 30\%\ h^{-1}$ and $k_{a,Hbu} = 40\%\ h^{-1}$, for HAc, HPr and HBu, respectively.
- Include additional state variables to keep track of the cumulative quantity of microbial biomass (cumMB), HAc (cumHac), HPr (cumHpr) and HBu (cumHbu) produced from the single meal.

After including these formulas in the SMART model, compile it and run it for a simulation period of 96 h to answer the questions below. Again, create a separate experiment for each question.

5. Check the change of microbial biomass and the quantity of HAc, HPr and HBu with time. Does it match your expectations? At what time do these variables reach peak values?
6. Can you explain why the peak value of microbial biomass is about 50% of that of HAc (both in g)? Is that what you expected, considering the threefold higher efficiency of conversion of degraded material into HAc compared with microbial biomass?
7. Now use straw instead of grass, adapting S, D, U and k_d as earlier (see question 2) and answer question 5 again. Compare and discuss the results.
8. Look at the total quantity of microbial biomass, HAc, HPr and HBu produced from the single meal of dried grass within 96 h. What proportion of the degraded material (see question 4) is actually converted into short-chain fatty acids and what proportion into microbial biomass?

Case Study 2. Simulating the Growing Pig: Post-absorptive Utilization of Amino Acids, Glucose and Fatty Acids (240 min)

Objective

The aim of this case study is to exercise the process of the partitioning of nutrients through intermediary metabolism into protein and fat retention (i.e. growth) or heat production. Special emphasis is on the use of carbohydrates versus fats as the main energy source. This case study connects well with basic principles of pig growth, biochemistry and energy metabolism.

Description of the system to be modelled

Please read this text carefully and complete the flow chart of the system to be modelled, presented in Fig. 25.1.

In this figure, pools (quantities, in g or kJ) are already present. Use arrows to indicate fluxes (rates, g day^{-1} or kJ day^{-1}). Digested nutrients are the starting point (top) and chemical body components are the end point (bottom). Pools or state variables are indicated in italics in the next paragraph.

After eating a meal, nutrients that are digested and absorbed are available for the pig. These nutrients (mainly glucose, fatty acids and amino acids) enter the systemic circulation and become available for metabolic processes. For the sake of simplicity, it is assumed that the concentration of nutrients in the blood is driving the various metabolic processes in the body directly, thus ignoring the well-known role of hormones in the partitioning of nutrients over various metabolic processes. Digested protein becomes available after absorption as *amino acids*. These amino acids can be used for body protein deposition or will be degraded, yielding glucose (gluconeogenesis), adenosine triphosphate (ATP) and urea. Digested starch becomes available as *glucose* and can be used for ATP production or, alternatively, be used to produce fatty acids (*de novo* fatty acid

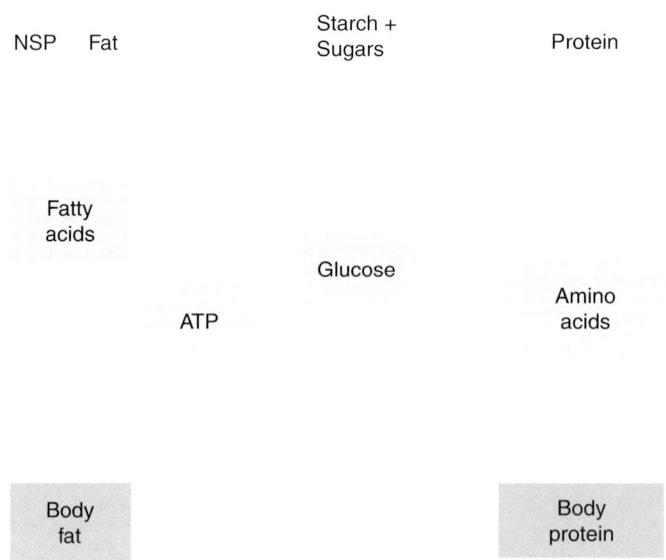

Fig. 25.1. Flow chart of the partitioning of macro nutrients in pigs. Complete this chart by drawing the appropriate arrows representing nutrient fluxes.

synthesis). Digested fat is assumed to consist of *fatty acids* only. In addition, fermentable non-starch polysaccharides (NSP) are assumed to appear post-absorptively as fatty acids. Fatty acids can be oxidized for ATP production or can be deposited as body fat. *ATP* is assumed to be the source of available energy to fuel the various energy-consuming processes in the pig. ATP is provided by the oxidation of glucose and fatty acids and is also formed during gluconeogenesis from amino acids. In addition, a part of the glucose used for *de novo* fatty acid synthesis inevitably goes to ATP. ATP is used for satisfying the maintenance energy needs, the energetic costs for body protein and body fat deposition, the energy costs of *de novo* fatty acid synthesis and the energy costs of urea production. *Body protein* and *body fat* are assumed as the main chemical components of the pig. They are deposited from amino acids and fatty acids, respectively. Body ash and body water are assumed to depend on the size of the body protein pool. Together, these body components add up to the empty body weight of the pig.

For simplicity...

- All metabolite and body compartment pools are in g, and the ATP pool is in kJ.
- All metabolite pools are anhydrous, i.e. the water molecules appearing during hydrolysis or disappearing during dehydration reactions are ignored.
- To ensure conservation of energy, fluxes between metabolite pools are calculated to be iso-energetic, i.e. the energy content of the (sum of) end products of each flux equals the energy content of the substrate used. The energy content of glucose, amino acids and fatty acids is assumed to be 17.5, 23.6 and 39.6 kJ g^{-1}, respectively.

Step-wise instructions to build this model in SMART

The text below should enable you to build the model you have represented schematically in your flow chart in SMART. The description is organized by pool (i.e. state variable). It is a good idea to follow this approach when building the model in SMART. A few hints:

- Open the model 'GrowPig' provided for you. In this model, all *Constants & Parameters* (mentioned in the text and summarized in Table 25.2) are already programmed to save you some typing time.
- Pools are represented as *State variables*. The rate of change of each pool with time (dPool/dt) should then be a simple summation of fluxes into and fluxes out of that pool. Variable names are already assigned to fluxes for you in the *Auxiliary variables* tab in the GrowPig model. Specify the formula of all fluxes according to the description below. Names of fluxes, as they are included in the GrowPig model, are indicated in the description below.
- Variable names can be quite long. To avoid typing errors, use the facility in SMART to click and drag variables into an equation. If you do not know how to do this, ask your instructor.
- Pay attention to the units and save the model regularly to avoid losing your work.

Table 25.2. Constants and parameters used in the model.

Name constant	Description	Default value	Unit
Dietary parameters:			
FeedIntake	Feed intake	0.888	kg day^{-1}
CPcontent	Crude protein content in the diet	171	g kg^{-1}
SScontent	Starch + sugar content in the diet	461	g kg^{-1}
CFcontent	Crude fat content in the diet	33	g kg^{-1}
NSPcontent	Non-starch polysaccharide content in the diet	150	g kg^{-1}
DCprotein	Digestion coefficient protein	0.85	g g^{-1}
DCss	Digestion coefficient starch + sugars	1.00	g g^{-1}
DCfat	Digestion coefficient fat	0.90	g g^{-1}
DCnsp	Digestion coefficient non-starch polysaccharides	0.50	g g^{-1}
Parameters Michaelis–Menten equations:			
VmaxAAdeg	Maximum rate of amino acid degradation	250	g day^{-1}
VmaxBPdep	Maximum rate of body protein deposition	150	g day^{-1}
VmaxGLox	Maximum rate of glucose oxidation	1000	g day^{-1}
VmaxFAsyn	Maximum rate of fatty acid synthesis	300	g day^{-1}
VmaxBFdep	Maximum rate of body fat deposition	200	g day^{-1}
AffinityBPdep	Affinity constant of amino acids for body protein deposition	2	g kg^{-1}
AffinityAAdeg	Affinity constant of amino acids for amino acid degradation	10	g kg^{-1}
AffinityGLox	Affinity constant of glucose for glucose oxidation	10	g kg^{-1}
AffinityFAsyn	Affinity constant of glucose for fatty acid synthesis	5	g kg^{-1}
AffinityBFdep	Affinity constant of fatty acids for body fat deposition	2	g kg^{-1}
InhibitionGL-forAAdeg	Inhibition constant of glucose for the degradation of amino acids	2	g kg^{-1}
Other parameters:			
kJgAA	ATP yield g^{-1} amino acid degraded	7.1[a]	kJ g^{-1}
kJgFA	ATP yield g^{-1} fatty acid oxidized	39.6	kJ g^{-1}
kJgGL	ATP yield g^{-1} glucose oxidized	17.5	kJ g^{-1}
EcostBP-deposition	ATP costs of body protein deposition	20	kJ g^{-1}
EcostBF-deposition	ATP costs of the deposition of fatty acids as body fat	5	kJ g^{-1}
EcostFA-synthesis	ATP costs for the use of glucose for fatty acid synthesis	3.3	kJ g^{-1}
EcostUREA-synthesis	ATP costs of urea synthesis	5.3	kJ g^{-1}

(Continued)

Table 25.2. *Continued.*

Name constant	Description	Default value	Unit
kJgGLforFA-syn	ATP yield from the use of glucose for fatty acid synthesis	5.8	kJ g^{-1}
gFAgGL	Yield of fatty acids g^{-1} of glucose used for fatty acid synthesis	0.3	g g^{-1}
gGLgAA	Yield of glucose g^{-1} of amino acid degraded	0.74	g g^{-1}
gUREAgAAdeg	Urea synthesis g^{-1} of amino acid degraded	0.34	g g^{-1}

[a]It is assumed that 1 g of amino acid degraded (23.7 kJ) yields 7.1 kJ ATP, 3.6 kJ urea and 13.0 kJ glucose.

Feeding the virtual pig

In this model, the starting weight of the pig is about 25 kg. A default diet, low in fat and high in starch, is included, supplying 14.17 kJ digestible energy per gram of feed, and is fed at a rate of 0.888 kg day^{-1}. Nutrient intake can be calculated from the feed intake, nutrient composition and digestion coefficients (constants, see Table 25.2). After the model is completed, experiments have to be conducted to run the model under various nutrient inputs to see the effects on nutrient partitioning. When simulating the high fat, low carbohydrate diet later, the constants representing diet composition can be changed when running an experiment.

The amino acid metabolite pool (AA, g)

- Initial pool size is 5 g.
- Dietary proteins are hydrolysed and absorbed as amino acids. The input into the amino acid pool (AA intake, g day^{-1}) can be calculated from the feed intake (see above), the dietary protein content and its digestibility. The crude protein content (CP content, g kg^{-1}) is 171 g kg^{-1} and the digestion coefficient for protein (DC protein, g g^{-1}) is 0.85.
- Amino acids can be used for body protein deposition (BPdep, g day^{-1}). This process is assumed to follow saturable enzyme kinetics, driven by the amino acid concentration in the blood, and can be represented by a Michaelis–Menten equation. For an explanation of this principle, see Box 25.1. Parameters for the Michaelis–Menten equation are included in Table 25.2 (Box 25.1 provides a generalized Michaelis–Menten equation that needs to be adapted and applied as required. For example, in body protein deposition, there is only one substrate and no end-product inhibition. The equation therefore becomes: BPdep = VmaxBPdep/(1 + (affinityBPdep/Aaconc)).) Calculate the blood amino acid concentration (AAconc, g kg^{-1}) from the AA pool size and the blood volume. Assume the blood volume to be 8% of the body weight of the pig (litres and kilograms can be considered equivalent). For the calculation of body weight, see the section on body weight below. Please add an auxiliary variable to calculate blood volume.

Box 25.1. Saturable enzyme kinetics.

The rate of substrate utilization often follows the behaviour of saturable enzyme kinetics. In such an approach, the concentration of a substrate stimulates and quite often the concentration of an end product inhibits the conversion of substrate into end product. The response of the fluxes to increasing substrate concentrations can be described by a Michaelis–Menten equation, of which a simplified version is presented below:

Rate of utilization of substrate S (g day^{-1}) = $V_{max}/(1+A/[S]+[E]/I)$,

In which

V_{max} = the maximum rate at which the substrate is utilized, in g day^{-1}
A = affinity constant, representing the affinity of substrate S for its utilization, g kg^{-1}
[S] = the substrate concentration in blood, g kg^{-1} blood
[E] = the concentration of end product in blood, g kg^{-1} blood
I = inhibition constant, representing the inhibition of end product E for the nutrient flux, g kg^{-1}

At low values for [S], the rate of utilization of S is low. With increasing [S], the rate of utilization increases up to a point at which it reaches V_{max}. Similarly, high [E] can inhibit the rate of substrate utilization (see figures below).

(Based on Gill *et al.*, 1989.)

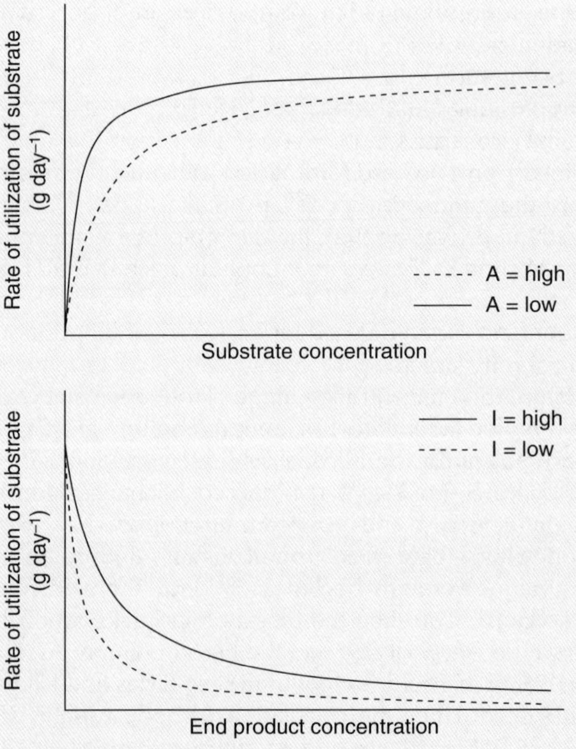

- Amino acids can also be degraded (AAdeg, g day^{-1}) to yield glucose, ATP and urea (it is assumed that 1 g of amino acid degraded (23.7 kJ) yields 7.1 kJ ATP, 3.6 kJ urea and 13.0 kJ glucose). This process is assumed to follow saturable enzyme kinetics, driven by the amino acid concentration in the blood. In addition, amino acid degradation is inhibited by high glucose concentration. Parameters for the Michaelis–Menten equation are presented in Table 25.2.
- Urea is the end product of the urea cycle, transferring amino-N to urine. The urea production rate is directly proportional to the amino acid degradation flux. Per gram amino acid degraded, 0.34 g urea is produced and excreted (gUREAgAAdeg = 0.34 g g^{-1}).

The glucose metabolite pool (GL, g)

- Initial pool size is 5 g.
- Dietary starch + sugars are hydrolysed and absorbed as glucose. The input into the glucose pool (Glintake, g day^{-1}) can be calculated from the feed intake (see above), the dietary starch + sugar content and its digestibility. The dietary starch + sugar content (SScontent, g kg^{-1}) is 461 g kg^{-1} and the digestibility can be assumed complete (DCSS = 1.0 g g^{-1}).
- Glucose can be produced from amino acids (GLfromAAdeg, g day^{-1}). Please note that, for every gram of amino acid degraded, 13.0 kJ is used for the production of glucose (see footnote to Table 25.2). This yields 13.0/17.5 = 0.74 g of glucose (gGLgAA = 0.74 g g^{-1}).
- Glucose can be used for the production of ATP (GLox, g day^{-1}). This process is assumed to follow saturable enzyme kinetics, driven by the glucose concentration in the blood. Parameters for the Michaelis–Menten equation are presented in Table 25.2. Calculate the glucose concentration (GLconc, g kg^{-1}) from the GL pool size and the blood volume.
- Glucose can be used for *de novo* fatty acid synthesis (GLforFAsyn, g day^{-1}). Like glucose oxidation, this process is assumed to follow saturable enzyme kinetics, driven by the glucose concentration in the blood. Parameters for the Michaelis–Menten equation are presented in Table 25.2.

The fatty acid metabolite pool (FA, g)

- Initial pool size is 5 g.
- Dietary fat is assumed to consist of fatty acids only (glycerol is ignored). After hydrolysis, fat is absorbed (mainly through lymph) and enters the fatty acid pool (FAintake, g day^{-1}). Furthermore, fermented dietary non-starch polysaccharides (NSPintake, g day^{-1}) are assumed to be converted into fatty acids (of course, this is not completely true). The input into the fatty acid pool can be calculated from the feed intake (see above). Dietary crude fat content (CFcontent) is 33 g kg^{-1} and the digestion coefficient (DCfat) = 0.90 g g^{-1}. The dietary non-starch polysaccharide content (NSPcontent) is 150 g kg^{-1} and its digestion coefficient (DCnsp) is 0.50. Seventy per cent of the digested non-starch polysaccharides is flowing into the fatty acid metabolite pool. The remainder (30%, please ignore in the model) is included in microbial biomass or is lost as fermentation heat.

- Fatty acids can be produced from glucose (FAsyn, g day^{-1}). The use of glucose for fatty acid synthesis is described in the section on the glucose metabolite pool. Please note that, because only four out of the six carbon atoms of glucose can be used for fatty acid synthesis, for every gram of glucose disappearing from the glucose pool, only 0.67 g will be used for fatty acid synthesis. Because this is a dehydration reaction, there is loss of mass. To ensure conservation of energy, it is assumed that this 0.67 g gives (0.67*17.5/39.6 = 0.3 g) fatty acids (gFAgGL = 0.3 g g^{-1}).
- Fatty acids can be oxidized to acetyl co-enzyme A, which yields ATP in the Krebs cycle (FAox, g day^{-1}). This flux is described in the section on the ATP pool. Assume this flux to be equal to ATPFAox (see below), but remember to convert it from kJ to g. It is assumed that 1 g of fatty acid oxidation gives 39.6 kJ ATP (kJgFA = 39.6 kJ g^{-1}).
- Fatty acids can be deposited as body fat (BFdep, g day^{-1}). This process is assumed to follow saturable enzyme kinetics, driven by the fatty acid concentration in the blood. Calculate the fatty acid concentration (FAconc, g kg^{-1}) from the fatty acid pool size and the blood volume. Parameters for the Michaelis–Menten equation are presented in Table 25.2.

The adenosine triphosphate metabolite pool (ATP, kJ)

- Initial pool size is 10 kJ.
- ATP is needed for maintaining vital life processes in the pig. The maintenance energy requirements are assumed constant when expressed as a function of metabolic body weight (ATPMaintenance = 450 kJ kg^{-1} body $weight^{0.75}$). For the calculation of body weight, see section 'Calculating body weight from body protein and body fat'. Calculate metabolic body weight from body weight. Note that the syntax in SMART for this calculation is 'pow(bodyweight, 0.75)'.
- ATP is needed for protein deposition (ATPBPdep, kJ day^{-1}) (peptide bond formation, protein turnover). It is assumed that this requirement is constant per gram of protein deposited (EcostBPdeposition = 20 kJ g^{-1}).
- ATP is needed for fat deposition (ATPBFdep, kJ g^{-1}) (esterification of fatty acids). It is assumed that this requirement is constant per gram of fat deposited (ECostBFdeposition = 5 kJ g^{-1}).
- ATP is needed for *de novo* fatty acid synthesis from glucose (ATPGLforFAsyn). It is assumed that this requirement is constant per gram of glucose used for fatty acid synthesis (EcostFAsynthesis = 3.3 kJ g^{-1} glucose used for fatty acid synthesis).
- ATP is needed for the urea cycle. The ATP costs per g urea produced are assumed to be 5.3 kJ g^{-1} (EcostUREAsynthesis = 5.3 kJ g^{-1}).
- ATP can be produced from degradation of amino acids (ATPAAdeg, kJ day^{-1}). Amino acid degradation is described in the section on the amino acid pool. It is assumed that, per gram amino acid degraded, 0.3 g is converted into ATP (kJgAA = 0.3*23.6 = 7.1 kJ g^{-1}). Refer to footnote to Table 25.2.

- ATP can be produced from the oxidation of glucose (ATPGLox, kJ day^{-1}). Glucose oxidation is described in the section on the glucose pool). Oxidation of glucose yields 17.5 kJ g^{-1} (kJgGL = 17.5 kJ g^{-1}).
- ATP will be a by-product of fatty acid synthesis from glucose (ATPGLFA, kJ day^{-1}). You can assume that two out of the six carbon atoms of glucose will be converted to ATP, yielding 0.33 × 17.5 kJ g^{-1} = 5.8 kJ g^{-1} glucose used for fatty acid synthesis (kJgGLforFAsyn = 5.8 kJ g^{-1}).
- ATP can be produced from the oxidation of fatty acids (ATPFAox, kJ day^{-1}). It is assumed this flux is used to close the gap between the total ATP requirements and the ATP produced in the transactions described above. First, compute the ATP requirements by summing the energy requirements for maintenance, body protein deposition, body fat deposition, fatty acid synthesis and urea production. Then, sum the ATP production from amino acid degradation, glucose oxidation and fatty acid synthesis from glucose. The ATP formed from fatty acid oxidation is calculated by the difference between the ATP requirements and the ATP produced. Note that the result will be that the rate of change of the ATP pool size will be 0 kJ day^{-1}. In other words, the size of the ATP pool is constant.

The body protein pool (BP, g)

- Initial pool size is 4000 g.
- Body protein is produced from amino acids only and is represented as a single flux from amino acids to body protein (BPdep, g day^{-1}). Note that, in reality, deposition is the difference between synthesis and breakdown. The amino acid flux for body protein deposition is described in the section about the amino acid pool. The energy costs for protein turnover are accounted for in the ATP pool section.

The body fat pool (BF, g)

- Initial pool size is 2500 g.
- Body fat is produced from fatty acids only and is represented as a single flux from fatty acids to body fat (BFdep, g day^{-1}). Note that, in reality, deposition is the difference between synthesis and breakdown.
- The contribution of the glucose pool to provide the glycerol part of the triglyceride is ignored.

Calculating body weight from body fat and body protein

- Body water can be calculated directly from body protein: BodyWater = 4.2 × body protein.
- Body ash can be calculated directly from body protein: BodyAsh = 0.2 × body protein.
- Body weight can be calculated by summation of body protein, body fat, body water and body ash. This summation has to be increased by 6% to account for the weight of the intestinal contents. Remember to divide by 1000, as body protein, fat, ash and water are in grams.

Calculating heat production

Heat production can be calculated by summation of all ATP-requiring processes, specified in the description of the ATP pool.

Save the model, check for syntax errors, compile it and run the model using SMART for a simulation period of 10 days to answer the questions below. Use the Runge–Kutta 4th order, fixed-step length algorithm (RK4fixed) with a time step of 0.01 day and an output interval of 1 day.

Questions

1. Run the model for 10 days on the high starch diet (this diet is included as the default in the model). Do you see big changes with time in the size of the pools (state variables) of metabolites (fatty acids, amino acids, glucose and ATP) and the body protein and body fat pool? Can you explain this?

2. What happens to the rate of body fat deposition and the heat production with time during the first 10 days? Can you explain this?

3. Record on the last day (day 10) of the simulation the following variables: body weight gain, protein deposition, fat deposition and heat production. Note that, as body weight gain is not a variable in your model, you have to compute it by the difference between body weights on days 10 and 9; protein deposition, fat deposition and heat production can be read directly on day 10 from the model output. Record your answers in Table 25.3. Save the experiment and run the model now on the high fat diet: FeedIntake = 0.790 kg day^{-1}; CPcontent = 192 g kg^{-1}; SScontent = 316 g kg^{-1}; CFcontent = 136 g kg^{-1}; NSPcontent = 168 g kg^{-1}. In addition, assume the digestion coefficients to be unaffected. The high fat diet provides 15.93 kJ digestible energy g^{-1} feed. Note that 790 g of the high fat diet provides equal amounts of digestible energy and of digestible protein, as does 888 g of the high starch diet (14.17 kJ DE g^{-1}; CPcontent 171 g kg^{-1}). Record the same variables at day 10 in Table 25.3 and compare the results. What do you observe? Does it confirm your expectations? Remember to save your experiment (under a different name for the high fat diet).

4. The same as question 2 but then record the fluxes to and from the glucose and fatty acid pool and record your answers in Table 25.4. What are the major shifts in intermediary metabolism when switching from a high carbohydrate to a high fat diet? Can you explain?

Table 25.3. Comparison of body weight gain, tissue deposition rates and heat production at day 10.

	High carbohydrate diet	High fat diet
Body weight gain, g day^{-1}		
Body protein deposition, g day^{-1}		
Body fat deposition, g day^{-1}		
Heat production, kJ day^{-1}		

Table 25.4. Comparison of inputs and outputs to and from the glucose and fatty acid pools at day 10.

	High carbohydrate diet	High fat diet
Glucose intake, g day^{-1}		
Glucose from amino acid oxidation, g day^{-1}		
Glucose used for fatty acid synthesis, g day^{-1}		
Glucose oxidation, g day^{-1}		
Fat intake, g day^{-1}		
NSP intake, g day^{-1}		
Fatty acids synthesized, g day^{-1}		
Fatty acids deposited as body fat, g day^{-1}		
Fatty acid oxidation, g day^{-1}		

Table 25.5. Effect of increased feeding level (10% increase in DE intake) on body weight gain, tissue deposition rates and heat production at day 10 for pigs fed a high carbohydrate or a high fat diet.

	Standard feeding level		10% increased DE intake	
	High carbohydrate diet	High fat diet	High carbohydrate diet	High fat diet
Body weight gain, g day^{-1}				
Body protein deposition, g day^{-1}				
Body fat deposition, g day^{-1}				
Heat production, kJ day^{-1}				

5. Run the model on both the high starch and the high fat diet at two feeding levels: 888 and 790 (standard DE intake) and 977 and 869 g day^{-1} (10% increase in DE intake). Record the effects on body weight gain (from day 9 to 10), body protein deposition rate, body fat deposition rate and heat production (the latter three at day 10) in Table 25.5. Is the increase in fat deposition (g day^{-1}) with increasing feeding level as big as the increase in protein deposition? Are the effects of increased feeding level the same for the high carbohydrate and high fat diets? Can you explain this?

References

Gill, M., Beever, D.E. and France, J. (1989) Biochemical basis needed for the mathematical representation of whole animal metabolism. *Nutrition Research Reviews* 2, 181–200.

Kramer, M.R. and Scholten, H. (2001) The Smart approach to modelling and simulation. In: Heemink, A.W., Dekker, L., Arons, H.d.S., Smit, I. and van Stijn, T.L. (eds) *Proceedings of Eurosim 2001, Shaping Future with Simulation, The 4th International*

EUROSIM Congress, in which is incorporated the 2nd Conference on Modelling and Simulation in Biology, Medicine and Biomedical Engineering. Technical University Delft, Delft, The Netherlands, 6 pages on CD-ROM, ISBN: 90-806441-1-0.

Further Reading

Rumen modelling

Baldwin, R.L. (1995) *Modelling Ruminant Digestion and Metabolism.* Chapman and Hall, London.

Dijkstra, J., Neal, H.D.St.C., Beever, D.E. and France, J. (1992) Simulation of nutrient digestion, absorption and outflow in the rumen: model description. *Journal of Nutrition* 122, 2239–2256.

Dijkstra, J., Forbes, J.M. and France, J. (2005) *Quantitative Aspects of Ruminant Digestion and Metabolism*, 2nd edn. CAB International, Wallingford, UK, 736 pp.

McDonald, I. (1981) A revised model for the estimation of protein degradability in the rumen. *Journal of Agricultural Science, Cambridge* 96, 251–252.

Pig growth modelling

Birkett, S. and Lange, K. de (2001) A computational framework for a nutrient flow representation of energy utilization by growing monogastric animals. *British Journal of Nutrition* 86, 661–674.

Halas, V., Dijkstra, J., Babinszky, L., Verstegen, M.W.A. and Gerrits, W.J.J. (2004) Modelling of nutrient partitioning in growing pigs to predict their anatomical body composition: 1. Model description. *British Journal of Nutrition* 92, 707–723.

Whittemore, C.T. and Fawcett R.H. (1976) Theoretical aspects of a flexible model to simulate protein and lipid growth in pigs. *Animal Production* 22, 87–96.

Answers to Questions of Case Study 1

Complete models for case study 1 are available as Rumen1 (part 1, questions 1–4) and Rumen2 (part 2, questions 5–8) at <http://www.uoguelph.ca/cnm/chapter25exercises>.

1. Look at the pool sizes at t = 20 h (preferably use Add Table option). At 20 h, there are 3.45E–18, 3.6788 and 2.1952 kg of S, D and U, respectively, which correspond to 0, 37 and 55% of the quantities of S, D and U initially present.

2. When switching to straw, the quantities of S, D and U present after 20 h are 1.15E–18, 4.9659 and 4.3905 kg, respectively, corresponding to 0, 50 and 55% of the quantities of S, D and U initially present. The difference with grass occurs mainly in the D fraction, which disappears from the rumen at a slower rate because of the lower k_d. The amount of U is lower with straw, but, when expressed as a percentage of the amount initially present, it remains the same.

This is because U disappears from the rumen only by passage and fractional passage rates have been assumed identical. In reality, they are not, of course, but, using this model, you can estimate the importance of changes in k_d.

3. Degradation and passage rates of grass at 20 h are 73.6 and 110.4 g h^{-1}, respectively. Doubling the fractional passage rate from 3 to 6% h^{-1} decreases this to 40.4 and 121.1 g h^{-1}, respectively. This is the result of simulating the fate of a single meal (i.e. pulse dose) and, at t = 20 h, pool sizes of S, D and U are reduced. As a consequence, the absolute amounts of D and U flowing out of the rumen at t = 20 h are decreased.

4. The cumulative amount of D and S degraded provides insight into the part of the single 20 kg meal that is actually degraded by the microorganisms. Cumulative quantities of D and S degraded at t = 96 h are 3.9671 and 5.7143 kg of D and S, which are 39.6 and 95.2% of the quantities initially present.

5. Patterns show an initial increase and subsequent decrease, and results from a balance between production and passage (microbial biomass pool), or from a balance between production, passage and absorption (short-chain fatty acid pools). The initial increase simply results from the production of biomass and short-chain fatty acids from degraded material. After the peak, total disappearance (passage for microbial biomass and passage + absorption for short-chain fatty acids) exceeds the production from degraded material. The peak in pool size of microbial biomass is later than for the short-chain fatty acids because it is not absorbed in the rumen. For the individual short-chain fatty acids, the time of peak inversely reflects the fractional absorption rates. Fractional absorption rates of short-chain fatty acids increase with an increasing lipophilic character of the acid, therefore increasing from HAc to HBu. For microbial biomass, peak in pool size occurs at 3.5 h. For HAc, HPr and HBu it is at 1.1, 1.0 and 0.9 h, respectively.

6. Peak pool sizes of microbial biomass and HAc are 0.87 and 1.96 kg, respectively. Efficiency of conversion of fermented material into microbial biomass is only 15%, whereas for acetic acid it is (0.7*0.65), or 45%. None the less, the peak pool size of HAc is not three times as high as that of microbial biomass, as the disappearance of HAc from the rumen is much faster (high passage and absorption rates).

7. Times at which maximum pool sizes are reached are virtually unchanged. The maximum pool sizes, however, are greatly reduced, due to the lower degradation rate and the higher U fraction of straw when compared with grass. For example, microbial biomass: 0.285 kg at 2.8 h versus 0.874 kg at 3.5 h for straw and grass, respectively; 0.65 kg at 1.1 h and 1.96 kg at 1.1 h for straw and grass, respectively.

8. The cumulative amount of D degraded = 3.97 kg (out of 10 kg potentially degradable material). Please note that, at $t = \infty$, this amount can be calculated also by: $k_d/(k_d + k_p)$*D (i.e. 4 kg for grass). The cumulative amount of S degraded = 5.71 kg (out of 6 kg potentially degradable material). At $t = \infty$, this can be calculated by: $(k_{dl}/(k_{dl} + k_l)$*S (i.e. 5.71 kg for grass). The cumulative amounts of microbial biomass, HAc, HPr and HBu at t = 96 h were 1.452, 4.405, 1.355 and 1.017 kg, respectively, adding up to 8.229 kg. This is very close to 85% of the cumulative amount of degraded material at $t = \infty$, i.e. an efficiency of 15% and 70% of converting degraded substrate into microbial biomass and short-chain fatty acids, respectively.

Answers to Questions of Case Study 2

The completed flow chart is presented in Fig. 25.2. The models belonging to this case study are available at <http://www.uoguelph.ca/cnm/chapter25exercises> under the names growpig (starting version for students) and growpig2 (completed version).

1. No. The big changes are in the body protein and body fat pool. Metabolite pools are relatively constant. The ATP pool is (because it is a 'zero-pool') by definition constant at 10 kJ. This is because total inputs are set to match total outputs. Fatty acid oxidation is used to cover the gap between total ATP requirements and the production from other substrates. In animals, blood concentrations are always maintained within a narrow range. Small changes in blood concentrations can have large effects on nutrient partitioning.
2. Heat production increases from 7904 on day 1 to 8587 on day 10, while feed intake (and therefore also energy intake) remains the same. As the pig grows, requirements for maintenance increase, which will be lost as heat. Consequently, body fat deposition decreases from day 1 to day 10.

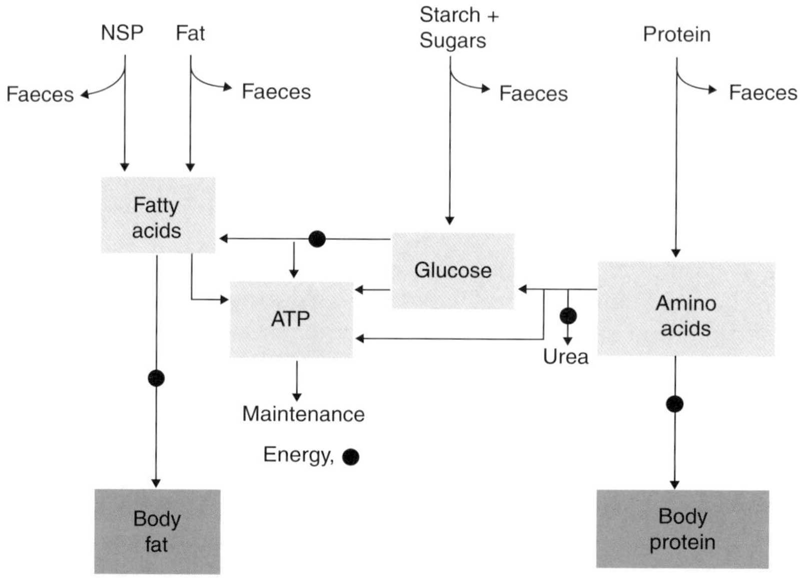

Fig. 25.2. Schematic representation of a flow chart representing the model simulating nutrient partitioning in growing pigs. Boxes represent state variables, arrows indicate nutrient fluxes. Fluxes requiring ATP are indicated by ●.

3. See data in Table 25.6. Body weight gain and body protein deposition are increased by 17 and 4.1 g day^{-1}, respectively (that is 3.0% and 4.8%), on the high carbohydrate diet. Body fat deposition is increased by 6.6 g day^{-1} (11.5%) on the high fat diet. Heat production is decreased by 208 kJ day^{-1} (2.4%) on the high fat diet. Although the decrease in body fat gain (6.6 g) on the high carbohydrate diet is larger than the increase in protein gain (4.1 g), the net result in body weight gain is still in favour of the high carbohydrate group. This is because body protein deposition is accompanied by body water. The increase in heat production on the high carbohydrate diet is because *de novo* fatty acid synthesis from glucose is increased (see question 4).

4. See the results in Table 25.7. On the high carbohydrate diet, about 68% of the total inputs (from the diet and from amino acid degradation) are oxidized to provide ATP and 32% is used for *de novo* fatty acid synthesis. On the high fat diet, clearly, intake is much lower. Of the total inputs, 66% is used for oxidation and 33% for *de novo* fatty acid synthesis. Inputs from amino acid degradation on the high fat diet are somewhat higher than on the high starch diet because of the end-product inhibition of glucose on amino acid degradation.

For the fatty acid pool: on the high carbohydrate diet, about 50% of the total input is oxidized and the remaining 50% is deposited as body fat. On the high fat diet, about 63% is oxidized and the remaining 37% is deposited as body fat. On the high carbohydrate diet, *de novo* fatty acid synthesis exceeds the intake from

Table 25.6. Comparison of body weight gain, tissue deposition rates and heat production at day 10.

	High carbohydrate diet	High fat diet
Body weight gain, g day^{-1}	578	561
Body protein deposition, g day^{-1}	90.2	86.1
Body fat deposition, g day^{-1}	57.3	63.9
Heat production, kJ day^{-1}	8587	8379

Table 25.7. Comparison of inputs and outputs to and from the glucose and fatty acid pools at day 10.

	High carbohydrate diet	High fat diet
Glucose intake, g day^{-1}	409	250
Glucose from amino acid oxidation, g day^{-1}	29	32
Glucose used for fatty acid synthesis, g day^{-1}	138	94
Glucose oxidation, g day^{-1}	300	187
Fat intake, g day^{-1}	26	97
NSP intake, g day^{-1}	47	46
Fatty acids synthesized, g day^{-1}	41	28
Fatty acids deposited as body fat, g day^{-1}	57	64
Fatty acid oxidation, g day^{-1}	57	108

Table 25.8. Effect of increased feeding level (10% increase in DE intake) on body weight gain, tissue deposition rates and heat production at day 10 for pigs fed a high carbohydrate or a high fat diet.

	Standard feeding level		10% increased DE intake	
	High carbohydrate diet	High fat diet	High carbohydrate diet	High fat diet
Body weight gain, g day^{-1}	578	561	652	627
Body protein deposition, g day^{-1}	90.2	86.1	100.0	94.2
Body fat deposition, g day^{-1}	57.3	63.9	73.6	82.1
Heat production, kJ day^{-1}	8587	8379	9012	8761

dietary fat (41 versus 26 g day^{-1}), whereas on the high fat diet intake exceeds *de novo* fatty acid synthesis (97 versus 28 g day^{-1}). In conclusion, compared with changes in body fat and body protein deposition, the effects of iso-energetic exchange of carbohydrates and fat (under iso-nitrogenous conditions) on intermediary metabolism (particularly fatty acid synthesis, glucose oxidation) are much larger.

5. See the results in Table 25.8. Similarly to question 3, the response to extra feed intake on the high carbohydrate diet, compared to the high fat diet, is higher for body weight gain and body protein deposition. The increase in body weight gain on the high carbohydrate diet was 74 g day^{-1} compared with 66 g day^{-1} for the high fat diet. The increases in body protein deposition were 9.8 and 8.1 g day^{-1}, respectively, and for body fat deposition the increases were 16.3 and 18.2 g day^{-1}. For an explanation, see the answer to question 3. The increases in fat deposition with increasing feed intake, on both diets, are much higher than the increase in protein deposition (17 versus 9 g day^{-1}). The reason for this effect is that extra feed intake at similar body weight will result in a dilution of the maintenance requirements. As the maintenance protein requirements are negligible compared with the maintenance energy requirements (maintenance protein requirements are ignored in the model), there will be more energy available for production, resulting in a large response in fat deposition.

Index